Edited by
Conor R. Caffrey

Parasitic Helminths

Titles of the Series "Drug Discovery in Infectious Diseases"

Selzer, P. M. (ed.)

Antiparasitic and Antibacterial Drug Discovery

From Molecular Targets to Drug Candidates

2009

ISBN: 978-3-527-32327-2

Becker, K. (ed.)

Apicomplexan Parasites

Molecular Approaches toward Targeted Drug Development

2011

ISBN: 978-3-527-32731-7

Forthcoming Topics of the Series

- Drug Discovery for Trypanosomatid Diseases
- Protein Phosphorylation in Parasites: Novel Targets for Antiparasitic Intervention

Related Titles

Gunn, A., Pitt, S. J.

Parasitology

An Integrated Approach

2012

ISBN: 978-0-470-68424-5

Scott, I., Sutherland, I.

Gastrointestinal Nematodes of Sheep and Cattle

Biology and Control

2009

ISBN: 978-1-4051-8582-0

Schwartz, E.

Tropical Diseases in Travelers

2009

ISBN: 978-1-4051-8441-0

Edited by Conor R. Caffrey

Parasitic Helminths

Targets, Screens, Drugs and Vaccines

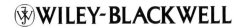

The Editors

Volume Editor:
Dr. Conor R. Caffrey
Sandler Center for Drug Discovery and Department of Pathology
University of California San Francisco
Byers Hall 501E
1700 4th Street
San Francisco, CA 94158-2330
USA
Conor.Caffrey@ucsf.edu

Series Editor:
Prof Dr. Paul M. Selzer
Intervet Innovation GmbH
MSD Animal Health
Molecular Discovery Sciences
Zur Propstei
55270 Schwabenheim
Germany
Paul.Selzer@msd.de

Cover

The cover depicts a phylogenetic tree based on the ligand binding regions of putative ligand-gated ion channel genes. Nematode, platyhelminth, insect and vertebrate sequences are shown in shades of green, yellow, purple and red, respectively. Some *C. elegans* and human subunits are indicated and the labels for proteins involved in drug susceptibility to levamisole, monepantel and ivermectin are colored in cyan, orange and blue, respectively (see Rufener *et al.*, PLoS Pathogens (2010) 6(9):e1001091; courtesy of R. Kaminsky; see Chapter 17 for details). Left inset: freshly hatched *Ascaridia galli* larva (courtesy of M. Uphoff, Intervet Innovation GmbH, MSD AH; see Chapter 9 for details). Right inset: ribbon representation of the crystal structure of the *Schistosoma mansoni* Sm14 fatty acid binding protein in complex with arachidonic acid that is shown in a space fill representation (PDB 1VYG). The image was prepared by R. Marhöfer, Intervet Innovation GmbH, MSD AH and based on an original adapted from Angelucci *et al.*, Biochemistry (2004) 43:13000-13011 that was kindly provided by M. Tendler (see Chapter 26 for details).

■ **Limit of Liability/Disclaimer of Warranty:** While the publisher and author have used their best efforts in preparing this book, they make no representations or warranties with respect to the accuracy or completeness of the contents of this book and specifically disclaim any implied warranties of merchantability or fitness for a particular purpose. No warranty can be created or extended by sales representatives or written sales materials. The Advice and strategies contained herein may not be suitable for your situation. You should consult with a professional where appropriate. Neither the publisher nor authors shall be liable for any loss of profit or any other commercial damages, including but not limited to special, incidental, consequential, or other damages.

Library of Congress Card No.: applied for

British Library Cataloguing-in-Publication Data
A catalogue record for this book is available from the British Library.

Bibliographic information published by the Deutsche Nationalbibliothek
The Deutsche Nationalbibliothek lists this publication in the Deutsche Nationalbibliografie; detailed bibliographic data are available on the Internet at http://dnb.d-nb.de.

© 2012 Wiley-VCH Verlag & Co. KGaA, Boschstr. 12, 69469 Weinheim, Germany

Wiley-Blackwell is an imprint of John Wiley & Sons, formed by the merger of Wiley's global Scientific, Technical, and Medical business with Blackwell Publishing

All rights reserved (including those of translation into other languages). No part of this book may be reproduced in any form – by photoprinting, microfilm, or any other means – nor transmitted or translated into a machine language without written permission from the publishers. Registered names, trademarks, etc. used in this book, even when not specifically marked as such, are not to be considered unprotected by law.

Composition Thomson Digital, Noida, India
Printing and Binding Markono Print Media Pte Ltd, Singapore
Cover Design Adam Design, Weinheim

Print ISBN: 978-3-527-33059-1
ePDF ISBN: 978-3-527-65283-8
oBook ISBN: 978-3-527-65296-9
epub ISBN: 978-3-527-65294-5

Printed in Singapore
Printed on acid-free paper

Foreword to *Parasitic Helminths: Targets, Screens, Drugs and Vaccines*

Peter Hotez

The last decade has witnessed a renewed interest in neglected diseases caused by parasitic helminths, especially for the high prevalence gastrointestinal nematode infections, filarial infections, schistosomiasis, food-borne trematodiases and larval cestode infections. A number of factors have contributed to this resurgent interest in helminthic infections as global health threats:

1) There is new information suggesting that parasitic helminthiases are the most common causes of infection among the "bottom billion", *i.e.*, the 1.4 billion world's poorest people who live below the World Bank poverty level in developing countries of Asia, Africa, and the Americas. The major helminthiases include 600–800 million people with one or more soil-transmitted helminth infection, 400–600 million with schistosomiasis, more than 100 million people filarial infections and tens of millions with food-borne trematode infections.
2) Additional studies have revealed that some of the most prevalent parasitic helminths may increase susceptibility to the "big three" diseases, *i.e.*, HIV/AIDS, malaria and tuberculosis or exacerbate the morbidities of the big three diseases.
3) According to some estimates the major parasitic helminth infections together cause a disease burden measured in disability adjusted life years that may rival or even exceed the big three conditions, while additional information indicates that these helminthiases may actually cause poverty through their deleterious effects on child growth and cognitive development, pregnancy outcome and agricultural worker productivity.

The global health community has responded to this public health threat by expanding efforts directed at mass drug administration (MDA). For example, using either diethylcarbamazine citrate or ivermectin together with albendazole, lymphatic filariasis (LF) has been eliminated as a public health problem in more than 20 countries, while through annual treatments with ivermectin, onchocerciasis has been eliminated in Senegal and Mali and may soon be eliminated from the Americas. Simultaneously, large scale financial support from the United States Agency for International Development (USAID), the British Department for International Development (DFID) and the non-profit Global Network for Neglected Tropical

Diseases has facilitated combining LF and onchocerciasis MDA efforts with MDA for soil-transmitted helminth infections and schistosomiasis to create "rapid impact" packages of anthelmintic interventions in national programs of helminth control in more than a dozen African countries, in addition to selected countries in Asia, Latin America and the Caribbean.

The promise of MDA for parasitic helminth infections has generated excitement among the international community that it might be possible to one day eliminate several helminthiases globally thereby achieving successes on this front that cannot yet be imagined for any of the big three diseases. However, there are warning signs that MDA with currently available drugs might fail to achieve such expectations: 1) high rates of mebendazole drug failure have been reported for hookworm infection caused by *Necator americanus* and trichuriasis, *i.e.*, two of the helminth infections with the greatest prevalence; 2) there is the looming specter of benzimidazole drug resistance among gastrointestinal nematodes of humans as has already occurred for nematode parasites of livestock, and 3) it has been shown that high rates of post-treatment re-infection occur for most of the major soil-transmitted helminth infections, schistosomiasis, and opisthorchiasis and other food-borne trematode infections.

Such concerns highlight the urgent need to develop and maintain a pipeline of new anthelmintic drugs in addition to anthelmintic vaccines to prevent infection or re-infection. Sadly, there is a glaring disconnect between the urgency for research and development (R&D) for new anthelmintic products and the global R&D budget for helminthiases. According to the global health think tank, *Policy Cures*, less than $100 million annually is spent on R&D for all human helminthiases compared to more than $3 billion spent annually on R&D for all the other neglected infections, including the big three diseases.

This volume summarizes the work of dedicated investigators in the medical and veterinary fields who are applying the latest technologies to discover the next generation of anthelmintic drugs and vaccines. Despite the difficulty in working with parasitic helminths in the laboratory, these investigators are overcoming significant hurdles in the study of the world's most important helminths affecting more than a billion people worldwide and countless livestock.

Their work is leading to a new generation of advances and represents the best in science and in the pursuit of humanitarian goals.

Peter Hotez MD PhD is Dean of the National School of Tropical Medicine and Professor of Pediatrics and Molecular Virology & Microbiology, Texas Children's Hospital and Baylor College of Medicine, Houston, Texas, USA

Contents

Foreword to *Parasitic Helminths: Targets, Screens, Drugs and Vaccines* V

Preface XI

List of Contributors XIII

Part One Targets *1*

1 Ligand-Gated Ion Channels as Targets for Anthelmintic Drugs: Past, Current, and Future Perspectives *3*
Kristin Lees*, Ann Sluder, Niroda Shannan, Lance Hammerland, and David Sattelle

2 How Relevant is *Caenorhabditis elegans* as a Model for the Analysis of Parasitic Nematode Biology? *23*
Lindy Holden-Dye* and Robert J. Walker

3 Integrating and Mining Helminth Genomes to Discover and Prioritize Novel Therapeutic Targets *43*
Dhanasekaran Shanmugam, Stuart A. Ralph, Santiago J. Carmona, Gregory J. Crowther, David S. Roos, and Fernán Agüero*

4 Recent Progress in Transcriptomics of Key Gastrointestinal Nematodes of Animals – Fundamental Research Toward New Intervention Strategies *61*
Cinzia Cantacessi, Bronwyn E. Campbell, Aaron R. Jex, Ross S. Hall, Neil D. Young, Matthew J. Nolan, and Robin B. Gasser*

5 Harnessing Genomic Technologies to Explore the Molecular Biology of Liver Flukes-Major Implications for Fundamental and Applied Research *73*
Neil D. Young*, Aaron R. Jex, Cinzia Cantacessi, Bronwyn E. Campbell, and Robin B. Gasser

6   RNA Interference: A Potential Discovery Tool for Therapeutic
    Targets of Parasitic Nematodes *89*
    Collette Britton

7   RNA Interference as a Tool for Drug Discovery in Parasitic
    Flatworms *105*
    Akram A. Da'dara and Patrick J. Skelly*

Part Two   Screens   *121*

8   Mechanism-Based Screening Strategies for Anthelmintic
    Discovery *123*
    Timothy G. Geary

9   Identification and Profiling of Nematicidal Compounds in Veterinary
    Parasitology *135*
    Andreas Rohwer, Jürgen Lutz, Christophe Chassaing, Manfred Uphoff,
    Anja R. Heckeroth, and Paul M. Selzer*

10 Quantitative High-Content Screening-Based Drug Discovery against
    Helmintic Diseases *159*
    Rahul Singh

11 Use of Rodent Models in the Discovery of Novel Anthelmintics *181*
    Rebecca Fankhauser, Linsey R. Cozzie, Bakela Nare, Kerrie Powell,
    Ann E. Sluder, and Lance G. Hammerland*

12 To Kill a Mocking Worm: Strategies to Improve *Caenorhabditis elegans*
    as a Model System for use in Anthelmintic Discovery *201*
    Andrew R. Burns and Peter J. Roy*

Part Three   Drugs   *217*

13 Anthelmintic Drugs: Tools and Shortcuts for the Long Road from
    Discovery to Product *219*
    Eugenio L. de Hostos* and Tue Nguyen

14 Antinematodal Drugs – Modes of Action and Resistance: And Worms
    Will Not Come to Thee (Shakespeare: *Cymbeline:* IV, ii) *233*
    Alan P. Robertson, Samuel K. Buxton, Sreekanth Puttachary,
    Sally M. Williamson, Adrian J. Wolstenholme, Cedric Neveu,
    Jacques Cabaret, Claude L. Charvet, and Richard J. Martin*

15 Drugs and Targets to Perturb the Symbiosis of *Wolbachia*
    and Filarial Nematodes *251*
    Mark J. Taylor*, Louise Ford, Achim Hoerauf, Ken Pfarr, Jeremy M. Foster,
    Sanjay Kumar, and Barton E. Slatko

16 Promise of *Bacillus thuringiensis* Crystal Proteins
as Anthelmintics   *267*
*Yan Hu and Raffi V. Aroian**

17 Monepantel: From Discovery to Mode of Action   *283*
Ronald Kaminsky and Lucien Rufener*

18 Discovery, Mode of Action, and Commercialization
of Derquantel   *297*
Debra J. Woods, Steven J. Maeder, Alan P. Robertson,
Richard J. Martin, Timothy G. Geary, David P. Thompson,
Sandra S. Johnson, and George A. Conder*

19 Praziquantel: Too Good to be Replaced?   *309*
Livia Pica-Mattoccia and Donato Cioli*

20 Drug Discovery for Trematodiases: Challenges
and Progress   *323*
Conor R. Caffrey, Jürg Utzinger, and Jennifer Keiser*

Part Four   Vaccines   *341*

21 Barefoot thru' the Valley of Darkness: Preclinical Development of a
Human Hookworm Vaccine   *343*
Jeffrey M. Bethony, Maria Victoria Periago, and Amar R. Jariwala*

22 Vaccines Linked to Chemotherapy: A New Approach to Control
Helminth Infections   *357*
Sara Lustigman, James H. McKerrow, and Maria Elena Bottazzi*

23 Antifilarial Vaccine Development: Present and Future
Approaches   *377*
Sara Lustigman, David Abraham, and Thomas R. Klei*

24 Proteases as Vaccines Against Gastrointestinal Nematode Parasites
of Sheep and Cattle   *399*
David Knox

25 Schistosomiasis Vaccines – New Approaches to Antigen Discovery
and Promising New Candidates   *421*
Alex Loukas, Soraya Gaze, Mark Pearson, Denise Doolan,
Philip Felgner, David Diemert, Donald P. McManus,
Patrick Driguez, and Jeffrey Bethony*

26 Sm14 *Schistosoma mansoni* Fatty Acid-Binding Protein: Molecular Basis for an Antihelminth Vaccine *435*
Miriam Tendler*, Celso Raul Romero Ramos, and Andrew J.G. Simpson

27 Mechanisms of Immune Modulation by *Fasciola hepatica*: Importance for Vaccine Development and for Novel Immunotherapeutics *451*
Mark W. Robinson*, John P. Dalton, Sandra M. O'Neill, and Sheila M. Donnelly

28 Prospects for Immunoprophylaxis Against *Fasciola hepatica* (Liver Fluke) *465*
Terry W. Spithill*, Carlos Carmona, David Piedrafita, and Peter M. Smooker

29 Vaccines Against Cestode Parasites *485*
Marshall W. Lightowlers*, Charles G. Gauci, Abdul Jabbar, and Cristian Alvarez

Index *505*

Preface

Parasitic helminths continue to plague the lives of billions of people, and those of farm and domestic animals. Their capacity to persist in the environment is infuriating, costly (health-wise and economically), and fascinating depending on one's perspective as a livestock farmer, medical provider, or research scientist. For the animal health industry, the intrinsic capacity of helminths to resist drug pressure drives the never-ending quest to bring new anthelmintic drugs to market. In recent years, we have seen the fruits of that industry with the registration of new drugs containing emodepside, monepantel, and derquantel. These drugs and other compounds in the pipeline are critical not just for staying "one up" on resistant parasites of animals, but also for their potential to cross-over to human medicine, as has occurred with earlier anthelmintics that have been of immeasurable value to improving global health. That contribution becomes all the more relevant today given the increasing concerns over the continued efficacy of many first-generation anthelmintic drugs relied upon to treat human helminthiases, not least the benzimidazoles and the "wonder drug" ivermectin, and the serious implications for public health should these drugs fail.

This volume is intended to showcase the state-of-the-art in the fields of drug and vaccine development for parasitic helminths as well as draw attention to the challenges associated with bringing such products to market. The book is Volume 3 in the series *Drug Discovery in Infectious Diseases* and expands on some of the themes raised in Volume 1, *Antiparasitic and Antibacterial Drug Discovery: From Molecular Targets to Drug Candidates*. Contributions from the animal health industry figure prominently with a focus on the discovery and development of new chemical entities. Importantly, however, the book also covers the increasingly relevant contribution of academia, not just in its traditional strengths of identifying new drug targets or understanding how drug resistance arises, but also in the ways and means of preclinical and translational drug discovery through highly collaborative and interdisciplinary research. Indeed, this exciting movement into the traditional domain of the pharmaceutical industry can be viewed as a natural consequence of the central importance and success of academia in the public–private consortia that currently maintain dynamic drug development portfolios for other global parasitic diseases such as malaria and the trypanosomatid diseases. The creativity and productivity of academic scientists are highlighted in the many chapters covering the development and expansion of genomics and functional genomic tools, and the application of automated screening technologies to prosecute anthelmintic drug discovery with rigor.

Finally, this volume discusses the need for, and the particular difficulties associated with, developing anthelmintic vaccines for both humans and animals – for many the "holy grail" in providing the tool (including in combination with chemotherapy) to ultimately control and, hopefully, eliminate helminth diseases. Great progress has been made in identifying a number of candidates with proven efficacy in target animal species or that are now entering human trials, thanks in part to the establishment of the necessary national and transnational institutional infrastructures.

To all of the authors, my sincere thanks for their time, insights, and patience in contributing to an important collection of on-topic discussions. My thanks also to the book series editor, Paul M. Selzer of Intervet Innovation GmbH, and to my colleagues at the Sandler Center for Drug Discovery at the University of California San Francisco for their constructive input.

March 2012 *Conor R. Caffrey*
San Francisco

List of Contributors

David Abraham
Thomas Jefferson University
Department of Microbiology and
Immunology
233 South 10th Street
Philadelphia, PA 19107
USA

Fernán Agüero[*]
Universidad de San Martín
Instituto de Investigaciones
Biotecnológicas
25 de Mayo y Francia
San Martín
B 1650 HMP, Buenos Aires
Argentina
E-mail: fernan@iib.unsam.edu.ar,
fcrnan.agucro@gmail.com

Cristian Alvarez
University of Melbourne
Veterinary Clinical Center
250 Princes Highway
Werribee
Victoria 3030
Australia

Raffi V. Aroian[*]
University of California San Diego
Section of Cell and Developmental
Biology
Division of Biological Sciences
9500 Gilman Dr
La Jolla, CA 92093-0322
USA
E-mail: raroian@ucsd.edu

Jeffrey M. Bethony[*]
George Washington University
Medical Center
Clinical Immunology Laboratory
Department of Microbiology,
Immunology and Tropical Medicine
2300 Eye Street, NW
Washington, DC 20052
USA
E-mail: mtmjmb@gwumc.edu

and

FIOCRUZ
Clinical Immunology Laboratory
Laboratório de Imunologia Celular e
Molecular
Centro de Pesquisas René Rachou
Av. Augusto de Lima 1715
Belo Horizonte
Minas Gerais 30190-002
Brazil

Maria Elena Bottazzi
National School of Tropical Medicine
Sabin Vaccine Institute and Texas
Children's Center for
Vaccine Development
Section of Pediatric Tropical Medicine
Baylor College of Medicine
1102 Bates St.
Houston, TX 77030
USA

Collette Britton[*]
University of Glasgow
Institute of Infection, Immunity
and Inflammation
College of Medical, Veterinary
and Life Sciences
Bearsden Road
Glasgow G61 1QH
UK
E-mail: Collette.Britton@glasgow.ac.uk

Andrew R. Burns
University of Toronto
Department of Molecular Genetics and
The Donnelly Centre for Cellular and
Biomolecular Research
160 College Street, Rm1202
Toronto
Ontario, M5S 1A8
Canada

Samuel K. Buxton
Iowa State University
Department of Biomedical Sciences
Ames, IA 50011
USA

Jacques Cabaret
INRA
UR1282 Infectiologie Animale et Santé
Publique
37380 Nouzilly
France

Conor R. Caffrey[*]
University of California San Francisco
Sandler Center for Drug Discovery and
the Department of Pathology
1700 4th Street
San Francisco, CA 94158-2330
USA
E-mail: conor.caffrey@ucsf.edu

Bronwyn E. Campbell
The University of Melbourne
Faculty of Veterinary Science
Corner Flemington Road and Park Drive
Parkville
Victoria 3010
Australia

Cinzia Cantacessi
The University of Melbourne
Faculty of Veterinary Science
Corner Flemington Road and Park Drive
Parkville
Victoria 3010
Australia

Carlos Carmona
Universidad de la República
Unidad de Biología Parasitaria
Instituto de Biología
Facultad de Ciencias
Av. A. Navarro 3051
CP 11600 Montevideo
Uruguay

Santiago J. Carmona
Universidad de San Martín
Instituto de Investigaciones
Biotecnológicas
25 de Mayo y Francia
San Martín
B 1650 HMP, Buenos Aires
Argentina

List of Contributors

Claude L. Charvet
INRA
UR1282 Infectiologie Animale et Santé Publique
37380 Nouzilly
France

Christophe Chassaing
Intervet Innovation GmbH
MSD Animal Health
Zur Propstei
55270 Schwabenheim
Germany

Donato Cioli
National Research Council
Cell Biology and Neurobiology Institute
32 Via Ramarini
Monterotondo
00015 Rome
Italy

George A. Conder
Pfizer Animal Health
Veterinary Medicine Research & Development
7000 Portage Road
Kalamazoo, MI 49001
USA

Linsey R. Cozzie
Merial Ltd
Clinical R&D Americas East
115 Transtech Drive
Athens, GA 30601
USA

Gregory J. Crowther
University of Washington
Department of Medicine
Division of Allergy and Infectious Diseases
1959 NE Pacific Street
Seattle, WA 98195-7185
USA

Akram A. Da'dara
Tufts University
Molecular Helminthology Laboratory
Division of Infectious Diseases
Department of Biomedical Sciences
Cummings School of Veterinary Medicine
200 Westboro Road
Grafton, MA 01536
USA

John P. Dalton
McGill University
Institute of Parasitology
21111 Lakeshore Road
St Anne de Bellevue
Quebec H9X 3V9
Canada

David Diemert
Sabin Vaccine Development PDP
723-D Ross Hall
2300 Eye Street NW
Washington, DC 20037
USA

Sheila M. Donnelly
University of Technology Sydney
ithree Institute
Level 6, Building 4
Corner of Thomas and Harris Street
Sydney
New South Wales 2007
Australia

Denise Doolan
Queensland Institute of Medical Research
Division of Infectious Diseases
300 Herston Rd
Brisbane
Queensland 4006
Australia

Patrick Driguez
Queensland Institute of Medical Research
Division of Infectious Diseases
300 Herston Rd
Brisbane
Queensland 4006
Australia

Rebecca Fankhauser
Merial Ltd
Clinical R&D Americas East
115 Transtech Drive
Athens, GA 30601
USA

Philip Felgner
University of California Irvine
School of Medicine
3052 Hewitt Hall
Irvine, CA 92697
USA

Louise Ford
Liverpool School of Tropical Medicine
Molecular and Biochemical Parasitology
Pembroke Place
Liverpool L3 5QA
UK

Jeremy M. Foster
New England Biolabs
Division of Molecular Parasitology
240 County Road
Ipswich, MA 01938
USA

Robin B. Gasser[*]
The University of Melbourne
Faculty of Veterinary Science
Corner Flemington Road and Park Drive
Parkville
Victoria 3010
Australia
E-mail: robinbg@unimelb.edu.au

Charles G. Gauci
University of Melbourne
Veterinary Clinical Center
250 Princes Highway
Werribee
Victoria 3030
Australia

Soraya Gaze
James Cook University
Queensland Tropical Health Alliance
McGregor Rd, Smithfield
Cairns
Queensland 4878
Australia

Timothy G. Geary[*]
McGill University
Institute of Parasitology
21111 Lakeshore Road
Ste-Anne-de-Bellevue
Quebec H9X 3V9
Canada
E-mail: timothy.g.geary@mcgill.ca

Ross S. Hall
The University of Melbourne
Faculty of Veterinary Science
Corner Flemington Road and Park Drive
Parkville
Victoria 3010
Australia

Lance G. Hammerland[*]
Merial Ltd
Pharmaceutical R&D
3239 Satellite Boulevard
Duluth, GA 30096
USA
E-mail: lance.hammerland@merial.com

Anja. R. Heckeroth
Intervet Innovation GmbH
MSD Animal Health
Zur Propstei
55270 Schwabenheim
Germany

Achim Hoerauf
University Clinic Bonn
Institute for Medical Microbiology,
Immunology, and Parasitology
Sigmund-Freud Strasse 25
53105 Bonn
Germany

Lindy Holden-Dye[*]
University of Southampton
Centre for Biological Sciences
University Road
Southampton SO17 1BJ
UK
E-mail: lmhd@soton.ac.uk

Eugenio L. de Hostos[*]
OneWorld Health
Suite 250
280 Utah Avenue
South San Francisco, CA 94080
USA
E-mail: edehostos@oneworldhealth.org

Peter Hotez[*]
National School of Tropical Medicine
Sabin Vaccine Institute and Texas
Children's Center for Vaccine
Development
Section of Pediatric Tropical Medicine
Baylor College of Medicine
1102 Bates St.
Houston, TX 77030
USA
E-mail: hotez@bcm.edu

Yan Hu
University of California San Diego
Section of Cell and Developmental
Biology
Division of Biological Sciences
9500 Gilman Dr
La Jolla, CA 92093-0322
USA

Abdul Jabbar
The University of Melbourne
Veterinary Clinical Center
250 Princes Highway
Werribee
Victoria 3030
Australia

Amar R. Jariwala
George Washington University
Medical Center
Clinical Immunology Laboratory
Department of Microbiology,
Immunology and Tropical Medicine
2300 Eye Street, NW
Washington, DC 20052
USA

Aaron R. Jex
The University of Melbourne
Department of Veterinary Science
Corner Flemington Road and Park Drive
Parkville
Victoria 3010
Australia

Sandra S. Johnson
Pfizer Animal Health
Veterinary Medicine Research &
Development
7000 Portage Road
Kalamazoo, MI 49001
USA

Ronald Kaminsky*
Novartis
Center de Recherche Santé Animale
Route de la Petite Glâne
1566 Saint Aubin
Switzerland
E-mail: ronald.kaminsky@novartis.com

Jennifer Keiser
Swiss Tropical and Public Health Institute
Department of Medical Parasitology and Infection Biology
PO Box
4002 Basel
Switzerland

Thomas R. Klei
Louisiana State University
School of Veterinary Medicine
Skip Bertman Drive
Baton Rouge, LA 70803
USA

David Knox*
Moredun Research Institute
Parasitology Division
Bush Loan
Penicuik EH26 0PZ
UK
E-mail: dave.knox@moredun.ac.uk

Sanjay Kumar
New England Biolabs
Division of Molecular Parasitology
240 County Road
Ipswich, MA 01938
USA

Kristin Lees*
University of Manchester
Faculty of Life Sciences
Oxford Road
Manchester M13 9PT
UK
E-mail: kristin.lees@manchester.ac.uk

Marshall W. Lightowlers*
University of Melbourne
Veterinary Clinical Center
250 Princes Highway
Werribee
Victoria 3030
Australia
E-mail: marshall@unimelb.edu.au

Alex Loukas*
James Cook University
Queensland Tropical Health Alliance
McGregor Rd, Smithfield
Cairns
Queensland 4878
Australia
E-mail: Alex.Loukas@jcu.edu.au

Sara Lustigman*
New York Blood Center
Laboratory of Molecular Parasitology
Lindsley F. Kimball Research Institute
310 East 67th Street
New York, NY 10065
USA
E-mail: slustigman@nybloodcenter.org

Jürgen Lutz
Intervet Innovation GmbH
MSD Animal Health
Zur Propstei
55270 Schwabenheim
Germany

Steven J. Maeder
Pfizer Animal Health
Veterinary Medicine Research & Development
38–42 Wharf Road West Ryde
Sydney
New South Wales 2114
Australia

Richard J. Martin*
Iowa State University
Department of Biomedical Sciences
Ames, IA 50011
USA
E-mail: rjmartin@iastate.edu

James H. McKerrow
University of California San Francisco
Sandler Center for Drug Discovery and
Department of Pathology
California Institute for Quantitative
Biosciences
1700 4th Street
San Francisco, CA 94158-2330
USA

Donald P. McManus
Queensland Institute of Medical
Research
Division of Infectious Diseases
300 Herston Rd
Brisbane
Queensland 4006
Australia

Bakela Nare
Scynexis Inc.
Department
3501C Tricenter Boulevard
Durham, NC 27713
USA

Cedric Neveu
INRA
UR1282 Infectiologie Animale et Santé
Publique
37380 Nouzilly
France

Tue Nguyen
OneWorld Health
Suite 250
280 Utah Avenue
South San Francisco, CA 94080
USA

Matthew J. Nolan
The University of Melbourne
Faculty of Veterinary Science
Corner Flemington Road and Park Drive
Parkville
Victoria 3010
Australia

Sandra M. O'Neill
Dublin City University
Parasite Immune Modulation Group
School of Nursing
Collins Avenue
Glasnevin
Dublin 9
Ireland

Mark Pearson
James Cook University
Queensland Tropical Health Alliance
McGregor Rd, Smithfield
Cairns
Queensland 4878
Australia

Maria Victoria Periago
George Washington University Medical
Center
Clinical Immunology Laboratory
Department of Microbiology,
Immunology and Tropical Medicine
2300 Eye Street, NW
Washington, DC 20052
USA

and

FIOCRUZ
Clinical Immunology Laboratory
Laboratório de Imunologia Celular e
Molecular
Centro de Pesquisas René Rachou
Av. Augusto de Lima 1715
Belo Horizonte
Minas Gerais 30190-002

Ken Pfarr
University Clinic Bonn
Institute for Medical Microbiology,
Immunology, and Parasitology
Sigmund-Freud Strasse 25
53105 Bonn
Germany

Livia Pica-Mattoccia[*]
National Research Council
Cell Biology and Neurobiology Institute
32 Via Ramarini
Monterotondo
00015 Rome
Italy
E-mail: lpica@ibc.cnr.it

David Piedrafita
Monash University
Biotechnology Research Laboratories
Wellington Road
Clayton
Victoria 3800
Australia

Kerrie Powell
Scynexis Inc.
Department
3501C Tricenter Boulevard
Durham, NC 27713
USA

Sreekanth Puttachary
Iowa State University
Department of Biomedical Sciences
Ames, IA 50011
USA

Stuart A. Ralph
University of Melbourne
Department of Biochemistry and
Molecular Biology
Bio21 Molecular Science and
Biotechnology Institute
30 Flemington Road
Parkville
Victoria 3010
Australia

Celso Raul Romero Ramos
FIOCRUZ
Laboratório de Esquistossomose
Experimental
Av. Brasil 4365
Manguinhos
Rio de Janeiro 21-045-900
Brazil

Alan P. Robertson
Iowa State University
Department of Biomedical Sciences
Ames, IA 50011
USA

Mark W. Robinson[*]
University of Technology Sydney
ithree Institute
Level 6, Building 4
Corner of Thomas and Harris Street
Sydney
New South Wales 2007
Australia
E-mail: mark.robinson@uts.edu.au

List of Contributors | XXI

Andreas Rohwer
Intervet Innovation GmbH
MSD Animal Health
Zur Propstei
55270 Schwabenheim
Germany

and

Roche Diagnostics Deutschland GmbH
Sandhofer Strasse 116
68305 Mannheim
Germany

David S. Roos
University of Pennsylvania
Department of Biology and Penn Genomics Institute
415 South University Ave
Philadelphia, PA 19104
USA

Peter J. Roy[*]
University of Toronto
Department of Molecular Genetics, The Donnelly Centre for Cellular and Biomolecular Research and the Collaborative Programme in Developmental Biology
160 College Street, Rm1202
Toronto
Ontario, M5S 1A8
Canada
E-mail: peter.roy@utoronto.ca

Lucien Rufener
Novartis
Center de Recherche Santé Animale
Route de la Petite Glâne
1566 Saint Aubin
Switzerland

David Sattelle
University of Manchester
Faculty of Life Sciences
Oxford Road
Manchester M13 9PT
UK

Dhanasekaran Shanmugam
Division of Biochemical Sciences
National Chemcial Laboratories
Dr. Homi Bhabha Road
Pune, 411008
India

Niroda Shannan
University of Manchester
Faculty of Life Sciences
Oxford Road
Manchester M13 9PT
UK

Paul M. Selzer[*]
Intervet Innovation GmbH
MSD Animal Health
Zur Propstei
55270 Schwabenheim
Germany
E-mail: Paul.Selzer@msd.de

Andrew J.G. Simpson
Ludwig Institute for Cancer Research
New York Branch at Memorial Sloan-Kettering Cancer Center
1275 York Avenue
New York, NY 10021
USA

Rahul Singh[*]
San Francisco State University
Department of Computer Science
1600 Holloway Avenue
San Francisco, CA 94132
USA
E-mail:rsingh@cs.sfusu.edu

Patrick J. Skelly*
Tufts University
Molecular Helminthology Laboratory
Division of Infectious Diseases
Department of Biomedical Sciences
Cummings School of Veterinary
Medicine
200 Westboro Road
Grafton, MA 01536
USA
E-mail: Patrick.Skelly@Tufts.edu

Barton E. Slatko
New England Biolabs
Division of Molecular Parasitology
240 County Road
Ipswich, MA 01938
USA

Ann E. Sluder
Scynexis Inc.
Department
3501C Tricenter Boulevard
Durham, NC 27713
USA

Peter M. Smooker
RMIT University
School of Applied Sciences
Plenty Road
Bundoora
Victoria 3083
Australia

Terry W. Spithill*
La Trobe University
Department of Agricultural Sciences
and Center for AgriBioscience
Kingsbury Drive
Bundoora
Victoria 3086
Australia
E-mail: t.spithill@latrobe.edu.au

Mark J. Taylor*
Liverpool School of Tropical Medicine
Molecular and Biochemical Parasitology
Pembroke Place
Liverpool L3 5QA
UK
E-mail: mark.taylor@liverpool.ac.uk

Miriam Tendler*
FIOCRUZ
Laboratório de Esquistossomose
Experimental
Av. Brasil 4365
Manguinhos
Rio de Janeiro 21-045-900
Brazil
E-mail: mtendler@ioc.fiocruz.br

David P. Thompson
Pfizer Animal Health
Veterinary Medicine Research &
Development
7000 Portage Road
Kalamazoo, MI 49001
USA

Manfred Uphoff
Intervet Innovation GmbH
MSD Animal Health
Zur Propstei
55270 Schwabenheim
Germany

Jürg Utzinger
Swiss Tropical and Public Health
Institute
Department of Epidemiology and Public
Health
PO Box
4002 Basel
Switzerland

Robert J. Walker
University of Southampton
Centre for Biological Sciences
University Road
Southampton SO17 1BJ
UK

Sally M. Williamson
University of Georgia
Department of Infectious Diseases &
Center for Tropical and Emerging
Global Disease
Athens, GA 30602
USA

Adrian J. Wolstenholme
University of Georgia
Department of Infectious Diseases &
Center for Tropical and Emerging
Global Disease
Athens, GA 30602
USA

Debra J. Woods[*]
Pfizer Animal Health
Veterinary Medicine Research &
Development
7000 Portage Road
Kalamazoo, MI 49001
USA
E-mail: debra.j.woods@pfizer.com

Neil D. Young[*]
The University of Melbourne
Faculty of Veterinary Science
Corner Flemington Road and Park Drive
Parkville, Victoria 3010
Australia
E-mail: nyoung@unimelb.edu.au

Part One
Targets

1
Ligand-Gated Ion Channels as Targets for Anthelmintic Drugs: Past, Current, and Future Perspectives

Kristin Lees, Ann Sluder, Niroda Shannan, Lance Hammerland, and David Sattelle*

Abstract

Ligand-gated ion channels (LGIC) are targets for anthelmintic drugs used in human health and veterinary applications. Given the diverse physiological roles of LGICs in neuromuscular function, the nervous system, and elsewhere, it is not surprising that random chemical screening programs often identify drug candidates targeting this superfamily of transmembrane proteins. Such leads provide the basis for further chemical optimization, resulting in important commercial products. Currently, members of three LGIC families are known to be targeted by anthelmintics. These include the nicotinic acetylcholine receptors gating cation channels, glutamate-gated chloride channels, and γ-aminobutyric acid-gated chloride channels. The recent impact of genomics on model invertebrates and parasitic species has been far-reaching, leading to the description of new helminth LGIC families. Among the current challenges for anthelmintic drug discovery are the assessment of newly discovered LGICs as viable targets (validation) and circumventing resistance when exploring further the well-established targets. Recombinant expression of helminth LGICs is not always straightforward. However, new developments in the understanding of LGIC chaperones and automated screening technologies may hold promise for target validation and chemical library screening on whole organisms or *ex vivo* preparations. Here, we describe LGIC targets for the current anthelmintics of commercial importance and discuss the potential impact of that knowledge on screening for new compounds. In addition, we discuss some new technologies for anthelmintic drug hunting, aimed at the discovery of novel treatments to control veterinary parasites and some neglected human diseases.

Introduction

Anthelmintic drugs are central to combating many human and veterinary disorders. One in four of the world's population is infected with a parasitic roundworm or nematode, with infestation being particularly severe in tropical and subtropical regions. The consequent debilitating effects on the workforce and the compounding

*Corresponding Author

Parasitic Helminths: Targets, Screens, Drugs and Vaccines, First Edition. Edited by Conor R. Caffrey.
© 2012 Wiley-VCH Verlag GmbH & Co. KGaA. Published 2012 by Wiley-VCH Verlag GmbH & Co. KGaA.

risk of other pathogenic infections represents a considerable social and economic burden. If we add to that a very high level of roundworm infestation among the world's farmed animals, and the devastating impact of trematode parasites in man and animals, then the need for adequate helminth control is transparent [1, 2].

The veterinary economic burden is reflected in the scale of the global animal health drug market (approximately US$11 billion/annum) [3]. The human health antiparasitic drug market is around US$0.5 billion/annum. However, it costs around US$40 million to develop a new drug that controls livestock nematodes, whereas it can cost US$800 million for a new drug for human use. Understandably, the cost barrier has limited progress, but the size of the global markets for antiparasitic drugs and chemicals make their pursuit of commercial interest as well as an important human and animal health priority.

Exciting new developments in research on vaccines targeting helminth parasites are underway and these, undoubtedly, will make important contributions in the future. However, at present, chemical approaches to helminth control predominate. For example, the world's three top-selling veterinary antiparasitic drugs (imidacloprid, fipronil, and ivermectin) and several others such as selamectin, levamisole, pyrantel, morantel, tribendimidine, piperazine, and amino-acetonitrile derivatives (AADs) act on Cys-loop ligand-gated ion channels (LGICs). These transmembrane receptor molecules facilitate the fast actions of neurotransmitter chemicals at nerve–nerve synapses and neuromuscular junctions (NMJs) in invertebrates. Often they offer rapid control of the pathogen. Much of our current knowledge of these important drug targets stems from the genetic model organism and free-living nematode, *Caenorhabditis elegans*, which possesses the most extensive known superfamily of Cys-loop LGICs, consisting of 102 subunit-encoding genes [4]. They include cation-permeable channels gated by acetylcholine (ACh) and γ-aminobutyric acid (GABA) as well as anion-selective channels gated by ACh, GABA, glutamate, 5-hydroxytryptamine (5-HT), dopamine, and tyramine [5–7]. Less than half of the genes in the *C. elegans* Cys-loop LGIC superfamily have been functionally characterized.

Unfortunately, many of the anthelmintic drugs in current use are under threat (Table 1.1). Important compounds such as ivermectin, which have given excellent service, are at the end of their patent life. Repeated use of effective chemicals leads to the development of pathogen resistance. Indeed, multidrug resistance against the three major classes of anthelmintics including macrocyclic lactones, which target glutamate-gated chloride channels (GluCls), has become a global problem for the treatment of gastrointestinal nematode parasites of farm animals [8–10]. The increasing development costs and poor return from conventional screening approaches are also problematic. Together, these factors bring a sense of urgency to the development of new, effective anthelmintics.

The life of a patent has always been finite, but as the time from discovery to market becomes protracted and the bar is raised for new, safer molecules with improved specifications on toxicity and environmental residues, the task of discovery becomes more difficult. The introduction of generic forms of a drug has the potential to lower the cost of treatment and make it available more widely, although this positive benefit

Table 1.1 Target sites for currently used anthelmintics.

Chemical group	Compound name	Site of action
Avermectins	ivermectin, moxidectin	GluCl channel
Imidazothiazole	levamisole, tetramisol	ACh cation channel
Tetrahydropyrimidines	pyrantel, morantel	ACh cation channel
Tribendimine	tribendimine	ACh cation channel
Benzimadazole	albendazole, triclabendazole	β-tubulin
Piperazine	piperazine	GABACl channel
AADs	monepantel	ACh cation channel
Oxindole alkaloids	paraherquamide, derquantel	ACh cation channel
Cyclo-octadepsipeptides	emodepside	voltage-gated potassium channel
Praziquantel	praziquantel	voltage-gated calcium channel[a]
Salicylanilide	niclosamide	ATPase activity (?)
Surmamin	germanin	ryanodine receptors
Diethylcarbamazine	hetrazan, carbilazine	arachidonic acid

a) Still under discussion [95].

may be offset by expediting the onset of resistance. Anthelmintic resistance is affected by the treatment frequency and dose, drug efficiency, the burden of adult worms, and the host immune reaction [6]. Monitoring drug resistance is expensive. The escalating challenges of drug development mean that new anthelmintic compounds have been added to the list of available treatments at the slow rate of just one per decade [11]. Thus, there is an urgent need to develop new, effective anthelmintics.

The Cys-loop LGICs form a receptor superfamily, rich in known targets for anthelmintics. Is there more mileage in these proven targets? Can new drugs be developed that act at a different locus on the same receptor without necessarily leading to cross-resistance? Are there new LGIC targets yet to be discovered and mined? Can the wealth of new data emerging from genomics [12], forward (e.g., chemistry-to-gene screens) and reverse (e.g., RNA interference (RNAi)) genetics, and functional studies on invertebrate model organisms such as *C. elegans* be harnessed to good effect in expediting anthelmintic drug discovery? Can parasite genome studies (completed or underway) also have a major impact? What can we learn from those parasite genomes already sequenced, following on from pioneering work on the first parasite genome, that of *Brugia malayi* [13]. Where there is no genome, valuable expressed sequence tag resources are sometimes available as starting points in the search for new LGIC targets. One important advance, which will undoubtedly accelerate anthelmintic drug discovery, is the recently reported crystal structure of the *C. elegans* GluCl complexed with its orthosteric ligand (glutamate), the allosteric ligand and anthelmintic drug (ivermectin), and a noncompetitive antagonist (picrotoxin) [14]. This is the first eukaryotic LGIC for which a crystal structure is available. Knowing where and how important drugs interact with a proven target from the LGIC superfamily is a major advance, and will assist in the targeting of other family members.

Finding and validating new targets among LGICs is crucial, and they need to be cloned and expressed so that their functions can be assayed (Figure 1.1). This has

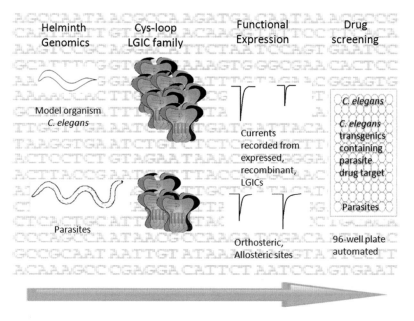

Figure 1.1 Schematic diagram showing some of the current approaches adopted to search for and characterize new anthelmintic drug targets ranging from genomics, via cell-based studies, to automated *in vivo* screening.

proved possible for some model organism LGICs using expression vehicles suited for low/medium-throughput screening; however, developing a platform of cell lines expressing a range of model organism and parasite LGICs is very much a future prospect, and assembling the prerequisite parasite LGIC drug targets remains a challenge. We need to meet this challenge in order to expedite anthelmintic drug discovery using the kinds of high-throughput screening methods deployed in the drug industry for developing new human therapies.

As well as developments in *in vitro* screening methods, developments in *in vivo* testing are urgently needed. Many assays rely on lethal end-points, but it may be that other assays can more sensitively detect important drug modifications of behavior *in vivo* that would be missed in such assays. It may not be necessary to kill worms to dislodge them or by other means prevent or reverse infestation. The difficulty of culturing parasites *ex vivo* remains a problem [15] and new approaches to improve such cultures would be welcomed. It may also be possible to exploit more effectively the recent development of transgenic *C. elegans*, which are easy to culture, in which a *C. elegans* LGIC target is replaced by a parasite ortholog [16]. Novel transgenic lines such as these used in conjunction with newly developed, plate-based, automated behavioral phenotyping may offer important opportunities for improved *in vivo* screening (Figure 1.1; see also Chapter 10 for a discussion on this topic with regard to parasitic helminths). This may even bring *in vivo* screening to bear on parasite species not hitherto considered feasible, where *ex vivo* culture is particularly difficult.

Thus, the emerging crisis of the shrinking pool of anthelmintic drug treatments at a time of growing need for control makes it timely to review the current state of anthelmintics targeting LGICs especially when placed alongside an examination of some emerging new approaches with the potential to expedite the discovery process.

Established LGIC Anthelmintic Drug Targets

Fast chemical neurotransmission at many synapses in humans is mediated by the actions of neurotransmitter molecules such as ACh, GABA, glycine, and 5-HT on specific receptors of the "Cys-loop" LGIC superfamily. These receptors play a crucial role in the function of synaptic signaling in the nervous system and NMJs. The structure of the *Torpedo marmorata* (marbled electric ray) electric organ nicotinic ACh receptor (nicotinic acetylcholine receptor nAChR) has been entirely resolved at 4.6 Å and in part at 4.0 Å [17]. Based on the structure of this prototypical nAChR, all LGICs are thought to be composed of five subunits arranged around a central ion channel. The well-characterized human LGICs are either permeable to cations (e.g., nAChRs and 5-HT$_3$Rs) or anions (e.g., GABA and glycine receptors) [18]. In nematodes there are, in addition, 5-HT-, glutamate-, ACh-, dopamine- and tyramine-gated anion channels, and GABA-gated cation channels, all of which are part of the Cys-loop LGIC superfamily. Other invertebrates, including *Drosophila melanogaster*, possess histamine-gated anion channels. Ligand-gated anion channels generally lead to rapid inhibitory synaptic responses, whereas ligand-gated cation channels mediate fast excitatory chemical transmission. Each subunit consists of an N-terminal, extracellular domain containing the Cys-loop (which is two disulfide-bond-forming cysteines separated by 13 residues) and six regions (loops A–F) that make up the ligand-binding site, as well as four transmembrane domains. Here, we review recent evidence from the invertebrate genetic model organism *C. elegans* as well as data from parasitic nematodes illustrating the rich diversity of LGICs present. The discovery of new receptor subtypes in helminths, some of which have no counterpart in mammals, may provide opportunities to develop a new generation of more selective, and hence safer, anthelmintics.

GluCls – Targets for Ivermectin

Several nematode GluCl subunits have been identified and for some their pharmacology has been characterized by expressing one or more subunits in *Xenopus laevis* oocytes. Cully et al. [19] showed that L-glutamate and ivermectin activate GluCls generated from heteromers of GluClα1 and GluClβ. Since then, other GluCl subunits have been identified in *C. elegans* [20]. These include GluClα1–4 and GluClβ. GluClα2 (AVR-15) and GluClβ are present in the pharynx of *C. elegans*, whereas GluClα3 (AVR-14) is only found in neurons [21]. Both GluClα2A and GluClα2B function in the inhibition of pharyngeal pumping [21–23], GluClα1–4 regulate locomotion [24], and GluClα4 functions in olfactory behavior [25].

A chemistry-to-gene screen in *C. elegans* for resistance to ivermectin confirmed the identity of GluCl subunits as drug targets [26]. Mutation of GluClα1–3 confers high resistance to ivermectin, whereas mutation of any two channel genes confers low-level or no resistance. Each of the three GluCl genes constitutes a parallel genetic pathway that contributes to ivermectin sensitivity in *C. elegans*. So, mutations affecting only one pathway will not confer resistance.

L-Type nAChRs –Targets for Levamisole, Pyrantel, Morantel, and Tribendimidine

Complete nAChR gene families have been described for both vertebrates and invertebrates. Mammals have 16 genes encoding nAChR subunits, whereas *C. elegans* possesses an extensive and diverse nAChR subunit family [27] with 29 subunits divided into five "core" groups based on sequence homology in addition to four ACh-gated chloride channels (acetylcholine-gated chloride channels AChCls) (Figure 1.2). Each of the core groups have been so named after the first of their number to be discovered. As part of exploring *C. elegans* as a model for genetic analysis, Sydney Brenner mutagenized worms with ethyl methane sulfonate and successfully isolated worm mutants resistant to the paralyzing effects of the anthelmintic, levamisole [28]. This is a classic example of a chemistry-to-gene screen that uncovers molecular components targeted by a drug [29]. Levamisole (a nicotine-like drug) when applied to nematodes triggers enhanced contraction followed by paralysis. Five resistance loci are genes encoding the nAChR subunits making up the levamisole receptor, LEV-1 [30–32], LEV-8 or ACR-13 (acetylcholine receptor) [33], UNC-29 [31], UNC-38 [31], and UNC-63 [32]. Consistent with the paralyzing effects of levamisole, all five subunits are expressed in body wall muscle and electrophysiological studies on neuromuscular preparations from important L-type nAChR mutants confirmed their contribution to levamisole-sensitive nAChRs [32, 33]. Heterologous expression in *X. laevis* oocytes show that UNC-38, UNC-29, UNC-63, LEV-1, and LEV-8 can coassemble in the presence of three other essential proteins, RIC-3 (resistant to inhibitors of cholinesterase), UNC-50, and UNC-74, to form functional recombinant levamisole-sensitive nAChRs [34].

nAChRs (DEG-3 Group) – Targets for AADs

Researchers at Cambria and Novartis identified a novel anthelmintic drug target from the large family of DEG-3-type (degeneration of certain neurons) nAChR subunits in *C. elegans* using a chemistry-to-gene screen. They discovered the AADs, a new chemical class of synthetic anthelmintics effective against various species of nematodes pathogenic in livestock [35]. These compounds have a novel mode of action involving DEG-3-type nAChRs, notably ACR-23. The AADs are well tolerated by host species and exhibit low toxicity to mammals. They also overcome resistance to the currently available anthelmintics. Their excellent host tolerance is such that they are being explored for their potential as possible human anthelmintics.

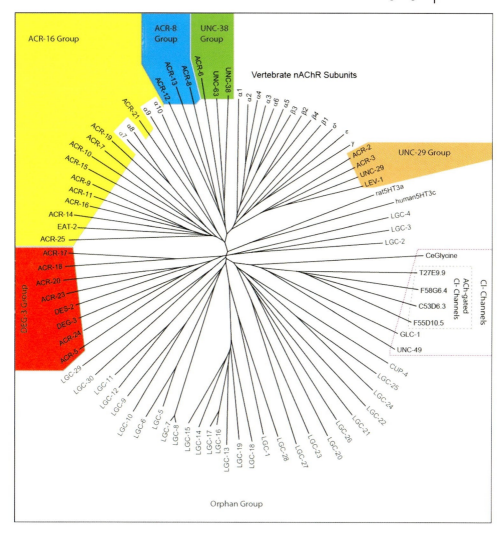

Figure 1.2 Tree showing the nAChR family of C. elegans. The worm nAChRs are divided into five core groups, whereas subunits showing substantial homology with other known nAChR subunits that do not fall within the core groups are designated orphan subunits. (Adapted by permission from Macmillan Publishers Ltd [29] © 2005.)

GABA-Gated Chloride Channels – Targets for Piperazine

GABA-gated chloride channels (γ-aminobutyric acid-gated chloride channel GABACls) have been described in C. elegans. Products of the unc-49 gene form a GABA-gated anion channel that mediates body muscle inhibition during locomotion [30]. The unc-49 gene is alternatively spliced with a single copy of a GABA receptor N-terminus, followed by three tandem copies of GABA receptor C-termini.

At least two of these subunits (UNC-49B and UNC-49C) are colocalized at the NMJ [36]. The UNC-49B subunit is also essential for receptor function and can form both homomeric and heteromeric receptors when co-expressed with UNC-49C in *X. laevis* oocytes [36, 37]. The application of GABA and the GABA receptor agonist muscimol to wild-type and *unc-49* mutant worms confirmed that the *unc-49* gene encodes the GABA receptors that control movement [30]. A separate study indicated that GABA receptors are found in *C. elegans* motor neurons and the ablation of these neurons induced defects in locomotion and defecation [38, 39]. Also, an inhibitory function for GABA receptors in body wall muscles has been shown [30]. There are four other subunits included in this group (Figure 1.3). With regard to other species, members of the UNC-49 group are most closely related to mammalian and insect GABA-gated anion channels [40]. *C. elegans* GAB-1 can contribute to functional GABA receptors when coexpressed in *X. laevis* oocytes with either HG1A or HG1E, which are putative GABA receptor subunits from the parasitic nematode *Haemonchus contortus* [41].

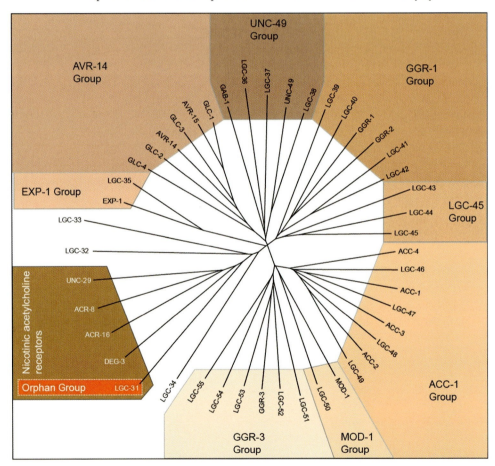

Figure 1.3 Tree showing the Cys-loop LGIC family of *C. elegans*. This figure focuses on Cys-loop LGICs other than nAChRs, although representative members of the nAChRs are shown (Adapted by permission from Springer [4] © 2008.)

Evaluating Possible Anthelmintic Targets for the Future

As our understanding of LGIC subgroups develops, more members come into the frame as candidate drug targets. Assessing the impact of gain- or loss-of-function mutants on nematode viability will be an important indicator of their potential utility as targets.

N-Type nAChRs

The *C. elegans* ACR-16 group, resembling vertebrate α7-like subunits, contains 11 members [42, 43]. ACR-16 is an essential component of the levamisole-insensitive N-type nAChR [44, 45]. ACR-16 forms functional homomeric channels when expressed in *X. laevis* oocytes [42, 46]. Similar α7-like subunits have also been found in the trematode *Schistosoma haematobium* [47] and arthropods [48], indicating an ancient lineage for this receptor subtype. They are sensitive to nicotine, not levamisole, and are designated N-type receptors.

Nematode-Specific nAChRs and Orphan nAChR-Like Subunits

The ACR-8 and DEG-3 groups appear to represent nematode-specific receptor subtypes [27]. In addition, there are 26 subunits, denoted orphan subunits (Figure 1.2), which show substantial homology to nAChRs, but do not fall within the five core groups. The orphan subunits CUP-4 and Y58G8A.1 are required for efficient endocytosis of fluids by coelomocytes [49].

GABA Receptor Cation Channels

This group contains EXP-1 (expulsion defective) and LGC-35 (ligand-gated ion channels of the Cys-loop superfamily) (Figure 1.3). EXP-1 is a GABA-gated channel that mediates muscle contraction [50]. When expressed in *Xenopus* oocytes, it forms a GABA receptor that is permeable to cations. EXP-1 lacks the PAR (Pro–Ala–Arg) motif preceding the second transmembrane domain (TM2) which is important for anion selectivity [51]. Instead, it possesses the residues ETE implicated in determining cation selectivity [51, 52]. LGC-35 has not been functionally expressed but also has a glutamate residue preceding TM2 and thus may also be a cation channel.

5-HT Channels

MOD-1 (modulation of locomotion defective) is a 5-HT-gated anion channel [53]. It is expressed in the *C. elegans* nervous system and modulates locomotor behavior [52]. LGC-50 is closely related to MOD-1.

ACh Chloride Channels

This group includes ACC-1 (acetylcholine-gated chloride channel), ACC-2, ACC-3, and ACC-4, which are ACh-gated anion channels [54] (Figure 1.3). ACC-1 and ACC-2 form homomeric channels in *X. laevis* oocytes. ACh and arecoline are agonists, but nicotine is not [54]. The ACh-binding domains of these AChCl subunits diverge substantially from the ACh-binding domain of nAChRs. Unlike ACh-gated anion channels of the snail, *Lymnaea stagnalis*, which appear to have evolved from cation channels through amino acid substitutions in the ion channel pore [55], the ACC-1 group may have arisen from substitutions in the ligand-binding domain of anion channels [54, 55].

GGR-1 Group

Six subunits make up this group, all of which remain to be functionally characterized (Figure 1.3). The neurotransmitters to which these subunits respond cannot easily be envisaged. The subunits most closely resemble glycine α-subunits (25%), whereas LGC-42 shows a 26% identity to insect histamine-gated anion channels [4, 40]. They are likely to be anion-selective as all possess the PAR motif [51]. Recently, LGC-40 was identified as a receptor for 5-HT, and it is also gated by choline and ACh [7].

GGR-3 Group

LGC-53 is a dopamine receptor gating a chloride channel, whereas LGC-55 is a tyramine-gated chloride channel [7, 56]. Both have been functionally expressed in *Xenopus* oocytes [7]. The remaining four subunits making up the GGR-3 group of *C. elegans* have not been characterized.

LGC-45 Group

LGC-43, LGC-44, and LGC-45 (Figure 1.3) remain to be functionally characterized. Like the GGR-1 group, the LGC-45 group members closely resemble human glycine α-subunits and insect histamine-gated anion channels [4]. However, unlike the GGR-1 group, the LGC-45 group subunits are likely to be cation-selective as they lack the PAR motif preceding M2 [51]. LGC-44 and LGC-45 possess a glutamic acid instead of the proline residue in the PAR motif, which is likely to result in a cation-selective channel [52]. LGC-44 also lacks a Cys-loop. The absence of a Cys-loop has also been reported in a bacterial proton-gated ion channel (from *Gloeobacter violaceus*) [57, 58]. Therefore, LGC-44 may represent an ancestral Cys-loop LGIC.

Ungrouped Subunits

The LGC-32, LGC-33, and LGC-34 subunits are highly divergent (Figure 1.3), showing up to 10, 10, and 15% identity, respectively, with other *C. elegans*, human, and *Drosophila melanogaster* Cys-loop LGICs [4]. These subunits have not been functionally characterized. Although these subunits contain some of the features common to Cys-loop LGICs, the Cys-loop is absent [59]. Thus, LGC-34 may also represent an ancestral Cys-loop LGIC.

Cys-Loop LGIC Superfamilies of Other Nematodes

Genome-sequencing projects are enabling the comparison of Cys-loop LGIC superfamilies from different nematode species. For example, *Caenorhabditis briggsae* [48, 60] also has an extensive Cys-loop LGIC gene superfamily, although comparative genomics suggest there appears to be an expansion in *C. elegans* within the nAChR orphan group. For example, there is only one homolog of LGC-28 in *C. briggsae*, whereas LGC-23, LGC-24, and LGC-28 are present in *C. elegans* [61].

The availability of genome sequence information for *B. malayi* and *Trichinella spiralis* (both smaller than the *C. elegans* genome) has facilitated the characterization of their Cys-loop LGICs (30 and 19 subunits, respectively). The Cys-loop LGICs of both parasites are orthologous with those of *C. elegans* with the exception of an nAChR subunit (ACR-26) that, to date, appears specific to *B. malayi*. Williamson *et al.* [62] propose that the difference in the Cys-loop LGIC family sizes may reflect a free-living versus a parasitic lifestyle in that a larger complement of subunits may be required to respond to many environmental cues not encountered by the parasites. Indeed, a study of over 30 nematode genomes (of varying completeness) [63] detected an average of 31 and 57 LGICs in parasitic and nonparasitic species, respectively. Sequencing and annotations are underway for other nematode parasites including *H. contortus*, *Teladorsagia circumcincta*, and the human hookworm, *Necator americanus*. Nomenclature can present problems [64]. Cys-loop LGIC genes have been identified from multiple nematode species, but relatively few have been cloned and expressed [62].

nAChRs in the body wall muscle of *Ascaris suum* have been investigated in detail. Excitatory actions of ACh [65, 66] and anticholinesterases potentiate the actions of ACh [65]. Also, morantel and pyrantel activate nAChRs [66]. Martin *et al.*, using patch-clamp recording from vesicles reconstituted from *Ascaris* muscles, showed the presence of at least two types of ACh-activated channels [67, 68]. Also, they showed that pyrantel is both an agonist and open channel blocker of nicotinic receptors in *A. suum* [69]. The nAChR antagonist, paraherquamide, a novel natural anthelmintic product, was employed to pharmacologically separate populations of *A. suum* muscle N-subtype (nicotine-sensitive) and L-subtype (levamisole-sensitive) nAChRs [70]. Later studies by Martin *et al.* have added a third muscle nAChR subtype, the B-type (bephenium-sensitive) receptor [71]. Williamson *et al.* have found that manipulating concentrations of *Ascaris unc-38* and *unc-29* RNA injected into *Xenopus* oocytes can generate heteromeric receptors that are more sensitive to levamisole or nicotine [72]. As genes encoding the LEV-1 and LEV-8 subunits are not present, this all points to a different composition for muscle nAChRs in *A. suum*. Levamisole-resistance in *Oesophagostomum dentatum* larvae is associated with a loss of L-subtype, but not the N-subtype receptors [73]. As more comparative physiology becomes available it will be of interest to establish whether these receptor subtypes are equivalent in different nematode phyla. For example, are the N-subtypes of *A. suum* and *O. dentatum* composed of homologs of ACR-16? Studies on muscle receptor subtypes of two parasitic species (*O. dentatum* and *A. suum*) confirm the continued utility of *C. elegans* as a model of parasitic nematodes in the search for new drug targets. *C. elegans* and

H. contortus belong to the same phylogenetic group (clade V), and their LGICs are now being extensively studied. There appears to be a large number of *C. elegans* homologs present in *H. contortus*. Neveu *et al.* have identified the L-subtype receptors and successfully functionally expressed these in *X. laevis* oocytes [74, 75]. Other LGICs have been identified, including GABA receptors (Hco-UNC-49B, Hco-UNC-49C) [76], and biogenic amine receptors including Hco-LGC-55 (tyramine) [77] and Hco-GGR-3 (dopamine) [78]. Multiple GluCls are present, including the alternatively spliced Hco-GBR/AVR-14 (Hco-GBR-2A and Hco-GBR-2B) [79], HcGluClα [80, 81], and HcGluClβ [82]. *C. elegans* has shown potential as a suitable system for studying parasitic nematode genes with the successful expression of Hco-AVR-14 in a *C. elegans* mutant line [16]. This method is showing promise as a high-throughput *in vivo* screen for novel anthelmintics. Studies on a *C. elegans* GGR-3 homolog in *H. contortus*, Hco-ggr-3 (84% similarity), showed that this subunit formed a homomeric receptor that responded primarily to dopamine [78]. A homolog of LGC-34 has been described in the parasitic roundworm, *Dirofilaria immitis*, that shows a 52% identity [59].

Genomics

WormBase (www.wormbase.org) is a major publically available dataset, initially created for the storage of *C. elegans* genomic information. It is now the central repository for nematode biology, containing complete genome sequences, gene predictions, and orthology assignments from a range of related nematodes. It relies on a manual curation pipeline ensuring that all data is consistent and of high quality. Genome sequence information and, recently, phylogenomics has been used to predict drug sensitivity in different species [63]. With the significant growth in the amount of sequence data available for nematodes, this has facilitated the prediction of potential drug targets using bioinformatics techniques. Hitherto, all antiparasitic drugs have been discovered by empirical screening in parasites or models such as *C. elegans* [83]. This remains an important and valid approach. Nevertheless, target-based screening has advantages as it generates structure–activity relationships and enables lead optimization at the target itself [84].

Chemistry-to-Gene Screens to Identify New Targets

Chemistry-to-gene screens that involve mutagenesis of *C. elegans* followed by screening for resistance to the chemical under investigation have a proven track record in target identification [29] and are likely to be equally useful in identifying gene targets for new compounds that have been shown to have anthelmintic activity, but for which the site of action is unknown. Double-stranded RNAi [85], a rapid method for individual gene silencing that is now applicable to the entire genome [86, 87], will also complement chemistry-to-gene studies in helping validate future candidate drug targets. The utility of chemistry-to-gene approaches is illustrated by the discovery that, as well as identifying genes encoding L-type nAChR subunits, the levamisole-resistance loci include genes encoding important proteins acting upstream or downstream of nAChRs (reviewed in [29]). These include: LEV-10, which is required for nAChR aggregation at the NMJ [88]; UNC-50, which is involved in the processing and assembly of receptors [89], for which the mammalian homolog was identified and found to function similarly [90]; LEV-11 and UNC-22, which regulate muscle contraction [90, 91]; and UNC-68 (a ryanodine receptor), which is involved in calcium signaling [92]. Interestingly, ryanodine itself has been used as a pesticide [93] and the receptor has recently been identified as the target of anthranilic diamides – an important new class of chemicals targeting invertebrate pests [94]. Thus, this study also identified a pesticide target that is functionally related to the primary target of levamisole (the L-type nAChR subunits). This suggests that molecular components functionally linked to Cys-loop LGICs and highlighted in chemistry-to-gene screens could also yield new animal health drug targets.

First Crystal Structure of a Cys-Loop LGIC Complexed with a Commercial Animal Health Drug

The first three-dimensional structure of a eukaryotic Cys-loop LGIC was reported in 2011 by Hibbs and Gouaux [14]. The *C. elegans* homomer-forming, anion-selective, GluClα subunit has been described at 3.3 Å resolution. The structure of the GluCl–Fab complex bound to ivermectin yields important insights into the interactions of a major animal health drug with its allosteric binding site. Ivermectin, which stabilizes the open pore conformation, binds in the transmembrane region, forming a wedge between the M1 and M3 helices, and also interacts with the M2–M3 loop. Other structures were obtained with the neurotransmitter L-glutamate docked in the orthosteric binding site. L-Glutamate binds to the agonist site at the interface between subunits. Arginine residues, in combination with neighboring cationic amino acids, provide the binding pocket with a strongly positive electrostatic potential. The α-amino nitrogen of L-glutamate is stabilized through a 3.8-Å cation–π interaction with Tyr200 on loop C, a hydrogen bond with the backbone carbonyl oxygen of Ser150, and a close interaction with the backbone carbonyl oxygen of Tyr151. Structures obtained with picrotoxin bound show that this open channel blocker binds to the cytoplasmic end of the pore. The tricyclic rings are directed extracellularly and near the 2′ Thr, whereas the isoprenyl tail points towards the cytoplasm and is close to the −2′ Pro residues. Thus, we can now visualize the binding of important orthosteric, allosteric, and channel blocking ligands and, not least, the important animal heath drug, ivermectin, to nematode Cys-loop LGICs.

Conclusions and Future Lines of Research

The adoption of a multigene family in the search for drug targets may be important. The evolution of drug resistance may be slower if several target genes have to be mutated simultaneously to confer resistance. This may account for the relatively slow onset of resistance to ivermectin. Research on nematode Cys-loop LGIC superfamilies, accelerated by genomics, is adding to our understanding of their rich diversity. This genomics-led expansion of our knowledge of the physiological spectrum of LGICs also exposes new candidate drug targets. The powerful genetic toolkit available in model organisms such as *C. elegans* is likely to remain useful in helping validate these candidate targets, even though the future holds the exciting prospect of access to many new parasite genomes.

From this brief overview it is evident that both forward and reverse genetic studies on *C. elegans* have contributed significantly to both identifying novel genes involved in nematode synaptic transmission and to determining the receptor subunits that form the molecular targets of antiparasitic drugs. Such approaches will continue to be to the fore when compounds with anthelmintic activity, but for which the target is unknown, are under development. Chemistry-to-gene screens, of the type that have focused attention on a small subset of subunits (from a very large family) as the targets for levamisole, have also proved useful in identifying functionally linked genes that include candidate targets for novel drugs with a quite different mechanism of action. In future, we can envisage generating improved selectivity for parasite over host by exploring further as drug targets those Cys-loop LGICs that are either parasite-specific or where host and parasite orthologs differ considerably in sequence. Studies on nematode parasites have shown that several types of chemistry with antiparasitic activity can act successfully on a single class of receptors such as nAChRs. Studies on laboratory-resistant strains have proved useful in understanding drug targets and synaptic function, and future studies on field-resistant strains will enhance our understanding of resistance mechanisms, which can imperil the longevity of a commercial antiparasitic product.

References

1 Garba, A., Toure, S., Dembele, R., Boisier, P., Tohon, Z., Bosque-Oliva, E., Koukounari, A., and Fenwick, A. (2009) Present and future Schistosomiasis control activities with support from the Schistosomiasis control initiative in west Africa. *Parasitology*, **136**, 1731–1737.

2 Kaplan, R.M. (2004) Drug resistance in nematodes of veterinary importance: a status report. *Trends Parasitol.*, **20**, 477–481.

3 Evans, T. and Chapple, N. (2002) The animal health market. *Nat. Rev. Drug Discov.*, **1**, 937–938.

4 Jones, A.K. and Sattelle, D.B. (2008) The cys-loop ligand-gated ion channel gene superfamily of the nematode, *Caenorhabditis elegans*. *Invert. Neurosci.*, **8**, 41–47.

5 Raymond, V. and Sattelle, D.B. (2002) Novel animal-health drug targets from ligand-gated chloride channels. *Nat. Rev. Drug Discov.*, **1**, 427–436.

6 Barnes, K.C., Grant, A.V., and Gao, P. (2005) A review of the genetic epidemiology of resistance to parasitic disease and atopic asthma: common variants for common phenotypes? *Curr. Opin. Allergy Clin. Immunol.*, **5**, 379–385.

7 Ringstad, N., Abe, N., and Horvitz, H.R. (2009) Ligand-gated chloride channels are receptors for biogenic amines in *C. elegans*. *Science*, **325**, 96–100.

8 Sutherland, I.A. and Leathwick, D.M. (2011) Anthelmintic resistance in nematode parasites of cattle: a global issue? *Trends Parasitol.*, **27**, 176–181.

9 Sargison, N.D., Jackson, F., Wilson, D.J., Bartley, D.J., Penny, C.D., and Gilleard, J.S. (2010) Characterisation of milbemycin-, avermectin-, imidazothiazole- and benzimidazole-resistant *Teladorsagia circumcincta* from a sheep flock. *Vet. Rec.*, **166**, 681–686.

10 VLA (2008) Suspected macrocyclic lactone resistance in common sheep nematodes. *Vet. Rec.*, **163**, 673–676.

11 McKellar, Q.A. and Jackson, F. (2004) Veterinary anthelmintics: old and new. *Trends Parasitol.*, **20**, 456–461.

12 *C. elegans* Sequencing Consortium (1998) Genome sequence of the nematode, *C. elegans*: a platform for investigating biology. *Science*, **282**, 2012–2018.

13 Ghedin, E., Wang, S., Foster, J.M., and Slatko, B.E. (2004) First sequenced genome of a parasitic nematode. *Trends Parasitol.*, **20**, 151–153.

14 Hibbs, R.E. and Gouaux, E. (2011) Principles of activation and permeation in an anion-selective cys-loop receptor. *Nature*, **474**, 54–60.

15 Brooks, D.R. and Isaac, R.E. (2002) Functional genomics of parasitic worms: the dawn of a new era. *Parasitol. Int.*, **51**, 319–325.

16 Glendinning, S.K., Sattelle, D.B., Buckingham, S.D., Wonnacott, S., and Wolstenholme, A.J. (2011) Glutamate-gated chloride channels of *Haemonchus contortus* restore drug sensitivity to ivermectin resistant *Caenorhabditis elegans*. *PLoS One*, **6**, e22390.

17 Unwin, N. (2005) Refined structure of the nicotinic acetylcholine receptor at 4A resolution. *J. Mol. Biol.*, **346**, 967–989.

18 Karlin, A. (2002) Emerging structure of the nicotinic acetylcholine receptors. *Nat. Rev. Neurosci.*, **3**, 102–114.

19 Cully, D.F., Paress, P.S., Liu, K.K., Schaeffer, J.M., and Arena, J.P. (1996) Identification of a *Drosophila melanogaster* glutamate-gated chloride channel sensitive to the antiparasitic agent avermectin. *J. Biol. Chem.*, **271**, 20187–20191.

20 Wolstenholme, A.J. and Rogers, A.T. (2005) Glutamate-gated chloride channels and the mode of action of the avermectin/milbemycin anthelmintics. *Parasitology*, **131**, S85–S95.

21 Dent, J.A., Davis, M.W., and Avery, L. (1997) Avr-15 encodes a chloride channel subunit that mediates inhibitory glutamatergic neurotransmission and ivermectin sensitivity in *Caenorhabditis elegans*. *EMBO J.*, **16**, 5867–5879.

22 Pemberton, D.J., Franks, C.J., Walker, R.J., and Holden-Dye, L. (2001) Characterization of glutamate-gated chloride channels in the pharynx of wild-type and mutant *Caenorhabditis elegans* delineates the role of the subunit GluCl-alpha2 in the function of the native receptor. *Mol. Pharmacol.*, **59**, 1037–1043.

23 Laughton, D.L., Lunt, G.G., and Wolstenholme, A.J. (1997) Alternative splicing of a *Caenorhabditis elegans* gene produces two novel inhibitory amino acid receptor subunits with identical ligand binding domains but different ion channels. *Gene*, **201**, 119–125.

24 Cook, A., Aptel, N., Portillo, V., Siney, E., Sihota, R., Holden-Dye, L., and Wolstenholme, A. (2006) *Caenorhabditis elegans* ivermectin receptors regulate locomotor behaviour and are functional orthologues of *Haemonchus contortus* receptors. *Mol. Biochem. Parasitol.*, **147**, 118–125.

25 Chalasani, S.H., Chronis, N., Tsunozaki, M., Gray, J.M., Ramot, D., Goodman, M.B., and Bargmann, C.I. (2007) Dissecting a circuit for olfactory behaviour in *Caenorhabditis elegans*. *Nature*, **450**, 63–70.

26 Dent, J.A., Smith, M.M., Vassilatis, D.K., and Avery, L. (2000) The genetics of ivermectin resistance in *Caenorhabditis elegans*. *Proc. Natl. Acad. Sci. USA*, **97**, 2674–2679.

27 Jones, A.K. and Sattelle, D.B. (2004) Functional genomics of the nicotinic acetylcholine receptor gene family of the nematode, *Caenorhabditis elegans*. *Bioessays*, **26**, 39–49.

28 Brenner, S. (1974) The genetics of *Caenorhabditis elegans*. *Genetics*, **77**, 71–94.

29 Jones, A.K., Buckingham, S.D., and Sattelle, D.B. (2005) Chemistry-to-gene screens in *Caenorhabditis elegans*. *Nat. Rev. Drug Discov.*, **4**, 321–330.

30 Richmond, J.E., and Jorgensen, E.M. (1999) One GABA and two acetylcholine receptors function at the *C. elegans* neuromuscular junction. *Nat. Neurosci.*, **2**, 791–797.

31 Fleming, J.T., Baylis, H.A., Sattelle, D.B., and Lewis, J.A. (1996) Molecular cloning and *in vitro* expression of *C. elegans* and parasitic nematode ionotropic receptors. *Parasitology*, (113 Suppl), S175–S190.

32 Culetto, E., Baylis, H.A., Richmond, J.E., Jones, A.K., Fleming, J.T., Squire, M.D., Lewis, J.A., and Sattelle, D.B. (2004) The *Caenorhabditis elegans unc-63* gene encodes a levamisole-sensitive nicotinic acetylcholine receptor alpha subunit. *J. Biol. Chem.*, **279**, 42476–42483.

33 Towers, P.R., Edwards, B., Richmond, J.E., and Sattelle, D.B. (2005) The *Caenorhabditis elegans lev-8* gene encodes a novel type of nicotinic acetylcholine receptor alpha subunit. *J. Neurochem.*, **93**, 1–9.

34 Boulin, T., Gielen, M., Richmond, J.E., Williams, D.C., Paoletti, P., and Bessereau, J.L. (2008) Eight genes are required for functional reconstitution of the *Caenorhabditis elegans* levamisole-sensitive acetylcholine receptor. *Proc. Natl. Acad. Sci. USA*, **105**, 18590–18595.

35 Kaminsky, R., Ducray, P., Jung, M., Clover, R., Rufener, L., Bouvier, J., Weber, S.S. et al. (2008) A new class of anthelmintics effective against drug-resistant nematodes. *Nature*, **452**, 176–180.

36 Bamber, B.A., Beg, A.A., Twyman, R.E., and Jorgensen, E.M. (1999) The *Caenorhabditis elegans unc-49* locus encodes multiple subunits of a heteromultimeric GABA receptor. *J. Neurosci.*, **19**, 5348–5359.

37 Bamber, B.A., Tyman, R.E., and Jorgensen, E.M. (2003) Pharmacological characterisation of the homomeric and heteromeric UNC-49 GABA receptors in *C. elegans*. *Br. J. Pharmacol.*, **138**, 883–893.

38 McIntire, S.L., Jorgensen, E., and Horvitz, H.R. (1993) Genes required for GABA function in *Caenorhabditis elegans*. *Nature*, **364**, 334–337.

39 McIntire, S.L., Jorgensen, E., Kaplan, J., and Horvitz, H.R. (1993) The GABAergic nervous system of *Caenorhabditis elegans*. *Nature*, **364**, 337–341.

40 Dent, J.A. (2006) Evidence for a diverse cys-loop ligand-gated ion channel superfamily in early bilateria. *J. Mol. Evol.*, **62**, 523–535.

41 Feng, X.P., Hayashi, J., Beech, R.N., and Prichard, R.K. (2002) Study of the nematode putative GABA type-A receptor subunits: evidence for modulation by ivermectin. *J. Neurochem.*, **83**, 870–878.

42 Ballivet, M., Alliod, C., Bertrand, S., and Bertrand, D. (1996) Nicotinic acetylcholine receptors in the nematode *Caenorhabditis elegans*. *J. Mol. Biol.*, **258**, 261–269.

43 Mongan, N.P., Jones, A.K., Smith, G.R., Sansom, M.S., and Sattelle, D.B. (2002) Novel alpha7-like nicotinic acetylcholine receptor subunits in the nematode *Caenorhabditis elegans*. *Protein Sci.*, **11**, 1162–1171.

44 Francis, M.M., Evans, S.P., Jensen, M., Madsen, D.M., Mancuso, J., Norman, K.R., and Maricq, A.V. (2005) The Ror receptor tyrosine kinase CAM-1 is required for ACR-16-mediated synaptic transmission at the *C. elegans* neuromuscular junction. *Neuron*, **46**, 581–594.

45 Touroutine, D., Fox, R.M., Von Stetina, S.E., Burdina, A., Miller, D.M. 3rd, and Richmond, J.E. (2005) Acr-16 encodes an essential subunit of the levamisole-resistant nicotinic receptor at the *Caenorhabditis elegans* neuromuscular junction. *J. Biol. Chem.*, **280**, 27013–27021.

46 Raymond, V., Mongan, N.P., and Sattelle, D.B. (2000) Anthelmintic actions on homomer-forming nicotinic acetylcholine receptor subunits: chicken alpha7 and ACR-16 from the nematode *Caenorhabditis elegans*. *Neuroscience*, **101**, 785–791.

47 Bentley, G.N., Jones, A.K., Parra, W.G.O., and Agnew, A. (2004) ShAR1 alpha and ShAR1 beta: novel putative nicotinic acetylcholine receptor subunits from the

platyhelminth blood fluke *Schistosoma*. *Gene*, **329**, 27–38.

48 Grauso, M., Reenan, R.A., Culetto, E., and Sattelle, D.B. (2002) Novel putative nicotinic acetylcholine receptor subunit genes, D alpha 5, D alpha 6 and D alpha 7 in *Drosophila melanogaster* identify a new and highly conserved target of adenosine deaminase acting on RNA-mediated A-to-I pre-mRNA editing. *Genetics*, **160**, 1519–1533.

49 Patton, A., Knuth, S., Schaheen, B., Dang, H., Greenwald, I., and Fares, H. (2005) Endocytosis function of a ligand-gated ion channel homolog in *Caenorhabditis elegans*. *Curr. Biol.*, **15**, 1045–1050.

50 Beg, A.A. and Jorgensen, E.M. (2003) EXP-1 is an excitatory GABA-gated cation channel. *Nat. Neurosci.*, **6**, 1145–1152.

51 Jensen, M.L., Schousboe, A., and Ahring, P.K. (2005) Charge selectivity of the cys-loop family of ligand-gated ion channels. *J. Neurochem.*, **92**, 217–225.

52 Wotring, V.E. and Weiss, D.S. (2008) Charge scan reveals an extended region at the intracellular end of the GABA receptor pore that can influence ion selectivity. *J. Gen. Physiol.*, **131**, 87–97.

53 Ranganathan, R., Cannon, S.C., and Horvitz, H.R. (2000) MOD-1 is a serotonin-gated chloride channel that modulates locomotory behaviour in *C. elegans*. *Nature*, **408**, 470–475.

54 Putrenko, I., Zakikhani, M., and Dent, J.A. (2005) A family of acetylcholine-gated chloride channel subunits in *Caenorhabditis elegans*. *J. Biol. Chem.*, **280**, 6392–6398.

55 van Nierop, P., Keramidas, A., Bertrand, S., van Minnen, J., Gouwenberg, Y., Bertrand, D., and Smit, A.B. (2005) Identification of molluscan nicotinic acetylcholine receptor (nAChR) subunits involved in formation of cation- and anion-selective nAChRs. *J. Neurosci.*, **25**, 10617–10626.

56 Pirri, J.K., McPherson, A.D., Donnelly, J.L., Francis, M.M., and Alkema, M.J. (2009) A tyramine-gated chloride channel coordinates distinct motor programs of a *Caenorhabditis elegans* escape response. *Neuron*, **62**, 526–538.

57 Bocquet, N., Prado de Carvalho, L., Cartaud, J., Neyton, J., Le Poupon, C., Taly, A., Grutter, T. *et al.* (2007) A prokaryotic proton-gated ion channel from the nicotinic acetylcholine receptor family. *Nature*, **445**, 116–119.

58 Tasneem, A., Iyer, L.M., Jakobsson, E., and Aravind, L. (2005) Identification of the prokaryotic ligand-gated ion channels and their implications for the mechanisms and origins of animal cys-loop ion channels. *Genome Biol.*, **6**, R4.

59 Yates, D.M. and Wolstenholme, A.J. (2004) *Dirofilaria immitis*: Identification of a novel ligand-gated ion channel-related polypeptide. *Exp. Parasitol.*, **108**, 182–185.

60 Stein, L.D., Bao, Z., Blasiar, D., Blumenthal, T., Brent, M.R., Chen, N., Chinwalla, A. *et al.* (2003) The genome sequence of *Caenorhabditis briggsae*: a platform for comparative genomics. *PLoS Biol.*, **1**, E45.

61 Jones, A.K., Davis, P., Hodgkin, J., and Sattelle, D.B. (2007) The nicotinic acetylcholine receptor gene family of the nematode *Caenorhabditis elegans*: an update on nomenclature. *Invert. Neurosci.*, **7**, 129–131.

62 Williamson, S.M., Walsh, T.K., and Wolstenholme, A.J. (2007) The cys-loop ligand-gated ion channel gene family of *Brugia malayi* and *Trichinella spiralis*: a comparison with *Caenorhabditis elegans*. *Invert. Neurosci.*, **7**, 219–226.

63 Rufener, L., Keiser, J., Kaminsky, R., Maser, P., and Nilsson, D. (2010) Phylogenomics of ligand-gated ion channels predicts monepantel effect. *PLoS Pathog.*, **6**, e1001091.

64 Beech, R.N., Wolstenholme, A.J., Neveu, C., and Dent, J.A. (2010) Nematode parasite genes: what's in a name? *Trends Parasitol.*, **26**, 334–340.

65 Rozhkova, E.K., Malyutina, T.A., and Shishov, B.A. (1980) Pharmacological characteristics of cholinoreception in somatic muscles of the nematode, *Ascaris suum*. *Gen. Pharmacol.*, **11**, 141–146.

66 Harrow, I.D. and Gration, K.A.F. (1985) Mode of action of the anthelmintics morantel, pyrantel and levamisole on muscle cell membrane of the nematode *Ascaris suum*. *Pestic. Sci.*, **16**, 662–672.

67 Pennington, A.J. and Martin, R.J. (1990) A patch-clamp study of acetylcholine-activated ion channels in *Ascaris suum* muscle. *J. Exp. Biol.*, **154**, 201–221.

68 Robertson, S.J. and Martin, R.J. (1993) Levamisole-activated single-channel currents from muscle of the nematode parasite *Ascaris suum*. *Br. J. Pharmacol.*, **108**, 170–178.

69 Robertson, S.J., Pennington, A.J., Evans, A.M., and Martin, R.J. (1994) The action of pyrantel as an agonist and an open channel blocker at acetylcholine receptors in isolated *Ascaris suum* muscle vesicles. *Eur. J. Pharmacol.*, **271**, 273–282.

70 Robertson, A.P., Clark, C.L., Burns, T.A., Thompson, D.P., Geary, T.G., Trailovic, S.M., and Martin, R.J. (2002) Paraherquamide and 2-deoxy-paraherquamide distinguish cholinergic receptor subtypes in *Ascaris* muscle. *J. Pharmacol. Exp. Ther.*, **302**, 853–860.

71 Trailovic, S.M., Clark, C.L., Robertson, A.P., and Martin, R.J. (2005) Brief application of AF2 produces long lasting potentiation of nAChR responses in *Ascaris suum*. *Mol. Biochem. Parasitol.*, **139**, 51–64.

72 Williamson, S.M., Robertson, A.P., Brown, L., Williams, T., Woods, D.J., Martin, R.J., Sattelle, D.B., and Wolstenholme, A.J. (2009) The nicotinic acetylcholine receptors of the parasitic nematode *Ascaris suum*: formation of two distinct drug targets by varying the relative expression levels of two subunits. *PLoS Pathog.*, **5**, e1000517.

73 Martin, R.J., Bai, G., Clark, C.L., and Robertson, A.P. (2003) Methyridine (2-[2-methoxyethyl]-pyridine]) and levamisole activate different ACh receptor subtypes in nematode parasites: a new lead for levamisole-resistance. *Br. J. Pharmacol.*, **140**, 1068–1076.

74 Boulin, T., Fauvin, A., Charvet, C., Cortet, J., Cabaret, J., Bessereau, J.L., and Neveu, C. (2011) Functional reconstitution of *Haemonchus contortus* acetylcholine receptors in *Xenopus* oocytes provides mechanistic insights into levamisole resistance. *Br. J. Pharmacol.*, **164**, 1421–1432.

75 Neveu, C., Charvet, C.L., Fauvin, A., Cortet, J., Beech, R.N., and Cabaret, J. (2010) Genetic diversity of levamisole receptor subunits in parasitic nematode species and abbreviated transcripts associated with resistance. *Pharmacogenet. Genomics*, **20**, 414–425.

76 Siddiqui, S.Z., Brown, D.D., Rao, V.T., and Forrester, S.G. (2010) An UNC-49 GABA receptor subunit from the parasitic nematode *Haemonchus contortus* is associated with enhanced GABA sensitivity in nematode heteromeric channels. *J. Neurochem.*, **113**, 1113–1122.

77 Rao, V.T., Accardi, M.V., Siddiqui, S.Z., Beech, R.N., Prichard, R.K., and Forrester, S.G. (2010) Characterization of a novel tyramine-gated chloride channel from *Haemonchus contortus*. *Mol. Biochem. Parasitol.*, **173**, 64–68.

78 Rao, V.T., Siddiqui, S.Z., Prichard, R.K., and Forrester, S.G. (2009) A dopamine-gated ion channel (HcGGR3*) from *Haemonchus contortus* is expressed in the cervical papillae and is associated with macrocyclic lactone resistance. *Mol. Biochem. Parasitol.*, **166**, 54–61.

79 Jagannathan, S., Laughton, D.L., Critten, C.L., Skinner, T.M., Horoszok, L., and Wolstenholme, A.J. (1999) Ligand-gated chloride channel subunits encoded by the *Haemonchus contortus* and *Ascaris suum* orthologues of the *Caenorhabditis elegans gbr-2 (avr-14)* gene. *Mol. Biochem. Parasitol.*, **103**, 129–140.

80 Cheeseman, C.L., Delany, N.S., Woods, D.J., and Wolstenholme, A.J. (2001) High-affinity ivermectin binding to recombinant subunits of the *Haemonchus contortus* glutamate-gated chloride channel. *Mol. Biochem. Parasitol.*, **114**, 161–168.

81 Forrester, S.G., Hamdan, F.F., Prichard, R.K., and Beech, R.N. (1999) Cloning, sequencing, and developmental expression levels of a novel glutamate-gated chloride channel homologue in the parasitic nematode *Haemonchus contortus*.

Biochem. Biophys. Res. Commun., **254**, 529–534.

82 Delany, N.S., Laughton, D.L., and Wolstenholme, A.J. (1998) Cloning and localisation of an avermectin receptor-related subunit from *Haemonchus contortus*. *Mol. Biochem. Parasitol.*, **97**, 177–187.

83 Woods, D.J. and Williams, T.M. (2007) The challenges of developing novel antiparasitic drugs. *Invert. Neurosci.*, **7**, 245–250.

84 Woods, D.J. and Knauer, C.S. (2010) Discovery of veterinary antiparasitic agents in the 21st century: a view from industry. *Int. J. Parasitol.*, **40**, 1177–1181.

85 Fire, A., Xu, S., Montgomery, M.K., Kostas, S.A., Driver, S.E., and Mello, C.C. (1998) Potent and specific genetic interference by double-stranded RNA in *Caenorhabditis elegans*. *Nature*, **391**, 806–811.

86 Fraser, A.G., Kamath, R.S., Zipperlen, P., Martinez-Campos, M., Sohrmann, M., and Ahringer, J. (2000) Functional genomic analysis of *C. elegans* chromosome I by systematic RNA interference. *Nature*, **408**, 325–330.

87 Gonczy, P., Echeverri, C., Oegema, K., Coulson, A., Jones, S.J., Copley, R.R., Duperon, J. *et al.* (2000) Functional genomic analysis of cell division in *C. elegans* using RNAi of genes on chromosome III. *Nature*, **408**, 331–336.

88 Gally, C., Eimer, S., Richmond, J.E., and Bessereau, J.L. (2004) A transmembrane protein required for acetylcholine receptor clustering in *Caenorhabditis elegans*. *Nature*, **431**, 578–582.

89 Lewis, J.A., Elmer, J.S., Skimming, J., McLafferty, S., Fleming, J., and McGee, T. (1987) Cholinergic receptor mutants of the nematode *Caenorhabditis elegans*. *J. Neurosci.*, **7**, 3059–3071.

90 Fitzgerald, J., Kennedy, D., Viseshakul, N., Cohen, B.N., Mattick, J., Bateman, J.F., and Forsayeth, J.R. (2000) UNCL, the mammalian homologue of UNC-50, is an inner nuclear membrane RNA-binding protein. *Brain Res.*, **877**, 110–123.

91 Benian, G.M., L'Hernault, S.W., and Morris, M.E. (1993) Additional sequence complexity in the muscle gene, *unc-22*, and its encoded protein, twitchin, of *Caenorhabditis elegans*. *Genetics*, **134**, 1097–1104.

92 Maryon, E.B., Coronado, R., and Anderson, P. (1996) Unc-68 encodes a ryanodine receptor involved in regulating *C. elegans* body-wall muscle contraction. *J. Cell Biol.*, **134**, 885–893.

93 Jenden, D.J. and Fairhurst, A.S. (1969) The pharmacology of ryanodine. *Pharmacol. Rev.*, **21**, 1–25.

94 Lahm, G.P., Selby, T.P., Freudenberger, J.H., Stevenson, T.M., Myers, B.J., Seburyamo, G., Smith, B.K. *et al.* (2005) Insecticidal anthranilic diamides: a new class of potent ryanodine receptor activators. *Bioorg. Med. Chem. Lett.*, **15**, 4898–4906.

95 Pica-Mattoccia, L., Orsini, T., Basso, A., Festucci, A., Liberti, P., Guidi, A., Marcatto-Maggi, A.L. *et al.* (2008) *Schistosoma mansoni*: lack of correlation between praziquantel-induced intra-worm calcium influx and parasite death. *Exp. Parasitol.*, **119**, 332–335.

2
How Relevant is *Caenorhabditis elegans* as a Model for the Analysis of Parasitic Nematode Biology?

Lindy Holden-Dye[*] and Robert J. Walker

Abstract

Due to the development of resistance to anthelmintics there is a continuous requirement to search for new anthelmintics that act at novel sites. Until now, new anthelmintics have been discovered through screens using parasitic nematodes. However, their mode of action has often been determined through experimental approaches utilizing the free-living nematode, *Caenorhabditis elegans*. In this chapter, the value of *C. elegans* as a surrogate parasite will be considered. The phylogenetic relationship between *C. elegans* and parasitic nematodes suggests that *C. elegans* may be a preferred model for some parasitic nematodes more than others, being particularly useful for those in the same clade. In this context an important achievement has been the sequencing of the *C. elegans* genome followed by the genomes of a number of parasitic nematodes. This has enabled the identification of homologous and orthologous genes between *C. elegans* and parasitic nematodes with two particular experimental advances: (i) the identification of genes in *C. elegans* that are orthologous to those genes key for normal function in parasitic nematodes and (ii) the expression of parasitic nematode genes in *C. elegans* to facilitate their functional characterization. Examples of both will be given here. The value of the experimental tractability of *C. elegans* is weighed against the extent to which it provides a reliable indicator for gene function in parasitic nematodes. Also, we review the value of *C. elegans* in elucidating the mode of action of anthelmintics with particular reference to anthelmintics acting on nicotinic acetylcholine receptors, glutamate-gated chloride channels, and calcium-activated potassium channels. The examples highlight the use of *C. elegans* as a model system to identify anthelmintic drug targets. Finally, the potential impact of newer technologies encompassing microfluidics, optogenetics, and imaging on the utility of *C. elegans* for high-throughput anthelmintic drug discovery is addressed.

[*] Corresponding Author

Parasitic Helminths: Targets, Screens, Drugs and Vaccines, First Edition. Edited by Conor R. Caffrey
© 2012 Wiley-VCH Verlag GmbH & Co. KGaA. Published 2012 by Wiley-VCH Verlag GmbH & Co. KGaA.

Introduction

Nematode infection in farm animals and small companion animals (pets) is widespread, requiring repeated treatment with anthelmintics to prevent reinfection. This has resulted in resistance to the major anthelmintics (i.e., benzimidazoles (fenbendazole), macrocyclic lactones (ivermectin), imidazothiazoles (levamisole), and tetrahydropyrimidines (pyrantel)) [1, 2]. Many of these same drugs are used in human tropical medicine and while the existence of drug resistance in parasitic nematodes of human is equivocal, there is a real possibility that it has already appeared or may appear in the near future [3]. Nematodes are also very damaging crop pests [4]. In this respect it is important to note that environmental toxicity of chemical agents used in crop protection against plant parasitic nematodes has prompted the tightening of the regulations that govern the use of compounds for this purpose. Overall, in the face of nematode anthelmintic resistance and in the context of more stringent demands for environmental safety from regulatory bodies, there is a clear need for basic research into compounds with efficacy against nematodes for use in agriculture, veterinary medicine, and human disease.

One of the problems of using parasitic nematodes for anthelmintic drug research is their complex life cycles, which make their use both time-consuming and expensive. An alternative is to use the model nematode *Caenorhabditis elegans*, which has a short and relatively simple life cycle. It was first proposed for anthelmintic drug screening 30 years ago [5]. At that time its positive attributes as a laboratory model included ease and economy of culture, and its established response to known anthelmintic agents [6]. It was gaining a reputation as a model genetic animal [7], although this was well in advance of its rise to fame as the first animal to have its genome sequenced [8]. Since 1998, the availability of a fully sequenced and annotated *C. elegans* genome [8, 9] (www.wormbase.org) has been followed by a detailed database of the structural anatomy (www.wormatlas.org) including the neural connectivity [10], a central resource for archiving and distributing strains (*Caenorhabditis elegans* Genetics Center), and the instigation of a program to provide knockouts for every one of the approximately 23 000 genes of the *C. elegans* genome (celeganskoconsortium.omrf.org). This wealth of resource, combined with the experimental tractability of *C. elegans*, in particular for transgenics and gene knockouts [11–13], has encouraged more researchers, including parasitologists, to adopt this nematode as an experimental animal. It is therefore important to consider whether or not *C. elegans* is a meaningful alternative to parasitic nematodes, particularly with regard to the discovery and development of new anthelmintics.

There have been a number of reviews on the value of *C. elegans* in parasitic nematode research [14–17]. Burglin *et al.* [14] list three ways in which *C. elegans* can provide a model for parasitic nematodes that encompass the analysis of the expression pattern and function of parasite genes. An important aspect is the use of the well-annotated genome information for *C. elegans* as a bioinformatic route to identifying similar genes in parasitic nematodes and subsequently defining their function. The review of Gilleard [16] is also pertinent since it considers the extent to which the basic biology and genome organization is conserved in nematodes in addition to the use of *C. elegans* as a surrogate expression system for gene function in parasitic nematodes.

Here, we discuss the evidence that *C. elegans* provides an informative and relevant model system for the study of parasitic nematodes. We highlight past successes, potential pitfalls, and future opportunities in adopting this experimental model.

Comparative Genome Analysis for the Phylum Nematoda

Using small subunit ribosomal DNA sequences from a range of nematodes, Blaxter *et al.* [18] proposed the division of nematodes into five clades. Parasitic nematodes occur in all five clades (Table 2.1), and these authors consider that parasitism in plant and animal nematodes has independently arisen 3 and 4 times, respectively. *C. elegans,* a member of the Rhabditida, is placed in clade V together with the Strongylida and Diplogasterida. From this, Blaxter *et al.* [18] conclude that *C. elegans* would be a good model for the order Strongylida. Clade V includes a number of key parasitic nematodes whose genomes are being sequenced, including *Haemonchus contortus, Necator americanus, Ostertagia osteragi, Ancylostoma duodenale,* and *Nippostrongylus brasiliensis* [19] (www.nematode.net). As this classification places the Strongyloides in clade IV, it is proposed that species of the free-living nematode, *Panagrellus,* would be a preferred model for this group. These authors also suggest

Table 2.1 Examples of nematode species classified in clades following a molecular evolutionary framework proposed by Blaxter *et al.* [18].

Clade	Species
I	*Longidorus elongatus*
	Xiphinema rivesi
II	*Trichodorus primitivus*
	Prismatolaimus intermedius
III	*Ascaris suum*
	Ascaridia galli
	Brugia malayi
	Onchocerca volvulus
IV	*Panagrellus redivivus*
	Heterodera glycines
	Strongyloides stercoralis
	Globodera pallida
	Meloidogyne arenaria
V	*Caenorhabditis elegans*
	Haemonchus contortus
	Necator americanus
	Ostertagia asteragi
	Ancylostoma duodenale
	Pristionchus pacificus
	Nippostrongylus brasiliensis

that the members of the family Cephalobidae (e.g., *Acrobeles* and *Zeldia*) would be good models for plant nematodes of the genera *Tylenchida* and *Meloidogyne*. This raises the interesting prospect in which initial studies could be undertaken using *C. elegans* and followed up using other free-living nematodes judiciously chosen from those that are most closely related to the target parasitic nematode – an approach that, to our knowledge, has not yet been adopted.

There is extensive evidence of genes that are unique to the phylum Nematoda. For example, Parkinson *et al.* [20] estimated from expressed sequence tag (EST) sequences that more than 50% of putative nematode genes occur only in this phylum. For certain gene families, such as the nicotinic acetylcholine receptor (nAChR) family, there are family members that do not appear to occur in other phyla [21] and, indeed, have provided novel anthelmintic targets (e.g., the nematode-specific ACR-23 nAChR subunit, which is the target of monepantel) [22]. Furthermore, and not surprisingly, there is evidence for nematode-specific genes that are associated with particular aspects of the parasitic lifestyle. A recent example of this is the abundance of genes encoding enzymes in plant parasitic nematodes that are likely important in the invasion of the host plant [23]. Within the phylum itself, there is also evidence for extensive divergence between the species. For example, Parkinson *et al.* [20] have estimated from EST sequences that 23% of genes are unique to each species.

One problem in identifying homologous genes between species is the variety of abbreviations used in the literature for genes from different species. It has been proposed that genes should be named following the convention applied to *C. elegans* [24]. For example, the ligand-gated anion channel protein gene from *H. contortus* originally named *RDL* would become *Hco-lgc-38*, where the first three letters designate the species, the next three letters designate the gene class followed by a gene number in order of discovery. In addition, there could be an optional paralog number, a spliced variant letter, and, finally, a capital letter for allele designation.

In a recent study comparing the transcriptome for intestinal tissue from *Ascaris suum*, *H. contortus*, and *C. elegans*, 241 gene families were identified that were represented in each of the three species [25]. This number represents about 20% of the total intestinal genes sampled from the three species and provides an indication of a cohort of genes that are responsible for the conserved physiological function of the nematode intestine. These genes in *C. elegans* could form the basis for studies to identify potential anthelmintics that might interfere with the function of the intestine in parasitic nematodes. In a comparative study between the genomes of *Brugia malayi* (clade III) and *C. elegans*, about 50% of the *B. malayi* genes have clear orthologs in *C. elegans* [26]. These authors found a reasonable number of orthologous genes between the two species in relation to molting, to Cys-loop receptors for ligand-gated ion channels, potassium channels, and in reproductive biology including germline development and gamete biology. They concluded these are areas where *C. elegans* could serve as a model in the development of novel anthelmintics. The draft genome of the necromenic nematode *Pristionchus pacificus* (clade V) has been published and subjected to a comparative analysis with *C. elegans* and *B. malayi* [27]. This reveals that 58% of predicted proteins for *P. pacificus* have a close match in *C. elegans*, while this figure is 73% for *B. malayi*. For *C. elegans* and *P. pacificus*, Dieterich *et al.* [27] noted clear differences in the relative numbers of genes falling into specific functional classes, as predicted from a protein domain analysis. For example, *P. pacificus* had a larger number of genes involved in metabolism of xenobiotics (perhaps consistent with its necromenic lifestyle, i.e., living in the corpse of a beetle) and ribosomal protein genes, whereas *C. elegans* had more seven-transmembrane receptor genes and more nuclear hormone receptor genes. The ease of culture of *P. pacificus* makes it an attractive laboratory model and genetic technology is also being applied. For example, a roller mutant of *P. pacificus*, based on the dominant behavioral marker gene *rol-6* of *C. elegans* [11], has been used as a marker to develop the transgenic technique in this nematode [28]. These results indicate a basis for developing further functional genomic models for parasitic nematodes [29].

At the genome level there are considerable differences between *Caenorhabditis* species [30]. For example, *C. elegans* and *Caenorhabditis briggsae* diverged from a common ancestor approximately 100 million years ago (although this figure may be considerably less [31]). In addition, fewer than 65% of *C. briggsae* genes could be assigned an ortholog in *C. elegans* [32]. Thus, nematodes that superficially appear similar (e.g., in terms of morphology) show considerable genomic variation. It is, therefore, essential to interpret the results carefully when comparing information or data between different species. Nonetheless, *C. elegans* and *C. briggsae* show 80% amino acid identity between orthologs [32]. For comparison, mice and humans show 78.5% amino acid identity between orthologs. Furthermore, based on 265 000 EST sequences, corresponding to 93 600 putative genes from 30 species, Parkinson *et al.* [20] found that parasitic nematodes from clade V had 50–70% of their ESTs in common with *C. elegans*. For clade IV, the percentage of ESTs in common with *C. elegans* was typically 50–60%, while for clade I and for some species from clade III, this figure was 45%. From these figures, Britton and Murray [33] conclude that *C. elegans* should not be discarded as a model for species in these clades.

Another important genetic analysis of the different nematode species is at the level of the temporal and spatial expression pattern of genes of interest. In his review, Gilleard [16] proposes that before *C. elegans* is used as a model to study the regulation of gene expression in a specific nematode, comparative studies should be undertaken to determine if these processes are sufficiently conserved to make the analysis meaningful. The ease of generating transgenic *C. elegans* expressing reporter constructs for genes of interest has led to this technology being avidly adopted in order to provide insight into the tissue-specific and developmental expression pattern of parasite genes. However, in using this approach it is important to know to what extent the expression pattern of the reporter gene, which utilizes the putative promoter region for the parasite gene to drive expression, faithfully reproduces the native expression pattern of the parasite gene. Evidence would suggest a good level of conservation of *cis*-regulatory elements that control tissue-specific expression between *C. elegans* and *H. contortus*, and probably other strongylid nematodes [16]. However, in this same review, it was noted that the evidence also suggests temporal regulation is not so well conserved. Insight into this is provided by the ongoing provision of sequence data for parasitic nematodes that will facilitate the identification of gene regulatory sequences. Work is in progress to extend the EST information for representative species of all the clades [19] (www.nematode.net).

The expression of three parasite nematode genes – a pepsinogen gene, *pep-1*, a cysteine protease gene, *AC2* (both from *H. contortus*), and a cuticular collagen gene, *colost-1* (from *Ostertagia circumcincta*) – was examined in *C. elegans* by transformation with putative parasite promoter/*lacZ* reporter constructs [24]. The report showed that parasitic nematode genes may be expressed in the same tissues of both the free-living and parasitic nematodes. This finding demonstrates that the genes probably have a similar role in both groups of nematodes and supports the use of *C. elegans* as a model for parasitic nematodes of clade V. In contrast, the timing of expression of the parasitic genes in *C. elegans* differs from the expression timing found in the parasitic nematodes themselves. This could indicate that the mechanisms regulating temporal expression of genes may vary between parasitic and free-living nematodes [34]. Britton *et al.* conclude that a greater knowledge of parasitic transcriptional regulators is required, including how they are controlled during development and interact with other factors to influence developmental event timing.

Functional Characterization of Parasite Genes by Heterologous Expression in *C. elegans*

The value of *C. elegans* for the expression and characterization of parasitic nematode genes is that all the facilities available for the analysis of gene function in *C. elegans* can be applied to the parasitic gene. The simplest way to do this is to express the parasitic nematode gene in a *C. elegans* mutant that lacks the homologous gene of interest. There have been a number of examples published using this technique (summarized in Table 2.2).

Table 2.2 Examples of parasitic nematode genes that have been expressed in *C. elegans*.

Parasitic nematode	Clade	Gene	Protein	Reference
H. contortus	V	*tub-1(iSE)*	β-tubulin	[35]
		tub-1(RU)	β-tubulin	
H. contortus	V	*pep-1 AC-2*	gut pepsinogen cysteine protease	[34]
O. circumcincta	V	*colost-1*	cuticular collagen	[34]
H. contortus	V	*elt-2*	GATA transcription factor	[37]
G. rostochiensis	IVb	*gpd*	GAPDH	[38]
H. contortus	V	*Hcavr-14 (HcGluClα3)*	GluCl subunit	[80]
O. volvulus	III	*Ov-GST-1a*	GST-1a	[102]
O. volvulus	III	*Ov-GST-3*	GST-3	[40]
S. stercoralis	IV	*fktf-1*	Forkhead transcription factor	[42]
B. malayi	III	*alt-1, alt-2*	abundant larval transcript	[103]
G. pallida	IVb	*ace-2*	acetylcholinesterase	[104]

An excellent example illustrating the value of *C. elegans* as a model for determining the mechanism of an anthelmintic is a study undertaken over 15 years ago [35]. In this paper the site of interaction between benzimidazoles and their target protein was investigated by generating *C. elegans* transgenic strains expressing *tub-1* from *H. contortus*. *tub-1* encodes the protein, β-tubulin. The *C. elegans* homolog *ben-1* is a nonessential gene that is required for benzimidazole sensitivity [36]. In their study, Kwa *et al*. took advantage of the *C. elegans ben-1* mutant as an experimental platform for functional analysis of parasite genes by expressing alleles of *tub-1* from benzimidazole-susceptible and -resistant strains of *H. contortus*. When the *H. contortus tub-1(iSE)* gene (from a drug-susceptible population) was used to transform a *C. elegans ben-1* mutant, the *C. elegans* became sensitive to thiabendazole. This demonstrated that a *H. contortus* gene was functional in *C. elegans*. In contrast, when *H. contortus tub-1(RU)*, which was isolated from a drug-resistant population, was used to transform *C. elegans*, the *ben-1* mutant remained resistant to thiabendazole. Further studies using *in vitro* mutagenesis of the *tub-1* gene prior to transformation of *C. elegans ben-1* indicated that a change from phenylalanine to tyrosine at position 200 was sufficient to confer resistance to benzimidazoles and thus provided robust identification of the drug target.

Another gene for which the function has been demonstrated in *C. elegans* is the *H. contortus* homolog of the *C. elegans* GATA transcription factor, *elt-2*, [37]. *elt-2* is a central regulator of endoderm development, being essential for gut development in *C. elegans* and Couthier *et al*. found that endodermal development in *H. contortus* was similar to that of *C. elegans*. These authors found that the temporal and spatial expression of the parasitic nematode gene was the same as that of *elt-2*. Interestingly, although the *H. contortus* ELT-2 polypeptide has only a 26.8% overall identity with *C. elegans* ELT-2 peptide, its ectopic expression in transgenic *C. elegans* activates a program of endodermal differentiation [37]. This approach, employing inducible promoters to drive ectopic overexpression of a parasite gene in *C. elegans*, while arguably not of direct physiological relevance, provides a powerful approach to obtain novel insight into potential downstream biochemical signaling pathways of the gene of interest.

Further evidence for the expression of parasitic genes in *C. elegans* comes from studies using a glyceraldehyde-3-phosphate dehydrogenase (GAPDH) gene, designated *gpd,* isolated from the plant nematode, *Globodera rostochiensis*. This has high homology with GAPDHs from *C. elegans* (about 80% identical at the amino acid level) [38]. The 5′-flanking region of this *gpd* gene was fused to a Green Fluorescent Protein (GFP) reporter gene to provide a promoter/reporter construct and used to transform *C. elegans*. In transgenic lines, GFP expression was observed in embryos and in the body wall muscle of different larval stages. *C. elegans gpd-2* and *gpd-3* are also expressed in body wall muscles during larval development [39]. These results suggest that though plant nematodes and *C. elegans* are only distantly related, *C. elegans* might act as a model system for the study of cyst nematode genes.

There have been a number of other studies in which the parasite genes have been expressed in *C. elegans* including the glutathione *S*-transferase (GST)-3 gene from *Onchocerca volvulus* (clade III), *Ov-GST-3* [40], the *Strongyloides stercoralis* (clade IV) *fktf-1* gene, an ortholog of *C. elegans daf-16* [41, 42], and the translationally controlled tumor protein gene, for which the *C. elegans* gene is *tct-1* and which occurs in 31 nematode species [43].

Thus, the evidence from the studies described above indicate that many parasitic nematode genes can be functionally expressed in *C. elegans*. As the genomes of more parasitic nematodes are sequenced, so more homologous genes between *C. elegans* and parasitic nematodes can be identified and expressed in *C. elegans*. This will enable identification of key genes for parasitic nematode viability that will provide potential novel loci for new generations of anthelmintics. These will include genes involved in development, reproduction, metabolism, cuticle formation, and the nervous system. An interesting area for further exploration is the role of the neuropeptides. These are a diverse family of signaling molecules in the nematode nervous system that have profound effects on behavior in *C. elegans* [44–46] and parasitic nematodes [47, 48]. While there are a large number of peptides and their receptors in nematodes [49], none has yet been identified as the target for an anthelmintic. However, in mammals, peptides have been developed to target a number of sites, including the immune system, the endocrine system, and cancer [50]. Also, in the mammalian system, neuropeptide analogs are being developed as therapeutic agents, suggesting that similar strategies could be used to develop peptide-derived anthelmintics [51], particularly as many nematode neuropeptides and their receptors do not occur in mammals.

Comparative Pharmacology of *C. elegans* and Parasitic Nematode Neurotransmitter Receptors

Another approach is to compare *C. elegans* and parasitic nematode receptors to determine to what extent their pharmacological profiles are sufficiently similar for *C. elegans* to be of value as a model in developing new anthelmintics. These studies typically employ expression of receptors in cell culture (e.g., HEK-293 cells) in order to make the functional analysis. A good example of this are studies conducted on receptors for biogenic amines [52]. Biogenic amines contribute to a number of important physiological processes in nematodes including feeding, locomotion, egg laying and various behaviors. A 5-hydroxytryptamine (5-HT) receptor, 5-HT$_{1Hc}$, has been cloned and sequenced from *H. contortus*, and its pharmacological profile investigated and compared with 5-HT receptors from *C. elegans* [53]. Recently, a tyramine-gated chloride channel, Hco-LGC-55, has been cloned and sequenced from *H. contortus* [54]. HcoLGC-55 is an ortholog of Cel-LGC-55 from *C. elegans* [55, 56]. Rao *et al.* [54] suggested that tyramine and other amine-gated chloride channels would be potential sites for the development of novel anthelmintics since these channels are absent in the host. The SER-2 tyramine receptor has also been the subject of another recent study that examined the actions of three monoterpenoids for anthelmintic activity [57]. Lei *et al.* [57] proposed their system might be developed as a platform for high-throughput compound screening for new anthelmintics.

C. elegans as a Tool to Understand the Mode of Action of Novel Anthelmintics

The precedent for this approach is well established, from the early studies that generated levamisole-resistant strains of C. elegans [58] through to more recent studies that have employed forward and reverse genetics to unpick the mode of action of the new anthelmintics monepantel [22] and emodepside [59].

For levamisole, pyrantel, and morantel, studies of the nAChRs of C. elegans have proven of great value [58, 60], although all three compounds were first shown to be agonists at nAChRs in A. suum [61] (for more information on nematode receptors, see Chapters 1 and 14). In C. elegans there are 29 subunits for nAChRs, which can be divided into five main groups: ACR-16, ACR-8, UNC-38, UNC-29, and DEG-3 [60]. There are five genes that encode nicotinic acetylcholine subunits that are expressed in the body wall muscle and are activated by levamisole: LEV-1, LEV-8/ACR-13, UNC-29, UNC-38, and UNC-63. Evidence would suggest that UNC-29 and LEV-1 can assemble with either UNC-38 or UNC-63 [60]. Null mutants of *unc-29*, *unc-38*, and *unc-63* are resistant to levamisole [58]. Certain amino acids, such as E153 of *unc-38* and Q57 of *unc-63*, are key for levamisole potency (Q57 in the case of pyrantel potency) [62]. In addition, there is evidence that three further genes – *ric-3*, *unc-50*, and *unc-74* – encode ancillary proteins that are involved in the assembly of the nAChRs [63].

The question is how to relate these levamisole-sensitive subunits identified in C. elegans to the situation in parasitic nematodes. Three types of nAChRs have been proposed for A. suum body wall muscle – nicotine-sensitive (N-subtype), levamisole-sensitive (L-subtype) and bephenium-sensitive (B-subtype) [64, 65]. There is evidence that C. elegans body wall muscle also contains levamisole-insensitive nAChRs, possibly composed of homo-oligomeric ACR-16 subunits [60]. These authors conclude that C. elegans muscle receptor subtypes resemble those from A. suum and also Oesophagostomum dentatum [66], which provides confirmation of its value as a model for parasitic nematodes. Qian et al. [67] summarized the properties of LEV-activated receptor channels for C. elegans and A. suum (Table 2.3).

Table 2.3 Summary of the properties of levamisole receptor channels in the body wall muscle of C. elegans and A. suum (data taken from [67]).

Animal	C. elegans	A. suum
Clade	V	III
Levamisole concentration (μM)	10–100	10–100
Conducts cesium	yes	yes
K_d at -75 mV for open channel block (μM)	13	46
Activation by nicotine	no	yes
Conductance (pS)	26–36	18–53
Mean open time (ms)	0.25–0.53	0.2–2.5
Rectification	yes	no

K_d is the equilibrium dissociation constant of levamisole for the receptor channel.

More recently, C. elegans has provided insight into the mode of action of the aminoacetonitrile derivatives (AADs) [22, 68]. These drugs also act through nAChRs, but in this case the receptors implicated belong to the DEG-3 family of channels, which is specific to the Nematoda. This discovery was facilitated by experiments in which AADs were effective against C. elegans mutants that were resistant to levamisole, indicating a novel mode of action. Subsequently, ACR-23 homologs have been identified in H. contortus and mutations in these channels (e.g., MPTL-1) are implicated in conferring reduced sensitivity to AADs [69]. This prompted a study to heterologously express H. contortus DEG-3/DES-2 channels and confirm them as targets for monepantel [70]. This latter study suggests that monepantel acts as a positive allosteric modulator of the heterologously expressed nAChR rather than gating channel opening and it will be interesting to discover whether or not this is also the case for the native channel. These authors have also extended their analysis to a bioinformatic interrogation of the genome sequence for a range of nematodes to test whether or not there is a correlation between monepantel sensitivity and the presence of ACR-23/MPTL-1 putative channel sequences in the genome [71]. This analysis indicated that *Pristionchus pacificus* and *Strongyloides ratti* lack an *acr-23/mptl-1* homolog. As these species are also insensitive to monepantel this is consistent with a role for these channels in mediating the drug effect.

In addition to monepantel, studies employing C. elegans have been most successful in the elucidation of the mode of action of the avermectins. Avermectins, together with the structurally related milbemycins, are macrocyclic lactones obtained from *Streptomyces* spp. These studies have been possible as C. elegans is very susceptible to avermectins [72]. In initial experiments, C. elegans poly(A)$^+$ RNA was injected into *Xenopus laevis* oocytes and currents recorded [73]. These currents were activated by avermectin with half-maximal activation obtained using 90 nM avermectin. This current was shown to be due to an increase in chloride conductance. Subsequently, it was shown that these chloride currents in C. elegans were gated by glutamate [74]. A labor-intensive expression cloning strategy eventually isolated two cDNA clones, pGluClα (subsequently termed GluClα1) and pGluClβ – the former was sensitive to avermectin, but not glutamate, while the latter was sensitive to glutamate, but not to avermectin. Prior to these experiments using C. elegans it was generally considered that avermectins interacted with γ-aminobutyric acid-gated chloride channels [75]. It is now clear that C. elegans expresses a family of glutamate-gated chloride channels (GluCls) and that these present the major site of action for ivermectin in nematodes [76]. In an early study, Dent et al. [77] identified *avr-15* as the gene responsible for the sensitivity of C. elegans pharynx to ivermectin. Further experiments that used intracellular recordings of C. elegans pharyngeal muscle to compare the effects of glutamate and ivermectin [78] showed that AVR-15/GluClα2 subunit is required for ivermectin sensitivity in the pharynx of C. elegans [78]. Thus, through its action on GluClα2, ivermectin inhibits pharyngeal pumping [77, 78], and so prevents feeding in C. elegans and, presumably, in other nematodes. A further analysis of GluCls in C. elegans [76] in conferring sensitivity to ivermectin revealed that three genes are pivotal. Thus, Dent et al. [79] found that the triple mutant, *avr-14/avr-15/glc-1*, was highly resistant to ivermectin. This analysis, involving the generation of viable strains of *C. elegans* harboring mutations in multiple genes, provides an excellent example of the power of genetic manipulation in *C. elegans* to address specific questions relating to drug mode of action.

How do these studies on the role of GluCls in the mode of action of ivermectin relate to parasitic nematodes? One of the *H. contortus* glutamate-gated chloride genes, *Hcavr-14* (*HcGluClα3*), which is involved in the action of ivermectin, has been expressed in *C. elegans* [80] where it rescues a motor deficit in the *avr-14* mutant. Holden-Dye and Walker [81] compared the actions of ivermectin on the pharyngeal muscle of *Ascaridia galli* and *C. elegans*. These authors found that ivermectin was over 1000 times less potent on the pharyngeal muscle of *A. galli* compared to the pharyngeal muscle of *C. elegans*. This lack of sensitivity of *A. galli* pharyngeal muscle to ivermectin was unexpected since the pharynxes of both *H. contortus* and *A. suum* are sensitive to low nanomolar ivermectin [82, 83]. The pharynxes also differed in their sensitivity to glutamate and glutamate agonists. These results emphasize the possibility that while the ivermectin receptor that directly binds the drug might be conserved between species of nematode, the tissues in which the receptor is expressed may differ, thus the key site of action of ivermectin and its subsequent impact on behavior might vary between different species of nematodes. This would suggest that avermectins act at a number of sites in nematodes and that this might be responsible for differences in sensitivity to avermectins in different nematodes (e.g., the main target organ might vary between nematode species).

The relationship between ivermectin resistance and increased expression of ABC transport proteins and P-glycoproteins has been investigated using *C. elegans* as a model system. Specifically, James and Davey [84] concluded that transport proteins are involved in ivermectin resistance, and they consider that their model is useful to investigate drug resistance and its reversal.

Insight into the mode of action of the cyclo-octadepsipeptide anthelmintic, emodepside, has also been provided from studies in *C. elegans*. These built on the earlier observations that the cyclo-octadepsipeptide, PF1022A, and emodepside might act on a latrophilin receptor in *H. contortus* [85]. It was shown that the *C. elegans* genome also contains genes that encode latrophilin-like proteins [85]. The gene *lat-1* is expressed in *C. elegans* pharynx [85] and it was shown that a low nanomolar concentration of emodepside inhibits pharyngeal pumping (i.e., feeding in a latrophilin-dependent manner) [86]. Furthermore, it was shown that both PF1022A and emodepside inhibited locomotion of *C. elegans* with IC_{50} values in the low nanomolar range [86]. The role of latrophilin in the mode of action of emodepside was investigated further in *C. elegans* using a functional null mutant for latrophilin (*lat-1*) [59]. The report found that, although emodepside was less active on the pharynx of this mutant, it still had an inhibitory effect on locomotion, indicating a possible second site of action for emodepside. There are two latrophilin genes in *C. elegans* – *lat-1* and *lat-2* – raising the possibility that this second target might be LAT-2. Generation of a strain carrying null mutations for both *lat-1* and *lat-2* permitted this hypothesis to be tested, and revealed that the double mutant was still inhibited by emodepside [59], indicating that there was a second, as yet undiscovered, mode of action for emodepside. A subsequent mutagenesis screen for emodepside resistance resulted in recovery of nine alleles of *slo-1* – a gene that encodes a large conductance calcium-activated potassium channel. [59]. Interestingly, *slo-1* mutants were very resistant to the inhibitory action of emodepside on both pharyngeal pumping and locomotion. *slo-1* is expressed widely through the nervous system of *C. elegans* and in body wall muscle, but not in pharyngeal muscle [87, 88]. Expression of *slo-1* either pan-neuronally or in body wall muscle restored the inhibitory effect of emodepside on locomotion although it was not as susceptible as wild-type [72]. However, expression of *slo-1* pan-neuronally resulted in a complete restoration of the emodepside effect on pharyngeal pumping. As noted above, native *slo-1* is not expressed in the pharyngeal muscle [87]; however, ectopic overexpression of *slo-1* in this muscle in the *slo-1* null mutant *js379* confers sensitivity to emodepside [89]. Taken together this suggests an intimate connection between the emodepside target and the SLO-1 channel, and is consistent with the proposal that emodepside signals through SLO-1 to inhibit feeding and motility. More recently, it has been shown that other biochemical pathways impinge on this channel and may regulate emodepside sensitivity [90].

Finally, it has been shown that *slo-1* orthologs cloned from the parasitic nematodes *H. contortus*, *Ancylostoma caninum*, and *Cooperia oncophora* confer sensitivity of the *C. elegans slo-1* null mutant to emodepside [91]. Taken together, these studies utilizing *C. elegans* as a model system have identified and confirmed SLO-1 as a new anthelmintic target.

C. elegans has also been employed to provide insight into the molecular basis of the selective toxicity of emodepside. The gene of the human ortholog of SLO-1 channel, KCNMA1, has been expressed in *slo-1* (*js379*) mutants of *C. elegans* [89]. Expression of *kcnma1* rescued the behavioral deficits observed in the *slo-1* mutant, indicating that the human channel can functionally replace the nematode SLO-1 channel. Interestingly, *C. elegans* expressing *kcnma-1* was 10–100 times less sensitive to emodepside than wild-type, suggesting that emodepside is selective for the nematode over the mammalian channel.

C. elegans as a Platform for Target Discovery

The above examples clearly demonstrate the value of *C. elegans* in determining the mode of action of anthelmintics. However, *C. elegans* was not employed in the identification of these compounds as potential anthelmintic drugs. Rather, this was achieved through the screening of compounds with efficacy in mammalian hosts infected with parasitic nematodes. Nonetheless, there are also ways in which *C. elegans* can contribute more directly to the drug discovery process and some examples are given below.

Recently, a novel anthelmintic has been identified using *C. elegans* as a screening system where 10 000 compounds were examined [92]. One compound, an aminoquinoline derivative, KSI-4088, inhibited egg hatching, larval development, and migration rate. These authors are currently defining the site of action of this compound, and it will be interesting to see if KSI-4088 has a novel site of action and if it can be developed as a commercial anthelmintic.

A novel approach has been to identify essential genes in *C. elegans* (i.e., those for which a loss of function results in death of the animal) and then to identify the homologous genes in a parasitic nematode (i.e., the soybean cyst nematode, *Heterodera glycines*) [93]. The aim of this approach is to introduce lethal RNA interference (RNAi) constructs into the host plant, the soybean, *Glycine max*, which are then ingested by *H. glycines*, resulting in the death of the cyst nematodes.

An important aspect in terms of considering the role of *C. elegans* in drug discovery is the impact that new technologies may have on this process. The technique of optogenetics, in which light-activated channels provide a means of remote, targeted activation or inhibition of specific cells, has been pioneered in *C. elegans* [94]. This exciting new approach provides a means to drive specific behaviors, such as body wall muscle [95] or pharyngeal muscle contraction [96], and to quantify the impact of drugs on these responses. In combination with this, a number of different genetically encoded sensors, particularly for calcium ions, provide a mechanism for imaging cellular activity [97]. These techniques for remote light-induced control of neural circuits and noninvasive imaging of cellular activity are now being incorporated into studies that deploy microfluidic technology both as a means to permit more detailed functional studies [98] and with a view to providing high-throughput analysis [99, 100]. Thus, there is an increasingly diverse "toolset" for the analysis of the physiology and pharmacology of *C. elegans*. Arguably, there should be the opportunity to adopt some of these approaches, in particular the use of microfluidics for the analysis of parasitic nematodes. Accordingly, *C. elegans* will serve, yet again, as the "trail-blazer" for functional analysis in the phylum.

Conclusions

C. elegans was first proposed as a model for anthelmintic drug discovery more than 30 years ago [5], and since then its utility for the purpose has gained added dimension from its tractability for RNAi and chemical biology approaches [101]. More recently, the application of imaging and optogenetics in combination with microfluidics [99] provides even more capability for a detailed and precise high-throughput analysis. Although, as discussed above, there are caveats to the use of *C. elegans* as a surrogate parasite, it remains the most experimentally tractable species in the phylum Nematoda. As such it will continue to provide an important platform for anthelmintic studies in the foreseeable future.

References

1 Coles, G.C. (1998) Drug-resistant parasites of sheep: an emerging problem in the UK? *Parasitol. Today*, **14**, 86–88.

2 Sutherland, I.A. and Leathwick, D.M. (2011) Anthelmintic resistance in nematode parasites of cattle: a global issue? *Trends Parasitol.*, **27**, 176–181.

3 Harhay, M.O., Horton, J., and Olliaro, P.L. (2010) Epidemiology and control of human gastrointestinal

parasites in children. *Expert Rev. Anti Infect. Ther.*, **8**, 219–234.

4 Bridge, J. and Starr, J.L. (2007) *Plant Nematodes of Agricultural Importance*, Manson, London.

5 Simpkins, K.G. and Coles, G.C. (1981) The use of *Caenorhabditis elegans* for anthelmintic screening. *J. Chem. Technol. Biotechnol.*, **31**, 66–69.

6 Lewis, J.A., Wu, C.-H., Berg, H., and Levine, J.H. (1980) The genetics of levamisole resistance in the nematode *Caenorhabditis elegans*. *Genetics*, **95**, 905–928.

7 Brenner, S. (1974) The genetics of *Caenorhabditis elegans*. *Genetics*, **77**, 71–94.

8 *C. elegans* Sequencing Consortium (1998) Genome sequence of the nematode, *C. elegans*: a platform for investigating biology. *Science*, **282**, 2012–2018.

9 Blaxter, M. (1998) *Caenorhabditis elegans* is a nematode. *Science*, **282**, 2041–2046.

10 White, J., Southgate, E., Thomson, J., and Brenner, S. (1986) The structure of the nervous system of the nematode *Caenorhabditis elegans*. *Philos. Trans. R. Soc. Lond. Biol. Sci.*, **B314**, 1–340.

11 Mello, C.C., Kramer, J.M., Stinchcomb, D., and Ambros, V. (1991) Efficient gene transfer in *C. elegans*: extrachromosomal maintenance and integration of transforming sequences. *EMBO J.*, **10**, 3959–3970.

12 Fire, A., Xu, S., Montgomery, M.K., Kostas, S.A., Driver, S.E., and Mello, C.C. (1998) Potent and specific genetic interference by double-stranded RNA in *Caenorhabditis elegans*. *Nature*, **391**, 806–811.

13 Zwaal, R.R., Broeks, A., van Meurs, J., Groenen, J.T., and Plasterk, R.H. (1993) Target-selected gene inactivation in *Caenorhabditis elegans* by using a frozen transposon insertion mutant bank. *Proc. Natl. Acad. Sci. USA*, **90**, 7431–7435.

14 Bürglin, T.R., Lobos, E., and Blaxter, M.L. (1998) *Caenorhabditis elegans* as a model for parasitic nematodes. *Int. J. Parasitol.*, **28**, 395–411.

15 Geary, T.G. and Thompson, D.P. (2001) *Caenorhabditis elegans*: how good a model for veterinary parasites? *Vet. Parasitol.*, **101**, 371–386.

16 Gilleard, J.S. (2004) The use of *Caenorhabditis elegans* in parasitic nematode research. *Parasitology*, **128**, S49–S70.

17 Holden-Dye, L. and Walker, R. (2007) Anthelmintic drugs, in *WormBook* (ed. The *C. elegans* Research Community), doi: 10.1895/wormbook.1.143.1.

18 Blaxter, M.L., De Ley, P., Garey, J.R., Liu, L.X., Scheldeman, P., Vierstraete, A., Vanfleteren, J.R. *et al.* (1998) A molecular evolutionary framework for the phylum Nematoda. *Nature*, **392**, 71–75.

19 Wylie, T., Martin, J.C., Dante, M., Mitreva, M.D., Clifton, S.W., Chinwalla, A., Waterston, R.H. *et al.* (2004) Nematode.net: a tool for navigating sequences from parasitic and free-living nematodes. *Nucleic Acids. Res.*, **32**, D423–D426.

20 Parkinson, J., Mitreva, M., Whitton, C., Thomson, M., Daub, J., Martin, J., Schmid, R. *et al.* (2004) A transcriptomic analysis of the phylum Nematoda. *Nat. Genet.*, **36**, 1259–1267.

21 Jones, A., Davis, P., Hodgkin, J., and Sattelle, D. (2007) The nicotinic acetylcholine receptor gene family of the nematode *Caenorhabditis elegans*: an update on nomenclature. *Invert. Neurosci.*, **7**, 129–131.

22 Kaminsky, R., Ducray, P., Jung, M., Clover, R., Rufener, L., Bouvier, J., Weber, S.S. *et al.* (2008) A new class of anthelmintics effective against drug-resistant nematodes. *Nature*, **452**, 176–180.

23 Bird, D.M., Williamson, V.M., Abad, P., McCarter, J., Danchin, E.G.J., Castagnone-Sereno, P., and Opperman, C.H. (2009) The genomes of root-knot nematodes. *Annu. Rev. Phytopathol.*, **47**, 333–351.

24 Beech, R.N., Wolstenholme, A.J., Neveu, C., and Dent, J.A. (2010) Nematode parasite genes: what's in a name? *Trends Parasitol.*, **26**, 334–340.

25 Yin, Y., Martin, J., Abubucker, S., Scott, A.L., McCarter, J.P., Wilson, R.K., Jasmer, D.P., and Mitreva, M. (2008) Intestinal transcriptomes of nematodes:

comparison of the parasites *Ascaris suum* and *Haemonchus contortus* with the free-living *Caenorhabditis elegans*. *PLoS Negl. Trop. Dis.*, **2**, e269.

26 Scott, A.L. and Ghedin, E. (2009) The genome of *Brugia malayi* – all worms are not created equal. *Parasitol. Int.*, **58**, 6–11.

27 Dieterich, C., Clifton, S., Schuster, L., Chinwalla, A., Delehaunty, K., Dinkelacker, I., Fulton, L. *et al.* (2008) The *Pristionchus pacificus* genome provides a unique perspective on nematode lifestyle and parasitism. *Nat. Genet.*, **40**, 1193–1198.

28 Schlager, B., Wang, X., Braach, G., and Sommer, R.J. (2009) Molecular cloning of a dominant roller mutant and establishment of DNA-mediated transformation in the nematode *Pristionchus pacificus*. *Genetics*, **47**, 300–304.

29 Lok, J.B. (2009) Transgenesis in parasitic nematodes: building a better array. *Trends Parasitol.*, **25**, 345–347.

30 Kiontke, K. and Fitch, D. (2005) The phylogenetic relationships of *Caenorhabditis* and other rhabditids, in *WormBook* (ed. The *C. elegans* Research Community), doi: 10.1895/wormbook.1.11.1.

31 Thomas, J.H. (2008) Genome evolution in *Caenorhabditis*. *Brief. Funct. Genomics Proteomics*, **7**, 211–216.

32 Stein, L.D., Bao, Z., Blasiar, D., Blumenthal, T., Brent, M.R., Chen, N., Chinwalla, A. *et al.* (2003) The genome sequence of *Caenorhabditis briggsae*: a platform for comparative genomics. *PLoS Biol.*, **1**, e45.

33 Britton, C. and Murray, L. (2006) Using *Caenorhabditis elegans* for functional analysis of genes of parasitic nematodes. *Int. J. Parasitol.*, **36**, 651–659.

34 Britton, C., Redmond, D.L., Knox, D.P., McKerrow, J.H., and Barry, J.D. (1999) Identification of promoter elements of parasite nematode genes in transgenic *Caenorhabditis elegans*. *Mol. Biochem. Parasitol.*, **103**, 171–181.

35 Kwa, M.S.G., Veenstra, J.G., Van Dijk, M., and Roos, M.H. (1995) β-Tubulin genes from the parasitic nematode *Haemonchus contortus* modulate drug resistance in *Caenorhabditis elegans*. *J. Mol. Biol.*, **246**, 500–510.

36 Driscoll, M., Dean, E., Reilly, E., Bergholz, E., and Chalfie, M. (1989) Genetic and molecular analysis of a *Caenorhabditis elegans* beta-tubulin that conveys benzimidazole sensitivity. *J. Cell Biol.*, **109**, 2993–3003.

37 Couthier, A., Smith, J., McGarr, P., Craig, B., and Gilleard, J.S. (2004) Ectopic expression of a *Haemonchus contortus* GATA transcription factor in *Caenorhabditis elegans* reveals conserved function in spite of extensive sequence divergence. *Mol. Biochem. Parasitol.*, **133**, 241–253.

38 Qin, L., Smant, G., Stokkermans, J., Bakker, J., Schots, A., and Helder, J. (1998) Cloning of a *trans*-spliced glyceraldehyde-3-phosphate-dehydrogenase gene from the potato cyst nematode *Globodera rostochiensis* and expression of its putative promoter region in *Caenorhabditis elegans*. *Mol. Biochem. Parasitol.*, **96**, 59–67.

39 Yarbrough, P.O. and Hecht, R.M. (1984) Two isoenzymes of glyceraldehyde-3-phosphate dehydrogenase in *Caenorhabditis elegans*. Isolation, properties, and immunochemical characterization. *J. Biol. Chem.*, **259**, 14711–14720.

40 Kampkötter, A., Volkmann, T.E., de Castro, S.H., Leiers, B., Klotz, L.-O., Johnson, T.E., Link, C.D., and Henkle-Dührsen, K. (2003) Functional analysis of the glutathione S-transferase 3 from *Onchocerca volvulus* (Ov-GST-3): a parasite GST confers increased resistance to oxidative stress in *Caenorhabditis elegans*. *J. Mol. Biol.*, **325**, 25–37.

41 Ogg, S., Paradis, S., Gottlieb, S., Patterson, G.I., Lee, L., Tissenbaum, H.A., and Ruvkun, G. (1997) The Forkhead transcription factor DAF-16 transduces insulin-like metabolic and longevity signals in *C. elegans*. *Nature*, **389**, 994–999.

42 Massey Jr, H.C., Bhopale, M.K., Li, X., Castelletto, M., and Lok, J.B. (2006) The fork head transcription factor FKTF-1b from *Strongyloides stercoralis* restores DAF-16 developmental function to

43 Meyvis, Y., Houthoofd, W., Visser, A., Borgonie, G., Gevaert, K., Vercruysse, J., Claerebout, E., and Geldhof, P. (2009) Analysis of the translationally controlled tumour protein in the nematodes *Ostertagia ostertagi* and *Caenorhabditis elegans* suggests a pivotal role in egg production. *Int. J. Parasitol.*, **39**, 1205–1213.

42 mutant *Caenorhabditis elegans*. *Int. J. Parasitol.*, **36**, 347–352.

44 Rogers, C.M., Walker, R.J., Burke, J.F., and Holden-Dye, L. (2001) Regulation of the pharynx of *Caenorhabditis elegans* by 5-HT, octopamine, and FMRFamide-like neuropeptides. *J. Neurobiol.*, **49**, 235–244.

45 Papaioannou, S., Marsden, D., Franks, C.J., Walker, R.J., and Holden-Dye, L. (2005) Role of a FMRFamide-like family of neuropeptides in the pharyngeal nervous system of *Caenorhabditis elegans*. *J. Neurobiol.*, **65**, 304–319.

46 Keating, C., Kriek, N., Daniels, M., Ashcroft, N., Hopper, N., Siney, E., Holden-Dye, L., and Burke, J. (2003) Whole-genome analysis of 60 G protein-coupled receptors in *Caenorhabditis elegans* by gene knockout with RNAi. *Curr. Biol.*, **13**, 1715–1720.

47 McVeigh, P., Geary, T.G., Marks, N.J., and Maule, A.G. (2006) The FLP-side of nematodes. *Trends Parasitol.*, **22**, 385–396.

48 Walker, R., Papaioannou, S., and Holden-Dye, L. (2009) A review of FMRFamide- and RFamide-like peptides in metazoa. *Invert. Neurosci.*, **9**, 111–153.

49 Li, C. and Kim, K. (2008) Neuropeptides, in *WormBook* (ed. The *C. elegans* Research Community), doi: 10.1895/wormbook.1.142.1.

50 Bellmann-Sickert, K. and Beck-Sickinger, A.G. (2010) Peptide drugs to target G protein-coupled receptors. *Trends Pharmacol. Sci.*, **31**, 434–441.

51 Geary, T.G., Woo, K., McCarthy, J.S., Mackenzie, C.D., Horton, J., Prichard, R.K., de Silva, N.R. *et al.* (2010) Unresolved issues in anthelmintic pharmacology for helminthiases of humans. *Int. J. Parasitol.*, **40**, 1–13.

52 Komuniecki, R.W., Hobson, R.J., Rex, E.B., Hapiak, V.M., and Komuniecki, P.R. (2004) Biogenic amine receptors in parasitic nematodes: what can be learned from *Caenorhabditis elegans*? *Mol. Biochem. Parasitol.*, **137**, 1–11.

53 Smith, M.W., Borts, T.L., Emkey, R., Cook, C.A., Wiggins, C.J., and Gutierrez, J.A. (2003) Characterization of a novel G-protein coupled receptor from the parasitic nematode *H. contortus* with high affinity for serotonin. *J. Neurochem.*, **86**, 255–266.

54 Rao, V.T.S., Accardi, M.V., Siddiqui, S.Z., Beech, R.N., Prichard, R.K., and Forrester, S.G. (2010) Characterization of a novel tyramine-gated chloride channel from *Haemonchus contortus*. *Mol. Biochem. Parasitol.*, **173**, 64–68.

55 Pirri, J.K., McPherson, A.D., Donnelly, J.L., Francis, M.M., and Alkema, M.J. (2009) A tyramine-gated chloride channel coordinates distinct motor programs of a *Caenorhabditis elegans* escape response. *Neuron*, **62**, 526–538.

56 Ringstad, N., Abe, N., and Horvitz, H.R. (2009) Ligand-gated chloride channels are receptors for biogenic amines in *C. elegans*. *Science*, **325**, 96–100.

57 Lei, J., Leser, M., and Enan, E. (2010) Nematicidal activity of two monoterpenoids and SER-2 tyramine receptor of *Caenorhabditis elegans*. *Biochem. Pharmacol.*, **79**, 1062–1071.

58 Fleming, J., Squire, M., Barnes, T., Tornoe, C., Matsuda, K., Ahnn, J., Fire, A., Sulston, J. *et al.* (1997) *Caenorhabditis elegans* levamisole resistance genes *lev-1*, *unc-29*, and *unc-38* encode functional nicotinic acetylcholine receptor subunits. *J. Neurosci.*, **17**, 5843–5857.

59 Guest, M., Bull, K., Walker, R.J., Amliwala, K., O'Connor, V., Harder, A., Holden-Dye, L., and Hopper, N.A. (2007) The calcium-activated potassium channel, SLO-1, is required for the action of the novel cyclo-octadepsipeptide anthelmintic, emodepside, in *Caenorhabditis elegans*. *Int. J. Parasitol.*, **37**, 1577–1588.

60 Brown, L.A., Jones, A.K., Buckingham, S.D., Mee, C.J., and Sattelle, D.B. (2006) Contributions from *Caenorhabditis elegans* functional genetics to antiparasitic drug target identification and validation: nicotinic acetylcholine receptors, a case study. *Int. J. Parasitol.*, **36**, 617–624.

61 Harrow, I.D. and Gration, K.A.F. (1985) Mode of action of the anthelmintics morantel, pyrantel and levamisole on the muscle cell membrane of the nematode *Ascaris suum*. *Pesticide Sci.*, **16**, 662–672.

62 Martin, R.J. and Robertson, A.P. (2007) Mode of action of levamisole and pyrantel, anthelmintic resistance, E153 and Q57. *Parasitology*, **134**, 1093–1104.

63 Boulin, T., Gielen, M., Richmond, J.E., Williams, D.C., Paoletti, P., and Bessereau, J.-L. (2008) Eight genes are required for functional reconstitution of the *Caenorhabditis elegans* levamisole-sensitive acetylcholine receptor. *Proc. Natl. Acad. Sci. USA*, **105**, 18590–18595.

64 Robertson, A.P., Clark, C.L., Burns, T.A., Thompson, D.P., Geary, T.G., Trailovic, S.M., and Martin, R.J. (2002) Paraherquamide and 2-deoxy-paraherquamide distinguish cholinergic receptor subtypes in *Ascaris* muscle. *J. Pharmacol. Exp. Ther.*, **302**, 853–860.

65 Trailovic, S.M., Clark, C.L., Robertson, A.P., and Martin, R.J. (2005) Brief application of AF2 produces long lasting potentiation of nAChR responses in *Ascaris suum*. *Mol. Biochem. Parasitol.*, **139**, 51–64.

66 Martin, R.J., Bai, G., Clark, C.L., and Robertson, A.P. (2003) Methyridine (2-[2-methoxyethyl]-pyridine]) and levamisole activate different ACh receptor subtypes in nematode parasites: a new lead for levamisole-resistance. *Br. J. Pharmacol.*, **140**, 1068–1076.

67 Qian, H., Robertson, A.P., Powell-Coffman, J.A., and Martin, R.J. (2008) Levamisole resistance resolved at the single-channel level in *Caenorhabditis elegans*. *FASEB J.*, **22**, 3247–3254.

68 Kaminsky, R., Gauvry, N., Schorderet Weber, S., Skripsky, T., Bouvier, J., Wenger, A., Schroeder, F. et al. (2008) Identification of the amino-acetonitrile derivative monepantel (AAD 1566) as a new anthelmintic drug development candidate. *Parasitol. Res.*, **103**, 931–939.

69 Rufener, L., Mäser, P., Roditi, I., and Kaminsky, R. (2009) *Haemonchus contortus* acetylcholine receptors of the DEG-3 subfamily and their role in sensitivity to monepantel. *PLoS Pathog.*, **5**, e1000380.

70 Rufener, L., Baur, R., Kaminsky, R., Mäser, P., and Sigel, E. (2010) Monepantel allosterically activates DEG-3/DES-2 channels of the gastrointestinal nematode *Haemonchus contortus*. *Mol. Pharmacol.*, **78**, 895–902.

71 Rufener, L., Keiser, J., Kaminsky, R., Mäser, P., and Nilsson, D. (2010) Phylogenomics of ligand-gated ion channels predicts monepantel effect. *PLoS Pathog.*, **6**, e1001091.

72 Schaeffer, J.M. and Haines, H.W. (1989) Avermectin binding in *Caenorhabditis elegans*. A two-state model for the avermectin binding site. *Biochem. Pharmacol.*, **38**, 2329–2338.

73 Arena, J.P., Liu, K.K., Paress, P.S., and Cully, D.F. (1991) Avermectin-sensitive chloride currents induced by *Caenorhabditis elegans* RNA in *Xenopus* oocytes. *Mol. Pharmacol.*, **40**, 368–374.

74 Cully, D.F., Vassilatis, D.K., Liu, K.K., Paress, P.S., Van der Ploeg, L.H.T., Schaeffer, J.M., and Arena, J.P. (1994) Cloning of an avermectin-sensitive glutamate-gated chloride channel from *Caenorhabditis elegans*. *Nature*, **371**, 707–711.

75 Turner, M.J. and Schaeffer, J.M. (1989) Mode of action of ivermectin, in *Ivermectin and Abamectin* (ed. W.C. Campbell), Springer, New York, pp. 73–88.

76 Wolstenholme, A. (2010) Recent progress in understanding the interaction between avermectins and ligand-gated ion channels: putting the pests to sleep. *Invert. Neurosci.*, **10**, 5–10.

77 Dent, J.A., Davis, M.W., and Avery, L. (1997) *avr-15* encodes a chloride channel subunit that mediates inhibitory glutamatergic neurotransmission and ivermectin sensitivity in *Caenorhabditis elegans*. *EMBO J.*, **16**, 5867–5879.

78 Pemberton, D., Franks, C., Walker, R., and Holden-Dye, L. (2001) Characterization of glutamate-gated chloride channels in the pharynx of wild-type and mutant *Caenorhabditis elegans* delineates the role of the subunit GluCl-alpha2 in the function of the native receptor. *Mol. Pharmacol.*, **59**, 1037–1043.

79 Dent, J., Smith, M., Vassilatis, D., and Avery, L. (2000) The genetics of ivermectin resistance in *Caenorhabditis elegans*. *Proc. Natl. Acad. Sci. USA*, **97**, 2674–2679.

80 Cook, A., Aptel, N., Portillo, V., Siney, E., Sihota, R., Holden-Dye, L., and Wolstenholme, A. (2006) *Caenorhabditis elegans* ivermectin receptors regulate locomotor behaviour and are functional orthologues of *Haemonchus contortus* receptors. *Mol. Biochem. Parasitol.*, **147**, 118–125.

81 Holden-Dye, L. and Walker, R.J. (2006) Actions of glutamate and ivermectin on the pharyngeal muscle of *Ascaridia galli*: a comparative study with *Caenorhabditis elegans*. *Int. J. Parasitol.*, **36**, 395–402.

82 Geary, T.G., Sims, S.M., Thomas, E.M., Vanover, L., Davis, J.P., Winterrowd, C.A., Klein, R.D. *et al.* (1993) *Haemonchus contortus*: ivermectin-induced paralysis of the pharynx. *Exp. Parasitol.*, **77**, 88–96.

83 Brownlee, D.J., Holden-Dye, L., and Walker, R.J. (1997) Actions of the anthelmintic ivermectin on the pharyngeal muscle of the parasitic nematode, *Ascaris suum*. *Parasitology*, **115**, 553–561.

84 James, C.E. and Davey, M.W. (2009) Increased expression of ABC transport proteins is associated with ivermectin resistance in the model nematode *Caenorhabditis elegans*. *Int. J. Parasitol.*, **39**, 213–220.

85 Saeger, B., Schmitt-Wrede, H.-P., Dehnhardt, M., Benten, W.P.M., Krücken, J., Harder, A., von Samson-Himmelstjerna, G. *et al.* (2001) Latrophilin-like receptor from the parasitic nematode *Haemonchus contortus* as target for the anthelmintic depsipeptide PF1022A. *FASEB J.*, **15**, 1332–1334.

86 Willson, J., Amliwala, K., Davis, A., Cook, A., Cuttle, M.F., Kriek, N., Hopper, N.A., O'Connor, V. *et al.* (2004) Latrotoxin receptor signaling engages the UNC-13-dependent vesicle-priming pathway in *C. elegans*. *Curr. Biol.*, **14**, 1374–1379.

87 Chiang, J., Steciuk, M., Shtonda, B., and Avery, L. (2006) Evolution of pharyngeal behaviors and neuronal functions in free-living soil nematodes. *J. Exp. Biol.*, **209**, 1859–1873.

88 Wang, Z.-W., Saifee, O., Nonet, M.L., and Salkoff, L. (2001) SLO-1 potassium channels control quantal content of neurotransmitter release at the *C. elegans* neuromuscular junction. *Neuron*, **32**, 867–881.

89 Crisford, A., Murray, C., O'Connor, V., Edwards, R.J., Kruger, N., Welz, C., von Samson-Himmelstjerna, G. *et al.* (2011) Selective toxicity of the anthelmintic emodepside revealed by heterologous expression of human KCNMA1 in *Caenorhabditis elegans*. *Mol. Pharmacol.*, **79**, 1031–1043.

90 Buxton, S.K., Neveu, C., Charvet, C.L., Robertson, A.P., and Martin, R.J. (2011) On the mode of action of emodepside: slow effects on membrane potential and voltage-activated currents in *Ascaris suum*. *Br. J. Pharmacol.*, **164**, 453–470.

91 Welz, C., Krüger, N., Schniederjans, M., Miltsch, S.M., Krücken, J., Guest, M., Holden-Dye, L.M. *et al.* (2011) SLO-1-channels of parasitic nematodes reconstitute locomotor behaviour and emodepside sensitivity in *Caenorhabditis elegans* slo-1 loss of function mutants. *PLoS Pathog.*, **7**, e1001330.

92 Kaewintajuk, K., Cho, P., Kim, S., Lee, E., Lee, H.-K., Choi, E., and Park, H. (2010) Anthelmintic activity of KSI-4088 against *Caenorhabditis elegans*. *Parasitol. Res.*, **107**, 27–30.

93 Alkharouf, N.W., Klink, V.P., and Matthews, B.F. (2007) Identification of *Heterodera glycines* (soybean cyst nematode [SCN]) cDNA sequences with high identity to those of *Caenorhabditis elegans* having lethal mutant or RNAi phenotypes. *Exp. Parasitol.*, **115**, 247–258.

94 Nagel, G., Brauner, M., Liewald, J.F., Adeishvili, N., Bamberg, E., and Gottschalk, A. (2005) Light activation of channelrhodopsin-2 in excitable cells of *Caenorhabditis elegans* triggers rapid behavioral responses. *Curr. Biol.*, **15**, 2279–2284.

95 Zhang, F., Wang, L.-P., Brauner, M., Liewald, J.F., Kay, K., Watzke, N., Wood, P.G. *et al.* (2007) Multimodal fast optical interrogation of neural circuitry. *Nature*, **446**, 633–639.

96 Franks, C., Murray, C., Ogden, D., O'Connor, V., and Holden-Dye, L. (2009) A comparison of electrically evoked and channel rhodopsin-evoked postsynaptic potentials in the pharyngeal system of *Caenorhabditis elegans*. *Invert. Neurosci.*, **9**, 43–56.

97 Kerr, R., Lev-Ram, V., Baird, G., Vincent, P., Tsien, R.Y., and Schafer, W.R. (2000) Optical imaging of calcium transients in neurons and pharyngeal muscle of *C. elegans*. *Neuron*, **26**, 583–594.

98 Chalasani, S.H., Chronis, N., Tsunozaki, M., Gray, J.M., Ramot, D., Goodman, M.B., and Bargmann, C.I. (2007) Dissecting a circuit for olfactory behaviour in *Caenorhabditis elegans*. *Nature*, **450**, 63–70.

99 Chung, K., Crane, M.M., and Lu, H. (2008) Automated on-chip rapid microscopy, phenotyping and sorting of *C. elegans*. *Nat. Methods*, **5**, 637–643.

100 Stirman, J.N., Brauner, M., Gottschalk, A., and Lu, H. (2010) High-throughput study of synaptic transmission at the neuromuscular junction enabled by optogenetics and microfluidics. *J. Neurosci. Methods*, **191**, 90–93.

101 Jones, A.K., Buckingham, S.D., and Sattelle, D.B. (2005) Chemistry-to-gene screens in *Caenorhabditis elegans*. *Nat. Rev. Drug Discov.*, **4**, 321–330.

102 Krause, S., Sommer, A., Fischer, P., Brophy, P.M., Walter, R.D., and Liebau, E. (2001) Gene structure of the extracellular glutathione *S*-transferase from *Onchocerca volvulus* and its overexpression and promoter analysis in transgenic *Caenorhabditis elegans*. *Mol. Biochem. Parasitol.*, **117**, 145–154.

103 Gomez-Escobar, N., Gregory, W.F., Britton, C., Murray, L., Corton, C., Hall, N., Daub, J. *et al.* (2002) Abundant larval transcript-1 and -2 genes from *Brugia malayi*: diversity of genomic environments but conservation of 5′ promoter sequences functional in *Caenorhabditis elegans*. *Mol. Biochem. Parasitol.*, **125**, 59–71.

104 Costa, J.C., Lilley, C.J., Atkinson, H.J., and Urwin, P.E. (2009) Functional characterisation of a cyst nematode acetylcholinesterase gene using *Caenorhabditis elegans* as a heterologous system. *Int. J. Parasitol.*, **39**, 849–858.

3
Integrating and Mining Helminth Genomes to Discover and Prioritize Novel Therapeutic Targets

Dhanasekaran Shanmugam, Stuart A. Ralph, Santiago J. Carmona, Gregory J. Crowther, David S. Roos, and Fernán Agüero[*]

Abstract

Diseases caused by helminth parasites remain the most neglected of tropical diseases. Consequently, discovery of new therapeutics, diagnostics, and vaccines for helminth parasites has been slow to progress. This is in part because anthelmintic discovery has relied upon biological screens – either genetic or chemical – in model as well as in parasitic worms and these approaches are limited in a number of ways. For example, genetic manipulation (such as RNA interference) is still not available for many helminth parasites, and, therefore, genomic-scale experimental target identification and validation studies remain challenging. Also, for many parasitic helminths, the life cycle of the parasite cannot be maintained *in vitro*, thus limiting experimental screens. To facilitate discovery of new targets, a genomics-based approach has been gaining traction and will be supported by the increasing numbers of complete genome sequences available for helminth parasites. The availability of these genome sequences is expected to support a wide variety of genomic-scale studies that will generate functional datasets regarding the expression, structure, phylogeny, essentiality, and validation of genes from parasite stages relevant to disease. In addition, target identification will be facilitated by mapping of functional data through orthology from model organisms like *Caenorhabditis elegans*. In order to realize the full potential of genomics-based target discovery, various functional datasets need to be integrated with genome sequence information in a structured format that can be easily accessed and mined for anthelmintic target discovery. This chapter discusses advances in genomics-driven target discovery for helminths, and highlights the increasing contribution of data repositories such as TDR Targets and WormBase to anthelmintic target discovery. The search strategies implemented in the TDR Targets database will be used to illustrate the utility of comparative genomics to discover potential helminth drug targets and identify missing functional datasets in helminth parasites that will greatly improve target identification.

[*] Corresponding Author

Introduction

In the era of genome sequencing, it is inevitable that comparative genomics plays a major role in driving biological and therapeutic discoveries. This is especially true for less-studied organisms, like the helminth parasites, that are not easily amenable to experimental manipulation in the laboratory. Helminth parasites (nematodes, cestodes, and trematodes) are a diverse group of invertebrate animals with complex life cycles during which they infect various animal hosts. The disease burden resulting from human helminth infections is enormous. Estimates from the World Health Organization (WHO) indicate that more than 2 billion people world-wide are at risk of acquiring such infections (http://www.who.int/tdr/svc/diseases/helminths). Few effective drugs are available to treat and control helminth infections [1, 2] (see also Chapters 14 and 20), and there are already a significant number of documented cases of resistance in veterinary helminths [3, 4]. In addition, recent reports suggest that resistance to some anthelmintic treatments in humans might be emerging [5, 6]; thus, alternate therapeutics are urgently required.

Although whole-organism (phenotypic) screening approaches have dominated the drug discovery landscape for helminth parasites, target-based approaches are gaining ground, being supported by a number of advances (see also Chapters 1 and 8). (i) There is the increased availability of genome sequence information for a number of helminth parasites, which is supported by parasitic helminth genome initiatives such as those of the Wellcome Trust Sanger Institute and Washington University's Genome Sequencing Center [7, 8]. (ii) There has been a steady increase in genome-wide studies on expression profiling (primarily by expressed sequence tag (EST) library sequencing and microarray analysis [9–12]), proteomics [13–15], and validation of function and phenotype (most often by RNA interference (RNAi) [16]; see also Chapters 6 and 7). In fact, recent advances in deep sequencing of both genomic and mRNA mean that there will not be a shortage of sequence data for helminth parasites. Rather, the focus is now shifting towards developing methods and tools to effectively integrate and use these datasets in order to understand the biology of helminths and support anthelmintic discovery.

Traditional genome repositories such as organism-specific genome databases and the National Center for Biotechnology Information GenBank [17] serve the essential function of hosting raw genome sequence data and associated genomic or gene-specific annotations, generated mostly by standardized computational pipelines. With the increasing availability of different types of genomic-scale experimental datasets, it is now standard practice by most genome servers to integrate these datasets and allow end-users to query the available data in order to retrieve desired genes. Moreover, genome servers such as GeneDB [18] and EuPathDB [19], which host genome data for various eukaryotic pathogens, have implemented tools to perform comparative genomics analysis of related species. Comparative genomics is especially important in the case of helminth pathogens for which the functional annotation of available genomes suffers from a relative lack of robust experimental tools. For example, the highly annotated genome sequence information available for *Caenorhabditis elegans* in WormBase [20] can be used to inform gene annotation for orthologs in parasitic helminths. In fact, this strategy has been already used to identify potential target genes in *Brugia malayi* [21] and *Schistosoma mansoni* [22]. Implementing a similar workflow, but as part of a curated database, will allow for the continual updating of underlying datasets.

We outline how *in silico* comparative genomics can be employed to enhance our understanding of helminth biology and assist in the discovery of novel drug and vaccine targets. Specifically, grouping proteins by orthology [23] has been useful to map functional genomic datasets such as metabolic pathways and genetic phenotypes from the model organism, *C. elegans*, to parasitic helminths. This chapter also reviews how genome-wide annotation that is integrated into genome databases can be used to identify and prioritize target genes. Finally, we provide a brief overview of the WHO's TDR Targets database [24], which integrates a number of datasets mapped to the genomes of different pathogens, including helminths, and provides the necessary informatics tools to prioritize target genes. Illustrative examples of target prioritization for *B. malayi*, *S. mansoni*, *Onchocerca volvulus*, and *Wuchereria bancrofti* will be demonstrated using the tools implemented in TDR Targets.

Availability of Genome Sequence Information for Parasitic Helminths

In addition to the model nematode, *C. elegans* [25], which was the first nematode genome to be sequenced, a handful of other parasitic worm genomes, including *B. malayi* [26], *S. mansoni* [27], and *Trichinella spiralis* [28], have been sequenced. Table 3.1 provides a list of worms, most of them parasitic in animals, which are currently under study by various sequencing centers. However, there are significant challenges ahead in terms of producing high quality genome annotation, making data accessible to the community, and enabling functional studies. Genome repositories and databases will be important here. For helminths, the Nematode.Net database [29] maintains a collection of sequences, both genomic and EST-based, and provides various functionalities such as functional classification, ortholog identification, and expression data analysis. Although this database also includes data for *C. elegans*, more sophisticated phenotype data (based on targeted gene disruption or RNAi studies) for *C. elegans* can be mined from WormBase [20] and used to identify potential targets in parasitic helminths (see Figure 3.1). Also, the GeneDB [18] and SchistoDB [30] databases provide access to genome sequence annotation for a number of *Schistosoma* species. The TDR Targets database contains genome information for *B. malayi* and *S. mansoni*, and integrates a variety of datasets (see below), including orthology-based mapping of *C. elegans* phenotype data, to aid in the identification of potential drug targets. The TDR Targets database will incorporate genome information for other parasitic worms as data become available.

Table 3.1 Sequence data availability for helminth organisms (as of March 2012).

Organism type	Number of species with EST data[a]	Number of species with genome sequence data[a]	Number of species with RNA sequence data[a]
Trematoda – flukes	3	2 (Sman; Sjap)	2 (Sman; Sjap)
Cestoda – tapeworm	2	4 (Egra; Emul; Hmic; Tsol)	3 (Egra; Emul; Hmic)
Nematoda – clade I	4	2 (Tspi; Tmur)	—
Nematoda – clade III	6	4 (Bmal; Asuu; Alum; Ovol)	1 (Asuu)
Nematoda – clade IV a/b	18	4 (Srat; Gpal; Minc; Hgly)	2 (Srat; Gpal)
Nematoda – clade V	13	13 (*Caenorhabditis* spp;[b] Acan; Acey; Aduo; Conco; Dviv; Name; Oden; Oost; Hcon; Nbra; Tcir; Ppac)	3 (*Caenorhabditis* spp;[b] Anca: Conc; Dviv; Hbac; Name; Nbra; Oden; Oost; Tcir; Tcol)

The table summarizes the various helminth species (both parasitic and nonparasitic) for which EST, genome, and RNA sequence data is either available or will soon be available. Sman, *Schistosoma mansoni*; Sjap, *Schistosoma japonicum*; Egra, *Echinococcus granulosus*; Emul, *Echinococcus multilocularis*; Hmic, *Hymenolepis microstoma*; Tsol, *Taenia solium*; Tspi, *Trichinella spiralis*; Tmur, *Trichuris muris*; Bmal, *B. malayi*; Asuu, *Ascaris suum*; Alum, *Ascaris lumbricoides*; Ovol, *Onchocerca volvulus*; Srat, *Strongyloides ratti*; Gpal, *Globodera pallida*; Minc, *Meloidogyne incognita*; Hgly, *Heterodera glycines*; Acan, Ancylostoma caninum; Acey, Ancylostoma ceylanicum; Aduo, Ancylostoma duodenale; Conco, Cooperia oncophora; Dviv, Dictyocaulus viviparus; Hbac, Heterorhabditis bacteriophora; Name, Necator americanus; Oden, Oesophagostomum dentatum; Oost, Ostertagia ostertagi; Tcir, Teladorsagia circumcincta; Tcol, Trichostrongylus colubriformis; Hcon, *Haemonchus contortus*; Nbra, *Nippostrongylus brasiliensis*; Tcir, *Teladorsagia circumcincta*; Ppac, *Pristionchus pacificus*.
a) Indicates both completed and projects in progress; data obtained from Nematode.Net, the Wellcome Trust Sanger Institute, the NCBI Genome and Gene Expression Omnibus Databases, and [8].
b) Includes multiple species of *Caenorhabditis*.

Overview of Genome Annotation Datasets that Aid Target Identification

In addition to storing the sequence information for any given genome, the respective genome databases also provide a collection of annotations describing several different features either on a genomic-scale or in a gene/protein-specific manner. Some of the annotations are gathered automatically (e.g., identification of open reading frames and their protein domains/properties to predict function), but many others are culled from experimental data and have to be constantly curated as the data become available. The latter set includes data that describe gene/protein expression and regulation, genetic variations, protein structure, gene essentiality, phenotypic/functional responses to genetic/chemical alterations of gene structure or function, ligand/inhibitor interactions, and any other relevant information (see Table 3.2 for a list of datasets that can be mapped to a sequenced genome). Although the data available from automated genome annotations are very similar in format and accessibility across various genomes, the quality and depth of coverage of experimental data varies widely between organisms. This is especially true for helminths in that the data available for *C. elegans* are much more comprehensive than those for parasitic worms. This is, in part, due to the patchy genome information available for parasitic worms, but also due to them

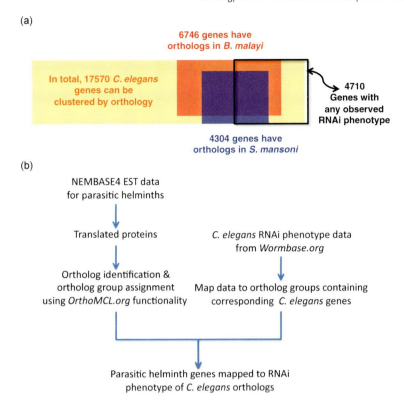

Figure 3.1 Mapping RNAi phenotype data using orthology. (a) The illustration shows how a significant number of C. elegans genes with orthologs in B. malayi and S. mansoni are also associated with at least one observed RNAi phenotype. Using this mapping information, desirable phenotypic data can be used to select for target genes from parasites. (b) General informatics pipeline used for transient mapping of phenotypic data from C. elegans to parasitic organisms.

being less experimentally tractable than C. elegans. Thus, it is useful to implement orthology-based transient mapping of annotation across closely related species to identify putative target genes, as described in the following section.

Orthology-Based Annotations and Comparative Genomics

Orthologs are defined as homologous proteins that are separated by a speciation event and are considered to be functionally conserved across species. Orthologous proteins may be estimated by reciprocal (two-way) best hits using BLAST. Precomputed ortholog pairs from more than 100 different species have been clustered into ortholog groups which can be accessed from the OrthoMCL database [23]. For example, Figure 3.1a illustrates how the RNAi phenotype data available for C. elegans genes can be mapped to orthologs in B. malayi and S. mansoni. Of the 4710 genes with observed RNAi phenotypes in C. elegans (available in WormBase [20]), 2242 are

Table 3.2 Genome annotation data made available through databases.

Annotation type	Annotated data
Automatic annotation and sequence based predictions	Gene ID
	Product name
	Gene/protein sequence
	Protein length in amino acids
	Molecular weight
	Isoelectric point
	Transmembrane domain
	Signal/transit sequences
	Protein domain by blast similarity
	Gene ontology predictions
	Pathway mapping and enzymes
	Metabolite mapping
	Protein structure model
	Phylogeny and orthology
	Druggability
Experimental evidence based annotation	Expression: anatomical and life cycle stage specificity
	Enzymatic activity and kinetics
	Metabolite and inhibitor ligand binding
	Recombinant availability
	Protein structure data
	Gene essentiality (knockout/down): life cycle stage specificity
	Phenotype (Genetic/Chemical): life cycle stage specificity

A variety of annotations, either from sequence-based prediction or based on experimental evidence, are made available through genome databases. For parasitic helminths in particular, the lack of genome wide experimental datasets needs to be addressed.

orthologous to 3064 *Schistosoma* genes and 3058 are orthologous to 3377 *Brugia* genes, with a large degree of overlap between orthologs of the two parasites. Similarly, the other annotations listed in Table 3.2 can be transiently mapped onto the genome of interest using information from a suitable model organism. However, the approach has some drawbacks. For example, whereas mapping enzymes and metabolic pathways using orthology is most likely to be correct, mapping genetic essentiality data can be misleading as a large proportion of these data tends to be organism-specific (see [31] and references therein). Therefore, in using such datasets, one needs to be familiar with the biology of each species and the suitability of the mapped data for a particular organism. Nevertheless, comparing orthologous genes across species is important when performing comparative genomics.

In addition to transient annotation of genomic-scale data as discussed above, the identification of orthologs enables phylogenetic profiling of the genome of interest. The presence or absence of genes in the host versus parasite genomes often provides a first-stage filter to narrow down the set of target genes of interest for further analysis [32]. As an example, one may want to select *B. malayi* genes that are absent from free-living nematodes, but are present in parasitic nematodes. Such a selection is likely to enrich for genes that are essential for parasitism and hence of interest as targets. Ortholog clustering also helps to identify gene duplications that can contribute to functional redundancy and genetic variation, sometimes even within different strains (isolates) of the same species [33]. Therefore, implementing orthology-based querying as part of database infrastructure can be of tremendous use to select target genes with the desired properties. TDR Targets implements this functionality making use of ortholog groupings already available in the OrthoMCL database. In the following sections, examples of target identification through orthology for various parasitic helminths are presented.

Predictions of Essentiality

A major task in the genome-wide prediction of promising drug targets for anthelmintics is the identification of essential genes [34, 35]. Essential targets are those for which inhibition of protein function is most likely to result in death, a severe phenotype(s), or a significant loss of fitness. These are not the only imaginable targets of anthelmintics. Indeed, chemical modulation of nonessential genes is a well-trodden path to eliminating helminths, such as agonists of nonessential genes that induce loss of muscle control and, therefore, worm expulsion (see Chapter 14 for examples). Identification of essential genes does enjoy one advantage in that resistance will not arise due to loss of function or deletion – resistance to some drugs in other pathogens involves deletion of nonessential genes including melarsaprol resistance in *Trypanosoma brucei* [36] and capreomycin resistance in *Mycobacterium tuberculosis* [37].

Although advances are being made in reverse genetics tools for pathogenic helminths, working either on a genome-wide scale or at the level of the individual gene, these are either lacking or rudimentary. Therefore, inference of essentiality through bioinformatic means is desirable and several potential methods are available, as discussed below. *C. elegans* has been employed as a model to suggest essentiality in important pathogenic nematodes, such as *B. malayi* [21], and it may also be useful to determine essentiality in *Onchocerca* spp. [38] and *Strongyloides* spp. [39]. Also, and as discussed above, TDR Targets allows the identification of *Brugia* genes with essential orthologs in *C. elegans*. The caveats to such inferences are that the parasitic lifestyle may allow these species to dispense with genes that are essential in free-living nematodes, whereas other molecules involved in host–pathogen interactions become newly essential. For helminths other than nematodes, it is less obvious whether essentiality can be inferred from functional data for *C. elegans* alone, and whether other animal models, such as the fruitfly, *Drosophila melanogaster*, can (should) be incorporated. A case in point is the analysis by Caffrey et al. [22] that filtered gene disruption data for *both C. elegans* and *D. melanogaster* to predict essential *S. mansoni* genes.

Helminth genes most likely to be essential are those that are shared by a greater number of evolutionarily diverse organisms [40]. One strategy, therefore, to determine essentiality in parasitic helminths is to focus on just these "essential" helminth genes that have orthologs in other phyla and are supported, where possible, by experimental data actually demonstrating essentiality. An unfortunate corollary of this is that helminth genes that are absent from the human host are less likely to be essential than those that are shared. Maximizing prediction of essentiality by choosing evolutionarily conserved proteins may therefore conflict with eventually developing ligands (inhibitors) that selectively target parasite proteins. In practice, therefore, these conflicting criteria must be balanced to identify targets that can be selectively drugged, but which are still likely to be essential. Also, as discussed by Caffrey et al. [22], it is often the case that selectivity and potency of any ligand eventually comes down to a range of parasitological and physiological factors, and smart medicinal chemistry to avoid "off-target" toxicity to the host.

An alternative to simply porting essentiality from experimentally characterized orthologs onto helminth genes is to rank essentiality based on gene product properties that are predictive of essentiality. One such approach is essentiality prediction from network connectivity. Proteins with larger numbers of interactions – called hubs – are more likely to be essential across several eukaryote groups [41, 42]. This observation informed the successful prediction and verification of essentiality in nematodes using highly connected genes in WormNet, which is a network that incorporates protein–protein interactions as well as other data types including coexpression, co-occurrence of gene names in text, and genetic interactions [43]. Future systems biology data from parasitic helminths could potentially be integrated into similar networks to improve and extend such network-based predictions.

Another property of gene products that can be used to infer essentiality is their position in metabolic networks. A number of genome-wide methods such as chokepoint analyses are available to predict essentiality and the curated *Schistosoma* metabolic network Schistocyc [30] or the NemaPath mapping of KEGG pathways [44] are useful starting templates for such analyses that will hopefully be replicated in other parasitic helminths.

Orthology-Based RNAi Phenotype Data Mapping Between *C. elegans* and Parasitic Helminths

C. elegans has been an important model organism to inform both experimental and comparative genomics studies with various parasitic helminths (see also Chapter 2). Examples of target identification for both *B. malayi* and *S. mansoni* using phenotype data available for *C. elegans* are published [20, 22, 45]. Here, we illustrate for *Onchocerca* spp. and *Wuchereria bancrofti* how this approach can be applied even in the absence of complete genome information (Figure 3.1b). In order to perform this analysis, EST data for various *Onchocerca* spp. and *W. bancrofti* were obtained from the NEMBASE4 database [46] that hosts EST data from more than 60 nematode species. The translated protein sequences for these ESTs were then used to identify the corresponding *C. elegans* orthologs using the ortholog identification pipeline implemented at the OrthoMCL database [23]. RNAi phenotypes for *C. elegans* genes obtained from the WormBase database were then mapped to the relevant ortholog groups of *Onchocerca* spp. and *W. bancrofti*. A supplementary file containing the results from this mapping exercise is available from TDR Targets using the link http://tdrtargets.org/static/shanmugam-helminth-genomes/Table-III.xlsx. This file lists all ortholog groups that contain at least one gene in *C. elegans* that has an observed RNAi phenotype and at least one gene in *Onchocerca* or *W. bancrofti*. From this list, parasite genes mapped to select RNAi phenotypes can be identified and pursued further as potential targets. As ever, downstream experimental work is required to validate the essentiality of these targets in these species. Once the genome sequence of these parasites becomes integrated into the TDR Targets database, genomic-scale mapping of the above exercise can be carried out. Using the workflow and functionalities implemented in TDR Targets (see Figure 3.2 and the discussion

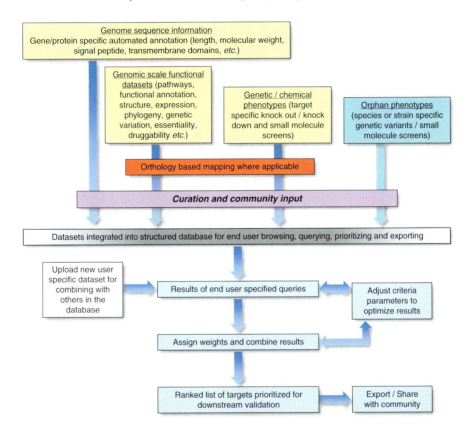

Figure 3.2 TDR Targets database structure and workflow for prioritizing genes. This scheme illustrates how various datasets integrated into the TDR Targets database can be used to identify and prioritize target genes. Note that mapping data from orthologous genes in other species, curation of published data, and community input on selected targets are key to making this process work. TDR Targets has implemented a user-friendly database infrastructure and easy-to-use informatics tools, all of which aid in target identification. For details of database functionality and case scenarios, see [24, 45].

below), we will next discuss the utility of genomic-scale datasets to identify targets of interest.

The TDR Targets Database

TDR Targets facilitates target identification for major tropical pathogens, including *B. malayi* and *S. mansoni* [24]. It contains genome information for all the pathogens listed in the target search page, and also integrates a variety of functional datasets (see Table 3.2) that facilitate the formulation of user-defined queries [45]. The various informatics tools provided via an open-access web interface, allow users to browse and query data, view and modify results, rank genes based on user-assigned weight values for selected criteria, export data and share results. TDR Targets obtains genome information for each species from various genome repositories like EuPathDB, GeneDB, WormBase, and GenBank. Functional annotations are obtained by a combination of methods, including orthology-based mapping of data across species, curation of literature information, and generating in-house datasets in collaboration with academic and industry partners. Figure 3.2 shows the general workflow of how one may carry out a target selection exercise using TDR Targets. First, the user searches for targets in the selected pathogen by formulating one or more queries based on the available datasets. The result of these queries can then be viewed as a list and exported as text or Excel files. The user can also manage queries from the *history* page by combining them using the *union* and *intersection* functions or *delete, export, rename*, and view the criteria used to formulate the queries. As an option, registered users can save the queries and publish the prioritized list of genes on the website to share with others.

Two different strategies can be employed to prioritize target genes using TDR Targets (Figure 3.3). The first is to use the *intersection* functionality to combine the results from multiple queries. As shown in Figure 3.3, five different hypothetical queries are displayed for a helminth genome. Combining in this manner is progressively restrictive because with the intersection of each query many genes are filtered away. Thus, starting from the whole genome of a helminth, which may contain more than 2×10^4 genes, one may end up with less than 100 genes. All genes contained in the resulting list will qualify for all of the criteria employed. Although this method helps to generate a list containing only the desired targets, it has the drawback of excluding genes that failed only one of the criteria used and does not provide the flexibility of modifying the target list without dramatically changing the query parameters or the query itself. One of the main issues affecting intersection-based strategies is the quality of the available genomes and their annotation. If resources allocated to manual curation of a genome are limited, or if the body of experimental evidence for any given genome is not sufficiently large or diverse, then it is more likely that many genes will fail to meet simple criteria that depend on the quality of annotation (e.g., "kinase" will not match a kinase that was annotated as "hypothetical protein"). Poor gene identification strategies (incorrect gene models that lead to the wrong identification of translational start sites and/or splicing sites)

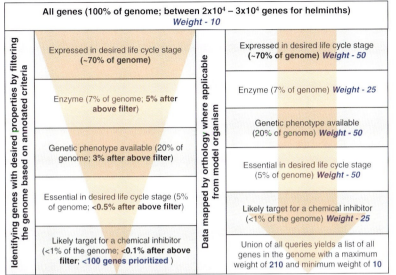

Figure 3.3 Examples of different strategies employed to prioritize targets using the TDR Targets database. The left side demonstrates the use of a more restrictive *intersection* (AND) functionality to run queries, whereas the right side demonstrates the *union* (OR) functionality. When using the *intersection* query, only genes that have qualified for all the selected criteria are obtained. In contrast, the *union* query facilitates a genome-wide ranking that is based on assigned weights for search criteria. For more details, see [24].

can also lead to failures of many downstream bioinformatics predictions (e.g., orthology detection, and domain and motif identification). For many helminth genomes available as drafts, alternative prioritization strategies may help to lower the impact of some of these knowledge gaps.

The second way to prioritize genes is to apply the *union* functionality in combination with weight assignments for individual queries. In Figure 3.3, this is demonstrated using the same queries used above with the intersection example. Note that for each query a *weight* value is assigned and when a gene qualifies for two or more query criteria, the individual weight values add up and provide a way to rank genes. Thus, in the example shown, genes that qualify for all of the selected criteria used to run the queries will receive the maximum weight value of 210 while other genes will receive lower weight values based on their qualifying criteria. The resulting list will contain all the genes from the genome ranked according to their weight values. The ranked target list can be easily modified by adjusting the weight values assigned to each criterion. The ranked list also provides users with a genome-wide perspective on how useful the chosen criteria are for the purpose of target selection. By default, TDR Targets performs a union of multiple queries run by users and provides a ranked list. Alternatively, users can manage and combine their queries in various ways using the functionalities available on the *history* page.

Target Prioritization in *B. malayi* and *S. mansoni* Using the TDR Targets Database

Genomic data for *B. malayi* and *S. mansoni* is integrated into the TDR Targets database and, based on orthology, their genes have been mapped to *C. elegans* phenotypic data. Using these data, examples of target prioritization were carried out for both these parasites [45] and the results are available for viewing and modification on the database site (*B. malayi*, http://tdrtargets.org/published/browse/361; *S. mansoni*, http://tdrtargets.org/published/browse/336). In these examples, targets have been prioritized based on a number of features; phenotype upon RNAi of the *C. elegans* ortholog, availability of structural models, availability of orthologs in *C. elegans*, predicted druggability, function as a catalyst (i.e., an enzyme), and assayability. The weights used for each criterion are heavily biased towards loss-of-fitness phenotypes with less weight for other features. Owing to the differences in the availability of data, but also because we wanted to illustrate the flexibility of the TDR Targets resource, we used somewhat different sets of criteria for each species. One of the main differences was the availability of gene expression data for *S. mansoni*. These data were derived from stage-specific EST sequencing projects available at SchistoDB [30] and were used to give an additional score to those gene products expressed in those life cycle stages relevant to infection in humans.

As a number of current anthelmintics modulate neuromuscular function [47], another useful prioritization strategy may take into account not just the timing of expression (developmentally regulated genes), but also the anatomical location of expression (spatially regulated genes). Genome-wide experimental datasets containing this information are currently lacking for parasitic helminths. Therefore, we used *C. elegans* expression data mapped to the corresponding orthologs of *B. malayi* and *S. mansoni*. These data, derived from a large compendium of microarray analyses (916 experiments from 53 datasets), were recently reanalyzed [48] to obtain subsets of genes that are differentially expressed in various tissues. The underlying hypothesis is that a gene that is expressed in a defined tissue (e.g., muscle) in one organism is more likely to have the same pattern of expression in another related organism. The evolutionary divergence of *B. malayi* and, especially, *S. mansoni* from *C. elegans* will need to be considered accordingly when weighting these criteria.

For this exercise, we used the same criteria and weights as before for *B. malayi* and *S. mansoni* [45], but added additional weights to those genes for which orthologs in *C. elegans* are expressed in nervous or muscular tissues. The results of these prioritizations are available from TDR Targets (*S. mansoni*, http://tdrtargets.org/published/browse/394; *B. malayi*, http://tdrtargets.org/published/browse/395). Although both the previous prioritization exercises and these latest revisions are very similar in displaying cytoskeleton and motor proteins, such as β-tubulin (the target of benzimidazole anthelmintics), dyneins, and myosins, at the top of these lists, a number of additional interesting targets emerge based on the criterion of tissue expression. For *S. mansoni*, among the 37 genes that were raised into the top 100 are a number of potentially druggable targets such as a putative Ras-like GTPase (Smp_146600), a putative calcium-dependent protein kinase (Smp_011660.2), and a putative tyrosine kinase (Smp_136300). For *B. malayi*, a similar approach led to higher scores for a number of potentially druggable targets, including a putative adenylate kinase (Bm1_24575), a Ser/Thr protein phosphatase family (Bm1_41290), and a short-chain dehydrogenase potentially involved in the metabolism of steroids (Bm_45995). Although these targets await further experimental validation, the underlying idea behind these computational exercises is that increased usage of experimental data providing information on different independent criteria (i.e., orthogonal, see [35]) should drive these prioritizations.

Currently Unavailable Genomic Datasets that will Improve Target Prioritization for Parasitic Helminths

A number of key datasets that would enhance the prioritization of targets in parasitic helminths are not yet available. Some of these datasets are high on the lists of priorities of many scientists and funding agencies, and, accordingly, deserve to be listed again. There is a notable lack of genomic-scale assessment of phenotypes caused by either targeted gene disruption or RNAi, particularly for flatworms, since *C. elegans* is not a perfect model of their biology. Targeted gene disruptions (e.g., knockouts) are a more reliable indicator of phenotype than RNAi, for which off-targeting is a real problem [22, 49]. Datasets that reveal the temporal and spatial expression of genes would also be highly valuable. Although substantial transcriptomic sequence information has become available for schistosomes over the last decade (cited in [16]; see also SchistoDB), and high-throughput sequencing has been (and will be) a boon for trematodes and nematode parasites (see also Chapters 4 and 5), the breadth and depth of these datasets requires further improvement. In addition, it is worth noting that protein structure information for these organisms is also limited. Although this is not strictly a validating criterion, knowledge of the structure of a target helps in a number of downstream analyses, such as the identification of potential ligand binding sites, the assessment of the likelihood of binding by small molecules and in the rational design of inhibitors. As of July 2011, the Protein Data Bank [50] carries the following structural data for helminths: Nematoda, 194 structures; Platyhelminths, 71 structures (Cestoda, two structures; Trematoda, 64 structures). Even when taking into account potential redundancies (several structures solved for the same protein), these figures are less than those for other parasites that cause neglected diseases (e.g., 552 and 564 structures available for trypanosomatids and apicomplexans, respectively). Finally, a recent addition to the TDR Targets database is the integration of chemical datasets (available as of Version 4) [51]. The availability of links between targets and compounds, manually curated from the literature, as well as the ability to perform similarity searches between compounds, opens the door to more comprehensive prioritizations. In this context, datasets from high-throughput chemical and whole-organism screens would be valuable as they would allow users to identify chemical scaffolds that are bioactive against helminths and that may then be linked by similarity to other compounds, and ultimately, to potential targets. Furthermore, the inclusion and integration of data for inactive compounds would be as important, not least in avoiding unnecessary duplication of effort. A comparison of the activity profile of any given compound against different parasitic helminths can help to shed light on the potential mode(s) of action of the compound.

Conclusions

Helminth infections are among the most neglected of human diseases relative to their global burden. Despite limited resources dedicated to either fundamental research or applied drug discovery for these organisms, recent whole-genome projects and transcriptomic surveys of many helminths offer promising starting points for chemotherapeutic or vaccine-based interventions. A challenge for these genome projects is that some of the respective organism-specific research communities are relatively small. This means that the human resources and biological technologies to fully exploit the data arising from some helminth genomes are quite limited. This has two important implications. (i) Limited resources make it all the more important to prioritize the most promising therapeutic targets from the myriad of potential macromolecules to work on. (ii) Where possible, relevant chemical and genetic data should be identified and ported from more thoroughly studied organisms. These tasks are limited by the appropriateness of the model organism and organism-specific features that can render cross-species inferences unsound. Nevertheless, genomics-based approaches will facilitate the process of identifying tractable drug targets and finding promising chemical leads for anthelmintic development. Informatic tools such as TDR Targets serve a useful function in organizing the genomic, phyletic, phenotypic, and chemical resources necessary for target identification. Also, cross-organism platforms that combine various individual genome projects (such as EuPathDB, GeneDB, and TDR Targets), assisted by comparative genomics, will certainly provide valuable insights into the biology of helminths and other parasites, particularly those outside the field of tropical diseases. Much remains to be done to alert such potential users to the significance of genomics in helminth drug development and to kindle their interest therein.

Acknowledgments

Development of the TDR Targets database is funded by the Special Programme for Research and Training in Tropical Diseases (WHO/World Bank/UNDP/UNICEF). S.A.R. is an Australian Research Council Future Fellow (FT0990350). S.J.C. and F.A. are fellows of the National Research Council (CONICET), Argentina.

References

1. Holden-Dye, L. and Walker, R.J. (2007) Anthelmintic drugs, in *WormBook* (ed. The *C. elegans* Research Community), doi: 10.1895/wormbook.1.143.1.
2. Nwaka, S. and Hudson, A. (2006) Innovative lead discovery strategies for tropical diseases. *Nat. Rev. Drug Discov.*, **5**, 941–955.
3. Prichard, R.K. (1990) Anthelmintic resistance in nematodes: extent, recent understanding and future directions for control and research. *Int. J. Parasitol.*, **20**, 515–523.
4. Kaplan, R.M. (2004) Drug resistance in nematodes of veterinary importance: a status report. *Trends Parasitol.*, **20**, 477–481.
5. Osei-Atweneboana, M.Y., Eng, J.K.L., Boakye, D.A., Gyapong, J.O., and Prichard, R.K. (2007) Prevalence and intensity of *Onchocerca volvulus* infection and efficacy of ivermectin in endemic communities in Ghana: a two-phase epidemiological study. *Lancet.*, **369**, 2021–2029.
6. Osei-Atweneboana, M.Y., Awadzi, K., Attah, S.K., Boakye, D.A., Gyapong, J.O., and Prichard, R.K. (2011) Phenotypic evidence of emerging ivermectin resistance in *Onchocerca volvulus*. *PLoS Negl. Trop. Dis.*, **5**, e998.
7. Berriman, M., Lustigman, S., and Mc Carter, J.P. (2007) Helminth initiative for drug discovery – report of the informal consultation, genomics and emerging drug discovery technologies. *Expert Opin. Drug Discov.*, **2**, S83–S89.
8. Brindley, P.J., Mitreva, M., Ghedin, E., and Lustigman, S. (2009) Helminth genomics: the implications for human health. *PLoS Negl. Trop. Dis.*, **3**, e538.
9. Parkinson, J., Anthony, A., Wasmuth, J., Schmid, R., Hedley, A., and Blaxter, M. (2004) Partigene – constructing partial genomes. *Bioinformatics*, **20**, 1398–1404.
10. Parkinson, J., Mitreva, M., Whitton, C., Thomson, M., Daub, J., Martin, J., Schmid, R., Hall, N. *et al.* (2004) A transcriptomic analysis of the phylum Nematoda. *Nat. Genet.*, **36**, 1259–1267.
11. Ramanathan, R., Varma, S., Ribeiro, J.M.C., Myers, T.G., Nolan, T.J., Abraham, D., Lok, J.B., and Nutman, T.B. (2011) Microarray-based analysis of differential gene expression between infective and noninfective larvae of *Strongyloides stercoralis*. *PLoS Negl. Trop. Dis.*, **5**, e1039.
12. Wasmuth, J., Schmid, R., Hedley, A., and Blaxter, M. (2008) On the extent and origins of genic novelty in the phylum Nematoda. *PLoS Negl. Trop. Dis.*, **2**, e258.
13. Marcilla, A., Sotillo, J., Pérez-Garcia, A., Igual-Adell, R., Valero, M.L., Sánchez-Pino, M.M., Bernal, D., Muñoz-Antolí, C. *et al.* (2010) Proteomic analysis of *Strongyloides stercoralis* l3 larvae. *Parasitology*, **137**, 1577–1583.
14. Mulvenna, J., Hamilton, B., Nagaraj, S.H., Smyth, D., Loukas, A., and Gorman, J.J. (2009) Proteomics analysis of the excretory/secretory component of the blood-feeding stage of the hookworm, *Ancylostoma caninum*. *Mol. Cell Proteomics*, **8**, 109–121.
15. Weinkopff, T., Atwood, J.A., Punkosdy, G.A., Moss, D., Weatherly, D.B., Orlando, R., and Lammie, P. (2009) Identification of antigenic *Brugia* adult worm proteins by peptide mass fingerprinting. *J. Parasitol.*, **95**, 1429–1435.
16. Stefanić, S., Dvořák, J., Horn, M., Braschi, S., Sojka, D., Ruelas, D.S., Suzuki, B., Lim, K. *et al.* (2010) RNA interference in *Schistosoma mansoni* schistosomula: selectivity, sensitivity and operation for larger-scale screening. *PLoS Negl. Trop. Dis.*, **4**, e850.
17. Benson, D.A., Karsch-Mizrachi, I., Lipman, D.J., Ostell, J., and Sayers, E.W. (2011) GenBank. *Nucleic Acids Res.*, **39**, D32–D37.
18. Hertz-Fowler, C., Peacock, C.S., Wood, V., Aslett, M., Kerhornou, A., Mooney, P., Tivey, A., Berriman, M. *et al.* (2004) GeneDB: a resource for prokaryotic and

18 eukaryotic organisms. *Nucleic Acids Res.*, **32**, D339–D343.
19 Aurrecoechea, C., Brestelli, J., Brunk, B.P., Fischer, S., Gajria, B., Gao, X., Gingle, A., Grant, G. et al. (2010) EuPathDB: a portal to eukaryotic pathogen databases. *Nucleic Acids Res.*, **38**, D415–D419.
20 Harris, T.W., Antoshechkin, I., Bieri, T., Blasiar, D., Chan, J., Chen, W.J., De La Cruz, N., Davis, P. et al. (2010) WormBase: a comprehensive resource for nematode research. *Nucleic Acids Res.*, **38**, D463–D467.
21 Kumar, S., Chaudhary, K., Foster, J.M., Novelli, J.F., Zhang, Y., Wang, S., Spiro, D., Ghedin, E. et al. (2007) Mining predicted essential genes of *Brugia malayi* for nematode drug targets. *PLoS One*, **2**, e1189.
22 Caffrey, C.R., Rohwer, A., Oellien, F., Marhöfer, R.J., Braschi, S., Oliveira, G., McKerrow, J.H., and Selzer, P.M. (2009) A comparative chemogenomics strategy to predict potential drug targets in the metazoan pathogen, *Schistosoma mansoni*. *PLoS One*, **4**, e4413.
23 Chen, F., Mackey, A.J., Stoeckert, C.J., and Roos, D.S. (2006) OrthoMCL-DB: querying a comprehensive multi-species collection of ortholog groups. *Nucleic Acids Res.*, **34**, D363–D368.
24 Agüero, F., Al-Lazikani, B., Aslett, M., Berriman, M., Buckner, F.S., Campbell, R.K., Carmona, S., Carruthers, I.M. et al. (2008) Genomic-scale prioritization of drug targets: the TDR Targets database. *Nat. Rev. Drug Discov.*, **7**, 900–907.
25 *C. elegans* Sequencing Consortium (1998) Genome sequence of the nematode, *C. elegans*: a platform for investigating biology. *Science*, **282**, 2012–2018.
26 Ghedin, E., Wang, S., Spiro, D., Caler, E., Zhao, Q., Crabtree, J., Allen, J.E., Delcher, A.L. et al. (2007) Draft genome of the filarial nematode parasite *Brugia malayi*. *Science*, **317**, 1756–1760.
27 Berriman, M., Haas, B.J., LoVerde, P.T., Wilson, R.A., Dillon, G.P., Cerqueira, G.C., Mashiyama, S.T., Al-Lazikani, B. et al. (2009) The genome of the blood fluke *Schistosoma mansoni*. *Nature*, **460**, 352–358.
28 Mitreva, M., Jasmer, D.P., Zarlenga, D.S., Wang, Z., Abubucker, S., Martin, J., Taylor, C.M., Yin, Y. et al. (2011) The draft genome of the parasitic nematode *Trichinella spiralis*. *Nat. Genet.*, **43**, 228–235.
29 Martin, J., Abubucker, S., Wylie, T., Yin, Y., Wang, Z., and Mitreva, M. (2009) Nematode.net update 2008: improvements enabling more efficient data mining and comparative nematode genomics. *Nucleic Acids Res.*, **37**, D571–D578.
30 Zerlotini, A., Heiges, M., Wang, H., Moraes, R.L.V., Dominitini, A.J., Ruiz, J.C., Kissinger, J.C., and Oliveira, G. (2009) SchistoDB: a *Schistosoma mansoni* genome resource. *Nucleic Acids Res.*, **37**, D579–D582.
31 Deng, J., Deng, L., Su, S., Zhang, M., Lin, X., Wei, L., Minai, A.A., Hassett, D.J. et al. (2011) Investigating the predictability of essential genes across distantly related organisms using an integrative approach. *Nucleic Acids Res.*, **39**, 795–807.
32 McCarter, J.P. (2004) Genomic filtering: an approach to discovering novel antiparasitics. *Trends Parasitol.*, **20**, 462–468.
33 Koonin, E.V. (2005) Orthologs, paralogs, and evolutionary genomics. *Annu. Rev. Genet.*, **39**, 309–338.
34 Wang, C.C. (1997) Validating targets for antiparasite chemotherapy. *Parasitology*, **114** (Suppl.), S31–S44.
35 Hardy, L.W. and Peet, N.P. (2004) The multiple orthogonal tools approach to define molecular causation in the validation of druggable targets. *Drug Discov. Today*, **9**, 117–126.
36 Carter, N.S. and Fairlamb, A.H. (1993) Arsenical-resistant trypanosomes lack an unusual adenosine transporter. *Nature*, **361**, 173–176.
37 Maus, C.E., Plikaytis, B.B., and Shinnick, T.M. (2005) Molecular analysis of cross-resistance to capreomycin, kanamycin, amikacin, and viomycin in *Mycobacterium tuberculosis*. *Antimicrob. Agents Chemother.*, **49**, 3192–3197.

38 Behm, C.A., Bendig, M.M., McCarter, J.P., and Sluder, A.E. (2005) RNAi-based discovery and validation of new drug targets in filarial nematodes. *Trends Parasitol.*, **21**, 97–100.

39 Viney, M.E. (2006) The biology and genomics of *Strongyloides*. *Med. Microbiol. Immunol.*, **195**, 49–54.

40 Doyle, M.A., Gasser, R.B., Woodcroft, B.J., Hall, R.S., and Ralph, S.A. (2010) Drug target prediction and prioritization: using orthology to predict essentiality in parasite genomes. *BMC Genomics*, **11**, 222.

41 Batada, N.N., Reguly, T., Breitkreutz, A., Boucher, L., Breitkreutz, B., Hurst, L.D., and Tyers, M. (2006) Stratus not altocumulus: a new view of the yeast protein interaction network. *PLoS Biol.*, **4**, e317.

42 Jeong, H., Mason, S.P., Barabási, A.L., and Oltvai, Z.N. (2001) Lethality and centrality in protein networks. *Nature*, **411**, 41–42.

43 Lee, I., Lehner, B., Crombie, C., Wong, W., Fraser, A.G., and Marcotte, E.M. (2008) A single gene network accurately predicts phenotypic effects of gene perturbation in *Caenorhabditis elegans*. *Nat. Genet.*, **40**, 181–188.

44 Wylie, T., Martin, J., Abubucker, S., Yin, Y., Messina, D., Wang, Z., McCarter, J.P., and Mitreva, M. (2008) NemaPath: online exploration of KEGG-based metabolic pathways for nematodes. *BMC Genomics*, **9**, 525.

45 Crowther, G.J., Shanmugam, D., Carmona, S.J., Doyle, M.A., Hertz-Fowler, C., Berriman, M., Nwaka, S., Ralph, S.A. *et al.* (2010) Identification of attractive drug targets in neglected-disease pathogens using an *in silico* approach. *PLoS Negl. Trop. Dis.*, **4**, e804.

46 Parkinson, J., Whitton, C., Schmid, R., Thomson, M., and Blaxter, M. (2004) NEMBASE: a resource for parasitic nematode ESTs. *Nucleic Acids Res.*, **32**, D427–D430.

47 Geary, T.G., Klein, R.D., Vanover, L., Bowman, J.W., and Thompson, D.P. (1992) The nervous systems of helminths as targets for drugs. *J. Parasitol.*, **78**, 215–230.

48 Chikina, M.D., Huttenhower, C., Murphy, C.T., and Troyanskaya, O.G. (2009) Global prediction of tissue-specific gene expression and context-dependent gene networks in *Caenorhabditis elegans*. *PLoS Comput. Biol.*, **5**, e1000417.

49 Jackson, A.L., Bartz, S.R., Schelter, J., Kobayashi, S.V., Burchard, J., Mao, M., Li, B., Cavet, G. *et al.* (2003) Expression profiling reveals off-target gene regulation by RNAi. *Nat. Biotechnol.*, **21**, 635–637.

50 Rose, P.W., Beran, B., Bi, C., Bluhm, W.F., Dimitropoulos, D., Goodsell, D.S., Prlic, A., Quesada, M. *et al.* (2011) The RCSB Protein Data Bank: redesigned web site and web services. *Nucleic Acids Res.*, **39**, D392–401.

51 Magariños, M.P., Carmona, S.J., Crowther, G.J., Ralph, S.A., Roos, D.S., Shanmugam, D., Van Voorhis, W.C., and Agüero, F. (2012) TDR Targets: a chemogenomics resource for neglected diseases. *Nucleic Acids Res.*, **40**, D1118–D1127.

4
Recent Progress in Transcriptomics of Key Gastrointestinal Nematodes of Animals – Fundamental Research Toward New Intervention Strategies

Cinzia Cantacessi, Bronwyn E. Campbell, Aaron R. Jex, Ross S. Hall, Neil D. Young, Matthew J. Nolan, and Robin B. Gasser[*]

Abstract

Much remains to be understood about the fundamental biology of parasitic nematodes that cause serious disease in animals and humans world-wide. Unlocking the biology of these parasites using "omic" technologies will yield new and crucial knowledge of their molecular biology and biochemistry on a global scale. Here, we review progress on the transcriptomics of gastrointestinal nematodes of major socioeconomic importance, focusing on massively parallel (next-generation) sequencing technologies and the latest bioinformatic approaches. We predict exciting prospects for future systems biological explorations of these parasites and for the design of new drugs and/or vaccines.

Introduction

Parasitic nematodes of the gastrointestinal tracts of humans and livestock are of major socioeconomic significance world-wide [1–4]. The soil-transmitted helminths (STHs) *Ancylostoma duodenale*, *Necator americanus*, *Ascaris* spp., and *Trichuris trichiura* are estimated to infect almost one-sixth of the global human population [4, 5]. Gastrointestinal parasites of livestock (including *Haemonchus contortus*, *Ostertagia ostertagi*, and *Trichostrongylus* spp.) cause economic losses estimated at billions of dollars per annum as a consequence of poor weight gain and lost productivity as well as the costs of repeated anthelmintic treatment [6]. In addition to the socioeconomic impact, resistance to the main classes of anthelmintics [7] continually drives the development of alternative intervention and control strategies. Despite the wealth of information on aspects of parasite taxonomy and systematics, biology, epidemiology, immunology, and anthelmintics [1, 2, 8–17], little is known at the molecular level regarding the mechanisms that govern essential biological processes in parasitic nematodes and their interactions with their animal hosts. Such information can underpin the discovery and development of novel methods of treatment and control.

Advances in sequencing technologies [18–21] are now providing unique opportunities for global molecular investigations. Indeed, the advent and integration of

[*] Corresponding Author

high-throughput "omics" technologies, such as genomics, transcriptomics, proteomics, metabolomics, glycomics, and lipidomics, are revolutionizing the way research in biology is performed and allows for the systems biology of organisms to be elucidated. In particular, studies of the "transcriptomes" of parasites (representing mRNA) [22] have become routine to gain insights into gene expression, regulation, and function [23, 24]. Here, we review recent advances in transcriptomics of gastrointestinal nematodes of socioeconomic significance; not least, the recent applications of massively parallel (next-generation, NGS) sequencing technologies and bioinformatic tools to large-scale investigations. We discuss the prospects and implications of these explorations for developing novel methods of intervention.

Recent Developments in the Bioinformatic Tools and Pipelines for the Analysis of Expressed Sequence Tag Data

The use of NGS [18–21] to yield transcriptomic datasets (Table 4.1) has been accompanied by a substantial expansion of bioinformatic tools for their analysis, both at the cDNA and protein levels. This expansion has resulted in the development of a number of web-based programs and/or integrated pipelines [25–28]. The principles, methods, and protocols for the analysis of expressed sequence tag (EST) data, together with currently available bioinformatic tools and pipelines, have been reviewed [23].

In brief, following the acquisition of sequence data, ESTs are first screened for sequence repeats, contaminants, and/or adapter sequences [23, 29], and "clustered" (assembled) into contiguous sequences (of maximum length) based on sequence similarity [23]. Long-reads (generated by Sanger sequencing or 454 technology; [18]) and short-reads (from the Illumina/HiSeq and SOLiD platforms; [19–21]) are assembled using the algorithms "overlap–layout–consensus" [30] and the "de Bruijn graph" [31], respectively. For the former algorithm, all pair-wise overlaps among reads are computed and stored in a graph. All graphs are then used to compute a layout of reads and consensus sequences of contigs (e.g., [25, 32, 33]). For the "de Bruijn graph" [31], reads are fragmented into short segments, termed "k-mers," where "k"

Table 4.1 Number of expressed sequence tags (ESTs) from selected gastrointestinal nematodes that were accessible from public sequence databases between 1995 and 2010.

Species	1995–2000	2001–2005	2006–2010
Ancylostoma caninum	4909	4448	1648206
Necator americanus	213	4595	116951
Haemonchus contortus	30	14153	207538
Trichostrongylus colubriformis	3	1	2674446
Oesophagostomum dentatum	12	7	1826446

Sources: http://www.ncbi.nlm.nih.gov/, http://www.ebi.ac.uk/embl/, and http://www.nematode.net/NN3_frontpage.cgi.

represents the number of nucleotides in each segment. Overlaps between or among *k*-mers are captured and stored in graphs, which are subsequently used to generate the consensus sequences [31–34].

Following assembly, the contigs and single reads (singletons) are compared with public sequence data using different types of BLAST [35] in order to assign a predicted identity to each query sequence, if significant matches are found [23]. In addition, assembled nucleotide sequences are conceptually translated into predicted proteins using algorithms that identify open reading frames (ORFs) from individual contigs [36, 37]. Once peptides are predicted, protein and protein domain identities are assigned using data and information in public databases [23, 38–40]. For ESTs, examples of these databases include UniGene [41] and the Sequence Read Archive (SRA) [42]. In addition to these general databases, there is a number of specialized collections. Examples include the databases for *Saccharomyces cerevisiae* (www.yeastgenome.org [43]), *Drosophila melanogaster* (www.flybase.org [44]), *Mus musculus* (www.informatics.jax.org [45]) and *Caenorhabditis elegans* (WormBase at www.wormbase.org [46]). WormBase is a comprehensive repository of information on *C. elegans* and related nematodes, including *Caenorhabditis briggsae* [46]. Here, information regarding classical genetics, cellular biology, and structural and functional genomics of these free-living nematodes is stored and meticulously curated [46].

Recently, a web-based bioinformatic pipeline (called ESTExplorer) was established to automate the analysis and annotation of EST datasets (both at the nucleotide and amino acid levels) [27]. The approach is faster than traditional database searches [47]. However, sequences generated by NGS are significantly shorter (400 bp for 454/Roche and 60 bp for Illumina/ABI SOLiD) than those determined by Sanger sequencing (0.8–1 kb), and this is challenging for assembly in the absence of a reference genome. In addition, the data files generated by these technologies are often gigabytes to terabytes in size, substantially increasing the demands placed on data transfer and storage, such that many web-based interfaces are not suited for large-scale analyses. To facilitate the *de novo* assembly and annotation of large datasets, Cantacessi *et al.* [48] developed a practical and integrated bioinformatic workflow system (Figure 4.1). The software is mainly derived from existing web-based application tools that are optimized using the Linux operational system and incorporated into pre-existing scripts, such as Perl, Python, and Unix shell. These tools are available for download at http://www.gasserlab.org [48] and can be readily employed by scientists with limited bioinformatic expertise. The workflow allows the display of biologically meaningful information (such as gene ontologies, pathway mapping, and the prediction of essential molecules) from NGS datasets.

Characterizing the Transcriptomes of Strongylid Nematodes

NGS platforms have helped explore the transcriptomes of different developmental stages and both sexes of the strongylid nematodes *T. colubriformis*, *H. contortus*, *N. americanus*, and *O. dentatum* [48–51] (Table 4.1). For example, the first study of the transcriptome of adult *T. colubriformis* employed 454 sequencing technology and the

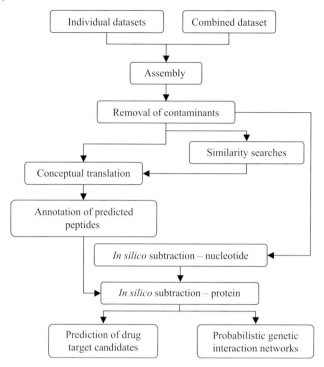

Figure 4.1 Example of an eight-step bioinformatic workflow system for the analyses of large-scale transcriptomic datasets generated by NGS. (Adapted by permission of Oxford University Press from [48] © 2010).

above-discussed bioinformatic analyses [49]. Highly represented were molecules associated with the nervous system (e.g., "transthyretin-like" and "neuropeptide-like" proteins), but also proteases and protease inhibitors, principally serine- and metalloproteases, and "Kunitz-type" protease inhibitors [49]. In strongylid nematodes, proteases are likely to be involved in the invasion of and establishment in the vertebrate host; specifically, tissue penetration, feeding, and immunoevasion by (i) digesting antibodies, (ii) cleaving cell surface receptors of cytokines, and (iii) directly lysing immune cells [52–54].

Likewise for *H. contortus*, 454 sequencing and bioinformatics were used to explore changes in gene transcription associated with the transition from the free-living (L3) to the parasitic third larval stage (xL3) and to predict the functions of transcripts linked to larval development [50]. This study revealed that "transthyretin-like" proteins and calcium-binding proteins are highly represented in the transcriptome of both *H. contortus* L3 and xL3, whereas collagens/ neuropeptides, and proteases are transcribed in L3 and xL3, respectively [50]. In nematodes, collagen synthesis is upregulated prior to molting [55]. Increased transcription of neuropeptides in the L3 stage might relate to axon guidance and synapse formation during transition to parasitism [50]. This statement is supported by the finding that the transition to xL3 is triggered by gaseous CO_2 (detected by amphid chemosensory neurons) that, in turn, leads to the secretion of noradrenaline [3]. Conversely, for *H. contortus* xL3, most transcripts encode proteases and other enzymes of catabolism, which supports the proposed involvement of proteases in the catabolism of globin, as is the case for *A. caninum* and *N. americanus* [56–58]. A similar spectrum of proteases and other molecules linked to catalytic activity is also represented in the transcriptomes of both *H. contortus* and *A. caninum* xL3 as compared with their respective L3 stages [50, 59]. This finding is, perhaps, not surprising, as both parasites have a similar pattern of development through the four larval stages to the adulthood [60] and both are hematophagic.

Although human hookworms are of major socioeconomic importance [1, 2, 5], genomic and molecular studies have mainly involved *A. caninum* [59, 61–63]. Recently, 454 sequencing and bioinformatic analyses were conducted to explore the global transcriptome of adult *N. americanus* [51]. The results showed that transcripts encoding proteases and Kunitz-type protease inhibitors were abundantly expressed, supporting their respective functions in host protein digestion [57, 58] and in the inhibition of homeostatic host proteases [64, 65], respectively. Using orthology mapping with the functional data available for *C. elegans*, Cantacessi *et al.* [51] predicted 18 potential drug targets in the transcriptome of adult *N. americanus* [51]. Among them were the mitochondrial-associated proteins identified known to be essential in *C. elegans* [66]. Accordingly, the information might provide a path for the discovery of compounds that target mitochondrial proteins in parasitic helminths [67].

To predict drug targets in *O. dentatum*, Cantacessi *et al.* [48] employed 454 sequencing and predictive algorithms to compare and contrast the transcriptomes of L3, fourth-stage larva (L4), and adult males and females [48]. Between 27 and 32% of the transcripts that encoded protein kinases and phosphatases were shared between the stages [48]. Recent studies have predicted that some phosphatases and kinases may represent nematocidal drug targets [68, 69]. The recent development of cantharidin and norcatharidin analogs [70, 71], as potent and selective inhibitors of PP1 and PP2A phosphatases, could be further explored to selectively inhibit essential serine/threonine phosphatase of parasitic nematodes [69].

Various molecules have also been proposed to play immunomodulatory roles in parasitic nematodes [72]. For example, proteins containing a "sperm-coating protein (SCP)-like extracellular domain" (InterPro: IPR014044), also called SCP/Tpx-1/Ag5/PR-1/Sc7 (SCP/TAPS; Pfam accession number no. PF00188) or *Ancylostoma*-secreted proteins (ASPs) [72], are well represented in the transcriptomes of *T. colubriformis*, *H. contortus*, *N. americanus*, and *O. dentatum* [48–51]. Due to their abundance in the excretory/secretory products of *A. caninum* serum-activated L3 (aL3) and their high transcriptional levels in *A. caninum* aL3 compared to non-activated ensheathed L3, ASPs might facilitate the transition from the free-living to the parasitic state [59, 73]. ASP homologs have been characterized in adult hookworms, and may assist in the initiation, establishment, and/or maintenance of the host–parasite relationship [59, 74, 75]. Being immunogenic, the *N. americanus* ASP (*Na*-ASP-2) is under investigation as a vaccine candidate against necatoriasis in humans [14, 76, 77].

Conclusions and Prospects

Knowing how genes are transcribed in the developmental stages of a given parasite will aid our understanding of the molecular mechanisms that govern essential biological processes and, ultimately, will identify new intervention strategies. Accurate bioinformatic analyses of transcriptomic and genomic data are crucial to providing meaningful biological information for parasitic nematodes. Until recently, detailed bioinformatics have been restricted largely to specialized laboratories with substantial computer and software capacities. The introduction of integrated bioinformatic systems such as Bio-cloud (cloud.genomics.cn) for the *de novo* assembly and annotation of sequence data could represent a turning point for transcriptomic and genomic research.

Recent transcriptomic studies have employed 454 sequencing of normalized cDNA libraries (e.g., [48–51]). Although the normalization process allows transcripts to be studied qualitatively, it does not allow quantitative differential profiling of gene expression. Future studies involving the sequencing of non-normalized cDNA libraries using Illumina technology [19] should address this aspect. However, the assembly and annotation of such short-read datasets will inevitably pose computational challenges to reliably predict alternatively spliced transcripts. In the absence of genomic sequence data, the combined use of the Illumina and 454 sequencing platforms should enable improved *de novo* assemblies of transcriptomic data through the of mapping short-read data to large scaffolds.

For added context, comparative analyses using the data held in public databases (e.g., [43–46]) will be necessary. Accurate annotation, particularly in the absence of a reference genome sequence, depends on routine software updates and dataset curation, as is the case with quality databases [46]. At present, however, the open-source programs and databases employed for bioinformatics of sequence data of parasitic nematodes are available through multiple portals, and this requires significant effort to maintain accurate and up-to-date assembly and annotation pipelines [78]. In addition, the rate at which public databases are updated and corrected differs considerably [79]. As a solution, the analyses and annotation of large-scale transcriptomic sequence datasets for parasitic nematodes could be facilitated through a centralized reference web site. Such a web site could provide regular releases of newly developed and validated bioinformatic pipelines. It could also provide links to (i) databases that are regularly updated and routinely employed to annotate new sequences, and (ii) a distinct, high-quality database of curated functional annotations, supported by experimental data from the peer-reviewed literature. In the future, the establishment of a consortium that shares and optimizes bioinformatic pipelines, and allows access to new sequence data, experimental protocols, and literature would be very useful.

The annotation of peptides inferred from the datasets analyzed [48–51] is usually performed by predicting biological function(s) employing the information available in public databases (e.g., WormBase, www.wormbase.org; InterPro, www.ebi.ac.uk/interpro/; Gene Ontology, www.geneontology.org; OrthoMCL, www.orthomcl.org; and BRENDA, www.brenda-enzymes.org). However, these predictions require experimental testing in either the parasites concerned and/or in a suitable surrogate organism. RNA interference (RNAi) has been tested in a number of parasitic nematodes of animals (orders Strongylida, Ascaridida, and Spirurida [80, 81]), but success has been relatively limited (see Chapter 6 for RNAi in parasitic nematodes). The indications are that a number of nematodes, including *H. contortus* and *B. malayi*, lack critical components of the RNAi machinery [80, 82]. Alternative transgenesis and gene complementation studies have shown some promise for evaluating gene function in parasitic nematodes [83, 84].

Comparative genomic analyses have been used to predict possible anthelmintic targets [85–87]. The approach involves "filtering" [88], and usually includes the inference of targets based on key principles and requirements [88]. First, target proteins should be essential to the parasite, such that the disruption of the protein will damage and/or kill the parasite. In the absence of functional data for most parasitic nematodes of animals, essentiality is inferred using extant information from *C. elegans*, *D. melanogaster*, *M. musculus*, and/or *S. cerevisiae* [48, 51, 85]. Also, candidate targets should be unique to the parasite or, at least, show significant differences in sequence and structure from host homologs, in order to avoid potential toxicity arising from chemical cross-reactivity between the parasite target host orthologs [89]. Finally, as drugs achieve activity by competing with endogenous small molecules for binding sites on the target protein [90], genes predicted to be essential should be screened for the presence of conserved ligand-binding domains [90, 91]. Using these filters, approximately 50% of the targets predicted for both *O. dentatum* [48] and *N. americanus* [51] were proteins belonging to the same categories, including zinc metalloproteases, aminopeptidases, guanosine triphosphatases, protein tyrosine kinases, as well as serine/threonine protein phosphatases and kinases [48, 51].

In the future, improved prediction and prioritization of potential drug targets in parasitic nematodes will depend on the availability of complete genome sequences. Repertoires of drug targets can then be inferred on a global scale. In addition, the successful integration of genomics, transcriptomics, and proteomics will assist the identification of potential drug targets. Clearly, NGS provides the efficiency and depth of coverage necessary to rapidly define the complete genomes of eukaryotic pathogens of socioeconomic importance. The transcriptomes for a number of parasitic nematodes are now available through www.ncbi.nlm.nih.gov and http://www.gasserlab.org, and these should be invaluable for the future assembly and annotation of the respective genomes.

Acknowledgments

Research in the Gasser Lab (http://www.gasserlab.org) is supported by grants from the Australian Research Council, Australian Academy of Science, Australian–American Fulbright Commission, National Health and Medical Research Council, and Melbourne Water Corporation. Other support from the Victorian Life Sciences

Computation Initiative, and its Peak Computing Facility at The University of Melbourne, and the IBM Research Collaboratory for Life Sciences – Melbourne is gratefully acknowledged.

References

1 de Silva, N.R., Brooker, S., Hotez, P.J., Montresor, A., Engels, D., and Savioli, L. (2003) Soil-transmitted helminth infections: updating the global picture. *Trends Parasitol.*, **19**, 547–551.

2 Bethony, J., Brooker, S., Albonico, M., Geiger, S.M., Loukas, A., Diemert, D., and Hotez, P.J. (2006) Soil-transmitted helminth infections: ascariasis, trichuriasis, and hookworm. *Lancet*, **367**, 1521–1532.

3 Nikolaou, S. and Gasser, R.B. (2006) Prospects for exploring molecular developmental processes in *Haemonchus contortus*. *Int. J. Parasitol.*, **36**, 859–868.

4 Harhay, M.O., Horton, J., and Olliaro, P.L. (2010) Epidemiology and control of human gastrointestinal parasites in children. *Expert Rev. Anti Infect. Ther.*, **8**, 219–234.

5 Hotez, P.J., Fenwick, A., Savioli, L., and Molyneux, D.H. (2009) Rescuing the bottom billion through control of neglected tropical diseases. *Lancet*, **373**, 1570–1575.

6 Sutherland, I. and Scott, I. (2010) *Gastrointestinal Nematodes of Sheep and Cattle: Biology and Control*, Wiley-Blackwell, Chichester.

7 Wolstenholme, A.J., Fairweather, I., Prichard, R., von Samson-Himmelstjerna, G., and Sangster, N.C. (2004) Drug resistance in veterinary helminths. *Trends Parasitol.*, **20**, 469–476.

8 Skrjabin, K.I., Sobolev, A.A., and Ivashkin, V.M. (1967) *Principles of Nematology*. Izdatel'sto Akademii Nauk SSSR/Israel Program for Scientific Translations, Washington, DC.

9 Blaxter, M.L., De Ley, P., Garey, J.R., Liu, L.X., Scheldeman, P., Vierstraete, A., Vanfleteren, J.R. *et al.* (1998) A molecular evolutionary framework for the phylum Nematoda. *Nature*, **392**, 71–75.

10 Knox, D.P. (2000) Development of vaccines against gastrointestinal nematodes. *Parasitology*, **120**, S43–S61.

11 Crompton, D.W. (2001) *Ascaris* and ascariasis. *Adv. Parasitol.*, **48**, 285–375.

12 Maizels, R.M. and Yazdanbakhsh, M. (2003) Immune regulation by helminth parasites: cellular and molecular mechanisms. *Nat. Rev. Immunol.*, **3**, 733–744.

13 Hotez, P.J., Brooker, S., Bethony, J., Bottazzi, M.E., Loukas, A., and Xiao, S. (2004) Hookworm infection. *N. Engl. J. Med.*, **351**, 799–807.

14 Loukas, A., Bethony, J., Brooker, S., and Hotez, P. (2006) Hookworm vaccines: past, present, and future. *Lancet Infect. Dis.*, **6**, 733–741.

15 Holden-Dye, L. and Walker, R.J. (2007) Anthelmintic drugs, in *WormBook* (ed. The *C. elegans* Research Community), doi: 10.1895/wormbook.1.143.1.

16 Pearson, M.S., Ranjit, N., and Loukas, A. (2010) Blunting the knife: development of vaccines targeting digestive proteases of blood-feeding helminth parasites. *Biol. Chem.*, **391**, 901–911.

17 Keiser, J. and Utzinger, J. (2010) The drugs we have and the drugs we need against major helminth infections. *Adv. Parasitol.*, **73**, 197–230.

18 Margulies, M., Egholm, M., Altman, W.E., Attlya, S., Bader, J.S., Bemben, L.A., Berka, J. *et al.* (2005) Genome sequencing in microfabricated high-density picolitre reactors. *Nature*, **437**, 376–380.

19 Bentley, D.R., Balasubramanian, S., Swerdlow, H.P., Smith, H.P., Smith, G.P., Milton, J., Brown, C.G. *et al.* (2008) Accurate whole human genome sequencing using reversible terminator chemistry. *Nature*, **456**, 53–59.

20 Harris, T.D., Buzby, P.R., Babcock, H., Beer, E., Bowers, J., Braslavsky, I., Causey, M. *et al.* (2008) Single-molecule

DNA sequencing of a viral genome. *Science*, **320**, 106–109.
21. Pandey, V., Nutter, R.C., and Prediger, E. (2008) Applied Biosystems SOLiD™ system: ligation-based sequencing, in *Next Generation Genome Sequencing: Towards Personalized Medicine* (ed. J.M. Milton), Wiley-VCH Verlag GmbH, Weinheim, pp. 29–41.
22. Adams, M.D., Kelley, J.M., Gocayne, J.D., Dubnick, M., Polymeropoulos, M.H., Xiao, H., Merril, C.R. *et al.* (1991) Complementary DNA sequencing: expressed sequence tags and human genome project. *Science*, **252**, 1651–1656.
23. Nagaraj, S.H., Gasser, R.B., and Ranganathan, S. (2007) A hitchhiker's guide to expressed sequence tag (EST) analysis. *Brief. Bioinfomatics*, **8**, 6–21.
24. Parkinson, J. and Blaxter, M. (2009) Expressed sequence tags: an overview. *Methods Mol. Biol.*, **533**, 1–12.
25. Huang, X. and Madan, A. (1999) CAP3: a DNA sequence assembly program. *Genome Res.*, **9**, 868–877.
26. Conesa, A., Gotz, S., Garcia-Gomez, J.M., Terol, J., Talon, M., Talón, M., and Robles, M. (2005) Blast2GO: a universal tool for annotation, visualization and analysis in functional genomics research. *Bioinformatics*, **21**, 3674–3676.
27. Nagaraj, S.H., Deshpande, N., Gasser, R.B., and Ranganathan, S. (2007) ESTExplorer: an expressed sequence tag (EST) assembly and annotation platform. *Nucleic Acids Res.*, **35**, W135–W147.
28. Soderlund, C., Johnson, E., Bomhoff, M., and Descour, A. (2009) PAVE: program for assembling and viewing ESTs. *BMC Genomics*, **10**, 400.
29. Falgueras, J., Lara, A.J., Fernandez-Poso, N., Canton, F.R., Perez-Trabado, G., and Claros, M. (2010) SeqTrim: a high throughput pipeline for pre-processing any type of sequence read. *BMC Bioinformatics*, **11**, 38.
30. Myers, E.W. (1995) Toward simplifying and accurately formulating fragment assembly. *J. Comput. Biol.*, **2**, 275–290.
31. Zerbino, D.R. and Birney, E. (2008) Velvet: algorithms for *de novo* short read assembly using de Bruijn graphs. *Genome Res.*, **18**, 821–829.
32. Scheibye-Alsing, K., Hoffmann, S., Frankel, A., Jensen, P., Stadler, P.F., Mang, Y., Tommerup, N. *et al.* (2009) Sequence assembly. *Comput. Biol. Chem.*, **33**, 121–136.
33. Miller, J.R., Koren, S., and Sutton, G. (2010) Assembly algorithms for next-generation sequencing data. *Genomics*, **95**, 315–327.
34. Li, R., Li, Y., Kristiansen, K., and Wang, J. (2008) SOAP: short oligonucleotide alignment program. *Bioinformatics*, **24**, 713–714.
35. Altschul, S.F., Gish, W., Miller, W., Myers, E.W., and Lipman, D.J. (1990) Basic local alignment search tool. *J. Mol. Biol.*, **215**, 403–410.
36. Iseli, C., Jongeneel, C.V., and Bucher, P. (1999) ESTScan: a program for detecting, evaluating, and reconstructing potential coding regions in EST sequences. *Proc. Int. Conf. Intell. Syst. Mol. Biol.*, **1**, 138–148.
37. Min, X.J., Butler, G., Storms, R., and Tsang, A. (2005) OrfPredictor: predicting protein-coding regions in EST-derived sequences. *Nucleic Acids Res.*, **33**, W677–W680.
38. Ashburner, M., Ball, C.A., Blake, J.A., Botstein, D., Butler, H. *et al.* (2000) Gene ontology: tool for the unification of biology. The Gene Ontology Consortium. *Nat. Genet.*, **25**, 25–29.
39. Bateman, A., Birney, E., Durbin, R., Eddy, S.R., Howe, K.L., and Sonnhammer, E.L. (2000) The Pfam protein families database. *Nucleic Acids Res.*, **28**, 263–266.
40. Hunter, S., Apweiler, R., Attwood, T.K., Bairoch, A., Bateman, A., Binns, D., Bork, P. *et al.* (2009) InterPro: the integrative protein signature database. *Nucleic Acids Res.*, **37**, D211–D215.
41. Wheeler, D.L., Church, D.M., Lash, A.E., Leipe, D.D., and Madden, T.L. (2001) Database resources of the National Center for Biotechnology Information. *Nucleic Acids Res.*, **29**, 11–16.
42. Shumway, M., Cochrane, G., and Sugawara, H. (2010) Archiving next generation sequencing data. *Nucleic Acids Res.*, **38**, D870–D871.
43. Cherry, J.M., Ball, C., Weng, S., Juvic, G., Schmidt, R., Adler, C., Dunn, B. *et al.*

(1997) Genetic and physical maps of *Saccharomyces cerevisiae*. *Nature*, **387**, 67–73.

44 Tweedie, S., Ashburner, M., Falls, K., Leyland, P., McQuilton, P., Marygold, S., Millburn, G. *et al.* (2009) FlyBase: enhancing *Drosophila* Gene Ontology annotations. *Nucleic Acids Res.*, **37**, D555–D559.

45 Bult, C.J., Epping, J.T., Kadin, J.A., Richardson, J.E., Blake, J.A., and Eppig, J.T. and Mouse Genome Database Group. (2008) The mouse genome database (MGD): mouse biology and model systems. *Nucleic Acids Res.*, **36**, D724–D728.

46 Harris, T.W., Antoshechkin, I., Bieri, T., Blasiar, D., Chan, J., Chen, W.J., De La Cruz, N. *et al.* (2010) WormBase: a comprehensive resource for nematode research. *Nucleic Acids Res.*, **38**, D463–D467.

47 Nagaraj, S.H., Gasser, R.B., Nisbet, A.J., and Ranganathan, S. (2008) In silico analysis of expressed sequence tags from *Trichostrongylus vitrinus* (Nematoda): comparison of the automated ESTExplorer workflow platform with conventional database searches. *BMC Bioinformatics*, **9**, S10.

48 Cantacessi, C., Jex, A.R., Hall, R.S., Young, N.D., Campbell, B.E., Joachim, A., Nolan, M.J. *et al.* (2010) A practical, bioinformatic workflow system for large data sets generated by next-generation sequencing. *Nucleic Acids Res.*, **38**, e171.

49 Cantacessi, C., Mitreva, M., Campbell, B.E., Hall, R.S., Young, N.D., Jex, A.R., Ranganathan, S., and Gasser, R.B. (2010) First transcriptomic analysis of the economically important parasitic nematode, *Trichostrongylus colubriformis*, using a next-generation sequencing approach. *Infect. Genet. Evol.*, **10**, 1199–1207.

50 Cantacessi, C., Campbell, B.E., Young, N.D., Jex, A.R., Hall, R.S., Presidente, P.J., Zawadzki, J.L. *et al.* (2010) Differences in transcription between free-living CO_2-activated third-stage larvae of *Haemonchus contortus*. *BMC Genomics*, **11**, 266.

51 Cantacessi, C., Mitreva, M., Jex, A.R., Young, N.D., Campbell, B.E., Hall, R.S., Doyle, M.A. *et al.* (2010) Massively parallel sequencing and analysis of the *Necator americanus* transcriptome. *PLoS Negl. Trop. Dis.*, **4**, e684.

52 Björnberg, F., Lantz, M., and Gullberg, U. (1995) Metalloproteases and serineproteases are involved in the cleavage of the two tumour necrosis factor (TNF) receptors to soluble forms in the myeloid cell lines U-937 and THP-1. *Scand. J. Immunol.*, **42**, 418–424.

53 Shaw, R.J., McNeill, M.M., Maass, D.R., Hein, W.R., Barber, T.K., Wheeler, M., Morris, C.A., and Shoemaker, C.B. (2003) Identification and characterisation of an aspartyl protease inhibitor homologue as a major allergen of *Trichostrongylus colubriformis*. *Int. J. Parasitol.*, **33**, 1233–1243.

54 Williamson, A.L., Brindley, P.J., Knox, D.P., Hotez, P.J., and Loukas, A. (2003) Digestive proteases of blood-feeding nematodes. *Trends Parasitol.*, **19**, 417–423.

55 Fetterer, R.H. (1996) Growth and cuticular synthesis in *Ascaris suum* larvae during development from third to fourth stage *in vitro*. *Vet. Parasitol.*, **65**, 275–282.

56 Pratt, D., Cox, G.N., Milhausen, M.J., and Boisvenue, R.J. (1990) A developmentally regulated cysteine protease gene family in *Haemonchus contortus*. *Mol. Biochem. Parasitol.*, **43**, 181–191.

57 Williamson, A.L., Lecchi, P., Turk, B.E., Choe, Y., Hotez, P.J., McKerrow, J.H., Cantley, L.C. *et al.* (2004) A multi-enzyme cascade of hemoglobin proteolysis in the intestine of blood-feeding hookworms. *J. Biol. Chem.*, **279**, 35950–35957.

58 Ranjit, N., Zhan, B., Hamilton, B., Stenzel, D., Lowther, J., Pearson, M., Gorman, J., Hotez, P., and Loukas, A. (2009) Proteolytic degradation of hemoglobin in the intestine of the human hookworm *Necator americanus*. *J. Infect. Dis.*, **199**, 904–912.

59 Datu, B.J., Gasser, R.B., Nagaraj, S.H., Ong, E.K., O'Donoghue, P., McInnes, R., Ranganathan, S., and Loukas, A. (2008) Transcriptional changes in the hookworm, *Ancylostoma caninum,* during the

transition from a free-living to a parasitic larva. *PLoS Negl. Trop. Dis.*, **2**, e130.

60 Cantacessi, C., Loukas, A., Campbell, B.E., Mulvenna, J., Ong, E.K., Zhong, W., Sternberg, P.W. *et al.* (2009) Exploring transcriptional conservation between *Ancylostoma caninum* and *Haemonchus contortus* by oligonucleotide microarray and bioinformatic analyses. *Mol. Cell. Probes*, **23**, 1–9.

61 Moser, J.M., Freitas, T., Arasu, P., and Gibson, G. (2005) Gene expression profiles associated with the transition to parasitism in *Ancylostoma caninum* larvae. *Mol. Biochem. Parasitol.*, **143**, 39–48.

62 Mitreva, M., McCarter, J.P., Arasu, P., Hawdon, J., Martin, J., Dante, M., Wylie, T. *et al.* (2005) Investigating hookworm genomes by comparative analysis of two *Ancylostoma* species. *BMC Genomics*, **26**, 58.

63 Abubucker, S., Martin, J., Yin, Y., Fulton, L., Yang, S.P., Hallsworth-Pepin, K., Johnston, J.S. *et al.* (2008) The canine hookworm genome: analysis and classification of *Ancylostoma caninum* survey sequences. *Mol. Biochem. Parasitol.*, **157**, 187–192.

64 Furmidge, B.A., Horn, L.A., and Pritchard, D.I. (1996) The anti-haemostatic strategies of the human hookworm *Necator americanus*. *Parasitology*, **112**, 81–87.

65 Milstone, A.M., Harrison, L.M., Bungiro, R.D., Kuzmic, P., and Cappello, M. (2000) A broad spectrum Kunitz type serine protease inhibitor secreted by the hookworm *Ancylostoma ceylanicum*. *J. Biol. Chem.*, **275**, 29391–29399.

66 Grad, L.I., Sayles, L.C., and Lemire, B.D. (2007) Isolation and functional analysis of mitochondria from the nematode *Caenorhabditis elegans*. *Methods Mol. Biol.*, **372**, 51–66.

67 Hu, M., Zhong, W., Campbell, B.E., Sternberg, P.W., Pellegrino, M.W., and Gasser, R.B. (2010) Elucidating ANTs in worms using genomic and bioinformatic tools – biotechnological prospects? *Biotechnol. Adv.*, **28**, 49–60.

68 Campbell, B.E., Boag, P.R., Hofmann, A., Cantacessi, C., Wang, C.K., Taylor, P., Hu, M., Sindhu, Z., Loukas, A., Sternberg, P.W., and Gasser, R.B. (2011) Atypical (RIO) protein kinases from *Haemonchus contortus* – promise as new targets for nematocidal drugs. *Biotechnol. Adv.*, **29**, 338–350.

69 Campbell, B.E., Hofmann, A., McCluskey, A., and Gasser, R.B. (2011) Serine/threonine phosphatases in socioeconomically important parasitic nematodes – prospects as novel drug targets? *Biotechnol. Adv.*, **29**, 28–39.

70 McCluskey, A., Keane, M.A., Walkom, C.C., Bowyer, M.C., Sim, A.T.R., Young, D.J., and Sakoff, J.A. (2002) The first two cantharidin analogues displaying PP1 selectivity. *Bioorg. Med. Chem. Lett.*, **12**, 391–393.

71 Hill, T.A., Stewart, S.G., Sauer, B., Gilbert, J., Ackland, S.P., Sakoff, J.A., and McCluskey, A. (2007) Heterocyclic substituted cantharidin and norcantharidin analogues – synthesis, protein phosphatase (1 and 2A) inhibition, and anti-cancer activity. *Bioorg. Med. Chem. Lett.*, **17**, 3392–3397.

72 Cantacessi, C., Campbell, B.E., Visser, A., Geldhof, P., Nolan, M.J., Nisbet, A.J., Matthews, J.B. *et al.* (2009) A portrait of the "SCP/TAPS" proteins of eukaryotes – developing a framework for fundamental research and biotechnological outcomes. *Biotechnol. Adv.*, **27**, 376–388.

73 Hawdon, J.M., Jones, B.F., Hoffman, D.R., and Hotez, P.J. (1996) Cloning and characterization of *Ancylostoma*-secreted protein. A novel protein associated with the transition to parasitism by infective hookworm larvae. *J. Biol. Chem.*, **271**, 6672–6678.

74 Zhan, B., Liu, Y., Badamchian, M., Williamson, A., Feng, J., Loukas, A., Hawdon, J.M., and Hotez, P.J. (2003) Molecular characterisation of the *Ancylostoma*-secreted protein family from the adult stage of *Ancylostoma caninum*. *Int. J. Parasitol.*, **33**, 897–907.

75 Mulvenna, J., Hamilton, B., Nagaraj, S., Smyth, D., Loukas, A., and Gorman, J. (2009) Proteomic analysis of the excretory/secretory component of the blood-feeding stage of the hookworm, *Ancylostoma caninum*. *Mol. Cell. Proteomics*, **8**, 109–121.

76 Mendez, S., D'Samuel, A., Antoine, A.D., Ahn, S., and Hotez, P. (2008) Use of the air pouch model to investigate immune responses to a hookworm vaccine containing the Na-ASP-2 protein in rats. *Parasite Immunol.*, **30**, 53–56.

77 Xiao, S., Zhan, B., Xue, J., Goud, G.N., Loukas, A., Liu, Y., Williamson, A. *et al.* (2008) The evaluation of recombinant hookworm antigens as vaccines in hamsters (*Mesocricetus auratus*) challenged with human hookworm, *Necator americanus*. *Exp. Parasitol.*, **118**, 32–40.

78 Coassin, S., Brandstatter, A., and Kronenberg, F. (2010) Lost in the space of bioinformatic tools: a constantly updated survival guide for genetic epidemiology. The GenEpi Toolbox. *Atherosclerosis*, **209**, 321–335.

79 Karp, P.D. (1998) What we do not know about sequence analysis and sequence databases. *Bioinformatics*, **14**, 753–754.

80 Geldhof, P., Visser, A., Clark, D., Saunders, G., Britton, C., Gilleard, J., Berriman, M., and Knox, D. (2007) RNA interference in parasitic helminths: current situation, potential pitfalls and future prospects. *Parasitology*, **134**, 609–619.

81 Samarasinghe, B., Knox, D.P., and Britton, C. (2011) Factors affecting susceptibility to RNA interference in *Haemonchus contortus* and *in vivo* silencing of an H11 aminopeptidase gene. *Int. J. Parasitol.*, **41**, 51–59.

82 Viney, M.E. and Thompson, F.J. (2008) Two hypotheses to explain why RNA interference does not work in animal parasitic nematodes. *Int. J. Parasitol.*, **38**, 43–47.

83 Hu, M., Lok, J.B., Ranjit, N., Massey, H.C. Jr, Sternberg, P.W., and Gasser, R.B. (2010) Structural and functional characterisation of the fork head transcription factor-encoding gene, *Hc-daf-16*, from the parasitic nematode *Haemonchus contortus* (Strongylida). *Int. J. Parasitol.*, **40**, 405–415.

84 Stepek, G., McCormack, G., and Page, A.P. (2010) Collagen processing and cuticle formation is catalysed by the astacin metalloprotease DPY-31 in free-living and parasitic nematodes. *Int. J. Parasitol.*, **40**, 533–542.

85 Doyle, M.A., Gasser, R.B., Woodcroft, B.J., Hall, R.S., and Ralph, S.A. (2010) Drug target prediction and prioritization: using orthology to predict essentiality in parasite genomes. *BMC Genomics*, **11**, 222.

86 Krasky, A., Rohwer, A., Schroeder, J., and Selzer, P.M. (2007) A combined bioinformatics and chemoinformatics approach for the development of new antiparasitic drugs. *Genomics*, **89**, 36–43.

87 Caffrey, C.R., Rohwer, A., Oellien, F., Marhofer, R.J., Braschi, S., Oliveira, G., McKerrow, J.H., and Selzer, P.M. (2009) A comparative chemogenomics strategy to predict potential drug targets in the metazoan pathogen, *Schistosoma mansoni*. *PLoS One*, **4**, e4413.

88 McCarter, J.P. (2004) Genomic filtering: an approach to discovering novel antiparasitics. *Trends Parasitol.*, **20**, 462–468.

89 Seib, K.L., Dougan, G., and Rappuoli, R. (2009) The key role of genomics in modern vaccine and drug design for emerging infectious diseases. *PLoS Genet.*, **5**, e1000612.

90 Hopkins, A.L. and Groom, C.R. (2002) The druggable genome. *Nature*, **1**, 727–730.

91 Chang, A., Scheer, M., Grote, A., Schomburg, I., and Schomburg, D. (2009) BRENDA, AMENDA and FRENDA the enzyme information system: new content and tools in 2009. *Nucleic Acids Res.*, **37**, D588–D592.

5
Harnessing Genomic Technologies to Explore the Molecular Biology of Liver Flukes-Major Implications for Fundamental and Applied Research

Neil D. Young*, Aaron R. Jex, Cinzia Cantacessi, Bronwyn E. Campbell, and Robin B. Gasser

Abstract

Liver flukes are socioeconomically important flatworms (Trematoda: Digenea) which parasitize the hepatobiliary systems of definitive mammalian hosts, including humans. Key representatives include *Opisthorchis viverrini*, *Clonorchis sinensis* (Opisthorchiidae), and *Fasciola gigantica* and *Fasciola hepatica* (Fasciolidae). Collectively, these parasites affect the health of tens of millions of humans and other animals throughout the world. *F. hepatica* and *F. gigantica* cause fascioliasis (= disease), leading to major production losses in livestock (mainly sheep and cattle) as a result of reduced weight gain and milk production, and mortality. Both fasciolids and opisthorchiids are important food-borne parasites in parts of the Middle East, Asia, and South America. In addition, *O. viverrini* and *C. sinensis* are carcinogenic parasites and can induce malignant cancer (cholangiocarcinoma) in chronically infected people. In spite of their impact, very little is known about liver flukes on an immunomolecular level, particularly their interplay with their mammalian hosts. Advances in "omics" technologies provide new opportunities for profound insights into the molecular biology, biochemistry, and physiology of these parasites as well as the diseases that they cause. Here, we review recent progress in the transcriptomics of liver flukes using high-throughput sequencing and bioinformatic technologies. We emphasize the unique prospects that transcriptomics provide for future explorations of the biology of these flukes and the development of new interventions.

Introduction

Liver flukes are food-borne parasitic flatworms (Trematoda: Digenea) of animals and humans, causing diseases that have broad adverse social and economic consequences, ranging from production losses in livestock [1–5] to chronic syndromes [6] and secondary complications, such as cancer in humans [7, 8]. As food-borne, zoonotic parasites, liver flukes are a serious public health problem in many parts of the Americas, Asia, Africa, and Europe [9–12], and cause some of the most neglected tropical diseases worldwide [13].

---

* Corresponding Author

Parasitic Helminths: Targets, Screens, Drugs and Vaccines, First Edition. Edited by Conor R. Caffrey
© 2012 Wiley-VCH Verlag GmbH & Co. KGaA. Published 2012 by Wiley-VCH Verlag GmbH & Co. KGaA.

Liver flukes are a diverse group of parasites and include members of the families Fasciolidae, Opisthorchiidae, and Dicrocoeliidae (Table 5.1). At the adult stage, they live in the hepatobiliary system of a definitive host. These flukes are dorsoventrally flattened, bilaterally symmetrical, hermaphroditic parasites with a typical digenean (indirect) life cycle, involving one or more invertebrate intermediate hosts, the first of which is a gastropod snail [5, 12, 14, 15]. There is significant variation among the life cycles of different species, which is reflected in major differences in their ecology and epidemiology. For instance, *Opisthorchis viverrini* and *Clonorchis sinensis* encyst in the tissues of freshwater fish (second intermediate host; Figure 5.1a), increasing the chances of being ingested by piscivorous animals, including humans, canids and felids [12, 15]. In contrast, the cercariae of fasciolid liver flukes, such as *Fasciola gigantica* and *Fasciola hepatica*, usually encyst directly as metacercariae on aquatic plants (Figure 5.1b), increasing the likelihood of being ingested by plant-eating animals, such as ruminants and humans [14, 16]. Once metacercariae have been ingested by the definitive host, the manifestation of disease relates to the species of parasite, the migration route taken by the developing parasite, the number of infective stages ingested, and also the immune response of the host. For example, fascioliasis is characterized by two phases. (i) The *acute* phase is associated with tissue damage caused by the migration of immature worms through the duodenal wall, peritoneum, and, then, the liver capsule and parenchyma (= traumatic hepatitis) [6, 17]. Associated clinical signs can include colic (abdominal pain), fever, anemia, hepatomegaly, diarrhea, and weight loss [17]. (ii) The *chronic* phase commences when juvenile flukes transmigrate from the liver parenchyma to and establish in the biliary ducts, and is characterized by progressive cholangitis, hyperplasia of the duct epithelium, and periductal fibrosis, which can result in cholestatic hepatitis, jaundice, diarrhea, ascites and/or edema (including "bottle jaw") [6, 17]. In contrast to fasciolids, the opisthorchiid flukes, *O. viverrini* and *C. sinensis*, are less destructive as the immature flukes do not undergo migration through tissues to cause traumatic hepatitis. Instead, following metacercarial excystation in the small intestine, the immature flukes migrate via the ampulla of Vater into the biliary ductal system and/or sometimes the pancreatic ducts, and establish as adults [12, 15]. Disease is mainly associated with chronic infections with relatively large numbers of parasites, leading to cholangitis, periductal fibrosis and/or cirrhosis [7]. Moreover, chronic opisthorchiasis/clonorchiasis in humans can lead to cholangiocarcinoma (CCA) in a significant proportion of patients in endemic regions [7, 8, 12]. For this reason, *O. viverrini* and *C. sinensis* are now recognized as carcinogens [18]. Chronic clonorchiasis/opisthorchiasis can predispose patients to CCA through an enhanced susceptibility to DNA damage, and is proposed to be associated with factors such as mechanical damage to the hepatobiliary system, inflammation, periductal fibrosis, and/or cellular responses to antigens from the infecting fluke [7].

Although efforts continue to develop anti-fluke vaccines (see Chapters 25–28), current control relies mainly on drugs, including triclabendazole (for fascioliasis) [19, 20] and praziquantel (for clonorchiasis/opisthorchiasis) [7, 12]. The excessive and widespread use of monotherapies comes with a risk that worm populations will

Table 5.1 Selected liver flukes of socioeconomic importance, and common clinical signs and pathological changes associated with infections/disease.

Family/species	Common clinical signs reported	Pathological changes	Geographical regions known to be affected (climatic zone)	References
Opisthorchiidae				
Clonorchis sinensis	abdominal pain, diarrhea, loss of appetite, indigestion	biliary occlusion, epithelial fibrosis of the biliary duct, cholangitis, cholelithiasis, cholangiocarcinoma	Asia (tropical/subtropical)	[12]
Opisthorchis viverrini	abdominal pain, weakness or malaise, flatulence, dyspepsia	biliary occlusion, fibrosis of the biliary tract, cholangitis, cholelithiasis, cholangiocarcinoma	Asia (tropical)	[95, 96]
Opisthorchis felineus	abdominal pain, fever, nausea, myalgia	biliary obstruction, fibrosis of the biliary tract, cholangitis	Europe/Asia (subtropical/temperate)	[97]
Metorchis conjunctus	abdominal pain, low-grade fever	no pathology documented	North America (temperate)	[98]
Fasciolidae				
Fasciola hepatica	abdominal pain, hepatomegaly, fever, anemia, diarrhea, urticaria, eosinophilia	hepatic fibrosis, cholangitis, hyperplasia of the bile duct epithelium, fibrosis of the biliary tract, cholecystitis, biliary occlusion, cholestatic hepatitis and secondary bacterial infection	Europe/Asia/Africa/North America/South America/Australia (subtropical/temperate)	[99, 100]
Fasciola gigantica	abdominal pain, hepatomegaly, fever, anemia, gastrointestinal disturbances, urticaria	hepatic fibrosis, cholangitis, hyperplasia of the bile duct epithelium, fibrosis of the biliary tract, cholecystitis, biliary occlusion and cholestatic hepatitis	Asia/Africa/Middle East (subtropical/tropical)	[16]
Fascioloides magna	anorexia, lethargy, weight loss	fibrosis and hemorrhaging in the liver parenchyma, fibrosis associated with the encapsulation of worms in the liver parenchyma, fibrosis of the biliary tract	North America/Europe (temperate)	[101, 102]
Dicrocoeliidae				
Dicrocoelium dendriticum	emaciation, anemia, edema	fibrosis and distention of the biliary duct, biliary occlusion and cholangitis	Europe/Asia/Africa/North America (tropical/subtropical)	[5]

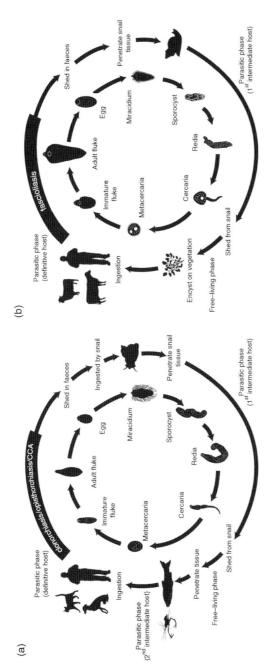

Figure 5.1 Life cycles of representative opisthorchiid and fasciolid liver flukes affecting animals and humans. (a) *O. viverrini* and *C. sinensis* (opisthorchiids) cause clonorchiasis and opisthorchiasis, respectively. Their life cycles begin with the infective metacercarial stage being ingested by a definitive mammalian host, such as a human, dog, or cat. The metacercaria undergoes excystation in the small intestine, releasing an immature fluke that passes through the ampulla of Vater and migrates and attaches to the extra- or intrahepatic bile duct wall. There, it matures as a hermaphroditic adult and produces eggs, which are released into the bile and pass, via the gall bladder and the bile duct, to the duodenum. From there, eggs pass with the feces into an aquatic environment. The eggs are ingested by an aquatic bithynid snail (Gastropoda; first intermediate host) and pass through the digestive tract of the snail where the miracidium hatches from the egg. The miracidium penetrates the intestinal wall and then transforms into a sporocyst from which rediae and cercariae propagate via polyembryony. The cercariae actively leave the snail and seek the second intermediate host, usually a freshwater cyprinid fish, or, in the case of *C. sinensis*, a freshwater fish and/or crustacean (shrimp) [93]. Cercariae penetrate the epidermis and encyst predominantly in the musculature of the second intermediate host. (b) *F. gigantica* and *F. hepatica* (fasciolids) are plant-borne pathogens that cause fascioliasis. Their life cycles begin when the definitive mammalian host ingests infective metacercariae encysted on plants, including watercress and legumes [94]. The metacercariae undergoes excystation, releasing a newly excysted juvenile, which penetrates the small intestinal wall and migrates to the peritoneal cavity. From there, the juvenile stage migrates through the liver capsule and parenchyma, after which it enters the bile ducts to become a sexually mature, hermaphroditic adult. Released eggs pass into the bile and, via the gall bladder and the bile duct, into the duodenum. From there, eggs pass with the feces into the environment. In a freshwater habitat, the miracidium hatches from the embryonated egg to infect a lymnaeid snail (Gastropoda), transforming into a sporocyst from which rediae and cercariae arise via polyembryony. The cercariae leave the snail and then swim to nearby vegetation where they then encyst and transform into metacercariae which are infective to the definitive host [61, 72].

develop resistance against the drug employed. Indeed, resistance to triclabendazole in *F. hepatica* of livestock has already been reported in Australia [21], Europe [22–25], and South America [26]. The search for new drugs to treat liver fluke infections has driven recent efforts to repurpose broad-spectrum anthelmintic (e.g., tribendimidine) or antimalaria (artemisinin) compounds [27–29], with some encouraging results [30, 31].

There is major potential for new drugs and/or vaccines to be developed, based on a profound understanding of the molecular biology of liver flukes themselves and their interplay with their mammalian hosts. Although the majority of molecular genetic and genomic investigations of trematodes has concentrated on blood flukes (schistosomes) of humans (i.e., *Schistosoma japonicum* and *Schistosoma mansoni*, e.g., [32–41]), genomic, transcriptomic, and proteomic resources for liver flukes have been limited [42–45]. However, recent advances in high-throughput sequencing and bioinformatic technologies [46–52] have provided an exciting platform for the rapid and detailed explorations of liver flukes. In the present chapter, we review recent progress in the transcriptomics of liver flukes of animal and human health importance using such technologies. We emphasize the unique prospects that this progress provides for future "omics" explorations, and the establishment of new intervention strategies to combat these flukes and the diseases that they cause.

Transcriptomic Studies of Liver Flukes Utilizing an Integrated High-Throughput Sequencing and Bioinformatic Platform

Recent "omics" investigations [53–59] have paved the way for the exploration of biological pathways in liver flukes. To provide the genomic infrastructure for future "omics" studies, our recent projects have employed Roche 454 or Illumina sequencing from cDNA libraries, and a semiautomated bioinformatic platform for the assembly and subsequent annotation of nonredundant transcriptomic datasets for *O. viverrini*, *C. sinensis*, *F. gigantica*, and *F. hepatica* [60–62] (Figure 5.2). Raw nucleotide sequences (from 500000 to more than 20 million reads per species) were assembled *de novo* and reclustered according to protein coding domains (Table 5.2). Usually redundancy was reduced by clustering sequences, if predicted proteins shared more than 95% amino acid sequence identity over 60% of their length. The interrogation of nucleotide and conceptually translated amino acid sequences using nonredundant (www.ensembl.org, http://schistodb.net/schistodb20, and http://life-center.sgst.cn/sjapathdb/data.html) [60–62] and other public (http://www.ncbi.nlm.nih.gov/est) databases identified orthologs in various eukaryotic organisms. Proteins were further annotated based on conservation in protein domains using the programs InterProScan [63], KOBAS [64], SignalP 3.0 [65], and TMHMM [66], and then classified according to gene ontology (GO), cellular location (intracellular, extracellular or transmembrane), and/or metabolic pathway mapping.

The results of these comparative analyses for *O. viverrini*, *C. sinensis*, *F. hepatica*, *F. gigantica*, *S. japonicum*, and *S. mansoni* indicate that the fasciolids and

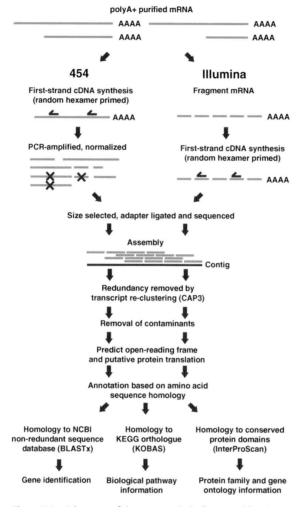

Figure 5.2 Schematic of the integrated platform used for the sequencing (using Roche 454 or Illumina technology) and bioinformatic annotation of the transcriptomes of selected liver flukes.

opisthorchiids share the highest level (29–31%) of protein sequence homology [60, 62]. Although approximately 90% of predicted proteins of liver flukes did not map to any known biological pathways, many proteins were associated with conserved cellular processing, genetic, and environmental information, and/or metabolic pathways [60–62]. This observation suggests that there are many presently unknown biological processes that are unique to these parasites and/or involved in specific parasite–host interactions. Interestingly, among liver flukes, the percentage of proteins with significantly greater homology to those of mammals (around 20%) than nematodes (around 15%) was in accordance with results for blood flukes [32, 33, 61, 62], and could reflect the ability of flukes to regulate immunological, biochemical, and/or molecular responses in their mammalian hosts [33, 67].

Table 5.2 Publicly available transcriptomic resources for liver flukes of socioeconomic importance.

	Opisthorchiidae		Fasciolidae	
	O. viverrini	C. sinensis	F. hepatica	F. gigantica
Raw sequence data				
NCBI EST/mRNA[a]	4194/15	2970/186	1677/161	8398/42
Roche 454 sequence data[b]	642918	574448	590927	NA
Illumina sequence data[b]	NA	NA	NA	21.9 million
Characterization of transcriptomic data[c]				
Coding domain GC content (%)	47.2 ± 4.1	47.5 ± 4.0	47.0 ± 14.1	46.0 ± 4.2
Contigs containing an open reading frame	61417	50769	44597	30513
Putative excretory/secretory proteins	1470	1143	1573	1543
InterPro conserved coding domains (sequences; InterPro terms)	11004; 4047	9564; 3932	9555; 3769	9326; 3535
GO terms predicted (sequences; GO terms)	7586; 1271	6580; 1250	6557; 1170	5183; 1124
KEGG biological pathway terms (sequences; terms)	5139; 249	4581; 242	4935; 241	4466; 225

NA, not applicable.
a) Data available from National Center for Biotechnology Information expressed sequence tag (EST) and nucleotide databases (www.ncbi.nlm.nih.gov; April, 2011).
b) Previously published sequence data for two fasciolid flukes, *F. gigantica* [62] and *F. hepatica* [61]; and two opisthorchiid flukes, *O. viverrini* and *C. sinensis* [60].
c) Summary of the adult transcriptome data, sequenced and assembled using the integrated sequencing platform described in Figure 5.2.

Exciting Prospects for "Omics" Research of Liver Flukes

Recent explorations give first insights into the transcriptomes of key fasciolid and opisthorchiid liver flukes [60–62]. Most sequences from these parasites are new, thus significantly expanding previous data and knowledge [42, 43, 45, 56, 57, 59], and providing a useful resource to molecular parasitologists investigating trematodes at the molecular and biochemical levels. The availability of these transcriptomes [60–62] provides a sound basis for exploring parasite development, reproduction, host–parasite interactions, and the pathogeneses of liver fluke diseases and associated complications, including biliary cancer [7, 42, 68, 69]. For example, parasite proteins, such as oncogene homologs and mitogens (e.g., granulin), are implicated in CCA induction and progression [53, 70, 71]. Human oncogene homologs in these parasites include: (i) Ras-related C3 botulinum toxin substrate 1 (RAC1), v-*raf* murine sarcoma viral oncogene homolog B1 (B-RAF), v-Ha-*ras* Harvey rat sarcoma viral oncogene GTPase (HRA), and growth factor receptor-binding protein 2 (GRB2) [72], the latter of which has been suggested to contribute to the development of *O. viverrini*-induced CCA [73]; and (ii) the cyclin-dependent kinase regulatory subunit CKS1. Clearly, these fluke proteins should be tested for their ability to induce uncontrolled proliferation of host cells *in vitro* and *in vivo* [69]. In addition, it would be very interesting to explore, in a comparative way, immunomolecular aspects of acute infections linked to the migration of juvenile flukes as well as the molecular mechanisms of bile duct epithelial hyperplasia and periductal fibrosis in animals with chronic disease.

Recent sequencing from cDNA libraries and the assembly of sequence datasets have yielded high-quality drafts of the transcriptomes of the adult stages of four liver flukes (*O. viverrini*, *C. sinensis*, *F. hepatica*, and *F. gigantica*) [60–62]. The assignment of predicted proteins to biological pathways and molecular functions has revealed major diversity, comparable with annotations inferred for *S. mansoni* [32]. Cysteine proteases, heat-shock proteins, and antioxidants are well represented in liver flukes [60–62]. Antioxidants appear to be involved in immune modulation in the mammalian host and are highly expressed throughout the life history of, for example, *F. hepatica* [59, 74]. These molecules include glutathione transferases, protein disulfide isomerase, peroxiredoxin, and thioredoxin, which are suggested to protect liver flukes from harmful reactive oxygen species (ROS) derived from the host [75, 76]. A protective function has also been reported for protein chaperones, such as heat-shock protein 70, which facilitates protein folding and appears to be induced by host immune responses against flukes [77]. Therefore, within their definitive host, adult liver flukes appear to express repertoires of molecules that protect cellular processes from ROS [78]. This protection is crucial, because juvenile flukes are susceptible to antibody-dependent cell-mediated cytotoxicity involving ROS [79].

The advances in transcriptomics of liver flukes will underpin future comparative "omics" studies. For example, short-read sequencing (Illumina), preferably in conjunction with proteomic and genomic analyses, could be used to quantitatively study transcription/expression profiles in key life cycle stages and distinct phenotypes. Although the transcriptomes of the adult stages of *O. viverrini*, *C. sinensis*, *F. gigantica*, and *F. hepatica* have been characterized, almost nothing is known about developmentally regulated transcription/gene expression in miracidia, sporocysts, rediae, cercariae, and juvenile stages of this parasite. Clearly, exploring transcription in all stages of these parasites should have important implications for understanding development, reproduction, parasite–host interactions, and disease at the molecular and biochemical levels. For such investigations, using short-read sequencing technology, it is possible that the abundance of related and, apparently, paralogous and/or alternatively spliced transcripts encoding some protein groups (e.g., cathepsins) could complicate assemblies from short-read data (even under stringent conditions) in the absence of a reference genome sequence. Combined assemblies and annotation of paired-end sequence data with medium to long sequences (e.g., 500–1000 nucleotides) generated using, for example, 454 technology (Roche) [47], might prevent this potential complication. This aspect needs further consideration in future work.

Quantitative transcriptomic datasets for liver flukes will also support studies of excretory/secretory, somatic, and tegumental proteins identified previously by proteomics [54, 56, 59], and future annotations of nuclear genomes, including the inference of genes, gene structures, and splicing mechanisms. The future sequencing and annotation of the genomes of fasciolids and opisthorchiids would provide major insights into their genetics and molecular biology. Comparative analyses of genomes to infer metabolic pathways, coupled to extensive transcriptomic and proteomic data sets for different developmental stages, should also facilitate functional genomic investigations of these parasites. Given that double-stranded RNA interference (RNAi) operates in *S. mansoni*, *F. hepatica* [38, 39, 80–82], and *O. viverrini* [83], there is some promise that this approach can help establish the functions of a variety of molecules in liver flukes of major socioeconomic significance. Looking ahead, it might also be possible to test gene functions using transgenesis [84] for some developmental stages. The integration of data from functional and comparative genomic studies will pave the way for the design of new intervention approaches, built on knowledge of essential genes or gene products linked to key biological pathways. For example, a homolog of thioredoxin glutathione reductase, a multifunctional and essential detoxifying enzyme in *S. mansoni* [85, 86], seems to be conserved among trematodes and thus represents a novel drug target candidate in trematodes [87]. Future functional and structural explorations of molecules (such as proteases and their inhibitors, neuropeptides, kinases, phosphatases, and selected structural proteins), which are conserved among fasciolids, opisthorchiids, and schistosomes, and/or predicted to be essential and druggable [88–91], could facilitate the design and development of new classes of trematocidal compounds.

Conclusions

Clearly, there are still major gaps in our knowledge of the fundamental biology and pathogenesis of liver flukes that cause considerable morbidity to millions of people and animals worldwide. A future focus should be on sequencing the genomes (predicted to be 0.5–2 Gb in size) from a number of food-borne flukes as a foundation for understanding their genetics, evolution, ecology, epidemiology, pathogenesis, and host–parasite relationships. A recent paper [92], describing the *de novo* sequencing and annotation of the giant panda genome (2.3 Gb in size) exclusively employing an Illumina-based approach, indicates the exciting prospect that fluke genomes could be sequenced using this direct approach. Knowledge of fluke genomes would provide a solid foundation for future, integrated studies of gene function and essentiality, employing tools such as transgenesis and RNAi. Unlocking the molecular biology of these neglected and globally important disease pathogens using "omics" technologies, particularly functional genomics, proteomics, and metabolomics, will provide entirely novel and unique insights into the development of digeneans, parasite–host interactions, liver fluke disease, and cancer associated with trematodes, and should underpin the design of new trematocidal drugs, vaccines, and diagnostic tools.

Acknowledgments

Neil Young is the grateful recipient of an Early Career Research Fellowship from the National Health and Medical Research Council (NHMRC). Research in the Gasser

Lab (http://www.gasserlab.org) is supported by grants from the Australian Research Council, Australian Academy of Science, NHMRC, and Melbourne Water Corporation. Other support from the Victorian Life Sciences Computation Initiative, its Peak Computing Facility at The University of Melbourne, and the IBM Research Collaboratory for Life Sciences – Melbourne is gratefully acknowledged.

References

1 Charlier, J., Duchateau, L., Claerebout, E., Williams, D., and Vercruysse, J. (2007) Associations between anti-*Fasciola hepatica* antibody levels in bulk-tank milk samples and production parameters in dairy herds. *Prev. Vet. Med.*, **78**, 57–66.

2 Mezo, M., Gonzalez-Warleta, M., Castro-Hermida, J.A., Muino, L., and Ubeira, F.M. (2011) Association between anti-*F. hepatica* antibody levels in milk and production losses in dairy cows. *Vet. Parasitol.*, **180**, 237–242.

3 Schweizer, G., Braun, U., Deplazes, P., and Torgerson, P.R. (2005) Estimating the financial losses due to bovine fasciolosis in Switzerland. *Vet. Rec.*, **157**, 188–193.

4 Borji, H. and Parandeh, S. (2010) The abattoir condemnation of meat because of parasitic infection, and its economic importance: results of a retrospective study in north-eastern Iran. *Ann. Trop. Med. Parasitol.*, **104**, 641–647.

5 Otranto, D. and Traversa, D. (2002) A review of dicrocoeliosis of ruminants including recent advances in the diagnosis and treatment. *Vet. Parasitol.*, **107**, 317–335.

6 Behm, C.A. and Sangster, N.C. (1999) Pathology, pathophysiology and clinical aspects, in *Fasciolosis* (ed. J.P. Dalton), CABI, Wallingford, United Kingdom, pp. 185–224.

7 Sripa, B., Kaewkes, S., Sithithaworn, P., Mairiang, E., Laha, T., Smout, M., Pairojkul, C. et al. (2007) Liver fluke induces cholangiocarcinoma. *PLoS Med.*, **4**, e201.

8 Shin, H.R., Oh, J.K., Masuyer, E., Curado, M.P., Bouvard, V., Fang, Y.Y., Wiangnon, S. et al. (2010) Epidemiology of cholangiocarcinoma: an update focusing on risk factors. *Cancer Sci.*, **101**, 579–585.

9 Mas-Coma, S., Valero, M.A., Bargues, M.D., Rollinson, D., and Hay, S.I. (2009) Chapter 2: *Fasciola*, lymnaeids and human fascioliasis, with a global overview on disease transmission, epidemiology, evolutionary genetics, molecular epidemiology and control. *Adv. Parasitol.*, **69**, 41–146.

10 Sripa, B., Bethony, J.M., Sithithaworn, P., Kaewkes, S., Mairiang, E., Loukas, A., Mulvenna, J. et al. (2010) Opisthorchiasis and Opisthorchis-associated cholangiocarcinoma in Thailand and Laos. *Acta Trop.*, **120** (Suppl. 1), S158–S168.

11 Kim, H.G., Han, J., Kim, M.H., Cho, K.H., Shin, I.H., Kim, G.H., Kim, J.S. et al. (2009) Prevalence of clonorchiasis in patients with gastrointestinal disease: a Korean nationwide multicenter survey. *World J. Gastroenterol.*, **15**, 86–94.

12 Lun, Z.R., Gasser, R.B., Lai, D.H., Li, A.X., Zhu, X.Q., Yu, X.B., and Fang, Y.Y. (2005) Clonorchiasis: a key foodborne zoonosis in China. *Lancet Infect. Dis.*, **5**, 31–41.

13 Hotez, P.J., Brindley, P.J., Bethony, J.M., King, C.H., Pearce, E.J., and Jacobson, J. (2008) Helminth infections: the great neglected tropical diseases. *J. Clin. Invest.*, **118**, 1311–1321.

14 Andrews, S.J. (1999) The life cycle of *Fasciola hepatica*, in *Fasciolosis* (eds J.P. Dalton), CABI, Wallingford, United Kingdom, pp. 1–30.

15 Kaewkes, S. (2003) Taxonomy and biology of liver flukes. *Acta Trop.*, **88**, 177–186.

16 Spithill, T., Smooker, P.M., and Copeman, B. (1999) *Fasciola gigantica*:

Epidemiology, control, immunology and molecular biology, in *Fasciolosis* (ed. J.P. Dalton), CABI, Wallingford, United Kingdom, pp. 465–525.

17 Marcos, L.A., Terashima, A., and Gotuzzo, E. (2008) Update on hepatobiliary flukes: fascioliasis, opisthorchiasis and clonorchiasis. *Curr. Opin. Infect. Dis.*, **21**, 523–530.

18 Bouvard, V., Baan, R., Straif, K., Grosse, Y., Secretan, B., El Ghissassi, F., Benbrahim-Tallaa, L. *et al.* (2009) A review of human carcinogens – part B: biological agents. *Lancet Oncol.*, **10**, 321–322.

19 Keiser, J., Engels, D., Büscher, G., and Utzinger, J. (2005) Triclabendazole for the treatment of fascioliasis and paragonimiasis. *Expert Opin. Investig. Drugs*, **14**, 1513–1526.

20 Fairweather, I. (2009) Triclabendazole progress report, 2005–2009: an advancement of learning? *J. Helminthol.*, **83**, 139–150.

21 Overend, D.J. and Bowen, F.L. (1995) Resistance of *Fasciola hepatica* to triclabendazole. *Aust. Vet. J.*, **72**, 275–276.

22 Coles, G.C., Rhodes, A.C., and Stafford, K.A. (2000) Activity of closantel against adult triclabendazole-resistant *Fasciola hepatica*. *Vet. Rec.*, **146**, 504–504.

23 Gaasenbeek, C.P.H., Moll, L., Cornelissen, J., Vellema, P., and Borgsteede, F.H.M. (2001) An experimental study on triclabendazole resistance of *Fasciola hepatica* in sheep. *Vet. Parasitol.*, **95**, 37–43.

24 Thomas, I., Coles, G.C., and Duffus, K. (2000) Triclabendazole-resistant *Fasciola hepatica* in southwest Wales. *Vet. Rec.*, **146**, 200.

25 Moll, L., Gaasenbeek, C.P.H., Vellema, P., and Borgsteede, F.H.M. (2000) Resistance of *Fasciola hepatica* against triclabendazole in cattle and sheep in the Netherlands. *Vet. Parasitol.*, **91**, 153–158.

26 Olaechea, F., Lovera, V., Larroza, M., Raffo, F., and Cabrera, R. (2011) Resistance of *Fasciola hepatica* against triclabendazole in cattle in Patagonia (Argentina). *Vet. Parasitol.*, **178**, 364–366.

27 Keiser, J., Duthaler, U., and Utzinger, J. (2010) Update on the diagnosis and treatment of food-borne trematode infections. *Curr. Opin. Infect. Dis.*, **23**, 513–520.

28 Keiser, J., Odermatt, P., and Tesana, S. (2009) Dose–response relationships and tegumental surface alterations in *Opisthorchis viverrini* following treatment with mefloquine *in vivo* and *in vitro*. *Parasitol. Res.*, **105**, 261–266.

29 Keiser, J., Shu-Hua, X., Jian, X., Zhen-San, C., Odermatt, P., Tesana, S., Tanner, M. *et al.* (2006) Effect of artesunate and artemether against *Clonorchis sinensis* and *Opisthorchis viverrini* in rodent models. *Int. J. Antimicrob. Agents*, **28**, 370–373.

30 Soukhathammavong, P., Odermatt, P., Sayasone, S., Vonghachack, Y., Vounatsou, P., Hatz, C., Akkhavong, K. *et al.* (2011) Efficacy and safety of mefloquine, artesunate, mefloquine–artesunate, tribendimidine, and praziquantel in patients with *Opisthorchis viverrini*: a randomised, exploratory, open-label, phase 2 trial. *Lancet Infect. Dis.*, **11**, 110–118.

31 Keiser, J., Shu-Hua, X., Chollet, J., Tanner, M., and Utzinger, J. (2007) Evaluation of the *in vivo* activity of tribendimidine against *Schistosoma mansoni*, *Fasciola hepatica*, *Clonorchis sinensis*, and *Opisthorchis viverrini*. *Antimicrob. Agents Chemother.*, **51**, 1096–1098.

32 Berriman, M., Haas, B.J., LoVerde, P.T., Wilson, R.A., Dillon, G.P., Cerqueira, G.C., Mashiyama, S.T. *et al.* (2009) The genome of the blood fluke *Schistosoma mansoni*. *Nature*, **460**, 352–358.

33 Liu, F., Zhou, Y., Wang, Z.Q., Lu, G., Zheng, H., Brindley, P.J., McManus, D.P. *et al.* (2009) The *Schistosoma japonicum* genome reveals features of host-parasite interplay. *Nature*, **460**, 345–351.

34 Gobert, G.N., Moertel, L., Brindley, P.J., and McManus, D.P. (2009) Developmental gene expression profiles of the human pathogen *Schistosoma japonicum*. *BMC Genomics*, **10**, 128.

35 Gobert, G.N., McManus, D.P., Nawaratna, S., Moertel, L., Mulvenna, J., and Jones, M.K. (2009) Tissue specific

profiling of females of *Schistosoma japonicum* by integrated laser microdissection microscopy and microarray analysis. *PLoS Negl. Trop. Dis.*, **3**, e469.

36 Fitzpatrick, J.M., Johnston, D.A., Williams, G.W., Williams, D.J., Freeman, T.C., Dunne, D.W., and Hoffmann, K.F. (2005) An oligonucleotide microarray for transcriptome analysis of *Schistosoma mansoni* and its application/use to investigate gender-associated gene expression. *Mol. Biochem. Parasitol.*, **141**, 1–13.

37 Ndegwa, D., Krautz-Peterson, G., and Skelly, P.J. (2007) Protocols for gene silencing in schistosomes. *Exp. Parasitol.*, **117**, 284–291.

38 Kalinna, B.H. and Brindley, P.J. (2007) Manipulating the manipulators: advances in parasitic helminth transgenesis and RNAi. *Trends Parasitol.*, **23**, 197–204.

39 Rinaldi, G., Morales, M.E., Alrefaei, Y.N., Cancela, M., Castillo, E., Dalton, J.P., Tort, J.F. *et al.* (2009) RNA interference targeting leucine aminopeptidase blocks hatching of *Schistosoma mansoni* eggs. *Mol. Biochem. Parasitol.*, **167**, 118–126.

40 Morales, M.E., Rinaldi, G., Gobert, G.N., Kines, K.J., Tort, J.F., and Brindley, P.J. (2008) RNA interference of *Schistosoma mansoni* cathepsin D, the apical enzyme of the hemoglobin proteolysis cascade. *Mol. Biochem. Parasitol.*, **157**, 160–168.

41 Brindley, P.J. and Pearce, E.J. (2007) Genetic manipulation of schistosomes. *Int. J. Parasitol.*, **37**, 465–473.

42 Laha, T., Pinlaor, P., Mulvenna, J., Sripa, B., Sripa, M., Smout, M., Gasser, R.B. *et al.* (2007) Gene discovery for the carcinogenic human liver fluke, *Opisthorchis viverrini*. *BMC Genomics*, **8**, 189.

43 Cho, P.Y., Kim, T.I., Whang, S.M., and Hong, S.J. (2008) Gene expression profile of *Clonorchis sinensis* metacercariae. *Parasitol. Res.*, **102**, 277–282.

44 Lee, J.S., Lee, J., Park, S.J., and Yong, T.S. (2003) Analysis of the genes expressed in *Clonorchis sinensis* adults using the expressed sequence tag approach. *Parasitol. Res.*, **91**, 283–289.

45 Cho, P.Y., Lee, M.J., Kim, T.I., Kang, S.Y., and Hong, S.J. (2006) Expressed sequence tag analysis of adult *Clonorchis sinensis*, the Chinese liver fluke. *Parasitol. Res.*, **99**, 602–608.

46 Pandey, V., Nutter, R.C., and Prediger, E. (2008) Applied Biosystems SOLiD™ system: ligation-based sequencing, in *Next Generation Genome Sequencing: Towards Personalized Medicine* (ed. J.M. Milton), Wiley-VCH Verlag GmbH, Weinheim, pp. 29–41.

47 Margulies, M., Egholm, M., Altman, W.E., Attiya, S., Bader, J.S., Bemben, L.A., Berka, J. *et al.* (2005) Genome sequencing in microfabricated high-density picolitre reactors. *Nature*, **437**, 376–380.

48 Bentley, D.R., Balasubramanian, S., Swerdlow, H.P., Smith, G.P., Milton, J., Brown, C.G., Hall, K.P. *et al.* (2008) Accurate whole human genome sequencing using reversible terminator chemistry. *Nature*, **456**, 53–59.

49 Zerbino, D.R. and Birney, E. (2008) Velvet: algorithms for *de novo* short read assembly using de Bruijn graphs. *Genome Res.*, **18**, 821–829.

50 Li, R., Zhu, H., Ruan, J., Qian, W., Fang, X., Shi, Z., Li, Y. *et al.* (2010) *De novo* assembly of human genomes with massively parallel short read sequencing. *Genome Res.*, **20**, 265–272.

51 Cantacessi, C., Jex, A.R., Hall, R.S., Young, N.D., Campbell, B.E., Joachim, A., Nolan, M.J. *et al.* (2010) A practical, bioinformatic workflow system for large data sets generated by next-generation sequencing. *Nucleic Acids Res.*, **38**, e171.

52 Nagaraj, S.H., Deshpande, N., Gasser, R.B., and Ranganathan, S. (2007) ESTExplorer: an expressed sequence tag (EST) assembly and annotation platform. *Nucleic Acids Res.*, **35**, W143–W147.

53 Kim, E.M., Kim, J.S., Choi, M.H., Hong, S.T., and Bae, Y.M. (2008) Effects of excretory/secretory products from *Clonorchis sinensis* and the carcinogen dimethylnitrosamine on the proliferation and cell cycle modulation of human

epithelial HEK293T cells. *Korean J. Parasitol.*, **46**, 127–132.

54 Mulvenna, J., Sripa, B., Brindley, P.J., Gorman, J., Jones, M.K., Colgrave, M.L., Jones, A. *et al.* (2010) The secreted and surface proteomes of the adult stage of the carcinogenic human liver fluke *Opisthorchis viverrini*. *Proteomics*, **10**, 1063–1078.

55 Gourbal, B.E., Guillou, F., Mitta, G., Sibille, P., Theron, A., Pointier, J.P., and Coustau, C. (2008) Excretory–secretory products of larval *Fasciola hepatica* investigated using a two-dimensional proteomic approach. *Mol. Biochem. Parasitol.*, **161**, 63–66.

56 Ju, J.W., Joo, H.N., Lee, M.R., Cho, S.H., Cheun, H.I., Kim, J.Y., Lee, Y.H. *et al.* (2009) Identification of a serodiagnostic antigen, legumain, by immunoproteomic analysis of excretory–secretory products of *Clonorchis sinensis* adult worms. *Proteomics*, **9**, 3066–3078.

57 Cancela, M., Ruetalo, N., Dell'Oca, N., da Silva, E., Smircich, P., Rinaldi, G., Roche, L. *et al.* (2010) Survey of transcripts expressed by the invasive juvenile stage of the liver fluke *Fasciola hepatica*. *BMC Genomics*, **11**, 227.

58 Wang, Y., Li, J.V., Saric, J., Keiser, J., Wu, J., Utzinger, J., and Holmes, E. (2010) Advances in metabolic profiling of experimental nematode and trematode infections. *Adv. Parasitol.*, **73**, 373–404.

59 Robinson, M.W., Menon, R., Donnelly, S.M., Dalton, J.P., and Ranganathan, S. (2009) An integrated transcriptomics and proteomics analysis of the secretome of the helminth pathogen *Fasciola hepatica*: proteins associated with invasion and infection of the mammalian host. *Mol. Cell. Proteomics*, **8**, 1891–1907.

60 Young, N.D., Campbell, B.E., Hall, R.S., Jex, A.R., Cantacessi, C., Laha, T., Sohn, W.M. *et al.* (2010) Unlocking the transcriptomes of two carcinogenic parasites, *Clonorchis sinensis* and *Opisthorchis viverrini*. *PLoS Negl. Trop. Dis.*, **4**, e719.

61 Young, N.D., Hall, R.S., Jex, A.J., Cantacessi, C., and Gasser, R.B. (2010) Elucidating the transcriptome of *Fasciola hepatica* – a key to fundamental and biotechnological discoveries for a neglected parasite. *Biotechnol. Adv.*, **28**, 222–231.

62 Young, N.D., Jex, A.R., Cantacessi, C., Hall, R.S., Campbell, B.E., Spithill, T.W., Tangkawattana, S. *et al.* (2011) A portrait of the transcriptome of the neglected trematode, *Fasciola gigantica* – biological and biotechnological implications. *PLoS Negl. Trop. Dis.*, **5**, e1004.

63 Zdobnov, E.M. and Apweiler, R. (2001) InterProScan – an integration platform for the signature-recognition methods in InterPro. *Bioinformatics*, **17**, 847–848.

64 Wu, J., Mao, X., Cai, T., Luo, J., and Wei, L. (2006) KOBAS server: a web-based platform for automated annotation and pathway identification. *Nucleic Acids Res.*, **34**, W720–W724.

65 Bendtsen, J.D., Nielsen, H., von Heijne, G., and Brunak, S. (2004) Improved prediction of signal peptides: SignalP 3.0. *J. Mol. Biol.*, **340**, 783–795.

66 Krogh, A., Larsson, B., von Heijne, G., and Sonnhammer, E.L. (2001) Predicting transmembrane protein topology with a hidden Markov model: application to complete genomes. *J. Mol. Biol.*, **305**, 567–580.

67 Han, Z.G., Brindley, P.J., Wang, S.Y., and Chen, Z. (2009) *Schistosoma* genomics: new perspectives on schistosome biology and host–parasite interaction. *Annu. Rev. Genomics Hum. Genet.*, **10**, 211–240.

68 Kim, Y.J., Choi, M.H., Hong, S.T., and Bae, Y.M. (2009) Resistance of cholangiocarcinoma cells to parthenolide-induced apoptosis by the excretory–secretory products of *Clonorchis sinensis*. *Parasitol. Res.*, **104**, 1011–1016.

69 Sripa, B., Mairiang, E., Thinkhamrop, B., Laha, T., Kaewkes, S., Sithithaworn, P., Tessana, S. *et al.* (2009) Advanced periductal fibrosis from infection with the carcinogenic human liver fluke *Opisthorchis viverrini* correlates with elevated levels of interleukin-6. *Hepatology*, **50**, 1273–1281.

70 Thuwajit, C., Thuwajit, P., Kaewkes, S., Sripa, B., Uchida, K., Miwa, M., and Wongkham, S. (2004) Increased cell

proliferation of mouse fibroblast NIH-3T3 *in vitro* induced by excretory/secretory product(s) from *Opisthorchis viverrini*. *Parasitology*, **129**, 455–464.

71 Smout, M.J., Laha, T., Mulvenna, J., Sripa, B., Suttiprapa, S., Jones, A., Brindley, P.J. *et al*. (2009) A granulin-like growth factor secreted by the carcinogenic liver fluke, *Opisthorchis viverrini*, promotes proliferation of host cells. *PLoS Pathog*., **5**, e1000611.

72 Young, N.D., Jex, A.R., Cantacessi, C., Campbell, B.E., Laha, T., Sohn, W.M., Sripa, B. *et al*. (2010) Progress on the transcriptomics of carcinogenic liver flukes of humans – unique biological and biotechnological prospects. *Biotechnol. Adv*., **28**, 859–870.

73 Prakobwong, S., Yongvanit, P., Hiraku, Y., Pairojkul, C., Sithithaworn, P., Pinlaor, P., and Pinlaor, S. (2010) Involvement of MMP-9 in peribiliary fibrosis and cholangiocarcinogenesis via Rac1 dependent DNA damage in a hamster model. *Int. J. Cancer*, **127**, 2576–2587.

74 Robinson, M.W., Hutchinson, A.T., Dalton, J.P., and Donnelly, S. (2010) Peroxiredoxin: a central player in immune modulation. *Parasite Immunol*., **32**, 305–313.

75 Cervi, L., Rossi, G., and Masih, D.T. (1999) Potential role for excretory–secretory forms of glutathione-S-transferase (GST) in *Fasciola hepatica*. *Parasitology*, **119**, 627–633.

76 Salazar-Calderon, M., Martin-Alonso, J.M., Ruiz de Eguino, A.D., and Parra, F. (2001) Heterologous expression and functional characterization of thioredoxin from *Fasciola hepatica*. *Parasitol. Res*., **87**, 390–395.

77 Smith, R.E., Spithill, T.W., Pike, R.N., Meeusen, E.N.T., and Piedrafita, D. (2008) *Fasciola hepatica* and *Fasciola gigantica*: cloning and characterisation of 70kDa heat-shock proteins reveals variation in HSP70 gene expression between parasite species recovered from sheep. *Exp. Parasitol*., **118**, 536–542.

78 Hewitson, J.P., Grainger, J.R., and Maizels, R.M. (2009) Helminth immunoregulation: the role of parasite secreted proteins in modulating host immunity. *Mol. Biochem. Parasitol*., **167**, 1–11.

79 Piedrafita, D., Estuningsih, E., Pleasance, J., Prowse, R., Raadsma, H.W., Meeusen, E.N.T., and Spithill, T.W. (2007) Peritoneal lavage cells of Indonesian thin-tail sheep mediate antibody-dependent superoxide radical cytotoxicity *in vitro* against newly excysted juvenile *Fasciola gigantica* but not juvenile *Fasciola hepatica*. *Infect. Immun*., **75**, 1954–1963.

80 Geldhof, P., De Maere, V., Vercruysse, J., and Claerebout, E. (2007) Recombinant expression systems: the obstacle to helminth vaccines? *Trends Parasitol*., **23**, 527–532.

81 McGonigle, L., Mousley, A., Marks, N.J., Brennan, G.P., Dalton, J.P., Spithill, T.W., Day, T.A. *et al*. (2008) The silencing of cysteine proteases in *Fasciola hepatica* newly excysted juveniles using RNA interference reduces gut penetration. *Int. J. Parasitol*., **38**, 149–155.

82 Rinaldi, G., Morales, M.E., Cancela, M., Castillo, E., Brindley, P.J., and Tort, J.F. (2008) Development of functional genomic tools in trematodes: RNA interference and luciferase reporter gene activity in *Fasciola hepatica*. *PLoS Negl. Trop. Dis*., **2**, e260.

83 Sripa, J., Pinlaor, P., Brindley, P.J., Sripa, B., Kaewkes, S., Robinson, M., Young, N.D. *et al*. (2011) RNA interference targeting cathepsin B of the carcinogenic liver fluke, *Opisthorchis viverrini*. *Parasitol. Int*., **60**, 283–288.

84 Kines, K.J., Morales, M.E., Mann, V.H., Gobert, G.N., and Brindley, P.J. (2008) Integration of reporter transgenes into *Schistosoma mansoni* chromosomes mediated by pseudotyped murine leukemia virus. *FASEB J*., **22**, 2936–2948.

85 Lea, W.A., Jadhav, A., Rai, G., Sayed, A.A., Cass, C.L., Inglese, J., Williams, D.L. *et al*. (2008) A 1,536-well-based kinetic HTS assay for inhibitors of *Schistosoma mansoni* thioredoxin glutathione reductase. *Assay Drug Dev. Technol*., **6**, 551–555.

86 Kuntz, A.N., Davioud-Charvet, E., Sayed, A.A., Califf, L.L., Dessolin, J.,

Arner, E.S., and Williams, D.L. (2007) Thioredoxin glutathione reductase from *Schistosoma mansoni*: an essential parasite enzyme and a key drug target. *PLoS Med.*, **4**, e206.

87 Salinas, G., Selkirk, M.E., Chalar, C., Maizels, R.M., and Fernandez, C. (2004) Linked thioredoxin-glutathione systems in platyhelminths. *Trends Parasitol.*, **20**, 340–346.

88 Verjovski-Almeida, S., DeMarco, R., Martins, E.A., Guimaraes, P.E., Ojopi, E.P., Paquola, A.C., Piazza, J.P. et al. (2003) Transcriptome analysis of the acoelomate human parasite *Schistosoma mansoni*. *Nat. Genet.*, **35**, 148–157.

89 Tran, M.H., Pearson, M.S., Bethony, J.M., Smyth, D.J., Jones, M.K., Duke, M., Don, T.A. et al. (2006) Tetraspanins on the surface of *Schistosoma mansoni* are protective antigens against schistosomiasis. *Nat. Med.*, **12**, 835–840.

90 Caffrey, C.R., Rohwer, A., Oellien, F., Marhöfer, R.J., Braschi, S., Oliveira, G., McKerrow, J.H. et al. (2009) A comparative chemogenomics strategy to predict potential drug targets in the metazoan pathogen, *Schistosoma mansoni*. *PLoS One*, **4**, e4413.

91 Crowther, G.J., Shanmugam, D., Carmona, S.J., Doyle, M.A., Hertz-Fowler, C., Berriman, M., Nwaka, S. et al. (2010) Identification of attractive drug targets in neglected-disease pathogens using an *in silico* approach. *PLoS Negl. Trop. Dis.*, **4**, e804.

92 Li, R., Fan, W., Tian, G., Zhu, H., He, L., Cai, J., Huang, Q. et al. (2010) The sequence and *de novo* assembly of the giant panda genome. *Nature*, **463**, 311–317.

93 Chen, D., Chen, J., Huang, J., Chen, X., Feng, D., Liang, B., Che, Y. et al. (2010) Epidemiological investigation of *Clonorchis sinensis* infection in freshwater fishes in the Pearl River Delta. *Parasitol. Res.*, **107**, 835–839.

94 Mas-Coma, S., Bargues, M.D., and Valero, M.A. (2005) Fascioliasis and other plant-borne trematode zoonoses. *Int. J. Parasitol.*, **35**, 1255–1278.

95 Sripa, B. and Pairojkul, C. (2008) Cholangiocarcinoma: lessons from Thailand. *Curr. Opin. Gastroenterol.*, **24**, 349–356.

96 Sithithaworn, P. and Haswell-Elkins, M. (2003) Epidemiology of *Opisthorchis viverrini*. *Acta Trop.*, **88**, 187–194.

97 Armignacco, O., Caterini, L., Marucci, G., Ferri, F., Bernardini, G., Natalini Raponi, G., Ludovisi, A. et al. (2008) Human illnesses caused by *Opisthorchis felineus* flukes, Italy. *Emerg. Infect. Dis.*, **14**, 1902–1905.

98 MacLean, J.D., Arthur, J.R., Ward, B.J., Gyorkos, T.W., Curtis, M.A., and Kokoskin, E. (1996) Common-source outbreak of acute infection due to the North American liver fluke *Metorchis conjunctus*. *Lancet*, **347**, 154–158.

99 Dalton, J.P. (ed.) (1999) *Fasciolosis*, CABI, Wallingford, United Kingdom.

100 Boray, J.C. (1969) Experimental fascioliasis in Australia. *Adv. Parasitol.*, **7**, 95–210.

101 Novobilsky, A., Horackova, E., Hirtova, L., Modry, D., and Koudela, B. (2007) The giant liver fluke *Fascioloides magna* (Bassi 1875) in cervids in the Czech Republic and potential of its spreading to Germany. *Parasitol. Res.*, **100**, 549–553.

102 Foreyt, W.J. and Todd, A.C.F.K. (1975) *Fascioloides magna* (Bassi, 1875) in feral swine from southern Texas. *J. Wildl. Dis.*, **11**, 554–559.

6
RNA Interference: A Potential Discovery Tool for Therapeutic Targets of Parasitic Nematodes

Collette Britton

Abstract

Although gene sequence data for parasitic nematodes have increased significantly in the last decade, there is currently no reliable method to test gene function and validate putative control targets. Gene silencing by RNA interference (RNAi) has proven successful in the free-living nematode *Caenorhabditis elegans* and the ease of this technique has allowed it to be adapted for high-throughput genome-wide screening of essential gene function. This success encouraged a number of RNAi studies on parasitic nematodes of animals and plants. Whereas RNAi in parasitic nematodes, as well as some free-living nematodes, is not as effective as it is in *C. elegans*, specific gene silencing has been observed for some target genes. Recent work with *Haemonchus contortus* suggests that the success of RNAi can be improved by targeting genes expressed in sites accessible to the environment such as the intestine, excretory/secretory system, or amphids. One of the genes robustly silenced in *H. contortus* encodes the aminopeptidase H11. RNAi of *H11* in larvae prior to oral infection resulted in significant reductions in worm burden and egg output, similar to vaccination with native H11 protein. This provides proof-of-principle that RNAi can be developed as a tool to identify essential gene function. Using current RNAi techniques, screening for essential genes as potential control targets may be limited by transcript accessibility to introduced double-stranded RNA. Optimization of double-stranded RNA delivery methods is discussed as enhanced uptake may allow RNAi to be fully exploited as a tool for both functional genomics and target discovery in parasitic nematodes.

Introduction

A significant problem facing livestock production is how to control parasitic helminth infections in the face of increasing anthelmintic resistance [1–3]. Possible solutions range from maintaining parasites in refugia (non-drug-treated) and drug rotation, to better husbandry, nutrition, and selective breeding of resistant animals [4]. Each approach has its advantages and disadvantages. In view of the reliance of livestock producers on drug control and the success so far of current anthelmintic treatments, development of new control therapies seems to be essential. This need has been met to some extent by the recent introduction of the amino-acetonitrile derivative monepantel (Zolvix®; Novartis Animal Health) – a new class of anthelmintic [5] (see also Chapter 17). However, the problem of resistance apparent for other anthelmintic classes has led to caution in the use of Zolvix, with the aim of prolonging its use. So how may new treatments be identified? Several reviews have highlighted the need for a better understanding of parasite physiology to identify and prioritize possible control targets [6, 7]. This is particularly important in the move by pharmaceutical companies away from whole-organism-based to mechanism-based drug screening, whereby effects on defined targets, such as receptors or enzymes, are searched for [6–8] (see also Chapter 8). For vaccine development, identification and validation of relevant targets also requires better knowledge of parasite biology and of target accessibility to immune effector mechanisms. Technologies, including genome sequencing and functional genomics, are and will be pivotal in advancing new parasite control therapies. So how close are these technologies to delivering novel targets of control?

From Sequence Data to Target Discovery

Over the last decade there has been a significant increase in the availability of sequence and expression data for parasitic nematode genes. Expressed sequence tag (EST) projects as well as microarray studies have identified genes temporally regulated at specific points of the parasite life cycle – those associated with reproduction and genes differentially expressed in different host environments [9–12]. With the decreasing cost and improving technologies associated with genome sequencing (and transcriptomics; see Chapter 4), we should soon have a complete picture of all genes present in different parasitic nematodes, how these are organized, and be able to identify genes unique to or divergent between parasitic species. Currently, draft genome data are available for several animal and plant parasitic nematodes [13–15], with significant coverage achieved for others, including *Haemonchus contortus* (http://www.sanger.ac.uk/resources/downloads/helminths). Although comparative analyses of this wealth of data can promote speculation on the possible functions and evolution of parasite genes, there is currently no reliable method to experimentally identify essential gene function in parasitic nematodes.

Functional Genomics Using *Caenorhabditis elegans*

Since the completion of the genome sequencing project for the free-living soil nematode *C. elegans* in 1998 [16], there has been increasing interest in using this model organism for studying parasitic nematodes and multicellular organisms in general (see also Chapters 1, 2 and 12). The *C. elegans* genome is approximately 100 Mb with around 19 000 protein-coding genes. The availability of parasitic nematode sequence data has allowed very useful comparisons of genes expressed in parasitic species with those of *C. elegans*. In addition to sequence information, for most *C. elegans* genes, data are available on site and stage of expression, interaction with other genes, identification of orthologs in other species, and phenotypes associated with gene mutation/deletion (www.wormbase.org). An array of *C. elegans* mutants has been generated and is used in forward genetics to identify mutations giving rise to specific phenotypes.

The discovery of RNA interference (RNAi) in *C. elegans* revolutionized functional genomics [17]. This mechanism of gene silencing is effective in a range of organisms, including insects, planarians, and mammals [18–20]. Silencing can be initiated in *C. elegans* by injection of double-stranded RNA into any site within the worm, with the silencing effect spreading to other tissues [17]. RNAi is also effective following soaking in double-stranded RNA solution [21] or feeding worms with *Escherichia coli* expressing double-stranded RNA [22]. The ease of the latter method has been exploited in high-throughput genome-wide RNAi screens [23–25] and the data are widely used as a first step in the functional analysis of putative orthologs from other organisms.

Conservation of gene function between *C. elegans* and other species, including parasitic nematodes, can be tested by rescue experiments in which the putative orthologous gene is expressed in *C. elegans* RNAi or genetic mutants and any reversion of phenotype examined [26]. Conservation of biological activity can also be demonstrated by overexpression or ectopic expression of parasite genes in wild-type *C. elegans*, as demonstrated for *Onchocerca volvulus* glutathione S-transferase [27] and *H. contortus* transcription factor ELT-2 [28]. Combining *C. elegans* RNAi data with comparative sequence information has been proposed as a screening step in identification of novel drug targets for helminth (including filarial) parasites [29–31]. However, the accessibility of the proposed target to immune effector mechanisms or to drug is an important factor. For example, a cathepsin L cysteine protease CPL-1 was shown by RNAi and mutant analysis to be essential for *C. elegans* embryonic development, specifically in the processing of egg yolk proteins [32]. The embryonic lethal phenotype could be efficiently rescued with the *cpl-1* gene from *H. contortus*, demonstrating conservation of function [33]. A recombinant version of *Hc*-CPL-1 was tested as a vaccine candidate for *H. contortus* in sheep, and effects on egg production and development examined. This showed that while CPL-1 may have an essential function, antibody generated to the vaccine did not access developing embryos within the gonad during infection and subsequently there was no protective effect [34]. Therefore, identifying potentially relevant control targets using RNAi-based methods is just one step in the process; target location to facilitate recognition by immune effector mechanisms or exposure to drug should also be evaluated when possible.

Drug Target Identification Using *C. elegans*

With a shift to target-based drug discovery programs [6–8], using functional data from *C. elegans* is a feasible and logical approach to identifying potential parasite control strategies. Screening for inhibitors of, for example, essential enzymes or transporters is conducive to mechanism-based screening. This approach has been successfully applied to screen for inhibitors of cyclin-dependent kinases that have been identified as targets for the control of trypanosomatid and apicomplexan protozoan parasites [35, 36], and for inhibitors of thioredoxin glutathione reductase in *Schistosoma mansoni* [37]. However, no currently available anthelmintic drugs have been developed using mechanism-based screening methods [8]. As mentioned above, accessibility of drug to target is required and the complexity of multicellular organisms increases the effort and risk involved in drug screens.

Interestingly, the current anthelmintics would not have been identified using RNAi in *C. elegans* as a screening tool for loss of or decreased gene function. With the exception of paraherquamide [38], all function to modulate or mimic target activity (agonists) rather than acting as antagonists [8]. The benzimadazoles, for example, bind to β-tubulin and interfere with microtubule formation [39]. However, mutation or deletion of *ben-1*, which encodes the only benzimadazole-sensitive β-tubulin in *C. elegans*, has no obvious effect on worm physiology [40]. This indicates likely functional redundancy with other β-tubulin genes of the nematode. Where *C. elegans* functional studies have been elegantly applied is in the identification of potential mechanisms of drug action and resistance. Loss or mutation of *C. elegans* β-tubulin *ben-1* results in benzimadazole resistance and, importantly, the same genetic mutation correlates with benzimadazole resistance in a number of parasitic nematode species [41, 42]. Similarly, RNAi or genetic mutation of the genes encoding *C. elegans* glutamate-gated chloride channels AVR-14 or AVR-15 results in no obvious abnormalities, except for a subtle increase in reverse movement frequency [43]. However, loss of both channels results in ivermectin resistance [44]. This raises the question of whether lack of essential function of current anthelmintic targets is a contributing factor in emergence of drug resistance. Nonessential targets can undergo deletion or mutation at drug-binding sites with no apparent fitness consequences to the nematode. This is less likely to occur with targets with essential functions. Would essential gene products be more stable targets for development of new drugs and can these be identified using an RNAi approach?

RNAi in Parasitic Nematodes – Story so Far

Although RNAi data from *C. elegans* can help identify the possible functional importance of parasitic nematode genes, direct application of RNAi in parasitic species would be a very valuable tool. This would also allow functional analysis of genes not conserved in *C. elegans*, which may be important for parasite survival within the host and/or influence host immune responses. The success of RNAi in *C. elegans* encouraged extension of this approach to parasitic nematodes and the first report of RNAi was published in 2002 for *Nippostrongylus brasiliensis* [45]. Subsequent studies reported RNAi effects in other nematode species including the filarial nematodes, *Brugia malayi* [46] and *Onchocerca volvulus* [47], and the sheep parasite, *Trichostrongylus colubriformis* [48] (detailed in Table 6.1). However, not all initial studies demonstrated a corresponding decrease in target transcript level, which is important for correlating any phenotypic effects with specific gene knockdown.

Table 6.1 RNAi in animal parasitic nematodes.

Species	Stage	Target gene(s)	Evaluation	Phenotype	Reference
Nippostrongylus brasiliensis	adult	acetylcholinesterase B	reduced activity	none	[45]
Brugia malayi	adult	β-tubulin (Bm-tub-1)	reduced transcript	death 24 h	[46]
		RNA polymerase II (Bm-ama-1)	reduced transcript	death 24 h	[46]
		microfilaria sheath protein (Bm-shp-1)	reduced transcript	reduced microfilaria release	[46]
	L2/L3*	cathepsin L (Bm-cpl-1)*	reduced transcript*	reduced motility and growth*	[71]
Onchocerca volvulus	L3	cathepsin L (Ov-cpl)	not tested	reduced molting	[47]
		cathepsin Z (Ov-cpz)	not tested	reduced molting	[47]
		protease inhibitors (Ov-spi-1 and -2)	reduced transcript and protein	reduced molting	[74]
Trichostrongylus colubriformis	L1	ubiquitin (Tc-ubq-1)	not tested	reduced development	[48]
Ascaris suum	L3	pyrophosphatase	reduced transcript and activity	reduced molting	[75]
Haemonchus contortus	L3/L4/adult	β-tubulin (isotypes-1 and -2)	reduced transcript	reduced development	[49, 76]
	L3	COPII component (Hc-sec-23)	reduced transcript (2/4 experiments)	none	[49]
		Ca^{2+}-binding protein	no reduction transcript	none	[49]
		heat-shock protein 70 (Hc-hsp-1)	no reduction transcript	none	[49]
		vacuolar ATPase (Hc-vha-10)	increased transcript	none	[49]
		cathepsin L (Hc-cpl-1)	no reduction transcript	none	[49]

(Continued)

Table 6.1 (Continued)

Species	Stage	Target gene(s)	Evaluation	Phenotype	Reference
		paramyosin (Hc-unc-15)	no reduction transcript	none	[49]
		superoxide dismutase (Hc-sod-1)	no reduction transcript	none	[49]
		intermediate filament (Hc-mua-6)	no reduction transcript	none	[49]
		collagen (Hc-let-2)	no reduction transcript	none	[49]
		GATA transcription factor (Hc-elt-2)	no reduction transcript	none	[49]
		aminopeptidase H11 (Hc-H11)	reduced transcript	none	[53]
		aminopeptidase H11 (Hc-H11)*	reduced activity*	reduced worms and eggs*	[53]
		L3 secretory proteins (Hc-asp-1)	reduced transcript	none	[53]
		aquaporin (Hc-aqp-2)	reduced transcript	none	[53]
		RNA helicase (Hc-phi-10)	reduced transcript	none	[53]
		chloride channel (Hc-exc-4)	no reduced transcript	none	[53]
		transcription factor (Hc-ceh-6)	increased transcript	none	[53]
		GTP cyclohydrolase (Hc-GTPch)	no reduction transcript	none	[53]
		signal peptidase (contig HCC00700)	no reduction transcript	none	[53]
		ribosomal gene (contig HCC00623)	no reduction transcript	none	[53]
		ribosomal gene (contig HCC00645)	no reduction transcript	none	[53]

Ostertagia ostertagi	L3	β-tubulin	none	reduced transcript (3/5 experiments)	[50]
		tropomyosin	none	reduced transcript (5/7 experiments)	[50]
		ATP-synthetase	none	reduced transcript (1/3 experiments)	[50]
		superoxide dismutase	none	reduced transcript (1/3 experiments)	[50]
		polyprotein allergen	none	reduced transcript (2/3 experiments)	[50]
		ubiquitin	none	no reduction transcript	[50]
		transthyretin-like protein	none	no reduction transcript	[50]
		17-kDa excretory/secretory protein	none	no reduction transcript	[50]
Litomosoides sigmodontis	adult	actin (Ls-act)	reduced motility	reduced transcript	[77]
Heligmosomoides polygyrus	adult	tropomyosin (Hp-tm-1)	increased aging	no reduction transcript	[52]

All evaluations and phenotypes are from *in vitro* RNAi soaking assays; those marked with an asterisk are from *in vivo* RNAi studies.

In addition, most studies focused on one or a small number of target genes. To determine whether RNAi could be widely applied as a functional genomics tool, two subsequent studies targeted a larger number of genes. L3 stages of *H. contortus* and *Ostertagia ostertagi* were soaked in double-stranded RNA and transcript levels measured after several days. These studies presented a less optimistic picture. Of 11 genes targeted in *H. contortus*, only one, encoding β-tubulin, was reproducibly silenced [49]. In *O. ostertagi*, five of eight genes could be silenced in some, but not all experiments [50]. The findings from RNAi studies to date suggest that an RNAi pathway functions in parasitic nematodes, and this is supported by the identification of Dicer and other pathway genes from genome data [51, 52]. However, target genes seem to vary in their susceptibility to RNAi. It seems unlikely, therefore, that large-scale screens to identify essential gene function, as applied to *C. elegans*, will be feasible using current methods.

So how can we improve on the success rate of RNAi and which genes are more likely to be amenable to silencing? Recent work on *H. contortus* suggests that site of gene expression influences susceptibility to RNAi. Of six genes selected based on their putative expression in the intestine, amphids, or excretory cell of the nematode, transcript levels of four were significantly reduced (up to 95%) following double-stranded RNA soaking [53]. Importantly, these results were reproducible. Therefore, genes expressed in sites accessible to the external environment are, more likely, better targets for RNAi, possibly as a result of greater uptake of double-stranded RNA into these cells This is consistent with RNAi studies in plant parasitic nematodes, in which genes expressed in the intestine, amphids, esophageal gland cells, and reproductive systems were effectively silenced, also suggesting uptake via external openings [54].

The transcripts that were effectively silenced in *H. contortus* L3 stage larvae encoded the intestinal aminopeptidase, H11 [55], the activation-associated secreted protein *Hc*-ASP-1 [56], an ortholog of a *C. elegans* aquaporin (*Ce*-AQP-2) that is expressed in the excretory cell, and an ortholog of *Ce*-PHI-10, an RNA helicase predominantly expressed in the excretory cell and intestine of *C. elegans* [53]. H11 and other intestinal proteases are associated with digestion of host proteins for nutrition, whereas ASPs are speculated to participate in the infection process and/or host immunomodulation (reviewed in [57]). Importantly, both proteins have received attention as potential control targets of *H. contortus* and other parasitic nematodes [55, 56, 58–60]. In addition to H11 and ASPs, other intestinal and excretory/secretory proteins are considered relevant targets for parasite control due to their interaction with the host environment. It will be important to widen the recent RNAi findings [53] to these and similar genes in other parasitic nematodes to better assess the contributory value of RNAi to the identification of control targets.

In Vivo RNAi

Despite the significant reductions in transcript levels following RNAi of the *H. contortus* genes described above [53], no phenotypic effects were observed in L3s maintained *in vitro*. This is, perhaps, not surprising given the limited development of parasite larvae in culture and the potential roles of the targeted genes within the host, particularly for *H11* and *Hc-asp-1*. H11 is a lead vaccine candidate for *H. contortus*, providing up to 90% reduction in egg output and 72% reduction in worm burden [55]. In addition, inhibition of aminopeptidase activity by antibody from vaccinated sheep correlates with protection [61]. In the absence of any *in vitro* phenotype, the effects of RNAi of *H11* on worm burden and egg production *in vivo* were examined [53]. As this was the first *in vivo* study of RNAi in an animal parasitic nematode, a pilot experiment was initially carried out to test whether pre-exposure of larvae to double-stranded RNA was inherently toxic and would, in itself, affect infection outcome. Incubation of *H. contortus* L3 larvae with control *C. elegans* double-stranded RNA prior to oral infection of sheep resulted in similar egg outputs compared to infection with untreated larvae, indicating no inherent toxicity of double-stranded RNA exposure. The *in vivo* effect of *H11* RNAi was, therefore, examined. Infective larvae were incubated in *H11* double-stranded RNA or control *C. elegans* double-stranded RNA for 24 h prior to oral infection of lambs. *H11* RNAi treatment resulted in reductions of 40% in adult worm burden and 57% in egg output relative to the control RNAi group. In addition, aminopeptidase activity in adult worms recovered from the *H11* double-stranded RNA group showed a corresponding decrease of 64% relative to control worms [53]. This was the first demonstration that RNAi of a parasitic nematode gene leads to effects *in vivo* and mimics those following vaccination. This provides proof-of-principle that RNAi can be applied to test effects of target gene knockdown.

Improving RNAi in Parasitic Nematodes

Knockdown of *H. contortus H11* transcript in larvae produced similar effects to vaccination with native H11 protein. Can RNAi be adapted to screen for new targets of parasite control? The recent findings from *H. contortus* strengthen the evidence that a functional RNAi pathway is active in parasitic nematodes [53]. However, efficient uptake of double-stranded RNA to effectively silence target genes remains a hurdle. Studies in *S. mansoni* have also reported variation in efficacy of target transcript knockdown, with reductions ranging from 40 to 80% [62–64] (see also Chapter 7). A detailed study targeting 11 different genes in *S. mansoni* schistosomula concluded that intestine and tegumental (surface)-expressed transcripts were more amenable to silencing [64], similar to the findings with *H. contortus* [53]. Electroporation as a means to deliver small interfering RNA (siRNA) to schistosomula or adult worms is reported to be more effective than soaking [63]. This method has been tried with parasitic nematodes; however, detrimental effects on worm survival have been reported in some studies [49, 52]. More extensive testing of different electroporation conditions may improve both RNAi success and survival. However, the impermeable nature of the nematode cuticle may make this challenging and alternative approaches should be considered.

Efficient delivery of siRNAs to mammalian cells for therapeutic purposes has been achieved using nanoparticles (diameter below 100 nm) and chemically modified

RNAs with increased stability [65]. The advantage of nanoparticles as a delivery vehicle is the large surface-to-volume ratio. These can also be modified to include targeting ligands to deliver siRNAs to specific cells or tissues. This was recently demonstrated using cyclodextrin-based siRNA-containing nanoparticles with surface-exposed transferrin to target cancer cells [66]. Nanoparticles, particularly polystyrene-based molecules, are taken up by the intestine, pharynx, and gonad of *C. elegans* with no apparent toxicity [67]. Also, chitosan nanoparticles effectively delivered double-stranded RNA to mosquito intestinal cells following feeding [68]. Nanoparticles have not yet been tested in parasitic nematodes.

Better culture methods for parasitic nematodes may improve uptake of double-stranded RNA as well as allow any RNAi effects to be monitored *in vitro*. This would be a significant advantage, in view of the expense and ethical considerations associated with *in vivo* testing. *In vitro* monitoring of phenotypes has been possible for some RNAi genes in *S. mansoni*, which can be maintained for several weeks in the appropriate culture medium. For example, RNAi of the cathepsin B gene, *SmCB1*, resulted in specific reductions in mRNA and enzyme activity, and significantly reduced parasite growth [69]. Similarly, *in vitro* RNAi of the leucine aminopeptidase genes *SmLAP1* or *SmLAP2* resulted in decreased hatching of eggs [70]. However, development of suitable culture systems for parasitic nematodes remains a challenge.

A recent study employed *in vivo* RNAi to examine transcript knockdown and effects on *B. malayi* L2 and L3 stage larvae within the mosquito [71]. Targeting of a cathepsin L cysteine protease gene, *Bm-cpl-1*, using double-stranded RNA or siRNA injected intrathoracically into infected mosquitoes resulted in an 83% reduction in target transcript levels. In addition, *Bm-cpl-1* RNAi reduced larval motility and migration to the mosquito head, thus reducing the potential for parasite transmission. Further development of this approach, such as the generation of transgenic mosquitoes [71] or transgenic parasite larvae [72], expressing double-stranded RNA to *B. malayi* genes of interest may allow larger-scale analysis. This would be important in identifying and characterizing genes involved in development either within a vector or mammalian host. Whereas delivery of double-stranded RNA or siRNA itself is unlikely to be exploited as a control approach, *in vivo* studies such as these will significantly progress identification and validation of novel drug or vaccine targets. Therefore, with further development and application, RNAi has the potential to be used as a first step in novel control development.

Conclusions

RNAi in *C. elegans* revolutionized functional genomics in this organism, and has greatly contributed to identifying possible functions of conserved genes in parasitic nematodes and other multicellular organisms. However, RNAi seems to function more effectively in *C. elegans* than in other nematode species, including *Caenorhabditis briggsae* [73]. Recent work has improved the success rate of RNAi in *H. contortus* by targeting genes expressed in sites accessible to the external environment, such as the intestine, amphids, and excretory system [53]. It will be important to test whether this approach can be extended to other parasitic nematodes. Also, experimental challenges remain regarding improving delivery of double-stranded RNA and developing better culture systems. This requirement is emphasized by the success of recent studies demonstrating the feasibility of *in vivo* RNAi in both mammalian and insect hosts to validate control targets [53, 71]. These recent findings with *H. contortus* and *B. malayi* encourage further research to more fully exploit RNAi as a functional genomics and discovery tool.

References

1 Sargison, N., Scott, P., and Jackson, F. (2001) Multiple anthelmintic resistance in sheep. *Vet. Rec.*, **149**, 778–779.

2 Kaplan, R.M. (2004) Drug resistance in nematodes of veterinary importance: a status report. *Trends Parasitol.*, **20**, 477–481.

3 Gasbarre, L.C., Smith, L.L., Lichtenfels, J.R., and Pilitt, P.A. (2009) The identification of cattle nematode parasites resistant to multiple classes of anthelmintics in a commercial cattle population in the US. *Vet. Parasitol.*, **166**, 281–285.

4 Jackson, F. and Miller, J. (2006) Alternative approaches to control – quo vadit? *Vet. Parasitol.*, **139**, 371–384.

5 Kaminsky, R., Ducray, P., Jung, M., Clover, R., Rufener, L., Bouvier, J., Schorderet Weber, S. *et al.* (2008) A new class of anthelmintics effective against drug-resistant nematodes. *Nature*, **452**, 176–181.

6 Geary, T.G., Thompson, D.P., and Klein, R.D. (1999) Mechanism-based screening: discovery of the next generation of anthelmintics depends upon more basic research. *Int. J. Parasitol.*, **29**, 105–112.

7 Geary, T.G., Condor, G.A., and Bishop, B. (2004) The changing landscape of antiparasitic drug discovery for veterinary medicine. *Trends Parasitol.*, **20**, 449–455.

8 Woods, D.J. and Williams, T.M. (2007) The challenges of developing novel antiparasitic drugs. *Invert. Neurosci.*, **7**, 245–250.

9 Datu, B.J., Gasser, R.B., Nagaraj, S.H., Ong, E.K., O'Donoghue, P., McInnes, R., Ranganathan, S., and Loukas, A. (2008) Transcriptional changes in the hookworm, *Ancylostoma caninum*, during the transition from free-living to a parasitic larva. *PLoS Negl. Trop. Dis.*, **2**, e130.

10 Li, B.W., Rush, A.C., Mitreva, M., Yin, Y., Spiro, D., Ghedin, E., and Weil, G.J. (2009) Transcriptomes and pathways associated with infectivity, survival and immunogenicity in *Brugia malayi* L3. *BMC Genomics*, **10**, 267.

11 Wang, Z., Abubucker, S., Martin, J., Wilson, R.K., Hawdon, J., and Mitreva, M. (2010) Characterizing *Ancylostoma caninum* transcriptome and exploring nematode parasitic adaptation. *BMC Genomics*, **11**, 307.

12 Li, B.W., Rush, A.C., Jiang, D.J., Mitreva, M., Abubucker, S., and Weil, G.J. (2011) Gender-associated genes in filarial nematodes are important for reproduction and potential intervention targets. *PLoS Negl. Trop. Dis.*, **5**, e947.

13 Ghedin, E., Wang, S., Spiro, D., Caler, E., Zhao, Q., Crabtree, J., Allen, J.E. *et al.* (2007) Draft genome of the filarial parasite *Brugia malayi*. *Science*, **317**, 1756–1760.

14 Abad, P., Gouzy, J., Aury, J.M., Castagnone-Sereno, P., Danchin, E.G., Deleury, E. Perfus-Barbeoch, L. *et al.* (2008) Genome sequencing of the metazoan plant-parasitic nematode *Meloidogyne incognita*. *Nat. Biotechnol.*, **26**, 909–915.

15 Mitreva, M., Jasmer, D.P., Zarlenga, D.S., Wang, Z., Abubucker, S., Martin, J., Taylor, C.M. *et al.* (2011) The draft genome

of the parasitic nematode *Trichinella spiralis*. *Nat. Genet.*, **43**, 228–235.

16 *C. elegans* Sequencing Consortium (1998) Genome sequence of the nematode, *C. elegans*: a platform for investigating biology. *Science*, **282**, 2012–2018.

17 Fire, A., Xu, S., Montgomery, M.K., Kostas, S.A., Driver, S.E., and Mello, C.C. (1998) Potent and specific genetic interference by double-stranded RNA in *Caenorhabditis elegans*. *Nature*, **391**, 806–811.

18 Kennerdell, J.R. and Carthew, R.W. (1998) Use of dsRNA-mediated genetic interference to demonstrate that frizzled and frizzled 2 act in the wingless pathway. *Cell*, **95**, 1017–1026.

19 Sanchez-Alvarado, A. and Newmark, P.A. (1999) Double-stranded RNA specifically disrupts gene expression during planarian regeneration. *Proc. Natl. Acad. Sci. USA*, **96**, 5049–5054.

20 Elbashir, S.M., Harborth, J., Lendeckel, W., Yalcin, A., Weber, K., and Tuschl, T. (2001) Duplexes of 21-nucleotide RNAs mediate RNA interference in mammalian cell culture. *Nature*, **411**, 494–498.

21 Tabara, H., Grishok, A., and Mello, C.C. (1998) RNAi in *C. elegans*: soaking in the genome sequence. *Science*, **282**, 430–431.

22 Fraser, A.G., Kamath, R.S., Zipperlen, P., Martinez-Campos, M., Sohrmann, M., and Ahringer, J. (2000) Functional genomic analysis of *C. elegans* chromosome I by systematic RNA interference. *Nature*, **408**, 325–330.

23 Kamath, R.S., Fraser, A.G., Dong, Y., Poulin, G., Durbin, R., Gotta, M., Kanapin, A. et al. (2003) Systematic functional analysis of the *Caenorhabditis elegans* genome using RNAi. *Nature*, **421**, 231–237.

24 Simmer, F., Moorman, C., van der Linden, A.M., Kuijk, E., van den Berghe, P.V., Kamath, R.S., Fraser, A.G. et al. (2003) Genome-wide RNAi of *C. elegans* using the hypersensitive *rrf-3* strain reveals novel gene functions. *PLoS Biol.*, **1**, E12.

25 Sönnichsen, B., Koski, L.B., Walsh, A., Marschall, P., Neumann, B., Brehm, M., Alleaume, A.M. et al. (2005) Full-genome RNAi profiling of early embryogenesis in *Caenorhabditis elegans*. *Nature*, **434**, 462–469.

26 Britton, C. and Murray, L. (2006) Using *Caenorhabditis elegans* for functional analysis of genes of parasitic nematodes. *Int. J. Parasitol.*, **36**, 651–659.

27 Kampkotter, A., Volkmann, T.E., de Castro, D.H., Leiers, B., Klotz, L.O., Johnson, T.E., Link, C.D., and Henkle-Duhrsen, K. (2003) Functional analysis of the glutathione S-transferase 3 from *Onchocerca volvulus* (Ov-GST-3): a parasite GST confers increased resistance to oxidative stress in *Caenorhabditis elegans*. *J. Mol. Biol.*, **325**, 25–37.

28 Couthier, A., Smith, J., McGarr, P., Craig, B., and Gilleard, J.S. (2004) Ectopic expression of a *Haemonchus contortus* GATA transcription factor in Caenorhabditis elegans reveals conserved function in spite of extensive sequence diversity. *Mol. Biochem. Parasitol.*, **133**, 241–253.

29 Behm, C.A., Bendig, M.M., McCarter, J.P., and Sluder, A.E. (2005) RNAi-based discovery and validation of new drug targets in filarial nematodes. *Trends Parasitol.*, **21**, 97–100.

30 Kumar, S., Chaudhary, K., Foster, J.M., Novelli, J.F., Zhang, Y., Wang, S., Spiro, D. et al. (2007) Mining predicted essential genes of *Brugia malayi* for nematode drug targets. *PLoS One*, **2**, e1189.

31 Crowther, G.J., Shanmugan, D., Carmona, S.J., Doyle, M.A., Hertz-Fowler, C., Berriman, M., Nwaka, S. et al. (2010) Identification of attractive drug targets in neglected-disease pathogens using an in silico approach. *PLoS Negl. Trop. Dis.*, **4**, e804.

32 Britton, C. and Murray, L. (2004) Cathepsin L protease (CPL-1) is essential for yolk processing during embryogenesis in *Caenorhabditis elegans*. *J. Cell Sci.*, **117**, 5133–5143.

33 Britton, C. and Murray, L. (2002) A cathepsin L protease essential for *Caenorhabditis elegans* is functionally conserved in parasitic nematodes. *Mol. Biochem. Parasitol.*, **122**, 21–33.

34 Murray, L., Geldhof, P., Clark, D., Knox, D.P., and Britton, C. (2007) Expression and purification of an active cysteine protease of *Haemonchus contortus* using *Caenorhabditis elegans*. *Int. J. Parasitol.*, **31**, 1117–1125.

35 Grant, K.M., Dunion, M.H., Yardley, V., Skaltsounis, A.L., Marko, D., Eisenbrand, G., Croft, S.L. et al. (2004) Inhibitors of *Leishmania mexicana* CRK3 cyclin-dependent kinase: chemical library screen and antileishmanial activity. *Antimicrob. Agents Chemother.*, **48**, 3033–3042.

36 Geyer, J.A., Prigge, S.T., and Waters, N.C. (2005) Targeting malaria with specific CDK inhibitors. *Biochim. Biophys. Acta*, **1754**, 160–170.

37 Kuntz, A.N., Davioud-Charvet, E., Sayed, A.A., Califf, L.L., Dessolin, J., Arner, E.S., and Williams, D.L. (2007) Thioredoxin glutathione reductase from *Schistosoma mansoni:* an essential parasite enzyme and a key drug target. *PLoS Med.*, **4**, e206.

38 Robertson, A.P., Clark, C.L., Burns, T.A., Thompson, D.P., Geary, T.G., Trailovic, S.M., and Martin, R.J. (2002) Paraherquamide and 2-deoxy-paraherquamide distinguish cholinergic receptor subtypes in *Ascaris muscle*. *J. Pharmacol. Exp. Ther.*, **302**, 853–860.

39 Lacey, E. (1988) The role of the cytoskeletal protein, tubulin, in the mode of action and mechanism of drug resistance to benzimadazoles. *Int. J. Parasitol.*, **18**, 885–936.

40 Driscoll, M., Dean, E., Reilly, E., Begholz, E., and Chalfie, M. (1989) Genetic and molecular analysis of a *Caenorhabditis elegans* beta-tubulin that conveys benzimidazole sensitivity. *J. Cell Biol.*, **109**, 2993–3003.

41 Kwa, M.S., Veenstra, J.G., Van Dijk, M., and Roos, M.H. (1995) Beta-tubulin genes from the parasitic nematode *Haemonchus contortus* modulate drug resistance in *Caenorhabditis elegans*. *J. Mol. Biol.*, **246**, 500–510.

42 Von Samson-Himmelstjerna, G., Blackhall, W.J., McCarthy, J.S., and Skuce, P.J. (2007) Single nucleotide polymorphism (SNP) markers for benzimidazole resistance in veterinary nematodes. *Parasitology*, **134**, 1077–1086.

43 Cook, A., Aptel, N., Portillo, V., Siney, E., Sihota, R., Holden-Dye, L., and Wolstenholme, A. (2006) *Caenorhabditis elegans* ivermectin receptors regulate locomoter behaviour and are functional orthologues of *Haemonchus contortus* receptors. *Mol. Biochem. Parasitol.*, **147**, 118–125.

44 Dent, J.A., Smith, M.M., Vassilatis, D.K., and Avery, L. (2000) The genetics of ivermectin resistance in *Caenorhabditis elegans*. *Proc. Natl. Acad. Sci. USA*, **97**, 2674–2679.

45 Hussein, A.S., Kichenin, K., and Selkirk, M.E. (2002) Suppression of secreted acetylcholinesterase expression in *Nippostrongylus brasiliensis* by RNA interference. *Mol. Biochem. Parasitol.*, **122**, 91–94.

46 Aboobaker, A.A. and Blaxter, M.L. (2003) Use of RNA interference to investigate gene function in the human filarial nematode parasite *Brugia malayi*. *Mol. Biochem. Parasitol.*, **129**, 41–51.

47 Lustigman, S., Zhang, J., Liu, J., Oksov, Y., and Hashmi, S. (2004) RNA interference targeting cathepsin L and Z-like cysteine proteases of *Onchocerca volvulus* confirmed their essential function during L3 molting. *Mol. Biochem. Parasitol.*, **138**, 165–170.

48 Issa, Z., Grant, W.N., and Shoemaker, C.B. (2005) Development of methods for RNA interference in the sheep gastrointestinal parasite *Trichostrongylus colubriformis*. *Int. J. Parasitol.*, **35**, 935–940.

49 Geldhof., P., Murray, L., Couthier, A., Gilleard, J.S., McLauchlan, G., Knox, D.P., and Britton, C. (2006) Testing the efficacy of RNA interference in *Haemonchus contortus*. *Int. J. Parasitol.*, **36**, 801–810.

50 Visser, A., Geldhof, P., de Maere, V., Knox, D.P., Vercruysse, J., and Claerebout, E. (2006) Efficacy and specificity of RNA interference in larval life-stages of *Ostertagia ostertagi*. *Parasitology*, **133**, 777–783.

51 Geldhof, P., Visser, A., Clark, D., Saunders, G., Britton, C., Gilleard, J.,

Berriman, M., and Knox, D.P. (2007) RNA interference in parasitic helminths: current situation, potential pitfalls and future prospects. *Parasitology*, **134**, 609–619.

52 Lendner, M., Doligalska, M., Lucius, R., and Hartmann, S. (2008) Attempts to establish RNA interference in the parasitic nematode *Heligmosomoides polygyrus*. *Mol. Biochem. Parasitol.*, **161**, 21–31.

53 Samarasinghe, B., Knox, D.P., and Britton, C. (2011) Factors affecting susceptibility to RNA interference in *Haemonchus contortus* and *in vivo* silencing of an H11 aminopeptidase gene. *Int. J. Parasitol.*, **41**, 51–59.

54 Rosso, M.N., Jones, J.T., and Abad, P. (2009) RNAi and functional genomics in plant parasitic nematodes. *Annu. Rev. Phytopathol.*, **47**, 207–232.

55 Smith, T.S., Munn, E.A., Graham, M., Tavernor, A.S., and Greenwood, C.A. (1993) Purification and evaluation of the integral membrane protein H11 as a protective antigen against *Haemonchus contortus*. *Int. J. Parasitol.*, **23**, 271–280.

56 Sharp,. PJ. and Wagland, B.M. (1998) US Patent 5734035.

57 Cantacessi, C., Campbell, B.E., Visser, A., Geldhof, P., Nolan, M.J., Nisbet, A.J., Matthews, J.B. *et al.* (2009) A potrait of the "SCP/TAPS" proteins of eukaryotes – developing a framework for fundamental research and biotechnological outcomes. *Biotechnol. Adv.*, **27**, 376–388.

58 Hawdon, J.M., Jones, B.F., Hoffman, D.R., and Hotez, P.J. (1996) Cloning and characterization of *Ancylostoma*-secreted protein. A novel protein associated with the transition to parasitism by infective hookworm larvae. *J. Biol. Chem.*, **271**, 6672–6678.

59 Tawe, W., Pearlman, E., Unnasch, T.R., and Lustigman, S. (2000) Angiogenic activity of *Onchocerca volvulus* recombinant proteins similar to vespid venom antigen. *Mol. Biochem. Parasitol.*, **109**, 91–99.

60 Bethony, J., Loukas, A., Smout, M., Brooker, S., Mendez, S., Plieskatt, J., Goud, G. *et al.* (2005) Antibodies against a secreted protein from hookworm larvae reduce the intensity of hookworm infection in humans and vaccinated laboratory animals. *FASEB J.*, **19**, 1743–1745.

61 Munn, E.A., Smith, T.S., Smith, H., James, F.M., Smith, F.C., and Andrews, S.J. (1997) Vaccination against *Haemonchus contortus* with denatured forms of the protective antigen H11. *Parasite Immunol.*, **19**, 243–248.

62 Krautz-Peterson, G., Radwanska, M., Ndegwa, D., Shoemaker, C.B., and Skelly, P.J. (2007) Optimizing gene suppression in schistosomes using RNA interference. *Mol. Biochem. Parasitol.*, **153**, 194–202.

63 Krautz-Peterson, G., Bhardwaj, R., Faghiri, Z., Tararam, C.A., and Skelly, P.J. (2010) RNA interference in schistosomes: machinery and methodology. *Parasitology*, **137**, 485–495.

64 Stefanić, S., Dvořák, J., Horn, M., Braschi, S., Sojka, D., Ruelas, D.S., Suzuki, B. *et al.* (2010) RNA interference in *Schistosoma mansoni* schistosomula: selectivity, sensitivity and operation for larger-scale screening. *PLoS Negl. Trop. Dis.*, **4**, e850.

65 Baker, M. (2010) RNA interference: homing in on delivery. *Nature*, **464**, 1225–1228.

66 Davis, M.E., Zuckerman, J.E., Choi, C.H.J., Seligson, D., Tolcher, A., Alabi, C.A., Yen, Y. *et al.* (2010) Evidence of RNAi in humans from systemically administered siRNA via targeted nanoparticles. *Nature*, **464**, 1067–1070.

67 Pluskota, A., Horzowski, E., Bossinger, O., and von Mikecz, A. (2009) In *Caenorhabditis elegans* nanoparticle-bio-interactions become transparent: silica-nanoparticles induce reproductive senescence. *PLoS One*, **4**, e6622.

68 Zhang, X., Zhang, J., and Zhu, K.Y. (2010) Chitosan/double-stranded RNA nanoparticle-mediated RNA interference to silence chitin synthase genes through larval feeding in the African malaria mosquito (*Anopheles gambiae*). *Insect Mol. Biol.*, **19**, 683–693.

69 Correnti, J.M., Brindley, P.J., and Pearce, E.J. (2005) Long-term suppression of cathepsin B levels by RNA interference

retards schistosome growth. *Mol. Biochem. Parasitol.*, **143**, 209–215.

70 Rinaldi, G., Morales, M.E., Alrefaei, Y.N., Cancela, M., Castillo, E., Dalton, J.P., Tort, J.F., and Brindley, P.J. (2009) RNA interference targeting leucine aminopeptidase blocks hatching of *Schistosoma mansoni* eggs. *Mol. Biochem. Parasitol.*, **167**, 118–126.

71 Song, C., Gallup, J.M., Day, T.A., Bartholomay, L.C., and Kimber, M.J. (2010) Development of an *in vivo* RNAi protocol to investigate gene function in the filarial nematode, *Brugia malayi*. *PLoS Pathog.*, **6**, e1001239.

72 Xu, S., Liu, C., Tzertzinis, G., Ghedin, E., Evans, C.C., Kaplan, R., and Unnasch, T.R. (2011) *In vivo* transfection of developmentally competent *Brugia malayi* infective larvae. *Int. J. Parasitol.*, **41**, 355–362.

73 Felix, M.-A. (2008) RNA interference in nematodes and the chance that favored Sydney Brenner. *J. Biol.*, **7**, 34.

74 Ford, L., Guiliano, D.B., Oksov, Y., Debnath, A.K., Liu, J., Williams, S.A., Baxter, M.L., and Lustigman, S. (2005) Characterization of a novel filarial serine protease inhibitor, Ov-SPI-1, from *Onchocerca volvulus*, with potential multifunctional roles during development of the parasite. *J. Biol. Chem.*, **280**, 40845–40856.

75 Islam, M.K., Miyoshi, T., Yamada, M., and Tsuji, N. (2005) Pyrophosphatase of the roundworm *Ascaris suum* plays an essential role in the worm's molting and development. *Infect. Immun.*, **73**, 1995–2004.

76 Kotze, A.C. and Bagnall, N.H. (2006) RNA interference in *Haemonchus contortus*: suppression of beta-tubulin gene expression in L3, L4 and adult worms *in vitro*. *Mol. Biochem. Parasitol.*, **145**, 101–110.

77 Pfarr, K., Heider, U., and Hoerauf, A. (2006) RNAi mediated silencing of actin expression in adult *Litomosoides sigmodontis* is specific, persistent and results in a phenotype. *Int. J. Parasitol.*, **36**, 661–669.

7
RNA Interference as a Tool for Drug Discovery in Parasitic Flatworms

*Akram A. Da'dara and Patrick J. Skelly**

Abstract

RNA interference (RNAi) is a post-transcriptional gene-silencing mechanism that involves the degradation of mRNA in a highly sequence-specific manner. The development of RNAi has changed the direction and speed of drug target discovery. RNAi has influenced strategies for the pharmacological treatment of many conditions including cancer and inflammatory disease, in addition to bacterial and viral infectious diseases. As reviewed here, the technology can likewise be applied to diseases caused by parasitic flatworms, including trematodes (schistosomes and liver flukes) and cestodes (tapeworms). Various successful methodologies have been employed to engender RNAi in different life cycle stages of a number of parasitic flatworms. Such methods include the use of long or short interfering, double-stranded RNAs, or the use of vectors encoding short hairpin RNAs, at various doses and delivered by soaking or via electroporation. In schistosomes, RNAi can be rapid, potent, and long-lasting. However, in some instances robust gene suppression yields no observable phenotype. This may be due to the presence of residual (perhaps long-lived) target protein and/or to functional redundancy in the gene being targeted. Genome sequence analysis has allowed the elucidation of potential molecular pathways that underscore RNAi in schistosomes. Variation in gene suppressibility is seen and this may be due to differences in target mRNA accessibility or to the fact that different tissues exhibit differences in double-stranded RNA uptake efficiency or variably express RNAi pathway components. Despite these caveats, RNAi has helped identify essential schistosome genes and candidate drug targets. These studies provide proof-of-concept that RNAi has value as a drug discovery tool for parasitic flatworms. Finally, the successful suppression of gene expression in schistosomes within infected experimental animals highlights the possibility of employing double-stranded RNAs directly as a therapy to treat parasitic flatworm infections.

* Corresponding Author

Platyhelminth Parasites

Members of the phylum Platyhelminthes are known commonly as flatworms. These are relatively simple, bilaterally symmetrical, soft-bodied, unsegmented invertebrates. Flatworms are triploblastic animals (i.e., they are composed of three fundamental cell layers) that are acoelomate (lacking a body cavity). Over half of all known flatworm species are parasites, including of humans, domestic animals, and wildlife. Foremost among these are members of the genus *Schistosoma*. These are intravascular parasites (blood flukes) that infect approximately 200 million people and are responsible for the debilitating disease schistosomiasis. Members of the genus *Fasciola* (liver flukes) infect several mammals, including humans, and cause economic losses world-wide, especially in ruminants. Other important flatworm parasites include members of the genus *Taenia*. These are tapeworms that, as adults, inhabit the gastrointestinal tract, causing taeniasis. Larval forms infect the internal tissues and may form cysts to cause cysticercosis. Members of the genus *Echinococcus* are significant tapeworm parasites of wildlife, livestock, and humans.

Few effective drugs currently exist to treat parasitic flatworm infections, and this is particularly true for schistosomiasis for which treatment and control have come to rely on a single drug, praziquantel. Concerns exist over the possible emergence and establishment of drug resistance [1, 2]. Therefore, it remains a priority to identify and develop novel chemical or immunological therapeutic interventions for schistosomiasis and other parasitic flatworm infections. A key challenge in this endeavor is the identification and validation of target molecules. In some cases, examination of genome and transcriptome sequence information has led to the *in silico* identification of potential targets [3, 4]. However, until recently, the lack of tools to, for example, genetically manipulate helminths and validate these targets has hindered the development of new drugs and vaccines. Against this background, the recent development of RNA interference (RNAi) in platyhelminths has emerged as an important tool to evaluate prospective therapeutic targets.

The premise of the approach is that suppression of gene expression through RNAi that results in parasite debility and/or death immediately points to the specific gene product as being of interest as a target for the development of antiparasitics. RNAi screening therefore should help to rapidly identify target molecules of interest and facilitate the development of new treatments. The technology has already influenced strategies for the pharmacological treatment of many conditions, including cancer, inflammatory disease, and bacterial and viral diseases [5–8]. Likewise for parasitic flatworm diseases, RNAi holds real potential.

Although RNAi is of proven utility to identify potential drug targets in flatworms (see below), its application in characterizing vaccine targets may be more limited. Specifically, gene products identified as essential through RNAi must, in addition, be accessible to immune effector mechanisms in order to be considered of interest as vaccine targets. This is true for gene products that are expressed in internal tissues as well as for those expressed in potentially immune-accessible sites such as the gut and tegument (outer surface). Accordingly, this chapter focuses on RNAi as a tool for drug discovery in parasitic flatworms with particular emphasis on the schistosomes – the most intensely studied of the group.

RNAi – Background

RNAi is a mechanism whereby gene-specific double-stranded RNA triggers degradation of homologous mRNA transcripts. The process can result in effective, sequence-specific, post-transcriptional gene silencing [9, 10]. RNAi was first discovered in the free-living nematode, *Caenorhabditis elegans*. It was observed that double-stranded RNA was at least 10-fold more potent in suppressing target gene expression than either sense or antisense RNA alone [11]. Silencing could be induced by injection or by feeding worms with either naked double-stranded RNA or bacteria that were engineered to express double-stranded RNA [9, 12]. In addition, silencing was both long lasting (sometimes being detected in the progeny of treated animals [13]) and potent [14, 15].

Since its discovery in *C. elegans*, RNAi has been described in organisms of diverse phylogeny, including plants, fungi, arthropods, African trypanosomes, and vertebrates [16–19]. However, the phenomenon is not universal; several organisms do not display RNAi. These include the unicellular parasites *Plasmodium falciparum*, *Babesia bovis*, *Leishmania major*, *Trypanosoma cruzi*, and the yeast, *Saccharomyces cerevisiae* [20–23]. Also, *C. elegans* is particularly sensitive to RNAi, yet other nematode species (including parasitic forms) seem less responsive [24–26].

RNAi in Platyhelminths

In flatworms, RNAi was first described in the free-living planarian, *Schmidtea mediterranea* [27]. As with *C. elegans*, RNAi could be induced by injecting or by feeding the planarian with either naked double-stranded RNA or bacteria expressing double-stranded RNA [27–29]. RNAi was used to target genes in a variety of cell types including secretory cells, cells of the gastrovascular system, and neurons [29]. Success with gene suppression in the nervous system stands in contrast to *C. elegans* in which mature neurons are refractory to RNAi [12].

For parasitic flatworms, RNAi was first described in two different life cycle stages of *Schistosoma mansoni* [30, 31]. Schistosomes have complex life histories with several distinct morphologies. Infectious freshwater larval forms called cercariae penetrate mammalian skin and transform into schistosomula. These grow and mature in the vasculature as adult male or female worms. The adults mate and lay eggs that are passed from the body. Larval forms called miracidia hatch from these eggs in freshwater and infect specific species of snails to transform into the intramolluscan parasitic stage known as the sporocyst. In the first experiments to suppress gene expression in schistosomes, cultured parasites were soaked in medium containing double-stranded RNA either during transformation of the miracidium to the sporocyst or the cercaria to the schistosomulum. It was thought that double-stranded

RNA entry during transformation might be optimal due to the considerable biochemical and morphological reorganization of the parasite, including of the outer membranes. For the miracidium-to-sporocyst transformation, timing does seem to be important in permitting RNAi. As the time between the initiation of miracidial transformation and the addition of double-stranded RNA increases, the effectiveness of RNAi decreases [31]. Interestingly, however, larval parasites exposed either at the start of transformation or 20 h later were able to take up labeled double-stranded RNA to a similar extent [31], suggesting that the variability of RNAi was not a consequence of a differential ability to take up double-stranded RNA.

No such time dependency is observed with intramammalian stage parasites. Parasites exposed to double-stranded RNA hours, or even days, after the commencement of transformation of cercariae to schistosomula (in addition to adult male and female parasites) are all susceptible to RNAi [32, 33]. Using fluorescent labeling, it has been shown that double-stranded RNA can enter schistosomula through the mouth [33, 34] and penetration glands [32]. For sporocysts (that lack a mouth) in the presence of labeled double-stranded RNA, approximately 39% was detected in excretory pores/flame cells and "parenchymal-like cells," whereas approximately 28% of the label was localized to the tegument [35].

RNAi in Schistosomes

Early experiments with RNAi in schistosomes involved soaking parasites in medium containing double-stranded RNA that had been generated from template polymerase chain reaction (PCR) products *in vitro*. Attempts to optimize RNAi using transfection reagents (liposomal or amine-based) were unsuccessful; in fact, many of these agents were directly toxic [33]. Electroporation has also been used as a delivery mechanism [36–38]. Electroporation was originally described as an approach for transgene expression in schistosomula [39] and was subsequently used to introduce double-stranded RNA into schistosomula [38]. Schistosomes are also susceptible to RNAi using chemically synthesized short-interfering RNA (siRNA). Electroporation has proven to be more efficient at delivering siRNA than soaking particularly at low RNA concentrations [40].

Exposure to relatively low concentrations of double-stranded RNA (below 10 μg/ml using electroporation [40] and as low as 1 μg/ml by soaking [41]) can elicit strong gene suppression in schistosomes, although most workers use more double-stranded RNA than this. Concentrations of 25–50 μg/ml double-stranded RNA have been used for electroporation [37, 40], whereas for soaking, approximately 90 μg/ml double-stranded RNA has been employed [34]. Soaking parasites in doses higher than this (150–200 μg/ml of double-stranded RNA) was shown to be directly toxic [34].

Vector-based RNAi that drives the expression of hairpin RNA in the parasite has also been tested [42, 43]. Hairpins are single-stranded RNA molecules that fold back on themselves due to engineered sequence complementarity and this allows the resultant double-stranded RNA to enter the RNAi pathway. Introducing a pseudotyped murine leukemia virus (MLV) transgene encoding a hairpin RNA targeting the *S. mansoni* cathepsin B1 gene decreases gene expression in the parasite by 80% [42]. In another study, a promoter-like element from the U6 gene of *S. mansoni* was used to drive transcription of short hairpin transcripts from plasmids delivered to schistosomula [43]. These approaches can theoretically lead to more sustained double-stranded RNA generation within cells.

Gene suppression in schistosomes is rapid; target mRNA levels begin to decline within hours of double-stranded RNA administration and may be substantially decreased within 24–48 h [34, 37]. Furthermore, suppression has been reported to be relatively long lasting in schistosomes (up to 3 weeks *in vivo* [38] and 40 days in culture [33]).

RNAi in intramammalian schistosomes appears to be target selective; off-target effects (i.e., mistargeting of double-stranded RNA to noncognate mRNA) have not been reported [34, 36]. This is the case even when two close homologs are targeted, such as the cathepsin B1 and B2 genes [34] or the glucose transporter protein SGTP 1 and 4 genes [36, 44]. With the intramolluscan sporocyst stage, however, RNAi has yielded phenotypes (predominantly stunted growth) without a concomitant alteration in the expression levels of the target gene – an outcome that might reflect off-targeting [35]. Finally, it is clear that more than one gene at a time can be efficiently targeted in schistosomes [34, 36, 45], indicating that the RNAi machinery is not overwhelmed by multiple exogenous double-stranded RNAs.

RNAi Pathway in Schistosomes

Among the important proteins in the canonical RNAi pathway is the RNase III enzyme Dicer, which acts to process long double-stranded RNA into less than 30-nucleotide siRNAs. Following this, siRNA is loaded into the RNA-induced silencing complex (RISC) [46]. The siRNA is then unwound in a strand-specific manner during RISC assembly and the resultant single-stranded RNA locates its cognate mRNA target by Watson–Crick base pairing. Gene silencing follows from the nucleolytic degradation of the targeted mRNA by the RNase H enzyme Argonaute (or Slicer) [46].

Given that schistosomes are sensitive to RNAi, it is not surprising that schistosome genome and transcriptome databases contain homologs of several RNAi pathway proteins [47, 48]. A single dicer homolog (SmDicer) has been characterized for *S. mansoni* [49]. SmDicer contains all the domains that are characteristic of metazoan dicers, including an amino-terminal helicase domain, DUF283 and PAZ domains, two RNase III domains, and an RNA-binding domain [49]. Four Argonaute protein homologs have been identified in *S. mansoni* (SmAgo1–4); SmAgo3 and 4 are splice variants [47]. Each SmAgo is approximately 900 amino acids in length, and all possess conserved PAZ and Piwi domains [47]. Finally, analysis of the schistosome transcriptome has revealed several other sequences with homology to additional components of the RNAi pathways from other organisms (e.g., accessory double-stranded RNA-binding proteins) [50].

A variety of functions have been proposed for the RNAi machinery in eukaryotic cells. These include suppressing potentially harmful segments of the genome such as transposons that might otherwise act as destabilizing insertional mutagens [51]. RNAi can also be part of a cell's antiviral defenses [52] and can participate in several gene regulatory pathways to control cellular differentiation [19, 53–57]. Over the past several years, small endogenous noncoding RNAs that enter silencing pathways have been described [57–60]. An example is microRNA (miRNA) that comprise short noncoding RNA that can form hairpin structures. miRNA can drive gene silencing by either destroying mRNA or suppressing protein synthesis [61]. Several miRNA molecules have been identified in schistosomes [62–64], and homologs of proteins known to generate and act upon miRNA have been identified in the schistosome genome [50]. For instance, a homolog of the RNase III enzyme, Drosha, has been identified in the *S. mansoni* genome (SmDrosha). By analogy with other systems, this would act to cleave nuclear precursor miRNA transcripts (pri-miRNA). Through alternative splicing, SmDrosha is predicted to generate two proteins, SmDrosha1 and 2, that comprise 1531 and 1577 amino acids, respectively, and contain conserved endonuclease domains and double-stranded RNA-binding motifs [47]. Drosha cleavage products, termed precursor miRNAs (pre-miRNAs), are 60–70 nucleotides in length and are exported to the cytoplasm via the carrier protein exportin 5. A potential exportin 5 homolog has been identified in the schistosome genome [47]. Once in the cytoplasm, the miRNA is free to enter RNAi pathways.

Gene silencing by RNAi can spread from the point of introduction of double-stranded RNA such that a targeted gene at a different site, or throughout the animal, can be suppressed [65]. In *C. elegans*, the *sid-1* gene encodes a multiple membrane-spanning protein [66] that functions as an energy-independent channel for importing double-stranded RNA into cells [67]. SID-1 is required for uptake of double-stranded RNA in *C. elegans* and is expressed in all cells sensitive to systemic RNAi [66, 68]. An examination of the *S. mansoni* genome reveals a SID-1 homolog (SmSID-1) of 1018 amino acids and predicted to contain the 11 conserved transmembrane domains, but also to possess an unusually large, extracellular amino-terminal domain [40]. This protein may facilitate double-stranded RNA uptake from the environment and/or the movement of RNA between schistosome cells.

RNAi as a Discovery Tool

The above discussion shows that RNAi is functional in schistosomes and may have application as a discovery tool for drug development. However, there are caveats. Foremost, perhaps, is that not all genes are equally susceptible to RNAi. With schistosomula and adult parasites, RNAi techniques that lead to the efficient suppression of some genes (e.g., *Schistosoma mansoni* aquaporin (SmAQP) and alkaline phosphatase (SmAP)) produce only modest suppression of other genes (e.g., permease 1 heavy chain (SPRM1hc) and inhibin/activin (SmInAct)) [40, 69, 70]. Even with the same approach in the same life cycle stage, gene responses to RNAi can vary [34]. Likewise with sporocysts, strong suppression (e.g., of the glutathione S-transferase-26 (GST-26) and thioredoxin peroxidase 1 (TPX1) genes) and weak knockdown (e.g., of the calpain and the mothers-against-decapentaplegic homolog 2 (Smad2) genes) have been reported using the same methodology in the same laboratory [71]. There are several possible reasons for this gene-to-gene variability:

- There is inherent parasite variability in the ability to take up double-stranded RNA, as has been shown for sporocysts soaked in fluorescently labeled double-stranded RNA [71]. Many parasites simply never acquire the labeled double-stranded RNA, whereas for others the localization of the label varied between the tegument, excretory pores/flame cells, and parenchyma [71].
- Some genes may be expressed in tissues that are not accessible to double-stranded RNA introduced either by electroporation or soaking [34].
- It is possible that, for certain tissues, key RNAi pathway proteins are not well expressed or RNAi pathway inhibitors are in effect. However, the notion that some tissues are refractory to RNAi or do not fully express RNAi pathway proteins does not explain gene knockdown variability in the same tissue type. For instance, the SPRM1hc gene and the SmAP gene are expressed in the parenchyma and tegument of schistosome adults [72–74], but the SmAP gene is routinely suppressed in excess of 90%, whereas expression of SPRM1hc is never decreased by more than 50% [72, 75, 76]. Perhaps this result indicates that parenchyma is not a uniform tissue type, but rather that genes are expressed in differing parenchymal cells that differ in their susceptibility to RNAi.
- Finally, the lower susceptibility of some gene targets to RNAi may be explained by mRNA secondary structure that impedes interaction with double-stranded RNA. To explore this in regard to the poorly suppressed SPRM1hc gene discussed above, three distinct siRNA molecules targeting different regions of the mRNA were tested. All gave a similar degree of suppression (around 50%) [74]. To ensure that the three siRNA molecules did not target inaccessible regions of the SPRM1hc mRNA, a 943-bp double-stranded RNA was generated by PCR and parasites were electroporated. This longer double-stranded RNA should be processed by SmDicer to generate an array of siRNA molecules. The expectation was that at least some of these siRNAs would interact with the SPRM1hc mRNA to effect strong suppression. This was not observed, however, and suppression remained at approximately 50% [74].

There are other considerations regarding transient RNAi and its application in schistosomes:

- Even robust gene suppression may not yield an obvious phenotype. This may be due to (i) transient RNAi not being absolute in its ability to "silence" gene expression (i.e., residual protein production may be sufficient to sustain normality), (ii) proteins with long half-lives that continue to provide nominal functionality even in the absence of nascent transcription, (iii) functional redundancy in the gene being targeted (e.g., members of the gut protease

network [34]), and (iv) the use of rich culture medium to support parasites that might otherwise succumb in the more physiologically challenging environment of the host.
- Obtaining sufficient numbers of parasites for double-stranded RNA treatments is never trivial; even for schistosomula derived from infected snails, the enterprise is labor-intensive and expensive.
- Thus far, there is no standard methodology for RNAi (see above discussions). Several diverse protocols work. Different research teams use different delivery methods employing PCR-derived double-stranded RNA or chemically synthesized siRNA over various concentrations and incubation times, and in different culture media. It is unclear whether a universal standardization is possible given the foregoing discussions; in this regard, permanent germline transgenesis, currently unavailable for schistosomes, may be a way forward.

RNAi-Induced Phenotypes and Identifying Essential Genes

The first report of RNAi eliciting a lethal phenotype in schistosomes involved the peroxiredoxin gene [77]. Peroxiredoxin functions in schistosome oxidative metabolism and may provide the main enzymatic activity to reduce H_2O_2 in the parasite. Silencing of peroxiredoxin in parasites cultured in 20% O_2 (or at the more physiologically relevant 5% O_2) caused significant increases in parasite mortality. Exogenous oxidative stress (200 μM H_2O_2) killed all of the double-stranded RNA-treated schistosomula in 4 days [77]. Genes encoding other schistosome redox proteins were subsequently subjected to RNAi, including, thioredoxin glutathione reductase (TGR), a unique selenium-containing enzyme [78]. After 3 days, TGR enzyme activity was reduced by about two-thirds in schistosomula cultured either anaerobically or aerobically (20% O_2). Approximately 90% of the parasites died 4 days after RNAi of TGR (in aerobic or anaerobic conditions) [78]. These RNAi data confirm the complementary biochemical evidence [77, 79, 80] of the essentiality of TGR and peroxiredoxin for schistosomes and their utility as drug targets (see also Chapter 20).

Note that incomplete gene knockdown does not eliminate the utility of RNAi. Even a modest diminution in expression may yield interesting and informative phenotypes. For instance, RNAi of schistosome SmInAct decreases mRNA levels only 40%. Nevertheless, eggs produced in such exposed female parasites fail to develop [69].

As pointed out above, not all RNAi experiments, even those yielding robust gene suppression, lead to such stark phenotypes as death. Often gene suppression leads to no observable change in parasite morphology or behavior and this can be the case even for genes predicted by bioinformatics to be essential for schistosomes [34]. When phenotypes are observed, the most common is growth stunting and this is, perhaps, not unexpected given that many biochemical pathways are associated with parasite growth [35, 37, 38, 71].

RNAi-Based Drugs

The application of RNAi thus far discussed involves RNAi as a tool to identify possible drug targets that are then prosecuted with chemical compounds to inhibit or impede that target. As an alternative, there is increasing interest in bypassing chemical drug development *per se* and instead using the interfering double-stranded RNA itself as a drug [5, 79, 80]. However, several hurdles must be overcome before using double-stranded RNA therapeutically [81]. Not least is that double-stranded RNA drugs need to survive in extracellular fluids that contain RNases. In addition, double-stranded RNA drugs need to target specific tissues and cells. Despite these obstacles, two studies have shown that double-stranded RNA drugs could, in principle, work for schistosomes. In the first study, the schistosome hypoxanthine–guanine phosphoribosyltransferase gene was targeted [82]. A hydrodynamic protocol was used to deliver siRNA to schistosome-infected mice. This single treatment reduced the number of parasites by approximately 27% at 6 days after siRNA delivery. Recovered parasites showed a 60% reduction in hypoxanthine–guanine phosphoribosyltransferase transcript [82]. In the second study, the effect of siRNA treatment was tested in *Schistosoma japonicum*-infected mice [83]. Here, siRNA targeting the gynecophoric canal protein was administered via intravenous injection in phosphate-buffered saline at different time points postinfection. The approach significantly reduced target gene expression and the proportion of paired parasites. Also, worm burdens were reduced by between 20 and 36% [83]. Both studies demonstrate the promise of siRNA oligonucleotides as therapeutics for treatment of schistosome infection. Nonetheless, clinical RNAi technology still faces obstacles related to delivery, potency, and stability that are being addressed for other diseases [84–86].

RNAi in Other Parasitic Platyhelminths

RNAi has also been successfully demonstrated in other trematodes, including the common liver fluke, *Fasciola hepatica* [87], and the Southeast Asian liver fluke, *Opisthorchis viverrini* [88] (see Chapter 28). In *F. hepatica*, genes encoding the cysteine proteases cathepsin B and L were effectively suppressed in the infective, newly excysted juvenile stage by soaking the parasites in target-specific double-stranded RNA. RNAi of either cathepsin gene resulted in marked reductions in target transcript levels and their respective proteins in the gut. Furthermore, suppression of either cathepsins B or L in juvenile parasites induced transient, abnormal locomotory phenotypes and significantly reduced penetration by the parasite of the rat intestinal wall *in vitro* [87]. *F. hepatica* leucine aminopeptidase has also been targeted using electroporation to deliver double-stranded RNA [45]. In *O. viverrini*, adult worms were electroporated with double-stranded RNA targeting a cathepsin B and this significantly reduced levels of mRNA and enzyme activity [88].

RNAi has been shown to operate in cestodes (tapeworms), specifically in the sheep tapeworm, *Moniezia expansa* [89], and in the fox tapeworm, *Echinococcus multilocularis* [90, 91]. With adult *M. expansa* worms, double-stranded RNA targeting the actin gene (delivered by electroporation or soaking) led to a 70% decrease in specific mRNA and decreased protein levels with a marked disruption of the tegument [89]. In contrast, the neuronal neuropeptide F (*Me-npf-1*) gene could not be consistently suppressed using the same methodology, suggesting that differences in the susceptibility to RNAi among tissues and/or genes exist in this parasite [89]. In the case of *E. multilocularis*, RNAi was first demonstrated in primary cell cultures [91]. In a second study, siRNA delivery via electroporation was used to suppress expression of the ezrin/radixin/moesin-like protein (*elp*) and *14-3-3* genes in *E. multilocularis* protoscoleces [90]. Expression levels of *elp* and *14-3-3* genes were reduced by 65 and 78%, respectively [90].

Conclusions

As reviewed here, RNAi clearly operates in flatworms, both free-living and parasitic [27, 30, 31]. Among the parasitic forms, RNAi has been demonstrated in trematodes (schistosomes and liver flukes) [34, 36, 45, 87, 88] and cestodes (tapeworms) [89–91]. Efforts to optimize RNAi have mainly involved *S. mansoni* [32, 34, 40]. Several different life stages of this parasite are susceptible to RNAi and much of the molecular machinery for RNAi has been identified in the schistosome genome [31, 32, 40, 47]. Further, RNAi can be achieved using several straightforward approaches that lead to rapid, specific, and long-lasting suppression [33, 34, 37]. However, it is clear that much remains to be understood with regard of the apparent differences in susceptibilities of genes and/or tissues to RNAi (as currently applied), and that might hinder a global RNAi screening approach. However, as so far employed on a case-by-case basis, RNAi has helped identify essential genes and candidate drug targets [77, 78, 92]. These studies provide proof-of-concept that RNAi has value as a drug discovery tool for parasitic flatworms.

Acknowledgments

This work was supported by grant AI-056273 from the National Institutes of Health National Institute of Allergy and Infectious Diseases.

References

1 Doenhoff, M.J. and Pica-Mattoccia, L. (2006) Praziquantel for the treatment of schistosomiasis: its use for control in areas with endemic disease and prospects for drug resistance. *Expert Rev. Anti Infect. Ther.*, **4**, 199–210.

2 Melman, S.D., Steinauer, M.L., Cunningham, C., Kubatko, L.S., Mwangi, I.N., Wynn, N.B., Mutuku, M.W. et al. (2009) Reduced susceptibility to praziquantel among naturally occurring Kenyan isolates of *Schistosoma mansoni*. *PLoS Negl. Trop. Dis.*, **3**, e504.

3 Caffrey, C.R., Rohwer, A., Oellien, F., Marhofer, R.J., Braschi, S., Oliveira, G., McKerrow, J.H., and Selzer, P.M. (2009)

A comparative chemogenomics strategy to predict potential drug targets in the metazoan pathogen, *Schistosoma mansoni*. *PLoS One*, **4**, e4413.

4 Fitzpatrick, J.M., Peak, E., Perally, S., Chalmers, I.W., Barrett, J., Yoshino, T.P., Ivens, A.C., and Hoffmann, K.F. (2009) Anti-schistosomal intervention targets identified by lifecycle transcriptomic analyses. *PLoS Negl. Trop. Dis.*, **3**, e543.

5 Petrocca, F. and Lieberman, J. (2011) Promise and challenge of RNA interference-based therapy for cancer. *J. Clin. Oncol.*, **29**, 747–754.

6 Nemunaitis, J., Rao, D.D., Liu, S.H., and Brunicardi, F.C. (2011) Personalized cancer approach: using RNA interference technology. *World J. Surg.*, **35**, 1700–1714.

7 Davidson, B.L. and McCray, P.B. Jr (2011) Current prospects for RNA interference-based therapies. *Nat. Rev. Genet.*, **12**, 329–340.

8 Hong-Geller, E. and Micheva-Viteva, S.N. (2010) Functional gene discovery using RNA interference-based genomic screens to combat pathogen infection. *Curr. Drug Discov. Technol.*, **7**, 86–94.

9 Tabara, H., Grishok, A., and Mello, C.C. (1998) RNAi in *C. elegans*: soaking in the genome sequence. *Science*, **282**, 430–431.

10 Hunter, C.P. (1999) Genetics: a touch of elegance with RNAi. *Curr. Biol.*, **9**, R440–R442.

11 Fire, A., Xu, S., Montgomery, M.K., Kostas, S.A., Driver, S.E., and Mello, C.C. (1998) Potent and specific genetic interference by double-stranded RNA in *Caenorhabditis elegans*. *Nature*, **391**, 806–811.

12 Timmons, L., Court, D.L., and Fire, A. (2001) Ingestion of bacterially expressed dsRNAs can produce specific and potent genetic interference in *Caenorhabditis elegans*. *Gene*, **263**, 103–112.

13 Grishok, A. and Mello, C.C. (2002) RNAi (nematodes: *Caenorhabditis elegans*). *Adv. Genet.*, **46**, 339–360.

14 Zamore, P.D. (2001) RNA interference: listening to the sound of silence. *Nat. Struct. Biol.*, **8**, 746–750.

15 Grishok, A., Pasquinelli, A.E., Conte, D., Li, N., Parrish, S., Ha, I., Baillie, D.L., Fire, A., Ruvkun, G., and Mello, C.C. (2001) Genes and mechanisms related to RNA interference regulate expression of the small temporal RNAs that control *C. elegans* developmental timing. *Cell*, **106**, 23–34.

16 Wianny, F. and Zernicka-Goetz, M. (2000) Specific interference with gene function by double-stranded RNA in early mouse development. *Nat. Cell Biol.*, **2**, 70–75.

17 Schoppmeier, M. and Damen, W.G. (2001) Double-stranded RNA interference in the spider *Cupiennius salei*: the role of Distal-less is evolutionarily conserved in arthropod appendage formation. *Dev. Genes. Evol*, **211**, 76–82.

18 Morris, J.C., Wang, Z., Drew, M.E., and Englund, P.T. (2002) Glycolysis modulates trypanosome glycoprotein expression as revealed by an RNAi library. *EMBO J.*, **21**, 4429–4438.

19 Shi, H., Djikeng, A., Tschudi, C., and Ullu, E. (2004) Argonaute protein in the early divergent eukaryote *Trypanosoma brucei*: control of small interfering RNA accumulation and retroposon transcript abundance. *Mol. Cell. Biol.*, **24**, 420–427.

20 Robinson, K.A. and Beverley, S.M. (2003) Improvements in transfection efficiency and tests of RNA interference (RNAi) approaches in the protozoan parasite *Leishmania*. *Mol. Biochem. Parasitol.*, **128**, 217–228.

21 DaRocha, W.D., Otsu, K., Teixeira, S.M., and Donelson, J.E. (2004) Tests of cytoplasmic RNA interference (RNAi) and construction of a tetracycline-inducible T7 promoter system in *Trypanosoma cruzi*. *Mol. Biochem. Parasitol.*, **133**, 175–186.

22 Ullu, E., Tschudi, C., and Chakraborty, T. (2004) RNA interference in protozoan parasites. *Cell Microbiol.*, **6**, 509–519.

23 Batista, T.M. and Marques, J.T. (2011) RNAi pathways in parasitic protists and worms. *J. Proteomics*, **74**, 1504–1514.

24 Samarasinghe, B., Knox, D.P., and Britton, C. (2011) Factors affecting susceptibility to RNA interference in *Haemonchus contortus* and *in vivo* silencing of an H11 aminopeptidase gene. *Int. J. Parasitol.*, **41**, 51–59.

25 Viney, M.E. and Thompson, F.J. (2008) Two hypotheses to explain why RNA interference does not work in animal

parasitic nematodes. *Int. J. Parasitol.*, **38**, 43–47.

26 Knox, D.P., Geldhof, P., Visser, A., and Britton, C. (2007) RNA interference in parasitic nematodes of animals: a reality check? *Trends Parasitol.*, **23**, 105–107.

27 Sanchez Alvarado, A. and Newmark, P.A. (1999) Double-stranded RNA specifically disrupts gene expression during planarian regeneration. *Proc. Natl. Acad. Sci. USA*, **96**, 5049–5054.

28 Orii, H., Mochii, M., and Watanabe, K. (2003) A simple "soaking method" for RNA interference in the planarian *Dugesia japonica*. *Dev. Genes. Evol.*, **213**, 138–141.

29 Newmark, P.A., Reddien, P.W., Cebria, F., and Sanchez Alvarado, A. (2003) Ingestion of bacterially expressed double-stranded RNA inhibits gene expression in planarians. *Proc. Natl. Acad. Sci. USA*, **100** (Suppl. 1), 11861–11865.

30 Skelly, P.J., Da'dara, A., and Harn, D.A. (2003) Suppression of cathepsin B expression in *Schistosoma mansoni* by RNA interference. *Int. J. Parasitol.*, **33**, 363–369.

31 Boyle, J.P., Wu, X.J., Shoemaker, C.B., and Yoshino, T.P. (2003) Using RNA interference to manipulate endogenous gene expression in *Schistosoma mansoni* sporocysts. *Mol. Biochem. Parasitol.*, **128**, 205–215.

32 Ndegwa, D., Krautz-Peterson, G., and Skelly, P.J. (2007) Protocols for gene silencing in schistosomes. *Exp. Parasitol.*, **117**, 284–291.

33 Krautz-Peterson, G., Radwanska, M., Ndegwa, D., Shoemaker, C.B., and Skelly, P.J. (2007) Optimizing gene suppression in schistosomes using RNA interference. *Mol. Biochem. Parasitol.*, **153**, 194–202.

34 Stefanic, S., Dvorak, J., Horn, M., Braschi, S., Sojka, D., Ruelas, D.S., Suzuki, B. et al. (2010) RNA interference in *Schistosoma mansoni* schistosomula: selectivity, sensitivity and operation for larger-scale screening. *PLoS Negl. Trop. Dis.*, **4**, e850.

35 Mourao, M.M., Dinguirard, N., Franco, G.R., and Yoshino, T.P. (2009) Phenotypic screen of early-developing larvae of the blood fluke, schistosoma mansoni, using RNA interference. *PLoS Negl. Trop. Dis.*, **3**, e502.

36 Krautz-Peterson, G., Simoes, M., Faghiri, Z., Ndegwa, D., Oliveira, G., Shoemaker, C.B., and Skelly, P.J. (2010) Suppressing glucose transporter gene expression in schistosomes impairs parasite feeding and decreases survival in the mammalian host. *PLoS Pathog.*, **6**, e1000932.

37 Faghiri, Z. and Skelly, P.J. (2009) The role of tegumental aquaporin from the human parasitic worm, *Schistosoma mansoni*, in osmoregulation and drug uptake. *FASEB J.*, **23**, 2780–2789.

38 Correnti, J.M., Brindley, P.J., and Pearce, E.J. (2005) Long-term suppression of cathepsin B levels by RNA interference retards schistosome growth. *Mol. Biochem. Parasitol.*, **143**, 209–215.

39 Correnti, J.M. and Pearce, E.J. (2004) Transgene expression in *Schistosoma mansoni*: introduction of RNA into schistosomula by electroporation. *Mol. Biochem. Parasitol.*, **137**, 75–79.

40 Krautz-Peterson, G., Bhardwaj, R., Faghiri, Z., Tararam, C.A., and Skelly, P.J. (2010) RNA interference in schistosomes: machinery and methodology. *Parasitology*, **137**, 485–495.

41 Tran, M.H., Freitas, T.C., Cooper, L., Gaze, S., Gatton, M.L., Jones, M.K., Lovas, E., Pearce, E.J., and Loukas, A. (2010) Suppression of mRNAs encoding tegument tetraspanins from *Schistosoma mansoni* results in impaired tegument turnover. *PLoS Pathog.*, **6**, e1000840.

42 Tchoubrieva, E.B., Ong, P.C., Pike, R.N., Brindley, P.J., and Kalinna, B.H. (2010) Vector-based RNA interference of cathepsin B1 in *Schistosoma mansoni*. *Cell Mol. Life Sci.*, **67**, 3739–3748.

43 Ayuk, M.A., Suttiprapa, S., Rinaldi, G., Mann, V.H., Lee, C.M., and Brindley, P.J. (2011) *Schistosoma mansoni* U6 gene promoter-driven short hairpin RNA induces RNA interference in human fibrosarcoma cells and schistosomules. *Int. J. Parasitol.*, **41**, 783–789.

44 Skelly, P., Cunningham, J., Kim, J., and Shoemaker, C. (1994) Cloning, characterization and functional expression of cDNAs encoding glucose

transporter proteins from the human parasite, *Schistosoma mansoni*. *J. Biol. Chem.*, **269**, 4247–4253.

45 Rinaldi, G., Morales, M.E., Alrefaei, Y.N., Cancela, M., Castillo, E., Dalton, J.P., Tort, J.F., and Brindley, P.J. (2009) RNA interference targeting leucine aminopeptidase blocks hatching of *Schistosoma mansoni* eggs. *Mol. Biochem. Parasitol.*, **167**, 118–126.

46 Pratt, A.J. and MacRae, I.J. (2009) The RNA-induced silencing complex: a versatile gene-silencing machine. *J. Biol. Chem.*, **284**, 17897–17901.

47 Gomes, M.S., Cabral, F.J., Jannotti-Passos, L.K., Carvalho, O., Rodrigues, V., Baba, E.H., and Sa, R.G. (2009) Preliminary analysis of miRNA pathway in *Schistosoma mansoni*. *Parasitol. Int.*, **58**, 61–68.

48 Luo, R., Xue, X., Wang, Z., Sun, J., Zou, Y., and Pan, W. (2010) Analysis and characterization of the genes encoding the Dicer and Argonaute proteins of *Schistosoma japonicum*. *Parasite Vectors*, **3**, 90.

49 Krautz-Peterson, G. and Skelly, P.J. (2008) *Schistosoma mansoni*: the dicer gene and its expression. *Exp. Parasitol.*, **118**, 122–128.

50 Verjovski-Almeida, S., DeMarco, R., Martins, E.A., Guimaraes, P.E., Ojopi, E.P., Paquola, A.C., Piazza, J.P. *et al.* (2003) Transcriptome analysis of the acoelomate human parasite *Schistosoma mansoni*. *Nat. Genet.*, **35**, 148–157.

51 Hannon, G.J. (2002) RNA interference. *Nature*, **418**, 244–251.

52 Song, L., Gao, S., Jiang, W., Chen, S., Liu, Y., Zhou, L., and Huang, W. (2011) Silencing suppressors: viral weapons for countering host cell defenses. *Protein Cell*, **2**, 273–281.

53 Djikeng, A., Shi, H., Tschudi, C., and Ullu, E. (2001) RNA interference in *Trypanosoma brucei*: cloning of small interfering RNAs provides evidence for retroposon-derived 24–26-nucleotide RNAs. *RNA*, **7**, 1522–1530.

54 Hu, W., Myers, C., Kilzer, J., Pfaff, S., and Bushman, F. (2002) Inhibition of retroviral pathogenesis by RNA interference. *Curr. Biol.*, **12**, 1301.

55 Zilberman, D., Cao, X., and Jacobsen, S.E. (2003) ARGONAUTE4 control of locus-specific siRNA accumulation and DNA and histone methylation. *Science*, **299**, 716–719.

56 Lejeune, E. and Allshire, R.C. (2011) Common ground: small RNA programming and chromatin modifications. *Curr. Opin. Cell Biol.*, **23**, 258–265.

57 Ketting, R.F. (2011) The many faces of RNAi. *Dev. Cell*, **20**, 148–161.

58 Ambros, V., Lee, R.C., Lavanway, A., Williams, P.T., and Jewell, D. (2003) MicroRNAs and other tiny endogenous RNAs in *C. elegans*. *Curr. Biol.*, **13**, 807–818.

59 Lagos-Quintana, M., Rauhut, R., Yalcin, A., Meyer, J., Lendeckel, W., and Tuschl, T. (2002) Identification of tissue-specific microRNAs from mouse. *Curr. Biol.*, **12**, 735–739.

60 Lai, E.C., Tomancak, P., Williams, R.W., and Rubin, G.M. (2003) Computational identification of *Drosophila* microRNA genes. *Genome Biol.*, **4**, R42.

61 Hutvagner, G. and Zamore, P.D. (2002) RNAi: nature abhors a double-strand. *Curr. Opin. Genet. Dev.*, **12**, 225–232.

62 Simoes, M.C., Lee, J., Djikeng, A., Cerqueira, G.C., Zerlotini, A., da Silva-Pereira, R.A., Dalby, A.R. *et al.* (2011) Identification of *Schistosoma mansoni* microRNAs. *BMC Genomics*, **12**, 47.

63 Copeland, C.S., Marz, M., Rose, D., Hertel, J., Brindley, P.J., Santana, C.B., Kehr, S. *et al.* (2009) Homology-based annotation of non-coding RNAs in the genomes of *Schistosoma mansoni* and *Schistosoma japonicum*. *BMC Genomics*, **10**, 464.

64 Xue, X., Sun, J., Zhang, Q., Wang, Z., Huang, Y., and Pan, W. (2008) Identification and characterization of novel microRNAs from *Schistosoma japonicum*. *PLoS One*, **3**, e4034.

65 Whangbo, J.S. and Hunter, C.P. (2008) Environmental RNA interference. *Trends Genet.*, **24**, 297–305.

66 Winston, W.M., Molodowitch, C., and Hunter, C.P. (2002) Systemic RNAi in *C. elegans* requires the putative

transmembrane protein SID-1. *Science*, **295**, 2456–2459.

67 Shih, J.D., Fitzgerald, M.C., Sutherlin, M., and Hunter, C.P. (2009) The SID-1 double-stranded RNA transporter is not selective for dsRNA length. *RNA*, **15**, 384–390.

68 Feinberg, E.H. and Hunter, C.P. (2003) Transport of dsRNA into cells by the transmembrane protein SID-1. *Science*, **301**, 1545–1547.

69 Freitas, T.C., Jung, E., and Pearce, E.J. (2007) TGF-beta signaling controls embryo development in the parasitic flatworm Schistosoma mansoni. *PLoS Pathog.*, **3**, e52.

70 Faghiri, Z., Camargo, S.M., Huggel, K., Forster, I.C., Ndegwa, D., Verrey, F., and Skelly, P.J. (2010) The tegument of the human parasitic worm schistosoma mansoni as an excretory organ: the surface aquaporin SmAQP is a lactate transporter. *PLoS One*, **5**, e10451.

71 Mourao Mde, M., Dinguirard, N., Franco, G.R., and Yoshino, T.P. (2009) Role of the endogenous antioxidant system in the protection of Schistosoma mansoni primary sporocysts against exogenous oxidative stress. *PLoS Negl. Trop. Dis.*, **3**, e550.

72 Krautz-Peterson, G., Camargo, S., Huggel, K., Verrey, F., Shoemaker, C.B., and Skelly, P.J. (2007) Amino acid transport in schistosomes: characterization of the permease heavy chain SPRM1hc. *J. Biol. Chem.*, **282**, 21767–21775.

73 Bhardwaj, R. and Skelly, P.J. (2011) Characterization of schistosome tegumental alkaline phosphatase (SmAP). *PLoS Negl. Trop. Dis.*, **5**, e1011.

74 Krautz-Peterson, G., Bhardwaj, R., Faghiri, Z., Tararam, C.A., and Skelly, P.J. (2010) RNA interference in schistosomes: machinery and methodology. *Parasitology*, **137**, 485–495.

75 Dusanic, D.G. (1959) Histochemical observations of alkaline phosphatase in Schistosoma mansoni. *J. Infect. Dis.*, **105**, 1–8.

76 Halton, D.W. (1967) Studies on phosphatase activity in trematoda. *J. Parasitol.*, **53**, 46–54.

77 Sayed, A.A., Cook, S.K., and Williams, D.L. (2006) Redox balance mechanisms in Schistosoma mansoni rely on peroxiredoxins and albumin and implicate peroxiredoxins as novel drug targets. *J. Biol. Chem.*, **281**, 17001–17010.

78 Kuntz, A.N., Davioud-Charvet, E., Sayed, A.A., Califf, L.L., Dessolin, J., Arner, E.S., and Williams, D.L. (2007) Thioredoxin glutathione reductase from Schistosoma mansoni: an essential parasite enzyme and a key drug target. *PLoS Med.*, **4**, e206.

79 Pecot, C.V., Calin, G.A., Coleman, R.L., Lopez-Berestein, G., and Sood, A.K. (2011) RNA interference in the clinic: challenges and future directions. *Nat. Rev. Cancer*, **11**, 59–67.

80 Walton, S.P., Wu, M., Gredell, J.A., and Chan, C. (2010) Designing highly active siRNAs for therapeutic applications. *FEBS J.*, **277**, 4806–4813.

81 Tiemann, K. and Rossi, J.J. (2009) RNAi-based therapeutics-current status, challenges and prospects. *EMBO Mol. Med.*, **1**, 142–151.

82 Pereira, T.C., Pascoal, V.D., Marchesini, R.B., Maia, I.G., Magalhaes, L.A., Zanotti-Magalhaes, E.M., and Lopes-Cendes, I. (2008) Schistosoma mansoni: evaluation of an RNAi-based treatment targeting HGPRTase gene. *Exp. Parasitol.*, **118**, 619–623.

83 Cheng, G., Fu, Z., Lin, J., Shi, Y., Zhou, Y., Jin, Y., and Cai, Y. (2009) In vitro and in vivo evaluation of small interference RNA-mediated gynaecophoral canal protein silencing in Schistosoma japonicum. *J. Gene Med.*, **11**, 412–421.

84 Seyhan, A.A. (2011) RNAi: a potential new class of therapeutic for human genetic disease. *Hum. Genet.*, **130**, 583–605.

85 Boudreau, R.L., Rodriguez-Lebron, E., and Davidson, B.L. (2011) RNAi medicine for the brain: progresses and challenges. *Hum. Mol. Genet.*, **20**, R21–R27.

86 Angaji, S.A., Hedayati, S.S., Poor, R.H., Madani, S., Poor, S.S., and Panahi, S. (2010) Application of RNA interference in treating human diseases. *J. Genet.*, **89**, 527–537.

87 McGonigle, L., Mousley, A., Marks, N.J., Brennan, G.P., Dalton, J.P., Spithill, T.W.,

Day, T.A., and Maule, A.G. (2008) The silencing of cysteine proteases in *Fasciola hepatica* newly excysted juveniles using RNA interference reduces gut penetration. *Int. J. Parasitol.*, **38**, 149–155.

88 Sripa, J., Pinlaor, P., Brindley, P.J., Sripa, B., Kaewkes, S., Robinson, M.W., Young, N.D. *et al.* (2011) RNA interference targeting cathepsin B of the carcinogenic liver fluke, *Opisthorchis viverrini*. *Parasitol. Int.*, **60**, 283–288.

89 Pierson, L., Mousley, A., Devine, L., Marks, N.J., Day, T.A., and Maule, A.G. (2010) RNA interference in a cestode reveals specific silencing of selected highly expressed gene transcripts. *Int. J. Parasitol.*, **40**, 605–615.

90 Mizukami, C., Spiliotis, M., Gottstein, B., Yagi, K., Katakura, K., and Oku, Y. (2010) Gene silencing in *Echinococcus multilocularis* protoscoleces using RNA interference. *Parasitol. Int.*, **59**, 647–652.

91 Spiliotis, M., Mizukami, C., Oku, Y., Kiss, F., Brehm, K., and Gottstein, B. (2010) *Echinococcus multilocularis* primary cells: improved isolation, small-scale cultivation and RNA interference. *Mol. Biochem. Parasitol.*, **174**, 83–87.

92 Bhardwaj, R., Krautz-Peterson, G., Da'dara, A., Tzipori, S., and Skelly, P.J. (2011) Tegumental phosphodiesterase SmNPP-5 is a virulence factor for schistosomes. *Infect. Immun.*, **79**, 4276–4284.

Part Two
Screens

8
Mechanism-Based Screening Strategies for Anthelmintic Discovery

Timothy G. Geary

Abstract

Until the late 1980s, anthelmintic discovery relied on whole-organism-based approaches. Methods employing nematodes or flatworms in culture were not very successful in identifying new compounds; a prominent drawback of many such screens was the high proportion of false-positives (compounds active in culture, but not in infected animals). This factor, along with the almost complete adoption of mechanism-based approaches in all other pharmaceutical operations, led to the development and incorporation of such strategies for anthelmintic discovery. The lack of suitable functional genomics platforms for parasitic nematodes made the choice of novel targets for screening a difficult step, as validation prior to screening could only be done in surrogate organisms and only for drugs that were inhibitors or antagonists of parasite proteins. Although no new anthelmintics have yet emerged from mechanism-based screens, relatively few attempts have been made with this strategy and it remains compelling. This chapter summarizes some attempts at anthelmintic discovery through high-throughput, mechanism-based screens and discusses possible solutions to problems that remain to be resolved to improve the success rate of this strategy.

Introduction

All available antiparasitic drugs, or at least the prototypes for all classes, were discovered in low-throughput screens that employed parasites (either target or surrogate species) in infected host animals or, less frequently, in culture. In the anthelmintic area, other than the screen for new drugs for human filariasis that led to the discovery of diethylcarbamazine [1], all the work that led to marketed drugs in this area over the past 50 years was pioneered in the animal health industry [2]. Considerable economic value is realized by drugs for use in livestock or companion animal species, unlike the case for human helminthiases, which benefited instead through the eventual transfer of some of those drugs into human medical applications [2]. Although undeniably productive [3], the infected-animal screening model for anthelmintic discovery was maintained as the primary strategy only from the 1950s until the 1980s, at which time it was supplemented or replaced with

Parasitic Helminths: Targets, Screens, Drugs and Vaccines, First Edition. Edited by Conor R. Caffrey.
© 2012 Wiley-VCH Verlag GmbH & Co. KGaA. Published 2012 by Wiley-VCH Verlag GmbH & Co. KGaA.

whole-organism screens that employed various life stages of target parasites or their surrogates, including the free-living nematode species *Caenorhabditis elegans*, in culture. The motivation for this switch was the desire to more efficiently identify lead compounds that could then be validated in infected-animal models, taking advantage of the development of increased industrial investment in burgeoning medicinal chemistry programs that were producing more compounds, and in lower amounts, than could be accommodated in the low-throughput infected animal models.

Whole-organism screens require much lower amounts of compounds, considerably less labor (depending on the species used for screening; some require expensive and laborious methods to maintain the life cycle), and less time for completion than infected animal models, and can operate at considerably higher throughput. In the nematode realm, many investigators chose *C. elegans* as a screening tool [4] (see also Chapters 2 and 12), while others used free-living larval stages of parasitic species such as *Haemonchus contortus* or another trichostrongylid species. This era of anthelmintic discovery began in the 1980s and although less productive than the infected-animal models that discovered almost all the marketed anthelmintic classes, the strategy is a useful compromise among factors such as throughput, compound requirements, and labor demand with the desire to retain a healthy degree of serendipity in the discovery process. A prominent disadvantage of these screens is the use of nontarget stages (such as free-living L3 stages of trichostrongylid species) or nonparasites (*C. elegans*). Also, because such screens are quite good at finding nonspecifically nematocidal substances, they must be accompanied by the sometimes onerous burden of identifying the most interesting leads by *in vivo* testing. Typically, thousands of hits can be found per year in an *in vitro* screen, of which only a very small number (often zero!) are active in a follow-up animal model. Due to the large number of initial hits, it is generally not possible to investigate reasons for inactivity *in vivo* of "interesting" *in vitro* hits (which may include relatively mundane clinical pharmacology factors). An *in vitro* hit that is not active in the next-step animal model may have intrinsic value as an anthelmintic lead, but will not be pursued because it fails to attain therapeutic concentrations at the site of infection for a sufficient duration ("exposure") to achieve detectable efficacy. Screening in animal models only finds actives that already exhibit some degree of pharmaceutical suitability, but the concerns about resource and throughput outlined above restrict broader use of these screens. An additional issue for *in vitro* screens is the recently realized possibility that this strategy may have missed useful compounds because they fail to accumulate in the test species in culture [5] (see also Chapter 12).

The "whole organism in culture" strategy for anthelmintic discovery was augmented or replaced in some anthelmintic discovery programs by high-throughput, mechanism-based screens beginning in the mid-1980s. In this strategy, a chemical collection is screened for interaction with (generally) a parasite protein that is known or predicted to be a target for chemotherapeutic intervention [6–8]. The premise behind this strategy is that compounds that affect the function of an essential parasite protein can lead to derivatives that kill the parasite in culture and in the host. This strategy became the method of choice for the discovery of drugs for most human diseases. Whereas subsequent genome-wide association studies have generally failed to confirm that single gene defects underlie some of the major target diseases for drug discovery and developmental pipelines have dried up across the industry, this concern is less significant for infectious diseases. Conceptually, it is much simpler to chemically interfere with function of an essential parasite protein than it is to restore normal function to a complex, multifactorial human system that is in disequilibrium. This principle is most clearly illustrated in the explosion of new anticancer drugs that are targeted to specific proteins essential for the growth of a particular tumor type, escaping the traditional model of cytotoxic drugs that could be applied to a variety of cancers.

Adoption of mechanism-based screens for anthelmintics was motivated by several factors [6–8]. As the human pharmaceutical industry adopted technology for high-throughput mechanism-based screening, chemical inventories became miniaturized and automated, and access to these samples became more restricted for initial screening. The ultrahigh throughput attainable with mechanism-based screens became the standard, and screens that operated at lower rates and demanded larger amounts of chemicals lost favor. Implementation of new medicinal chemistry processes such as combinatorial chemistry necessitated roboticized, miniaturized screening platforms, which are difficult to adopt for helminths. A drive to reduce labor costs in favor of depreciable instruments also limited acceptance of biology-based screens. Finally, the rapid turnaround time for mechanism-based screens was highly favored over the long duration employed for whole-organism screens (often 1 week of exposure, e.g., with *C. elegans*).

The primary advantage of mechanism-based anthelmintic screens relates to the necessity of focusing investment in chemistry around new leads. The limiting resource in drug discovery is the ability to provide close analogs around a hit compound to generate higher-value derivatives for development that exhibit better intrinsic potency and/or improved pharmaceutical properties. As noted, the hit rate in whole-organism screens was too high to allow chemical investigation of even a small percentage of them and no good way to prioritize the hits. Investigating a compound with a known mechanism of action permits a series of hypothesis-based experiments to validate it as a lead. Proof of high affinity against the target can be followed up with whole-organism assays that include a measurement of compound permeation into the test organism (measuring exposure of the target *in situ*) and consequent changes in target function. If the effect of the compound on the target is detected, but the viability or behavior of the organism is unchanged, a conclusion can be drawn that the target is not suitable and attention can be directed to other series. Infected animal screens can include a pharmacodynamic component to ensure that adequate exposure is attained *in vivo*. If adequate exposure is attained (based on *in vitro* results), but efficacy is not observed, a conclusion can be reached that normal function of the target is not required for survival in the host and again the investment may be redirected with confidence that a hidden gem has not been overlooked.

This chapter does not address in depth issues of anthelmintic discovery based on drug design via *in silico* screening of chemicals in virtual operations, computationally analyzing docking of three-dimensional molecules to putative receptor sites in parasite proteins [9]. This process uses estimates of fit (deduced in various ways with emphasis on various parameters) to prioritize hundreds of thousands of compounds, and then select those to be tested in target-based assays and whole-organism screens. Although this strategy has proven valuable in other areas of chemotherapy, only a few programs for helminth target proteins have advanced to the published literature. One screen focused on purine nucleoside phosphorylase in *Schistosoma mansoni* [10]. A collection of over 850 000 commercially available compounds was virtually screened, leading to the identification of several hits with IC_{50} values against this enzyme in the low micromolar range. Whether any was active against parasites in culture or in animals, or was selective for the parasite enzyme, has not been reported.

Similarly, this chapter does not address the topics of anthelmintic target identification or validation, which are covered in other chapters in this volume.

Mechanism-Based Screens for Anthelmintics: Examples

Public disclosure of screens is not routine in the pharmaceutical industry, although recent examples in malaria screening are a welcome development (see https://www.ebi.ac.uk/chemblntd), so it is not possible to provide a comprehensive review of such efforts. Based on the published literature and some patents, however, an instructive overview of the kinds of programs undertaken illuminates the potential utility of the approach.

Screens for Enzyme Inhibitors

An early example of this strategy is embodied in a series of screens for inhibitors of nematode enzymes that employed recombinant microbes as hosts for their functional expression. Screens based on this technology have been developed for a number of enzyme targets in protozoa and helminths [11, 12]. Employing deletion mutants of *Escherichia coli* or *Saccharomyces cerevisiae* complemented with the parasite (in this case, *H. contortus*) homolog, a nutrient-dependent viability approach was used to screen for inhibitors of nematode phosphofructokinase (PFK), phosphoenolpyruvate carboxykinase (PEPCK), and ornithine decarboxylase (ODC) [13–15]. The principle of the assay for glycolytic enzyme inhibitors involves exposure of the recombinant microbe to test compounds in the presence of an essential nutrient that requires the action of the parasite enzyme for utilization (for PFK, a hexose such as mannitol); hits are then retested in medium that contains a nutrient that bypasses the requirement for the parasite enzyme (glycerol) [11]. Hits that are active in the first medium, but not the second, are candidate enzyme inhibitors and are further investigated in enzyme assays to verify the site of action. A slightly different paradigm was used in a screen for inhibitors of *H. contortus* ODC in a medium devoid of exogenous polyamines; test compounds were assayed for inhibition of growth of an ODC null mutant of *S. cerevisiae* functionally complemented with an *H. contortus* gene encoding this enzyme [12, 15]. Positives were then retested in the presence of 10 μM spermidine. Compounds for which toxicity was reversed by the presence of spermidine were considered candidate ODC inhibitors and were tested in enzyme assays. A screen of more than 90 000 synthetic compounds [15] revealed a single polyamine-dependent positive, stilbamidine, which was subsequently identified to be an inhibitor of S-adenosylmethionine decarboxylase – an enzyme in the polyamine pathway.

An alternative strategy for the use of recombinant microbes involves screening for selective inhibition of parasite versus host enzymes in microbes complemented with a gene encoding the target enzyme from either organism. An early example of this approach was a screen for selective inhibitors of hypoxanthine phosphoribosyl transferase in strains of E. coli complemented with the homologous enzyme from S. mansoni, several protozoan parasites, and humans [16]. Relatively selective purine derivatives were identified by screening a modest number of compounds.

In a more recent embodiment, this strategy was used to devise a screen for compounds that inhibit Wolbachia enzymes involved in heme synthesis [17]. Wolbachia is a bacterial symbiont in many filariid parasites and possesses a metabolic pathway of essential importance to the nematode – heme synthesis. Indeed, heme synthesis genes are absent from the phylum Nematoda. A series of recombinant strains of E. coli expressing the homologous enzyme from Wolbachia or mammals permits screening for selective inhibitors of the former through detection of differential toxicity.

Screens that employ recombinant microbes provide several advantages [11, 12], including the fact that an initial indication of selectivity is attained, since compounds that act indiscriminately on proteins will not be detected. In addition, since multiple kinds of targets (enzymes, nuclear receptors, ion channels, G-protein-coupled receptors (GPCRs), etc.) can be accommodated in recombinant microbes, a wide variety of targets can be screened in a constant format (measuring microbial viability and growth). Recombinant microbe platforms have particular value in resource-poor settings, since assays of microbial viability are very simple and do not require expensive or demanding technology suites.

In more typical approaches, screens have been performed with purified recombinant helminth enzymes. Of recent interest are reports of inhibitors of S. mansoni thioredoxin glutathione reductase (TGR) in a novel assay for inhibitors of schistosome redox metabolism [18] (see also Chapter 20). The format measured the transfer of reducing equivalents from NADPH to H_2O_2 through the activity of TGR coupled to schistosome peroxiredoxin. Actives included the known compound auranofin [19], which has been used in the treatment of rheumatoid arthritis in human and is also reported to be an inhibitor of PFK [20]. A novel series of oxadiazoles was also discovered; these compounds appear to act as NO donors to inhibit the target enzyme [21]. Potent derivatives with *in vivo* activity in mice have been reported and provide the most promising anthelmintic leads derived from mechanism-based high-throughput screening (HTS) to date.

A recombinant form of an S. mansoni surface protein, termed NAD^+-catabolizing enzyme (SmNACE), has been subjected to a screen of around 14 000 synthetic chemicals and natural products [22]. This enzyme is postulated to play a role in managing the host NAD-dependent immune response, and is structurally and mechanistically distinct from host NAD-catabolizing enzymes. It is therefore a potential antischistosomal drug target. The screen was based on changes in NAD concentration measured by a fluorescent reporter. Several natural products in the flavonoid class were identified as hits, most notably cyanidin and delphinidin, with IC_{50} values in the micromolar range [22]. Whether any compound or derivative in this class can be optimized as a selective inhibitor of SmNACE, in addition to demonstrating antischistosomal activity *in vitro* or *in vivo*, remains to be seen.

An HTS campaign has also been run for *Brugia malayi* asparaginyl-tRNA synthetase using Malachite Green to form a product with phosphate liberated from the pyrophosphate generated during the reaction [23]. Screening a large collection of microbial fermentation extracts led to the identification of tirandamycins as inhibitors of this enzyme; the best compound had an IC_{50} value of 30 µM and proved lethal to adult *B. malayi* in culture with an IC_{50} value of around 1 µM [24]. This compound is reported to be about 10-fold selective for the nematode enzyme versus the host synthetase, but the class is known to have other biological activities as well. Further work will reveal their potential as leads for chemotherapy of filariasis.

Another example in the area of filariasis is a screen for inhibitors of *Onchocerca volvulus* chitinase, using an enzyme assay to test a collection of around 1500 licensed drugs [25]. Chitinase expression is linked to molting in larval development and may have other functions in worm biology. The known anthelmintic closantel was found to inhibit chitinase with an IC_{50} value of around 1 µM; it inhibited molting of L3 larvae of *O. volvulus* at 100 µM in culture [25]. This molecule is known to have protonophoric activity and a small medicinal chemistry campaign was subsequently able to generate derivatives that had selective activity as protonophores or chitinase inhibitors. Both mechanisms had antifilarial activity in culture [26]. The compounds have relatively low potency in these assays and whether a useful drug can emerge from this template, or against this target (molting), will only be clear with additional research.

Work has also been done with extracts or subcellular fractions of helminths as enzyme substrates for HTS. The Kitasato Institute in Japan employed submitochondrial particles isolated from *Ascaris suum* to identify natural products that inhibit the unusual nematode electron transport pathway, with a focus on fumarate reductase. Nafuredin, produced by a strain of *Aspergillus niger*, is a potent inhibitor of this complex with remarkable selectivity for the nematode pathway compared to host mitochondria [27]. This molecule was active and safe in sheep infected with *H. contortus* at a dose of 2 mg/kg, but its further development as an anthelmintic has not been reported. Subsequent work from the same group identified additional inhibitors of this complex, including verticipyrone, produced by *Verticillium* sp. FKI-1083 [28]. This compound inhibited *A. suum* fumarate reductase with an IC_{50} value below 1 nM and was highly selective for the nematode complex compared to mammalian electron transport. It is modestly potent against *C. elegans* in culture and possible advantages over nafuredin as an anthelmintic have not been reported.

Additional examples of helminth enzymes that are good candidate drug targets are readily available, although few have been expressed or prepared in a format suitable for HTS. A target that could easily be subjected to HTS is heat-shock protein Hsp90 from *B. malayi* [29], using an assay that measures competition for binding of radiolabeled geldanomycin to Hsp90 in extracts of *B. malayi*; results from such a screen have not yet been reported.

Neuromuscular Targets in HTS

The second category of important anthelmintic targets includes receptors and ion channels that function in the neuromuscular system (see also Chapters 1, 2 and 14). Such proteins are the targets of most of the commercially available anthelmintics. Several kinds of assays have been employed to identify candidate anthelmintic leads that act on these receptors. A considerable effort has been devoted to discovering nonpeptide agonists or antagonists for receptors for a family of neuropeptides related to FMRFamide (FMRFamide-like peptides (FLPs)) that are exceptionally broadly distributed in invertebrates, but almost absent from vertebrates [30–32]. The first example of an assay for this target used a ligand displacement strategy to detect nonpeptide ligands for binding sites (receptors) for [^{125}I]KHEYLRFamide (AF2) on *A. suum* muscle membrane preparations [33, 34]. This assay identified several different lead series with modest affinity for this binding site, but none has been reported to have entered into development.

A more intensive effort in this area targeted a family of GPCRs cloned from *C. elegans* which have FLP ligands [25–37]. This strategy utilizes recombinant *C. elegans* FLP-GPCRs expressed in mammalian cells or in a strain of *S. cerevisiae* that enables HTS in a microbial growth format [38, 39]. No lead identified in these campaigns has been reported to have entered development [40]. However, a platform based on recombinant yeast strains expressing nematode FLP-GPCRs has been adapted for on-site screening of natural products collections in Africa (T.G. Geary, unpublished observations). The platform enjoys the same benefits outlined above for other recombinant microbe-based screens for low-resource settings: robust and simple end-points with minimal technical requirements for operation. The same system has been used to express helminth GPCRs that recognize classical neurotransmitters, broadening the potential range of anthelmintic targets that can be screened in this platform [41, 42].

Another example in this area is a screen for ligands of a *H. contortus* serotonin (5-hydroxytryptamine (5-HT)) receptor that is expressed in mammalian or insect cells [43]. A limited screen identified a known 5-HT ligand, *p*-amino-phenethyl-*m*-trifluoromethylphenyl piperazine (PAPP), as a potent ligand for this receptor with subnanomolar affinity. PAPP is a selective ligand for mammalian 5-HT$_{1A}$ receptors and was only modestly selective for the nematode GPCR compared to the mammalian target. However, the compound was active (at high doses) against some trichostrongylid species in sheep [44]. It did not exhibit the breadth of spectrum typically required for anthelmintics marketed for this indication and whether further analogs were developed to enhance clinical activity has not been reported.

Finally, it has been postulated for some time that nematodes and arthropods are phylogenetically related [45] – a relationship evident in the cross-phylum activity of macrocyclic lactone endectocides such as ivermectin [46]. In this context, a screen for ligands that bind to a cockroach ryanodine receptor in membrane preparations identified the natural product verticilide, produced by *Verticillium* sp. FKI-1033 [47]. This compound was reported to be active against *C. elegans* at relatively high concentrations [47]; however, its evaluation as an anthelmintic has not been reported.

Challenges and Prospects for Anthelmintic HTS

The ultimate validation of a putative anthelmintic drug target is provided by a chemical that acts through that protein to significantly reduce parasite viability in culture and/or in an infected animal. Selecting from among a plethora of anthelmintic candidates to screen is not a simple matter and considerations of essentiality can only be easily addressed in model organisms such as *C. elegans*, which reflect the biology of parasitic species in their hosts to an uncertain degree [4]. As parasite genomes become more readily available, spectrum becomes an important variable for analysis spectrum: is the target protein highly conserved among helminth species of therapeutic importance? Convenience of assay is another important variable for prioritization, including both initial screening and follow-up in whole-organism models, especially those that employ the target parasite species. The biological activity of initial hits must be evaluated in a pharmacodynamic context, measuring exposure of the target (internal helminth concentrations) at therapeutic levels in culture [48] to ensure that the activity of the compound is mediated only through the target protein. Specificity of action makes the interpretation of subsequent toxicological data simpler, validates medicinal chemistry around the target, and prevents investment of resources in a low-value series with a nonspecific mechanism of action. This analysis should include a time-to-kill (or affect) analysis; compounds that require several days of exposure to higher than $10\,\mu M$ concentrations to cause a detectable effect are unlikely to be efficacious in animal models given the challenge of maintaining such high plasma concentrations for prolonged periods via convenient dosing regimens. An early medicinal chemistry program (or otherwise obtaining a large set of close analogs) may be indicated to identify related compounds with intrinsic affinity for the target below $1\,\mu M$ prior to evaluation in infected animal models.

Choice of a chemical collection to screen is also crucially important. Virtual collections of commercially available compounds have evident value, as the screening laboratory can (usually) purchase sufficient amounts of hit compounds for follow-up evaluation. Even in such cases, chemical validation of the compound is an important criterion to ensure authenticity. An underutilized compound source that has generated abundant antiparasitic drugs is natural products derived from botanical and microbial origins. These kinds of compounds have particularly rich history in all areas of chemotherapy, but have not usually been favored for other indications and are no longer often included in industrial or commercial screening sets. Mechanism-based screens for anthelmintics should include such compound resources as a priority for the same reasons noted above: detection of an extract as active in such a screen is more than sufficient justification for the investment of the chemistry resources needed to identify the active compound(s) and prepare enough of it for follow-up evaluation.

Despite the inability of target-based HTS programs to deliver the quantity and quality of new drugs needed to sustain large pharmaceutical companies, there are few reasons to believe that another major paradigm shift in drug discovery is on the horizon. The strategy has clear advantages for conditions and diseases that are amenable to single-target intervention, and helminth chemotherapy remains a viable opportunity. Difficulties in performing truly HTS using helminths in culture mean that the mechanism-based approach remains a valued alternative. However, the optimal strategy is an integrated approach that uses both whole-organism screens to assay specific compound sets and mechanism-based HTS to sample larger collections. In either case, incisive, rapid, and thorough secondary testing of hits is necessary for efficiency in decision making, allowing the discovery team to intensively focus on truly promising hits as early in the process as possible.

References

1 Santiago-Stevenson, D., Oliver-Gonzalez, J., and Hewitt, R.I. (1947) Treatment of filariasis bancrofti with 1-diethylcarbamyl-4-methylpiperazine hydrochloride ("Hetrazan"). *J. Am. Med. Assoc.*, **135**, 708–712.

2 Geary, T.G., Woo, K., McCarthy, J.S., Mackenzie, C.D., Horton, J., Prichard, R.K., de Silva, N.R. *et al.* (2010) Unresolved issues in anthelmintic pharmacology for helminthiases of humans. *Int. J. Parasitol.*, **40**, 1–13.

3 Woods, D.J., Lauret, C., and Geary, T.G. (2007) Anthelmintic discovery and development in the animal health industry. *Expert Opin. Drug Discov.*, **2** (Suppl. 1), S25–S33.

4 Geary, T.G. and Thompson, D.P. (2001) *Caenorhabditis elegans*: how good a model for veterinary parasites? *Vet. Parasitol.*, **101**, 371–386.

5 Ruiz-Lancheros, E., Viau, C., Walter, T.N., Francis, A., and Geary, T.G. (2011) Activity of novel nicotinic anthelmintics in cut preparations of *C. elegans*. *Int. J. Parasitol.*, **41**, 455–461.

6 Thompson, D.P., Klein, R.D., and Geary, T.G. (1996) Prospects for rational approaches to anthelmintic discovery. *Parasitology*, **113**, S217–S238.

7 Witty, M.J. (1999) Current strategies in the search for novel antiparasitic agents. *Int. J. Parasitol.*, **29**, 95–103.

8 Geary, T.G., Thompson, D.P., and Klein, R.D. (1999) Mechanism-based screening: discovery of the next generation of anthelmintics depends upon more basic research. *Int. J. Parasitol.*, **29**, 105–112.

9 Guido, R.V.C. and Oliva, G. (2009) Structure-based drug discovery for tropical diseases. *Curr. Top. Med. Chem.*, **9**, 824–843.

10 Postigo, M.P., Guido, R.V.C., Oliva, G., Castilho, M.S., Pitta, I.daR., de Albuquerque, J.F.C., and Andricopulo, A.D. (2010) Discovery of new inhibitors of *Schistosoma mansoni* PNP by pharmacophore-based virtual screening. *J. Chem. Inf. Model.*, **50**, 1693–1705.

11 Klein, R.D. and Geary, T.G. (1997) Recombinant microorganisms as tools for high-throughput screening for non-antibiotic compounds. *J. Biomol. Screen.*, **2**, 41–49.

12 Geary, T.G. (2001) Screening for parasiticides using recombinant microorganisms, in *Enzyme Technology for Pharmaceutical and Biotechnological Applications* (eds H.A. Kirst, W.-K. Yeh, M. Zmijewski, and

13 Klein, R.D., Olson, E.R., Favreau, M.A., Winterrowd, C.A., Hatzenbuhler, N.T., Shea, M.H., Nulf, S.C., and Geary, T.G. (1991) Cloning of a cDNA encoding phosphofructokinase from *Haemonchus contortus*. *Mol. Biochem. Parasitol.*, **48**, 17–26.

14 Klein, R.D., Winterrowd, C.A., Hatzenbuhler, N.T., Shea, M.H., Favreau, M.A., Nulf, S.C., and Geary, T.G. (1992) Cloning of a cDNA encoding phosphoenolpyruvate carboxykinase from *Haemonchus contortus*. *Mol. Biochem. Parasitol.*, **50**, 285–294.

15 Klein, R.D., Favreau, M.A., Alexander-Bowman, S.J., Nulf, S.C., Vanover, L., Winterrowd, C.A., Yarlett, N., Martinez, M., Keithly, J.S., Zantello, M.A., Thomas, E.M., and Geary, T.G. (1997) *Haemonchus contortus*: cloning and functional expression of a cDNA encoding ornithine decarboxylase and development of a screen for inhibitors. *Exp. Parasitol.*, **87**, 171–184.

16 Eakin, A.E., Nives-Alicea, R., Tosado-Acevedo, R., Chin, M.S., Wang, C.C., and Craig, S.P. III (1995) Comparative complement selection in bacteria enables screening for lead compounds targeted to a purine salvage enzyme of parasites. *Antimicrob. Agents Chemother.*, **39**, 620–625.

17 Wu, B., Novelli, J., Foster, J., Vaisvila, R., Conway, L., Ingram, J., Ganatra, M., Rao, A.U., Hamza, I., and Slatko, B. (2009) The heme biosynthetic pathway of the obligate *Wolbachia* symbiont of *Brugia malayi* as a potential anti-filarial drug target. *PLoS Negl. Trop. Dis.*, **3**, e45.

18 Simeonov, A., Jadhav, A., Sayed, A.A., Wang, Y., Nelson, M.E., Thomas, C.J., Inglese, J., Williams, D.L., and Austin, C.P. (2008) Quantitative high-throughput screen identifies inhibitors of the *Schistosoma mansoni* redox cascade. *PLoS Negl. Trop. Dis.*, **2**, e127.

19 Angelucci, F., Sayed, A.A., Williams, D.L., Boumis, G., Brunori, M., Dimastrogiovanni, D., Miele, A.E. et al. (2009) Inhibition of *Schistosoma mansoni* thioredoxin-glutathione reductase by auranofin. Structural and kinetic aspects. *J. Biol. Chem.*, **284**, 28977–28985.

20 Anderson, R., Van Rensburg, C.E., Joone, G.K., and Lessing, A. (1991) Auranofin inactivates phosphofructokinase in human neutrophils, leading to depletion of intracellular ATP and inhibition of superoxide generation and locomotion. *Mol. Pharmacol.*, **40**, 427–434.

21 Sayed, A.A., Simeonov, A., Thomas, C.J., Inglese, J., Austin, C.P., and Williams, D.L. (2008) Identification of oxadiazoles as new drug leads for the control of schistosomiasis. *Nat. Med.*, **14**, 407–412.

22 Kuhn, I., Kellenberger, E., Said-Hassane, F., Villa, P., Rognan, D., Lobstein, A., Haiech, J. et al. (2010) Identification by high-throughput screening of inhibitors of *Schistosoma mansoni* NAD^+ catabolizing enzyme. *Biorg. Med. Chem.*, **18**, 7900–7910.

23 Danel, F., Caspers, P., Nuoffer, C., Hartlein, M., Kron, M.A., and Page, M.G.P. (2011) Asparaginyl-tRNA synthetase pre-transfer editing assay. *Curr. Drug Discov. Technol.*, **8**, 66–75.

24 Yu, Z., Vodanovic-Jankovic, S., Ledeboer, N., Huang, S.-X., Rajski, S.R., Kron, M., and Shen, B. (2011) Tirandamycins from *Streptomyces* sp. 17944 inhibiting the parasite *Brugia malayi* asparagine tRNA synthetase. *Org. Lett.*, **13**, 2034–2037.

25 Gloeckner, C., Garner, A.L., Mersha, F., Oksov, Y., Trichoche, N., Eubanks, L.M., Lustigman, S., Kaufmann, G.F., and Janda, K.D. (2010) Repositioning of an existing drug for the neglected tropical disease Onchocerciasis. *Proc. Natl. Acad. Sci. USA*, **107**, 3424–3429.

26 Garner, A.L., Gloeckner, C., Tricoche, N., Zakhari, J.S., Samje, M., Cho-Ngwa, F., Lustigman, S., and Janda, K.D. (2011) Design, synthesis and biological activities of closantel analogues: structural promiscuity and its impact on *Onchocerca volvulus*. *J. Med. Chem.*, **54**, 3963–3972.

27 Ōmura, S., Miyadera, H., Ui, H., Shiomi, K., Yamaguchi, Y., Masuma, R., Nagamitsu, T. et al. (2001) An

anthelmintic compound, nafuredin, shows selective inhibition of complex I in helminth mitochondria. *Proc. Natl. Acad. Sci. USA*, **98**, 60–62.

28 Ui, H., Shiomi, K., Suzuki, H., Hatano, H., Morimoto, H., Yamaguchi, Y., Masuma, R. *et al.* (2006) Verticipyrone, a new NADH-fumarate reductase inhibitor, produced by *Verticillium* sp. FKI-1083. *J. Antibiot.*, **59**, 785–790.

29 Taldone, T., Gillan, V., Sun, W., Rodina, A., Patel, P., Maitland, K., O'Neill, K. *et al.* (2010) Assay strategies for the discovery and validation of therapeutics targeting *Brugia malayi* Hsp90. *PLoS Negl. Trop. Dis.*, **4**, e714.

30 Maule, A.G., Mousley, A., Marks, N.J., Day, T.A., Thompson, D.P., Geary, T.G., and Halton, D.W. (2002) Neuropeptide signaling systems – potential drug targets for parasite and pest control. *Curr. Top. Med. Chem.*, **2**, 733–758.

31 Greenwood, K., Williams, T., and Geary, T. (2005) Nematode neuropeptide receptors and their development as anthelmintic screens. *Parasitology*, **131**, S169–S177.

32 Woods, D.J., Butler, C., Williams, T., and Greenwood, K. (2010) Receptor-based discovery strategies for insecticides and parasiticides: A review, in *Neuropeptide Systems as Targets for Parasite and Pest Control* (eds T.G. Geary and A.G. Maule), Landes Bioscience, Austin, TX, pp. 1–9.

33 Geary, T.G., Bowman, J.W., and Friedman, A.R. (1999) Method for discovering novel anthelmintic compounds. US Patent 5,859,188.

34 Lee, B.H., Dutton, F.E., Clothier, M.F., Thomas, E.W., Bowman, J.W., Davis, J.P., Johnson, S.S. *et al.* (1999) Synthesis and biological activity of anthelmintic thiadiazoles using an AF-2 receptor binding assay. *Bioorg. Med. Chem. Lett*, **9**, 1727–1732.

35 Lowery, D.E., Geary, T.G., Kubiak, T.M., and Larsen, M.J. (2007) G protein-coupled receptor-like receptors and modulators thereof. US Patent 7,208,591.

36 McVeigh, P., Geary, T.G., Marks, N.J., and Maule, A.G. (2006) The FLP-side of nematodes. *Trends Parasitol.*, **22**, 385–396.

37 Husson, S.J., Mertens, I., Janssen, T., Lindemans, M., and Schoofs, L. (2007) Neuropeptidergic signaling in the nematode *Caenorhabditis elegans*. *Prog. Neurobiol.*, **82**, 33–55.

38 Wang, Z.X., Broach, J.R., and Peiper, S.C. (2006) Functional expression of CXCR4 in *Saccharomyces cerevisiae* in the development of powerful tools for the pharmacological characterization of CXCR4. *Methods Mol. Biol.*, **332**, 115–127.

39 Minic, J., Sautel, M., Salesse, R., and Pajot-Augy, E. (2005) Yeast system as a screening tool for the pharmacological assessment of G protein coupled receptors. *Curr. Med. Chem.*, **12**, 961–969.

40 Geary, T.G., Woods, D.J., Williams, T., and Nwaka, S. (2009) Target identification and mechanism-based screening for anthelmintics: application of veterinary antiparasitic research programmes to search for new antiparasitic drugs for human indications, in *Drug Discovery in Infectious Diseases* (ed. P.M. Selzer), Wiley-VCH Verlag GmbH, Weinheim, pp. 1–16.

41 Taman, A. and Ribeiro, P. (2009) Investigation of a dopamine receptor in *Schistosoma mansoni*: functional studies and immunolocalization. *Mol. Biochem. Parasitol.*, **168**, 24–33.

42 El-Shehabi, F. and Ribeiro, P. (2010) Histamine signaling in *Schistosoma mansoni*: immunolocalisation and characterisation of a new histamine-responsive receptor (SmGPR-2). *Int. J. Parasitol.*, **40**, 1395–1406.

43 Smith, M.W., Borts, T.L., Emkey, R., Cook, C.A., Wiggins, C.J., and Gutierrez, J.A. (2003) Characterization of a novel G-protein coupled receptor from the parasitic nematode *H. contortus* with a high affinity for serotonin. *J. Neurochem.*, **86**, 255–266.

44 White, W.H., Gutierrez, J.A., Naylor, S.A., Cook, C.A., Gonzalez, I.C., Wisehart, M.A., Smith, C.K. II, and Thompson, W.A. (2007) In vitro and in vivo characterization of *p*-amino-phenethyl-*m*-trifluoromethylphenyl piperazine (PAPP), a novel serotonergic agonist with anthelmintic activity against *Haemonchus contortus*, *Teladorsagia circumcincta* and *Trichostrongylus colubriformis*. *Vet. Parasitol.*, **146**, 58–65.

45 Aguinaldo, A.M., Turbeville, J.M., Linford, L.S., Rivera, M.C., Garey, J.R., Raff, R.A., and Lake, J.A. (1997) Evidence for a clade of nematodes, arthropods and moulting animals. *Nature*, **387**, 489–493.

46 Geary, T.G. and Moreno, Y. (2011) Macrocyclic lactone anthelmintics: spectrum of activity and mechanism of action. *Curr. Pharm. Biotechnol.*, Epub ahead of print.

47 Shiomi, K., Matsui, R., Kakei, A., Yamaguchi, Y., Masuma, R., Hatano, H., Arai, N., Isozaki, M., Tanaka, H., Kobayashi, S., Turberg, A., and Ōmura, S. (2010) Verticilide, a new ryanodine-binding inhibitor, produced by *Verticillium* sp. FKI-1033. *J. Antibiot.*, **63**, 77–82.

48 Ho, N.F.H., Sims, S.M., Vidmar, T.J., Day, J.S., Barsuhn, C.L., Thomas, E.M., Geary, T.G., and Thompson, D.P. (1994) Theoretical perspectives on anthelmintic drug discovery: interplay of transport kinetics, physicochemical properties and *in vitro* activities of anthelmintic drugs. *J. Pharm. Sci.*, **83**, 1052–1059.

9
Identification and Profiling of Nematicidal Compounds in Veterinary Parasitology

Andreas Rohwer, Jürgen Lutz, Christophe Chassaing, Manfred Uphoff, Anja R. Heckeroth, and Paul M. Selzer*

Abstract

Infections with parasitic nematodes are responsible for a significant part of the parasitic burden in humans, animals, and plants. They cause devastating diseases and drastic economic losses in agriculture. Several anthelmintic drugs are on the market to combat the parasites and to treat the respective diseases. Although those drugs have been effective in eliminating nematodes, increasing drug resistance makes their continued use of less value. Therefore, the development of novel anthelmintic drugs is essential. Here, we review several physiology-based nematode assays, which are important for the identification and profiling of novel nematicidal compounds in veterinary medicine. Using these bioassays, we screened approximately 160 000 compounds, and identified 61 structural compound classes and 171 singleton hits that were active against gastrointestinal nematodes. Many of these compounds cause distinct phenotypic changes with respect to morphology and locomotion of the treated nematodes. By discovering the specific mode of action (MoA) of several compounds, we were able to link the compound's activity to the related phenotype and consider this a genotype-to-compound-to-phenotype correlation. One compound class and its MoA is linked to a specific phenotype and has now been transferred via our lead optimization process to a nematicidal drug candidate. From our experience, we conclude that a combination of physiology- and target-based approaches will increase drug discovery output.

Introduction

Parasitic diseases caused by protozoa, worms, and arthropods affect billions of people world-wide, particularly in developing countries [1]. Of these diseases, it is estimated that almost half of all people living in developing countries are infected by helminths [2]. The term "helminth" is derived from the Greek "hélmins" (English "worm") and describes worms classified as parasites, mainly parasitic tapeworms (cestodes), roundworms (nematodes), and flukes (trematodes) (http://en.

---

* Corresponding Author

wikipedia.org/wiki/Parasitic_worm). Therefore, helminths are an accumulation of organisms belonging to different phyla. Like all parasites, helminths live almost completely at the expense of their particular host – plants, animals, and humans – and the main parasitic life stages of helminths reside within host tissue [3].

Parasitic nematodes include pathogens in humans, animals (Table 9.1), and plants. In humans, parasitic worms are still a major health concern, particularly in developing countries. Globally, more than 120 million people are infected with filarial nematodes like *Onchocerca volvulus*, *Brugia malayi*, and *Wuchereria bancrofti*, and approximately 1 billion people are at risk of infection [4]. Similarly, nematode infections in livestock are a major factor for losses in agricultural productivity [5]. For example, the barber pole worm, *Haemonchus contortus*, is a highly pathogenic nematode that can infect a large number of wild and domesticated ruminant species, and is the most economically important parasite of sheep and goats world-wide. It causes economic losses of billions of dollars per annum due to lost production and drug costs (http://www.sanger.ac.uk/resources/downloads/helminths/haemonchus-contortus.html) [3, 6]. In industrialized nations, infections with parasitic nematodes are routinely treated with anthelmintic drugs. Several anthelmintics are on the market, and the most important classes are the benzimidazoles (e.g., fenbendazole), imidazothiazoles (e.g., levamisole), and macrocyclic

Table 9.1 Examples of important nematodes in animals.

Category	Helminth	Main host	Current Treatment	Resistance reported in (for example)
Filaria	*Dirofiliaria immitis*	dog, cat	ML	[84]
	Dirofiliaria repens	dog, cat	ML	
Roundworm	*Ascaris suum*	pig	BZ	
	Toxocara/Toxascaris spp.	dog, cat	BZ, ML, IT	
	Parascaris equorum	horse	BZ, ML, IT	[85, 86]
Hookworm	*Ancylostoma caninum*	dog, cat	BZ, ML, IT	[87]
	Uncinaria stenocephala	dog, cat	BZ, IT	
Whipworm	*Trichuris suis*	pig	BZ	
	Trichuris vulpis	dog	BZ, ML, IT	
Strongyles	*Trichostrongylus* spp.	small ruminants, cattle	BZ, ML, IT	[85, 88, 89]
	Haemonchus contortus	small ruminants	BZ, ML, IT	[85, 88, 89]
	Ostertagia spp.	small ruminants, cattle	BZ, ML, IT	[85, 88, 89]
	Cooperia spp.	cattle	BZ, ML, IT	[85, 89]
	Cyathostomes	horse	BZ, ML, IT	[85, 90]
Nodular worm	*Oesophagostomum* spp.	pig	BZ	[91]

ML, macrocyclic lactones; BZ, benzimidazoles; IT, imidazothiazoles.

lactones (e.g., ivermectin) [7]. All these products are highly effective against nematodes, and have a wide margin of safety for livestock and companion animals. Unfortunately, resistance against all major anthelmintic classes has been reported [8, 9]. This makes the proper application of anthelmintics complex. Even worse, multiresistant strains insensitive to common drugs are reported [10]. Therefore, the search for new anthelmintics with a novel mode of actions (MoAs) was intensified in the animal health industry and academia [11]. This led to the development of three new anthelmintic classes: paraherquamides (e.g., derquantel; see also Chapter 18.) [12], amino-acetonitrile derivatives (e.g., monepantel; see also Chapter 17) [13], and depsipeptides (e.g., emodepside) [14, 15]. Monepantel and emodepside are described as resistance-breaking substances [16], whereas in the case of derquantel this seems to be questionable [17]. Although these relatively new drugs were market-registered recently, the limitations of the current treatment possibilities make the identification and development of new anthelmintics absolutely essential [16].

Drug Discovery Approaches for New Anthelmintics

The drug discovery process for the identification of new anthelmintic drugs has changed significantly in the last few decades [18]. In general, all available anthelmintic products on the market were discovered by screening synthetic or natural compounds against intact parasites either in animal models or in bioassays, also known as physiology-based assays [19, 20]. In these assays, the parasites are cultured *in vitro* in the presence of candidate compounds, and phenotypic parameters such as the viability, motility, and/or growth of the worms recorded. If bioactivity is detected, this implies that the compounds possess physicochemical properties that allow them to penetrate membrane barriers of the parasite and reach their molecular targets [21]. The identification of bioavailable compounds is a major advantage of physiology-based assays as the optimization of lead compounds towards bioavailability is one of the major hurdles in the drug discovery process [22]. However, screening intact parasites has the drawback that molecular targets of bioactive compounds are mostly unknown. Therefore, many compounds possibly active at antiparasitic target sites but inactive in bioassays were, in the past, discarded [18, 23]. More recently, along with novel high-throughput technologies, alternative target- or mechanism-based drug screening strategies have been established and implemented in modern drug discovery workflows towards the discovery and development of anthelmintics [19, 20, 24].

The target-based approach starts with the identification and validation of a target protein, which is subsequently used to search for new active compounds in *in vitro* and/or *in silico* screens (lead discovery phase) [25–27]. Promising lead compounds move then into the lead optimization phase, including medicinal chemistry and *in vitro* and *in vivo* profiling activities. The final goal is to identify drug candidates active in a model or target animal system. Through further testing, drug candidates may then lead to clinical candidates and, if successful, to the market [18]. However, in many parasitological fields, the target-based approach has not lived up to expectations. In helminthology, this is due to three main issues: (i) incomplete genome information or gene/protein-related phenotype information available in contrast to model organisms like *Caenorhabditis elegans* and *Drosophila melanogaster*; (ii) genetic modification and validation technologies like knockouts or RNA interference for relevant life cycle stages of most helminths are not routinely available or limited (see also Chapter 6); and (iii) optimized compounds are very active on isolated target molecules, but are not able to penetrate the parasite tegument and membranes and lack bioactivity.

Therefore, in order to increase drug discovery output, it seems sensible to combine the benefits and technologies of the physiology- and target-based approaches. It is known that the connection of specific worm phenotypes in bioassays with molecular target molecules and pathways is highly beneficial [28, 29]. Indeed, the knowledge of a molecular target and its corresponding phenotype is an ideal starting point for the optimization of antiparasitic activity and bioavailability of compounds. It enables an accurate and effective lead optimization and the generation of anthelmintic drug candidates. Knowledge of the compound interaction with a target protein also allows the utilization of protein crystallography followed by structure-based drug design strategies, where protein structures and computer models guide lead optimization [18, 23, 30]. Today, it is widely accepted that these technologies accelerate the drug discovery process and improve the likelihood of discovering successful drugs [23, 31, 32].

At present, we are far from having all these tools at our fingertips. Bioassays are still the main starting point for the discovery of novel anthelmintics. However, by increasing our set of screening data points, we are able to connect compound information with activity data and observed phenotypes. In addition, in several cases, through the discovery of the particular compound's MoA we can also make a link between phenotype and protein–target complex, which can be considered a genotype-to-compound-to-phenotype relationship. The converse is also true where an observed phenotype will give insight into the potential MoA of a compound class. By gaining more knowledge for more compound classes, respective MoA, and phenotypes, a more complete picture of the genotype-to-compound-to-phenotype relationship can be developed. Here, we review our first steps towards that goal by describing useful nematode *in vitro* assays, the detection of active compounds, and their resultant phenotypes. Finally, we describe an example of a successful lead optimization project that led to a novel anthelmintic drug candidate.

Physiology-Based Nematode Assays in Veterinary Parasitology

Various physiology-based parasitic nematode bioassays have been published [33, 34]. They are mainly used to identify and profile new anthelmintic substances or monitor for the development of resistance. The egg hatch test (EHT) [35], larval development test (LDT) [36], and larval migration inhibition test (LMIT) [36, 37] are widely accepted as standard nematode test systems.

EHT

The EHT, first described by Le Jambre in 1976 [38], is a technically demanding, but accurate and rapid *in vitro* test for gastrointestinal nematodes of ruminants, horses, and pigs, such as *H. contortus*, *Teladorsagia circumcincta* and *Trichostrongylus colubriformis* [34]. The EHT is mainly utilized for resistance monitoring, research applications like MoA studies, and the evaluation of novel drugs against veterinary gastrointestinal nematodes. Despite being an important and well-established standard assay in veterinary laboratories for many years, the EHT generates variable results and not always reproducible data [35]. Therefore, the World Association for the Advancement of Veterinary Parasitology established a standardized and simplified protocol for the EHT in 1992 [39].

As the name implies, the EHT compares the proportion of eggs that fail to hatch in the absence or presence of anthelmintic drugs. The test is mainly employed for the analysis of benzimidazoles – a class of anthelmintics known to bind to tubulin monomers. These prevent tubulin polymerization and the assembly of microtubules, and kill the eggs of many helminth species [35]. Therefore, the EHT is the optimal assay for screening of resistance towards benzimidazoles [33].

A prerequisite for the assay is the availability of fresh eggs recovered from feces (no older than 3 h postshedding from the host). If this is not feasible, the isolated eggs are stored under anaerobic conditions until the EHT is performed, because the benzimidazole-based suppression of egg development requires anaerobic conditions [34]. Under aerobic conditions, the larvae become insensitive to the ovicidal activity of benzimidazoles [33]. Another important requirement for the successful implementation of the EHT is the parallel application of comprehensive and adequate control experiments. This is necessary because only a fraction of untreated and susceptible eggs will hatch [33].

The test can also be employed to screen for novel anthelmintics with ovicidal properties or, alternatively, to verify the MoA of already identified anthelmintics [33]. We routinely employ the EHT to investigate the potential MoA of anthelmintic compounds, especially those with structural similarities to benzimidazoles. Although benzimidazoles are very successful in treating helminthic infections, the development of resistance is a major threat for this compound class and potentially for novel drugs with a similar MoA [8, 40]. Therefore, we try to exclude anthelmintics that have a similar MoA to benzimidazoles. In our experience, most compounds postulated to be tubulin inhibitors, due to structural similarities to benzimidazoles, also inhibited egg hatching and thus were excluded from further hit-to-lead evaluations. Interestingly, a set of well-known tubulin formation inhibitors, including colchicine, do not inhibit egg hatching, but demonstrate anthelmintic activity against parasitic larval stages [41]. This indicates that egg hatch inhibition can be confounded by insufficient absorption through the eggshell and result in "false negatives" in the assay.

LDT

The LDT is a nematode assay that enables resistance monitoring and efficacy studies of compounds, drugs, and drug combinations irrespective of their MoA. Nematode eggs or free-living larvae 1 (L1) and larvae 2 (L2) are transferred into microtiter plates filled with respective media. The development of the larvae to the infective stage 3 (L3) is monitored in the presence of test compounds, including positive and negative controls [42]. Substances are categorized as anthelmintic if larvae fail to develop to the L3. Furthermore, effects on the pharyngeal muscle and finally starvation of the larvae can be monitored [36]. The LDT is also widely used for monitoring of resistance. Worms are categorized resistant when a significant proportion of the parasites develop to L3 in the presence of anthelmintic drugs. The LDT can also be used in cases of multiple worm infections. As different nematode species have morphologically distinct larvae, the LDT allows distinguishing different species by visual inspection [33]. In addition, the age of eggs is, in contrast to the EHT, not as important for the assay, which makes the test easier to perform [34, 36, 43].

The LDT has been developed for different parasites comprising the major ruminant gastrointestinal nematodes such as *H. contortus*, *Ostertagia ostertagi*, *Cooperia oncophora*, as well as for the small cyathostomin strongyles of equids [36, 44, 45]. Two major LDT variations have been described, the main difference being the use of liquid culture or solid agar media. The liquid-based LDT was introduced in 1988 [46]. Here, the larvae develop in wells containing water and *Escherichia coli* or yeast extract as nutrient. Alternatively, in the micro agar larval development test (MALDT), the eggs or larvae are placed on an agar matrix with or without anthelmintics [34, 44]. Utilizing agar has the advantage of eliminating solubility issues with ivermectin [44]. Comparing the liquid culture media and solid agar-based tests, both produced similar and reliable results, but the liquid assay is less time-consuming, less labor-intensive, and technically easier to perform than the MALDT [47]. The MALDT is, however, available in a commercial and ready-to-use version named DrenchRite® (www.scsrpc.org). It is a standardized assay to measure both compound efficacy against and resistance in gastrointestinal helminths [45].

Physiology-Based Assays on L3 and Adult Helminths

Several bioassays based on inhibition of motility or migration of infective L3 are available including the larval paralysis test (LPT) [48] and the LMIT [49]. These bioassays are reproducible and correlate well with other bioassays [50]. They are relatively easy to perform and costs are moderate. As L3 do not have a functional pharynx and do not feed, the tests are thought to act on body muscles [36]. The major advantage of these assays is the use of L3 – a homogenous, robust parasite development stage that is relatively easy to isolate from fecal collections and can be stored in the refrigerator for extended periods [37].

The LPT was used to detect the efficacy of and resistance to levamisole and morantel tartrate in cattle infected with *Ostertagia* species [48]. The measurement of motility is based on visual inspection and scored by specific criteria within a relative mobility ranking [51]. However, as visual scoring is subjective, a micromotility meter was developed that allows the quantitative measurement of movement by photodetectors [52]. Movement of the worms causes a variation of reflected light and the signals are converted into a motility index that represents an estimation of worm motility [42].

The LMIT permits objective assessment of the inhibition of migration of L3 [49]. The larvae and the test compounds are cast in agar blocks, and the numbers of worms that migrate out of the blocks are counted. A well-established variation of the test uses sieves in migration chambers where the larvae have to pass through the mesh [53]. The mesh has to be smaller than the cross-diameter of the L3. This causes the larvae to penetrate actively through the mesh – a dynamic phenomenon thought to resemble the worm penetration of the gut mucosa and mucus [50]. In addition, this leads to a physical separation of motile and nonmotile larvae, and has the advantage that motility can be quantified directly by using a microscope rather than judging if individual larvae are paralyzed [50]. The LMIT is employed to detect resistance to many anthelmintic drugs and has been established for many helminths, including gastrointestinal nematodes of ruminants [37]. It is also suited for drug screening [54, 55].

In vitro motility tests are not only available for L3, but also for adult worms. Adult worm motility (AWM) assays have been established for *H. contortus* [56] and *B. malayi* [57], and it is thought that AWMs allow for a more realistic evaluation of *in vivo* nematicidal activity [58]. Recently, a new bioassay for drug screening and resistance diagnosis that is based on parasite motility in *H. contortus* has been developed [59]. The authors used a real-time cell-monitoring device (xCELLigence; Roche) to assess objectively anthelmintic effects by measuring parasite motility in real-time. This method has the potential to be used for automated high-throughput screens and is amenable to other purposes where motility is monitored, such as gene silencing or antibody-mediated killing [59].

Physiology-Based Screening Assays Using Parasitic Nematode Stages

In addition to the aforementioned physiology-based assays, we developed several highly standardized *in vitro* model assay systems, which are optimized for screening of potential anthelmintic compounds. Prior to the screening, the relevant parasitic stage is grown *in vitro* at low oxygen concentration and at body temperature of the respective animal host to mimic the physiological situation within the host. Thus, the parasite is forced to change its gene/protein expression pattern to resemble that of a parasite within the host rather than of environmental larval stages.

A prerequisite for screening is the availability of large batches of high-quality parasite material. We have chosen *Ascaridia galli* and *Oesophagostomum dentatum* as model parasites for physiology-based assays, as these parasites are relatively easy to maintain. For the supply of *A. galli*, chickens are orally infected with embryonated parasite eggs and upon the subsequent shedding of eggs, they are necropsied and

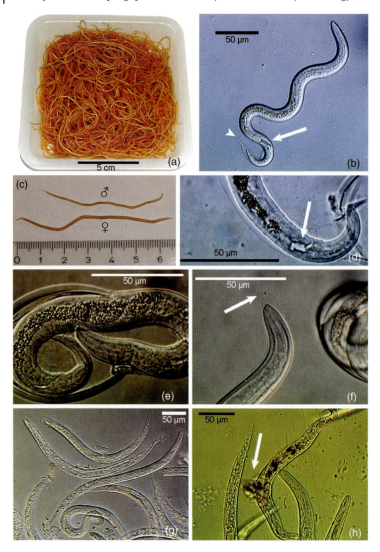

Figure 9.1 A. galli. (a) A. galli, adult worms, isolated from small intestine of chicken. (b) A. galli, larva freshly hatched from embryonated egg. Arrowhead: larva is sheathed, which is a characteristic for L3. Arrow: crystal-like structure in the sheath is always observed in L3. However, its function is not fully understood. (c) A. galli, adult worms, male and female. (d) A. galli, hatched L3. Arrow: crystal-like structure as in (b). (e) A. galli, L3 hatching from embryonated egg. (f) A. galli, hatched L3. Arrow: sheath with cemented area of the stoma. (g) A. galli, L3 in culture, treated with ivermectin at day 5. Larvae are paralyzed in the middle; head and tail region are mobile. (h) A. galli, L3 in culture, treated with screening substance. Arrow: larva is disrupted in the middle.

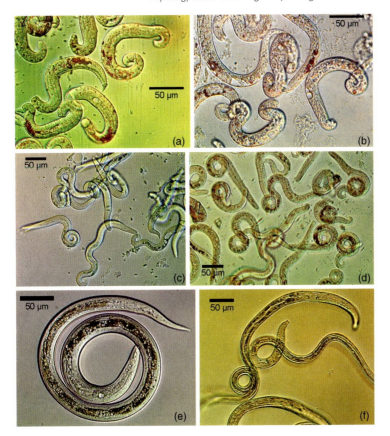

Figure 9.2 A. galli and H. contortus. (a) A. galli, L3, incubated with propoxur at day 5. Larvae appear cramped, shortened, and swollen, and motility is drastically reduced. Neutral Red uptake is strongly increased. (b) A. galli, L3, incubated with levamisole at day 5. Larvae show same phenotype as in (a). (c) A. galli, L3, incubated with paraherquamide E. Larvae have reduced motility, the posterior end of larvae appear coiled. (d) A. galli, L3, incubated with screening substance. Larvae present the distinctive phenotype as in (c), anterior part straight with greatly reduced motility. (e) H. contortus, exsheathed L3 in culture, untreated. (f) H. contortus, L4 in culture at day 5, untreated. Enormous increased growth compared to L3. Strong activity of the esophagus.

adult female *A. galli* worms are collected from the small intestine (Figure 9.1a). The female worms are cut into pieces and squashed, then suspended in buffer solution and the *A. galli* eggs are purified by differential washing steps. The eggs are then incubated until complete embryonation and stored in the refrigerator. They can be used for screening up to 6 month after collection.

To collect *O. dentatum*, pigs are orally infected with infectious L3. Once the pigs start shedding eggs, feces are collected on a regular basis, mixed with saw dust, and maintained for approximately 10 days [60]. Within that time, larvae hatch from the eggs, develop into the infectious L3, and migrate out of the fecal culture. They are then collected and transferred into tap water for storage. The patent period of *O. dentatum* in pigs is quite long, thus only a few pigs continuously shedding eggs over months, without any health issues, are required to maintain a supply of the parasite.

For both parasites, we developed *in vitro* culture systems to obtain the respective parasitic larval stages. In a shaking water bath at 38 °C, *A. galli* L3 are released from eggs (Figure 9.1e) using sodium hypochlorite in a saturated CO_2 atmosphere. Vital L3 (Figure 9.1d and f) are separated using the Baermann–Wetzel technique [60] and are then incubated in a modified KW-2 medium [61] at 41 °C, 10% CO_2, and 95% relative humidity before screening. L3 are identified by their sheath (Figure 9.1b and f) and a typical crystalline structure which appears in the head region after hatching that disappears after incubation (Figure 9.1b and d).

O. dentatum L3 (Figure 9.3b) derived from the fecal culture represent the environmental stage and are still sheathed. To obtain parasitic L3 necessary for screening, they are exsheathed using sodium hypochlorite, and the vital larvae are separated as described above and incubated at 38.5 °C, 10% CO_2, and 95% relative humidity in a modified KW-2 medium [61] before use in the assay. To obtain the L4 (Figure 9.3c), *O. dentatum* L3 have to be maintained for an additional 8 days under the same conditions.

In vitro culture systems for gastrointestinal nematodes of ruminants such as *H. contortus* (Figure 9.2e and f) are currently in development. The robustness of the *H. contortus* assay is hampered because the parasite material (i.e., sheathed L3) collected from feces of infected sheep is more sensitive to long-term storage than, for example, *O. dentatum*. Moreover, parasitic L3 and L4 of *H. contortus* develop at lower rates, and thus allow low-throughput assays only. Therefore, this assay is only used to confirm the anthelmintic activity of hits derived from our screening cascade (Figure 9.4).

Compound Screening for Novel Anthelmintics

In primary screening, compounds are tested at a single concentration on *A. galli* L3 because it is the most sensitive organism. In secondary screening, positive compounds are tested against both *A. galli* L3 (control verification) and *O. dentatum* L4 (activity extension). Compounds that pass both screenings are subsequently tested in a tertiary screening using *A. galli* L3, *O. dentatum* L4, and *O. dentatum* L3 (extension of larval spectrum). In addition, a dose titration is performed in order to evaluate the potency (minimal effective concentration (MEC)) of the respective compounds (Figure 9.4). Precultivated parasites are incubated in the presence of compounds for up to 5 days, and morphology, motility, damage, mortality as well as uptake of Neutral Red as a vitality test are recorded (Figures 9.1–9.3). The most promising compounds are further evaluated in additional helminth assays and finally move into MoA studies.

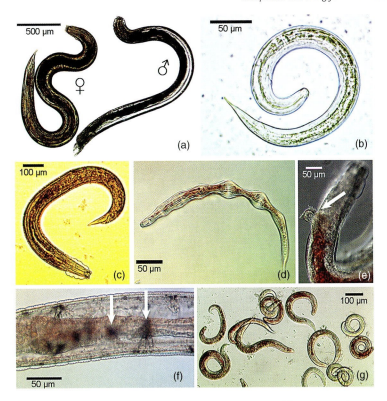

Figure 9.3 *O. dentatum*. (a) *O. dentatum*, adult worms in culture, female and male. (b) *O. dentatum*, exsheathed L3 in culture at day 1, untreated; (c) *O. dentatum*, L4 untreated at day 8. Large increase in size, esophagus bulb and intestine well developed, complete development of the alae at the head, permanent contractions of the esophagus. (d) *O. dentatum*, L3, incubated with screening substance. Larvae appear moniliform. (e) *O. dentatum*, L4 in culture, incubated with screening substance. Arrow: larva is disrupted in the middle similar to Figure 9.1h. (f) *O. dentatum*, L4 in culture, incubated with screening substance. Arrow: needle-shaped crystals are visible inside the larva. (g) *O. dentatum*, exsheathed L3 in culture, incubated with levamisole. Larvae are shortened and thickened.

Over the last decade, we have screened about 160 000 compounds in anthelmintic bioassays. An average hit rate of about 5% was determined in primary screens. In the subsequent secondary and tertiary screens, these hits were narrowed down to yield a final average hit rate of 0.3% (Figure 9.4). All identified hits were clustered into structural compound classes. Compounds not matching any structural class were classified as "singletons." Compounds not suitable for a hit-to-lead evaluation due to known toxicity or high reactivity were excluded at this stage. Thus far, we have collected 61 structural compound classes and 171 singletons. These hits were annotated using all of the available scientific information, including literature and patent information, biological activity and spectrum, MEC, on-target activity, potential MoA, and parasite phenotype and parasite motility data.

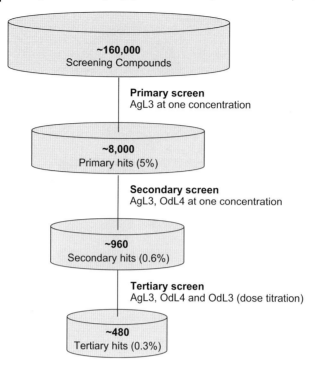

Figure 9.4 Screening cascade for anthelmintic bioassays. A.g. = *A. galli*; O.d. = *O. dentatum*.

Biological Activity and Phenotype Correlation

All data, including the anthelmintic activity, are vital to assess the potential of novel structural compound classes. Relying only on MEC data could easily lead to a misinterpretation of a compound's potential. In our screens, avermectins show activity in the low nanomolar range, whereas imidazothiazoles such as levamisole possess relatively high MEC values at around 1 μM. Therefore, instead of just following the most active hit structures based on MEC, one should also consider compounds showing additional interesting features in the observed phenotype and behavior of the parasite. Nevertheless, a certain activity threshold has to be reached in order to prove the potential of such "initially lower activity compounds" because lead optimization campaigns exclusively based on anthelmintic screening require a minimum level of activity to deduce reliable structure–activity relationships (SARs). Knowing the MoA of a compound class, however, would considerably extend the lead optimization and SAR possibilities because compounds could be optimized on the target protein itself [18, 32].

In addition to the determination of the MECs, the full examination of phenotype is of vital importance for the total assessment of the potential of a compound class. Not only direct damage and mortality, but also characteristic morphological and motility changes at different compound concentrations can be observed, such as changes in locomotion, paralysis of the pharynx, changes in appearance, or characteristic distortions (Figures 9.1–9.3). Such phenotypic effects of anthelmintics have been frequently investigated with adult and immature parasitic nematodes [62–65] as well as with the model organism *C. elegans* [28, 66, 67]. Similar procedures have been recently developed for the trematode parasite, *Schistosoma mansoni* [68, 69] (see also Chapter 20).

Of interest, phenotypic changes can often be connected to specific classes of compounds and their respective MoA (genotype-to-compound-to-phenotype correlation). A well-known example is represented by the "levamisole phenotype" where treated *A. galli* L3 are extremely coiled, shortened, and thickened with significantly reduced motility. Further, they show significantly higher uptake of Neutral Red, a viability marker, compared to nontreated larvae (Figure 9.2b). Treated *O. dentatum* L3 show an identical phenotype and development to the L4 is arrested (Figure 9.3g). The characteristic phenotype of levamisole is caused by the activation of the acetylcholine signaling cascade as the compound acts as a nicotinic acetylcholine receptor agonist [70]. Consistent with this compound-to-phenotype correlation, anthelmintic drugs, such as imidazothiazoles, tetrahydropyrimidines, and tribendimidines, also known to act on the nicotinic acetylcholine receptor, generate very similar phenotypes [29, 70]. Moreover, compounds acting on other proteins of the cholinergic pathway often cause the same phenotype. Examples are acetylcholine esterase inhibitors such as physostigmine [71] or propoxur [72] (Figure 9.2a), which lead to an increase of the acetylcholine concentration in the synaptic cleft. Consequently, novel compounds showing the "levamisole phenotype" can be considered to act on the cholinergic pathway, but may not easily be linked to a single target protein. Therefore, interesting compound classes causing a "levamisole phenotype" have to be further characterized in *in vitro* target protein assays in order to define their possible MoA.

Another example of a strong phenotype-to-molecule class correlation is the "ivermectin phenotype," which can be detected by treating parasites with macrocyclic lactones. Ivermectin inhibits pharyngeal pumping and causes flaccid paralysis [63, 73, 74]. In *A. galli* L3, ivermectin leads to uncoordinated movement after 5 days of treatment. The middle of the larval body seems to be paralyzed, while synchronous obsessive movements of the head and tail region can be observed (Figure 9.1g). The MoA of ivermectin is well studied; the glutamate-gated chloride channel being the primary molecular protein target [74]. Very recently, a protein crystal structure of this channel with the bound allosteric agonist ivermectin was solved, giving deeper insight into the interaction of both molecules and opening great potential for new structure-based approaches [75].

Based on our screening experiments, of the 61 identified structural compound classes and the 171 singletons, we can currently describe 13 distinct phenotypes within the different larvae of *A. galli*, *O. dentatum*, and *H. contortus*, and we are continuing to extend that list in terms of compound classes, phenotypes, and organisms. Once a new phenotype is detected, we routinely test in an on-target assay panel to determine the respective MoA. In addition, common cytotoxicity and genotoxicity assays are applied to be able to distinguish between compounds acting on particular targets or showing a general toxicity profile. For some compounds, the phenotype of a single organism can change as a function of compound concentration. This may indicate that those compounds are acting on more than one target. Interesting phenotypes with to some extent unidentified MoAs include the "disrupted phenotype" (Figures 9.1h and 9.2e), the "coiled phenotype" (Figure 9.2d), the "moniliform phenotype" (Figure 9.3d), and the "needle-shaped precipitation phenotype" (Figure 9.3f).

Lead Optimization Towards a Drug Candidate

In contrast to human drug discovery for which most functional screening is based on cellular assays [76, 77], whole organisms are available for testing in the field of veterinary anthelmintic drug discovery. Consequently, lead compounds identified from screening campaigns based on such assays not only possess sufficient intrinsic activity, but also physicochemical properties enabling efficient uptake by the parasitic species [21]. In addition, the knowledge accumulated on a repertoire of distinct phenotypes that have been associated with target families allows for proposing a tentative MoA for an active compound and for following the evolution of this phenotype along the lead optimization process.

This process begins with the optimization of the anthelminthic *in vitro* profile of the initial lead compound. Here, the objective is to rapidly define which structural components of the lead compound are driving the biological activity and concurrently to determine optimal ranges for the relevant physicochemical parameters. This goal is achieved by systematically modifying as many elements of the lead as possible and by interpreting the resultant effects on the biological activity in order to build a SAR [22]. In parallel, physicochemical parameters such as lipophilicity ($\log P$) and polar surface area (PSA) are calculated for each compound entering a screening campaign in order to eventually relate these parameters to variations in functional activity. As an illustrative example, compound **1** was identified as a lead compound after screening for anthelmintic activity (Figure 9.5). The observed phenotype was the "disrupted phenotype" similar to that shown in Figures 9.1h and 9.3e. It was also discovered that compound **1** inhibits the respiratory chain. Subsequently, compound **1** was the starting point for a lead optimization process towards the discovery of a new drug candidate.

First, compound **1** was divided into five components that were sequentially investigated: the terminal end aromatic rings on both sides (Figure 9.5, components **a** + **e**), the diamines on both sides (Figure 9.5, components **b** + **d**), and the central dicarboxylic acid (Figure 9.5, component **c**). Drastic changes in the structure were first performed in order to determine which key structural features of compound **1** were essential for the functional activity. For example, the replacement of the central part of the molecule (Figure 9.5, component **c**) leading to compounds of type **2** or the desymmetrization of the molecule resulting in compounds of type **3** were investigated (Figure 9.5). This revealed that the replacement of the central part (Figure 9.5, component **c**) of compound **1** by various dicarboxylic acids was well tolerated and eventually led to an increase in functional activity.

As illustrative examples, compounds derived from 1,5-pentanedioic acid (Figure 9.6f) or from 1,3-cyclohexandioic acid (Figure 9.6g) were on average more

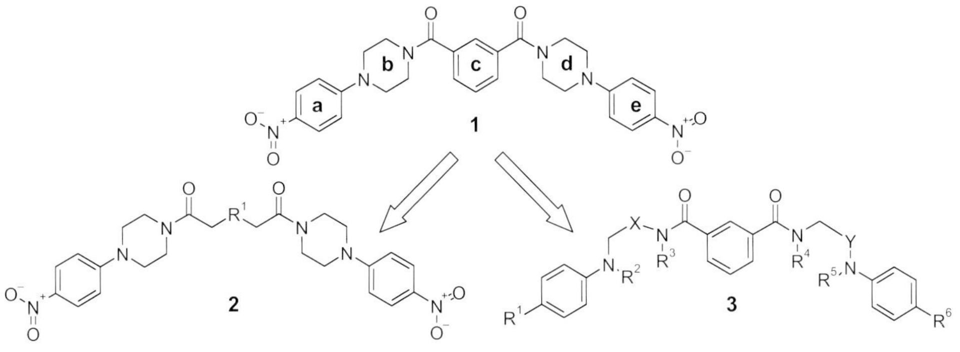

Lead Optimization Towards a Drug Candidate | 149

Figure 9.5 Lead compound **1** and first optimization focus.

active when compared to compounds derived from 1,3-benzenedioic acid (Figure 9.6h) as was the case for the starting compound **1**. In contrast, derivatives of *trans*-1,4-butenedioic acid (Figure 9.6i) were found to be less active than compounds of type 1 (Figure 9.5).

The desymmetrization of compound **1** was achieved either by functionalizing the central dicarboxylic acid element by two unlike primary or secondary amines (Figure 9.5, components **b** + **d**) or by omitting one of the two carbonyl groups or the diacid (Figure 9.5, component **c**). As in the case of the work focused on the diacid moiety, it was not only possible to demonstrate that the symmetry was not a key element for maintaining the biological activity, but a set of amines leading to an increase in activity was identified. The substitution of the original 4-nitrophenyl component of compound **1** with a 4-nitro-3-trifluoromethylphenyl group, leading to amine **j** (Figure 9.6j), optionally combined with the replacement of the piperazine by a 4-aminopiperidine and resulting in amine **k** (Figure 9.6k), led to compounds possessing increased functional activity. In contrast, compounds derived from 4-nitrophenylpiperidine (Figure 9.6m) were poorly active.

By combining the introduction of two unlike aromatic amines with the replacement of the diacid by a monoacid, it was also demonstrated that the orientation of the remaining carbonyl group is triggering the functional activity (Figure 9.7).

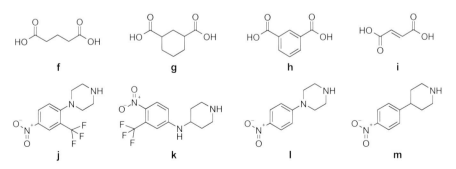

Figure 9.6 Building blocks selected for synthesizing derivatives of lead compound **1**.

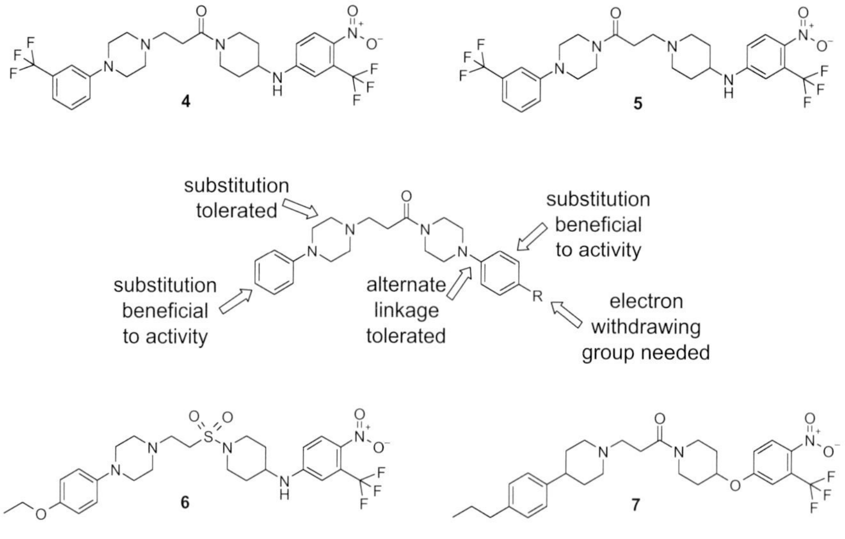

Figure 9.7 SAR – illustrative examples.

For example, compound **4** and analogs thereof were on average more active than compounds derived from compound **5**. Following the first phase of the optimization, based on profound structural modifications of the original compound **1**, more subtle changes such as changes in the types of substituents on each component or of the position of such substituents were then investigated. It was shown that substitutions of both aromatic rings present in compounds of type **4** were contributing to an increase in the functional activity. It was also confirmed that the presence of an electron-withdrawing group on the aromatic moiety shown on the right-hand side of the structure **4** is required for a high level of activity. Other changes such as substitution of the left-hand side diamine or the modification of the linkage of the other diamine to the attached aromatic ring were tolerated, but had no significant influence on the functional activity (Figure 9.7). As a result, compounds such as **6** and **7**, possessing a high level of anthelmintic activity against all species, were obtained (Figure 9.7). As described earlier, the optimization work was not solely dedicated to the identification of SARs, but also to property–activity correlations. As a prerequisite to such investigations, the design of the compounds to be synthesized and screened needs to be guided in such a way that they will collectively cover a large enough physicochemical property space (or diversity space). This is usually ensured by generating the physicochemical parameters of all new planned derivatives and by looking at their distribution. In case the distribution of one or more physicochemical parameter does not follow the intended profile, corrections can be implemented in the planned structures until this objective is fulfilled. Once the screening results are available, it is then possible to determine which physicochemical parameters influence functional activity and the optimal values for these parameters, and, ultimately, adapt the design of new compounds towards these values. As already demonstrated in the case of anthelmintic benzimidazoles [78, 79], the work

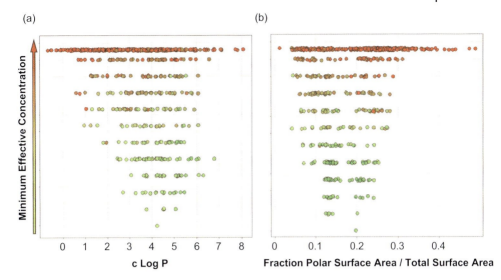

Figure 9.8 Lipophilicity and PSA: influence on the biological activity. Each spot corresponds to an individual compound. Green spots represent highly active compounds (effective at low concentrations), whereas red spots represent poorly active compounds (only effective at high concentrations).

performed on the optimization of compound **1** showed that an increase in lipophilicity is generally beneficial to the biological activity. As shown in Figure 9.8a, a large majority of the most active compounds had a $\log P$ value greater than 3.5 with an optimum around 4–4.5.

Interestingly, we discovered that the ratio of the PSA to the total surface of the compounds also correlates with the functional activity, which corroborates the observations on lipophilicity (Figure 9.8b). Thus, in cases where the PSA exceeds a quarter of the total surface, a dramatic drop in activity is observed.

Once established, these types of correlations are very helpful tools for distinguishing negative results that are a consequence of a lack of intrinsic efficacy or from those that can be attributed to a suboptimal set of physicochemical parameters. However, it should be noted that such correlations are not valid in a reverse manner. Compounds having a $\log P$ value of about 4 and/or a PSA not exceeding a quarter of their total surface will not necessarily possess high anthelmintic activity (Figure 9.8). As stated by the "Rule-of-Five" [80], the correlations should be understood and used as

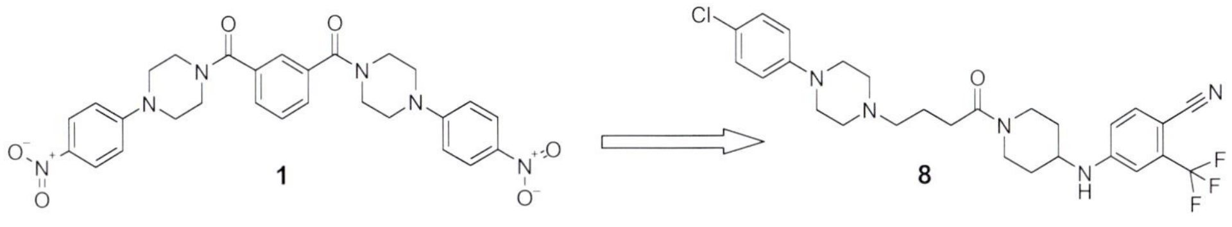

Figure 9.9 Structural evolution from lead compound **1** to a drug candidate **8**.

deselecting rather than selecting tools (i.e., compounds not fulfilling the identified criteria have a lower probability of eliciting biological activity).

As a result of the lead optimization process described above, compounds possessing a high level of activity on a broad range of parasitic species were obtained. Due to the intrinsic propensity of functional assays to select for biocidal compounds, the *in vitro* optimization process is usually continued by the deselection of compounds with potential toxicity to the hosts. This is done by testing the compounds in a panel of assays (e.g., cytotoxicity, genotoxicity) from which a small fraction qualifies for further investigation in a rodent infection model. The first part of the *in vivo* optimization is then dedicated to the confirmation of the nontoxic character of the compounds by determining the acute toxicity in rodents. When no toxicity is observed in rodents, the optimization process is concluded by the determination of the anthelmintic efficacy, first in rodents and then in target animals to arrive at drug candidates.

In the context of optimizing lead compound **1**, a set of drug candidates could be identified from which compound **8** (Figure 9.9) showed high anthelmintic efficacy against *H. contortus* when given orally to sheep [81–83].

Conclusions

Due to the development of resistance and unmet needs, veterinary and human medicine depends on novel nematicidal drugs. It is clear that the productivity of recent drug discovery efforts focusing solely on single approaches has not been as anticipated. We believe that a sensible combination of target-based and physiology-based drug discovery approaches will boost the number of drug candidates. From mid- and long-term perspectives, this will most likely lead to an increase of marketed drugs and the availability of alternative treatment options.

Acknowledgments

We thank Dr Richard J. Marhöfer (Intervet Innovation GmbH, Germany) for his technical support in generating Figures 9.1–9.3. We are also grateful to Dr Graham Cox (Merck Animal Health, Elkhorn, NE) for critical discussions and comments.

References

1 Renslo, A.R. and McKerrow, J.H. (2006) Drug discovery and development for neglected parasitic diseases. *Nat. Chem. Biol.*, **2**, 701–710.

2 Hall, A., Horton, S., and de Silva, N. (2009) The costs and cost-effectiveness of mass treatment for intestinal nematode worm infections using different treatment thresholds. *PLoS Negl. Trop. Dis.*, **3**, e402.

3 Mehlhorn, H. (2008) *Encyclopedia of Parasitology*, Springer, Heidelberg.

4 Taylor, M.J., Hoerauf, A., and Bockarie, M. (2010) Lymphatic filariasis and onchocerciasis. *Lancet*, **376**, 1175–1185.

5 Tsotetsi, A.M. and Mbati, P.A. (2003) Parasitic helminths of veterinary importance in cattle, sheep and goats on communal farms in the northeastern free state, South Africa. *J. S. Afr. Vet. Assoc.*, **74**, 45–48.

6 Tasawar, R., Ahmad, S., Lashari, M.H., and Hayat, C.S. (2010) Prevalence of *Haemonchus contortus* in sheep at research centre for conservation of sahiwal cattle (RCCSC) jehangirabad district Khanewal, Punjab, Pakistan. *Pakistan J. Zool.*, **42**, 735–739.

7 Holden-Dye, L. and Walker, R.J. (2007) CT Anthelmintic drugs, in *WormBook* (ed. The *C. elegans* Research Community), doi: 10.1895/wormbook.1.143.1.

8 Gilleard, J.S. (2006) Understanding anthelmintic resistance: the need for genomics and genetics. *Int. J. Parasitol.*, **36**, 1227–1239.

9 von Samson-Himmelstjerna, G., Wolstenholme, A.J., and Prichard, R. (2009) CT Anthelmintic resistance as a guide to the discovery of new drugs?, in *Antiparasitic and Antibacterial Drug Discovery: From Molecular Targets to Drug Candidates* (ed. P.M. Selzer), Wiley-VCH Verlag GmbH, Weinheim, pp. 17–32.

10 Chandrawathani, P., Waller, P.J., Adnan, M., and Höglund, J. (2003) Evolution of high-level, multiple anthelmintic resistance on a sheep farm in Malaysia. *Trop. Anim. Health Prod.*, **35**, 17–25.

11 Woods, D.J., Vaillancourt, V.A., Wendt, J.A., and Meeus, P.F. (2011) Discovery and development of veterinary antiparasitic drugs: past, present and future. *Future Med. Chem.*, **3**, 887–896.

12 Zinser, E.W., Wolfe, M.L., Alexander-Bowman, S.J., Thomas, E.M., Davis, J.P., Groppi, V.E., Lee, B.H. et al. (2002) Anthelmintic paraherquamides are cholinergic antagonists in gastrointestinal nematodes and mammals. *J. Vet. Pharmacol. Ther.*, **25**, 241–250.

13 Kaminsky, R., Gauvry, N., Schorderet Weber, S., Skripsky, T., Bouvier, J., Wenger, A., Schroeder, F. et al. (2008) Identification of the amino-acetonitrile derivative monepantel (AAD 1566) as a new anthelmintic drug development candidate. *Parasitol. Res.*, **103**, 931–939.

14 Harder, A. and von Samson-Himmelstjerna, G. (2002) Cyclooctadepsipeptides – a new class of anthelmintically active compounds. *Parasitol. Res.*, **88**, 481–488.

15 Welz, C., Krüger, N., Schniederjans, M., Miltsch, S.M., Krücken, J., Guest, M., Holden-Dye, L. et al. (2011) SLO-1 channels of parasitic nematodes reconstitute locomotor behaviour and emodepside sensitivity in *Caenorhabditis elegans* slo-1 loss of function mutants. *PLoS Pathog.*, **7**, e1001330.

16 Keiser, J. and Utzinger, J. (2010) The drugs we have and the drugs we need against major helminth infections. *Adv. Parasitol.*, **73**, 197–230.

17 Kaminsky, R., Bapst, B., Stein, P.A., Strehlau, G.A., Allan, B.A., Hosking, B.C., Rolfe, P.F., and Sager, H. (2011) Differences in efficacy of monepantel, derquantel and abamectin against multi-resistant nematodes of sheep. *Parasitol. Res.*, **109**, 19–23.

18 Rohwer, A., Marhöfer, R.J., Caffrey, C.R., and Selzer, P.M. (2011) CT Drug discovery approaches toward antiparasitic agents, in *Apicomplexan Parasites: Molecular Approaches toward Targeted Drug Development* (ed. K. Becker) Wiley-VCH Verlag GmbH, Weinheim, pp. 3–20.

19 Woods, D.J. and Williams, T.M. (2007) The challenges of developing novel antiparasitic drugs. *Invert. Neurosci.*, **7**, 245–250.

20 Geary, T.G., Woods, D.J., Williams, T., and Nwaka, S. (2009) CT Target identification and mechanism-based screening for anthelmintics: application of veterinary antiparasitic research programs to search for new antiparasitic drugs for human indications, in *Antiparasitic and Antibacterial Drug Discovery: From Molecular Targets to Drug Candidates* (ed. P. Selzer), Wiley-VCH Verlag GmbH, Weinheim, pp. 3–15.

21 Gassel, M., Cramer, J., Kern, C., Noack, S., and Streber, W. (2009) CT Lessons learned from target-based lead discovery, in *Antiparasitic and Antibacterial*

Drug Discovery: From Molecular Targets to Drug Candidates (ed. P.M. Selzer), Wiley-VCH Verlag GmbH, Weinheim, pp. 99–115.

22 Chassaing, C. and Sekljic, H. (2009) CT Approaches towards antiparasitic drug candidates for veterinary use, in Antiparasitic and Antibacterial Drug Discovery: From Molecular Targets to Drug Candidates (ed. P.M. Selzer), Wiley-VCH Verlag GmbH, Weinheim, pp. 117–133.

23 Klebe, G. (2012) Drug Design: Methodology, Concepts, and Mode-of-Action, Springer, Heidelberg.

24 Geary, T.G., Thompson, D.P., and Klein, R.D. (1999) Mechanism-based screening: discovery of the next-generation of anthelmintics depends upon more basic research. Int. J. Parasitol., 29, 105–112.

25 Selzer, P.M., Marhöfer, J.R., and Rohwer, A. (2008) Applied Bioinformatics, Springer, Heidelberg.

26 Krasky, A., Rohwer, A., Marhöfer, R., and Selzer, P.M. (2009) CT Bioinformatics and chemoinformatics: key technologies in the drug discovery process, in Antiparasitic and Antibacterial Drug Discovery: From Molecular Targets to Drug Candidates (ed. P.M. Selzer), Wiley-VCH Verlag GmbH, Weinheim, pp. 45–57.

27 Engels, K., Beyer, C., Suárez Fernández, M.L., Bender, F., Gassel, M., Unden, G., Marhöfer, R.J., Mottram, J.C., and Selzer, P.M. (2010) Inhibition of Eimeria tenella CDK-related kinase 2: from target identification to lead compounds. Chem. Med. Chem., 5, 1259–1271.

28 Ardelli, B.F., Stitt, L.E., Tompkins, J.B., and Prichard, R.K. (2009) A comparison of the effects of ivermectin and moxidectin on the nematode Caenorhabditis elegans. Vet. Parasitol., 165, 96–108.

29 Hu, Y., Xiao, S.-H., and Aroian, R.V. (2009) The new anthelmintic tribendimidine is an L-type (levamisole and pyrantel) nicotinic acetylcholine receptor agonist. PLoS Negl. Trop. Dis., 3, e499.

30 Andricopulo, A.D., Salud, L.B., and Abraham, D.J. (2009) Structure-based drug design strategies in medicinal chemistry. Cur. Top. Med. Chem., 9, 771–790.

31 Guido, R.V. and Oliva, G. (2009) Structure-based drug discovery for tropical diseases. Curr. Top. Med. Chem., 9, 824–843.

32 Marhöfer, R.J., Oellien, F., and Selzer, P.M. (2011) Drug discovery and the use of computational approaches for infectious diseases. Future Med. Chem., 3, 1011–1025.

33 Johansen, M.V. (1989) An evaluation of techniques used for the detection of anthelmintic resistance in nematode parasites of domestic livestock. Vet. Res. Commun., 13, 455–466.

34 Coles, G.C., Jackson, F., Pomroy, W.E., Prichard, R.K., von Samson-Himmelstjerna, G., Silvestre, A., Taylor, M.A., and Vercruysse, J. (2006) The detection of anthelmintic resistance in nematodes of veterinary importance. Vet Parasitol., 136, 167–185.

35 von Samson-Himmelstjerna, G., Coles, G.C., Jackson, F., Bauer, C., Borgsteede, F., Cirak, V.Y., Demeler, J. et al. (2009) Standardization of the egg hatch test for the detection of benzimidazole resistance in parasitic nematodes. Parasitol. Res., 105, 825–834.

36 Demeler, J., Küttler, U., and von Samson-Himmelstjerna, G. (2010) Adaptation and evaluation of three different in vitro tests for the detection of resistance to anthelmintics in gastro intestinal nematodes of cattle. Vet. Parasitol., 170, 61–70.

37 Demeler, J., Küttler, U., El-Abdellati, A., Stafford, K., Rydzik, A., Varady, M., Kenyon, F. et al. (2010) Standardization of the larval migration inhibition test for the detection of resistance to ivermectin in gastro intestinal nematodes of ruminants. Vet. Parasitol., 174, 58–64.

38 Le Jambre, L.F. and Whitlock, J.H. (1976) Changes in the hatch rate of Haemonchus contortus eggs between geographic regions. Parasitology, 73, 223–238.

39 Coles, G.C., Bauer, C., Borgsteede, F.H., Geerts, S., Klei, T.R., Taylor, M.A., and Waller, P.J. (1992) World Association for the Advancement of Veterinary Parasitology (W.A.A.V.P.) methods for the detection of anthelmintic resistance in

nematodes of veterinary importance. *Vet. Parasitol.*, **44**, 35–44.

40 Köhler, P. and Marhöfer, R. (2009) CT Selective drug targets in parasites, in *Antiparasitic and Antibacterial Drug Discovery: From Molecular Targets to Drug Candidates* (ed. P.M. Selzer), Wiley-VCH Verlag GmbH, Weinheim, pp. 45–57.

41 Lutz, J. and Uphoff, M. (2008) Utilizing the egg hatch test of *Oesophagostumum dentatum* for the evaluation of endo-active screening compounds. 23rd Annual Meeting of The German Society for Parasitology, Hamburg.

42 Taylor, M.A., Hunt, K.R., and Goodyear, K.L. (2002) Anthelmintic resistance detection methods. *Vet. Parasitol.*, **103**, 183–194.

43 Várady, M., Cudeková, P., and Corba, J. (2007) In vitro detection of benzimidazole resistance in *Haemonchus contortus*: egg hatch test versus larval development test. *Vet. Parasitol.*, **149**, 104–110.

44 Lacey, E., Redwin, J.M., Gill, J.H., Demargheriti, V.M., and Waller, P.J. (1991) CT A larval development assay for the simultaneous detection of broad spectrum anthelmintic resistance, in *Resistance of Parasites to Antiparasitic Drugs* (ed. J.C. Boray), MSD AGVET, Rahway, NJ, pp. 177–184.

45 Tandon, Z. and Kaplan, R.M. (2004) Evaluation of a larval development assay (DrenchRite®) for the detection of anthelmintic resistance in cyathostomin nematodes of horses. *Vet. Parasitol.*, **121**, 125–142.

46 Coles, G.C., Tritschler, J.P. 2nd, Giordano, D.J., Laste, N.J., and Schmidt, A.L. (1988) Larval development test for detection of anthelmintic resistant nematodes. *Res. Vet. Sci.*, **45**, 50–53.

47 Várady, M., Corba, J., Letková, V., and Kovác, G. (2009) Comparison of two versions of larval development test to detect anthelmintic resistance in *Haemonchus contortus*. *Vet. Parasitol.*, **160**, 267–271.

48 Martin, P.J. and Le Jambre, L.F. (1979) Larval paralysis as an *in vitro* assay of levamisole and morantel tartrate resistance in *Oslertagia*. *Vet. Sci. Commun.*, **3**, 159–164.

49 Douch, P.G., Harrison, G.B., Buchanan, L.L., and Greer, K.S. (1983) *In vitro* bioassay of sheep gastrointestinal mucus for nematode paralysing activity mediated by substances with some properties characteristic of SRS-A. *Int. J. Parasitol.*, **13**, 207–212.

50 Rabel, B., McGregor, R., and Douch, P.G. (1994) Improved bioassay for estimation of inhibitory effects of ovine gastrointestinal mucus and anthelmintics on nematode larval migration. *Int. J. Parasitol.*, **24**, 671–676.

51 Kiuchi, F., Miyashita, N., Tsuda, Y., Kondo, K., and Yoshimura, H. (1987) Studies on crude drugs effective on visceral larva migrans. I. Identification of larvicidal principles in betel nuts. *Chem. Pharm. Bull.*, **35**, 2880–2886.

52 Bennett, J.L. and Pax, R.A. (1986) Micromotility meter: an instrument designed to evaluate the action of drugs on motility of larval and adult nematodes. *Parasitology*, **93**, 341–346.

53 Wagland, B.M., Jones, W.O., Hribar, L., Bendixsen, T., and Emery, D.L. (1992) A new simplified assay for larval migration inhibition. *Int. J. Parasitol.*, **22**, 1183–1185.

54 O'Grady, J. and Kotze, A.C. (2004) *Haemonchus contortus*: in vitro drug screening assays with the adult life stage. *Exp. Parasitol.*, **106**, 164–172.

55 Kotze, A.C., Le Jambre, L.F., and O'Grady, J. (2006) A modified larval migration assay for detection of resistance to macrocyclic lactones in *Haemonchus contortus*, and drug screening with Trichostrongylidae parasites. *Vet. Parasitol.*, **137**, 294–305.

56 Hounzangbe-Adote, M.S., Paolini, V., Fouraste, I., Moutairou, K., and Hoste, H. (2005) *In vitro* effects of four tropical plants on three life-cycle stages of the parasitic nematode, *Haemonchus contortus*. *Res. Vet. Sci.*, **78**, 155–160.

57 Tompkins, J.B., Stitt, L.E., and Ardelli, B.F. (2010) *Brugia malayi*: in vitro effects of ivermectin and moxidectin on adults and microfilariae. *Exp. Parasitol.*, **124**, 394–402.

58 Marie-Magdeleine, C., Udino, L., Philibert, L., Bocage, B., and Archimede, H. (2010) *In vitro* effects of

Cassava (*Manihot esculenta*) leaf extracts on four development stages of *Haemonchus contortus*. *Vet. Parasitol.*, **173**, 85–92.

59 Smout, M.J., Kotze, A.C., McCarthy, J.S., and Loukas, A. (2010) A novel high throughput assay for anthelmintic drug screening and resistance diagnosis by real-time monitoring of parasite motility. *PLoS Negl. Trop. Dis.*, **4**, e885.

60 Eckert, J., Friedhoff, K.T., Zahner, H., and Deplazes, P. (2008) *Lehrbuch der Parasitologie für die Tiermedizin*, 2nd edn, Enke, Stuttgart.

61 Douvres, F.W. and Urban, J.F. (1983) Factors contributing to the *in vitro* development of *Ascaris suum* from second-stage larvae to mature adults. *J. Parasitol.*, **69**, 549–558.

62 Boisvenue, R.J., Brandt, M.C., Galloway, R.B., and Hendrix, J.C. (1983) The *in vitro* activity of various anthelmintic compounds against *Haemonchus contortus* larvae. *Vet. Parasitol.*, **13**, 341–347.

63 Geary, T.G., Sims, S.M., Thomas, E.M., Vanover, L., Davis, J.P., Winterrowd, C.A., Klein, R.D. et al. (1993) *Haemonchus contortus*: ivermectin-induced paralysis of the pharynx. *Exp. Parasitol.*, **77**, 88–96.

64 Gill, J.H. and Lacey, E. (1993) In vitro activity of paraherquamide against the free-living stages of *Haemonchus contortus*, *Trichostrongylus colubriformis* and *Ostertagia circumcincta*. *Int. J. Parasitol.*, **23**, 375–381.

65 Courtney, C.H. and Robertso, E.L. (1995) CT Chemotherapy of parasitic diseases, in *Veterinary Pharmacology and Therapeutics* (ed. H.R. Adams), Iowa State University Press, Ames, IA, pp. 904–908.

66 Bull, K., Cook, A., Hopper, N.A., Harder, A., Holden-Dye, L., and Walker, R.J. (2007) Effects of the novel anthelmintic emodepside on the locomotion, egg-laying behaviour and development of *Caenorhabditis elegans*. *Int. J. Parasitol.*, **37**, 627–636.

67 Schindelman, G., Fernandes, J.S., Bastiani, C.A., Yook, K., and Sternberg, P.W. (2011) Worm Phenotype Ontology: integrating phenotype data within and beyond the *C. elegans* community. *BMC Bioinformatics*, **12**, 32.

68 Maha-Hamadien, A., Ruelas, D.S., Wolff, B., Snedecor, J., Lim, K.-C., Xu, F., Renslo, A.R. et al. (2009) Drug discovery for schistosomiasis: hit and lead compounds identified in a library of known drugs by medium-throughput phenotypic screening. *PLoS Negl. Trop. Dis.*, **3**, e478.

69 Singh, R., Pittas, M., Heskia, I., Xu, F., McKerrow, J.H., and Caffrey, C.R. (2009) Automated image-based phenotypic screening for high-throughput drug discovery. IEEE Symposium on Computer-Based Medical Systems, Albuquerque, NM.

70 Martin, R.J., Robertson, A.P., and Bjorn, H. (1997) Target sites of anthelmintics. *Parasitology*, **114** (Suppl.), S111–S124.

71 Robinson, B. (1971) Alkaloids of the calabar bean. *Alkaloids*, **13**, 213–226.

72 Tomlin, C.D.S. (2010) *The e-Pesticide Manual V5.0*, British Crop Production Council, Alton; www.pesticidemanual.com.

73 Kass, I.S., Wang, C.C., Walrond, J.P., and Stretton, A.O. (1980) Avermectin B1a, a paralyzing anthelmintic that affects interneurons and inhibitory motoneurons in *Ascaris*. *Proc. Natl. Acad. Sci. USA*, **77**, 6211–6215.

74 Omura, S. (2008) Ivermectin: 25 years and still going strong. *Int. J. Antimicrob. Agents*, **31**, 91–98.

75 Hibbs, R.E. and Gouaux, E. (2011) Principles of activation and permeation in an anion-selective Cys-loop receptor. *Nature*, **474**, 54–60.

76 Moore, K. and Rees, S. (2001) Cell-based versus isolated target screening: how lucky do you feel? *J. Biomol. Screen.*, **6**, 69–74.

77 Hughes, J.P., Rees, S., Kalindjian, S.B., and Philpott, K.L. (2011) Principles of early drug discovery. *Br. J. Pharm.*, **162**, 1239–1249.

78 Mottier, L., Alvarez, L., Ceballos, L., and Lanusse, C. (2006) Drug transport mechanisms in helminth parasites: passive diffusion of benzimidazole anthelmintics. *Exp. Parasitol.*, **113**, 49–57.

79 Alvarez, L.I., Lourdes Mottier, M., and Lanusse, C.E. (2007) Drug transfer into

target helminth parasites. *Trends Parasitol.*, **23**, 97–104.

80 Lipinski, C.A., Lombardo, F., Dominy, B.W., and Feeney, P.J. (1997) Experimental and computational approaches to estimate solubility and permeability in drug discovery and development settings. *Adv. Drug Deliv. Rev.*, **23**, 3–25.

81 Chassaing, C.P.A., Schroeder, J., Ilg, T.S., Uphoff, M, and Meyer, T. (2009) Preparation of 4-aminocyclohexanol derivatives as anthelmintic agents. World Patent WO2009077527.

82 Chassaing, C.P.A. and Meyer, T. (2010) Heterocyclylethanone derivatives as anthelmintic agents and their preparation, pharmaceutical compositions and use in the treatment of helminth infection. World Patent WO2010146083.

83 Chassaing, C.P.A. and Meyer, T. (2010) Piperidine derivatives and related compounds as anthelmintic agents and their preparation. World Patent WO2010115688.

84 Blagburn, B.L., Dillon, A.R., Arther, R.G., Butler, J.M., and Newton, J.C. (2011) Comparative efficacy of four commercially available heartworm preventive products against the MP3 laboratory strain of *Dirofilaria immitis*. *Vet. Parasitol.*, **176**, 189–194.

85 Kaplan, R.M. (2004) Drug resistance in nematodes of veterinary importance: a status report. *Trends Parasitol.*, **20**, 477–481.

86 Reinemeyer, C.R. (2009) Diagnosis and control of anthelmintic-resistant *Parascaris equorum*. *Parasit. Vectors*, **2** (Suppl. 2), S8.

87 Kopp, S.R., Kotze, A.C., McCarthy, J.S., Traub, R.J., and Coleman, G.T. (2008) Pyrantel in small animal medicine: 30 years on. *Vet. J.*, **178**, 177–184.

88 Jabbar, A., Iqbal, Z., Kerboeuf, D., Muhammad, G., Khan, M.N., and Afaq, M. (2006) Anthelmintic resistance: the state of play revisited. *Life Sci.*, **79**, 2413–2431.

89 Sutherland, I.A. and Leathwick, D.M. (2011) Anthelmintic resistance in nematode parasites of cattle: a global issue? *Trends Parasitol.*, **27**, 176–181.

90 Kaplan, R.M., Klei, T.R., Lyons, E.T., Lester, G., Courtney, C.H., French, D.D., Tolliver, S.C. et al. (2004) Prevalence of anthelmintic resistant cythostomes on horse farms. *J. Am. Vet. Med. Assoc.*, **225**, 903–910.

91 Bauer, C. and Gerwert, S. (2002) Characteristics of a flubendazole resistant isolate of *Oesophagostomum dentatum* from Germany. *Vet. Parasitol.*, **103**, 89–97.

10
Quantitative High-Content Screening-Based Drug Discovery against Helmintic Diseases
Rahul Singh

Abstract

At the state-of-the-art, high-throughput and high-content screening (HTS/HCS) have become key technologies in modern drug discovery. These highly automated techniques allow rapid analysis of a large number of drug molecules and selection of candidates for lead optimization. Drug discovery for helmintic diseases, however, presents significant challenges to the standard HTS/HCS framework as well as opportunities for its further development. The central problem lies in the fact that discovery of efficacious leads against helminths often requires screening molecules against the entire parasite. Ideally, the effect of a drug needs to be studied in terms of effects on the parasite morphology, motility, and behavior, in addition to measuring often oversimplistic end-points for parasite death. Such an enhanced approach to screening can help in forming a more holistic understanding of the drug–parasite interactions and ensure that molecules that do not lead to immediate death, yet perturb the parasite's ability to survive, are not missed. The tasks of data acquisition, processing, and analysis in such settings require addressing technical problems that are different and arguably richer than those underlying the corresponding stages in both molecular-target-based HTS, as well as cell-based screening. In the first part of this chapter, using the specific context of two diseases, schistosomiasis and filariasis, the key problems that confront further development of HTS/HCS, especially in the context of its applicability against helmintic diseases, are identified and analyzed. This is followed by an introduction to the basics of automated image analysis using a typical image analysis workflow for HTS as the backdrop. Next, we briefly review the progress to date in quantitative whole-organism phenotyping and screening. Finally, we present results from our own research on segmentation and automated phenotyping, which provide a detailed perspective on how some of the critical challenges in this area can be addressed.

Introduction

Neglected tropical diseases (NTDs) constitute the most common infections of the world's poorest people. Various studies, as reviewed in contributions to this volume, indicate them to be the prime factors behind depriving the affected populations, especially women and children, of their health and economic potential. The search for new therapeutics against these diseases is consequently of significance; success in this area can be transformative to our civilization – in terms of scientific as well as economic and societal progress.

This chapter takes an interdisciplinary perspective on the problem of developing high-throughput screening (HTS) methods against NTDs. We seek to present a unified view of how efforts in biological sciences can be combined with engineering and computational methods to address some of the most challenging problems in screening drugs against parasitic diseases. The technical focus of this chapter is specifically driven by two such diseases: schistosomiasis, which is caused by several species of trematodes of the genus *Schistosoma*, and filariasis, which is caused by several nematodes of the superfamily Filarioidea. To understand the impact of these diseases, one may note that schistosomiasis ranks second only behind malaria in terms of socioeconomic and public health impact in developing countries. This disease inflicts at least 200 million people (with 20 million suffering severe effects) and places over 600 million people at risk. Filariasis infects more than 120 million people and puts over 1 billion people at risk of infection [1–4].

At the state-of-the-art, drug screening against these two NTDs is typically conducted using whole-organism screens. In whole-organism settings, one or more pathogens are simultaneously exposed to the drug being tested. Subsequently, observations are made at regular time intervals to assess the effect of the drug on the pathogen(s). This approach is distinct from the classical molecular biology-driven strategy, where, a molecular target is first identified, then functionally verified, and finally purified to be screened against. Thus, in whole-organism screening, a drug is studied in terms of the cumulative systemic effects it introduces in the pathogen(s), rather than just in terms of how it interacts with a specific protein or enzyme in isolation. Clearly, this situation is very different and much more complex than classical screening for hit-and-lead identification.

Specifically, we have to work with the following issues. (i) Drug–pathogen interactions are expressed through multiple indicators, such as changes in the shape, appearance (color and/or texture), motion patterns, and behavioral patterns of the pathogen. Thus, the potential measurements are multidimensional in nature. Reducing them to a single end-point measurement of "live or dead" (e.g., LD_{50} value) can arguably be oversimplistic, and exclude significant information from subsequent decision making and lead optimization. In this context, it is important to note that for parasitic helminths, and certainly gastrointestinal nematodes, perturbation of normal behavior through modulation of neuromuscular activity is a successful therapeutic strategy that does not necessarily demand outright death. More fundamentally, such multidimensional information is incompatible with the types of single end-point assays that are common to biochemical target-based or single-cell HTS phenotypic screens [5]. (ii) The effect of the drug can vary over time and may contain patterns of significance, such as cause–effect relationships between states of the pathogen, which once identified can provide crucial inputs on the mechanistic effects of a drug at the systemic level. (iii) The response of individual parasites may show significant variations due to genetic or environmental factors.

Such variability may significantly exceed what is expected in molecular target-level HTS, and requires new approaches to understand and assimilate.

To date, attempts to develop quantitative whole-organism screens for schistosomes and filarids have employed end-point observations based on vital "live/dead" color and fluorescent dyes, and real-time measurements of motility and heat exchange as a result of exposure to drug (reviewed in Chapter 20). Manual phenotyping [6], although expedient in classifying deviations from the "normal worm," nevertheless limits throughput, introduces subjectivity into measurements, is inherently nonquantitative, and, consequently, cannot be subjected to rigorous analysis. Furthermore, the nonquantitative nature of manual phenotyping complicates structure–activity modeling and lead optimization. The alternate approaches listed above are quantitative and real-time. However, they rely on single-dimensional outputs (motility or heat exchange) and cannot cover the totality of responses that are possible with complex pathogens. Thus, the design of algorithmic techniques for quantification and analysis of complex and dynamic phenotypic effects that constitute the system response of the pathogen to a drug molecule is imperative. To date, significant research has been conducted in the behavioral analysis of model organisms such as *Caenorhabditis elegans* [7, 8], *Danio rerio* [9, 10], *Drosophila melanogaster* [11, 12], *Mus musculus* [13, 14], and *Manduca sexta* [15–17]. Although generally relevant to our problem, the above methods do not deal with the issues that are critical for drug screening, such as statistical quantification of phenotypes and their variations, challenges arising from miniaturization and screen throughput, and phenotypic analysis that is useful towards constructing structure–activity relationship (SAR) models.

Although the focus of this chapter is on computational problems and solutions for high-throughput phenotypic screening, it should be noted that there are a number of biological and technological challenges to interfacing the etiological agents of helminth NTDs with an HTS format [18, 19] (see also Chapter 20). Consider the case of schistosomes as an example, which like other parasitic helminths do not proliferate in culture. Therefore, the entire life cycle, including the snail vector and small mammals (hamsters or mice) as intermediate and final hosts, respectively, must be maintained in order to supply sufficient biological material for screening. Furthermore, being relatively large, the adult and immature schistosomulum stages sediment quickly out of solution. The parasites are also prone to physical damage that complicates automated dispensation into microtiter culture plates (conversations with Jim McKerrow (2008) and Conor Caffrey (2009)). Finally, the traditional screening focus has been on adult parasites. This has hampered throughput as adults can only be grown to maturity in small mammals and in low numbers (e.g., around 50–100 worms per mouse). Also, direct evaluation of compound efficacy in animal disease models requires at least 40 days between infection of small mammals (typically mice) and maturity of the model *Schistosoma mansoni* parasite.

This chapter begins with a brief overview of the necessary background and terminology of biological image analysis, which is a cornerstone for automated phenotyping. Next, we review the current state-of-the-art in terms of automated phenotypic analysis, based especially on the model organism *C. elegans*. Of the commonly studied model organisms, *C. elegans* is somewhat similar (in terms of visual analysis) to the etiological agents of schistosomiasis and filariasis. Finally, we present results from our ongoing research that seeks to develop automated HTS technologies based on rigorous quantification of phenotypes.

Basic Concepts of Biological Image Analysis for Quantitative Phenotyping

In this section, we give an overview of the basic concepts of automated biological image analysis. Using examples obtained from time-lapse bright-field image capture of *S. mansoni* and *Brugia malayi*, a typical screening workflow is presented and the basic problem formulations explained. As part of our narrative, we review the foundations of image analysis. Using these ideas, it is possible to capture and quantify the effect of a compound in terms of the phenotypic responses of the pathogen. It should be noted that this is but an introductory treatment of biological image analysis. The interested reader is referred to more comprehensive reviews and texts on image processing for details [20–24]. For online resources on biological image analysis, we refer the reader to [25].

We begin by outlining the steps in a typical image analysis workflow as applied to drug screening. The workflow is illustrated in Figure 10.1 and consists of the following parts:

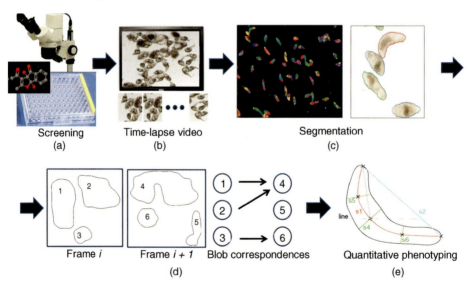

Figure 10.1 Image analysis workflow for drug screening. The main stages of the workflow are as follows. (a) HTS of compound libraries. (b) The information capture is typically done using time-lapse video recordings of the parasite appearance, activity, and/or behavior. Each video can be thought as a structure that contains a temporally ordered sequence of still images. (c) Segmentation, consisting of the separation of parasites from the background and identification of individual parasites. (d) Tracking individual parasites across the video. (e) Quantitative phenotyping by measuring characteristics of individual parasites.

i) **Screening**: Medium- and high-throughput screens are typically conducted using 24/96/384-well plates used in conjunction with partially or fully automated systems for parasite handling and dispensation that can place a defined number of parasites to each well of the plate. Automated systems are then used to add drug molecules at predefined concentrations to the wells of the plate.

ii) **Image capture**: An imaging system is next used to capture a visual recording of the response of the pathogen to the drug. The imaging system can be a high-content screening (HCS) system. Examples include the likes of the InCell Analyzer™ series from GE healthcare, the Opera™ confocal microplate imaging reader system from PerkinElmer, and the Cellomics ArrayScan™ from ThermoScientific. Alternatively, the imaging system can be as simple as an inverted microscope outfitted with a video camera. It is typical to take time-lapse videos or still images. A digital camera divides its field of view into a discrete grid of pixels. Each pixel in this grid is characterized by its intensity value, which defines the intensity of light received by the camera at this point. For an 8-bit image, the range of intensity values that can be represented consists of 256 distinct values varying from 0 to 255 (2^8-1). Similarly, the commonly used 12-bit image formats in HCS can represent 4096 distinct intensity values. If different channels are imaged (e.g., for different fluorescent wavelengths) then each channel is represented by one such grid. As video recordings provide information on both non-time-varying characteristics and motion-based characteristics of the pathogens, in the following discussion we will assume video data capture. A video can be thought of as a series of still images (alternatively called frames) taken over a specific period of time. The number of frames captured per second defines the video sampling frequency and is called the frame rate of the video. For a given video, its frame rate is denoted by the abbreviation fps (frames per second). In HCS, frame rates typically vary in the range of 10–30 fps. In deciding the appropriate frame rate, it is important to account for the Nyquist rate, which is defined as twice the bandwidth of a band-limited signal [26]. The Nyquist rate gives the lower bound of the sampling rate (in this case the frame rate) for alias-free sampling of the signal. Operationally, this implies that the frame rate should be at least twice the frequency of a phenotype that is being studied.

iii) **Image segmentation**: The goal of image segmentation is to determine all the pixels in the image that belong to each specific entity (parasite) in the field of view. That is, we want to partition the image such that regions representing different objects are explicitly marked. Image segmentation is one of the most complex problems in biological image analysis. There are two classes of methods that can partition an image into regions: region-based segmentation and edge detection. *Regions* and *edges* constitute two of the fundamental concepts of image analysis. A region in an image is a group of connected pixels with similar properties [21]. Ideally an object, such as a parasite, in an image will have a one-to-one correspondence with a region in that image. However, due to segmentation errors the correspondence between regions and objects may not be perfect. The notions of connectivity and neighborhood are central to the definition of a region. In a digital image represented on a square grid, a pixel is spatially close to several other pixels. Specifically, a pixel shares a common boundary with four of its neighboring pixels and shares a corner with four additional pixels. Two pixels are called 4-neighbors if they share a common boundary. Analogously, two pixels are called 8-neighbors if they share at least one corner. Note, that the 4-neighborhod of a pixel is contained in its 8-neighborhood. In a region R, any two pixels p and q can be connected by a path that consists entirely of pixels in R such that any two pixels in this path are either 4-neighbors or 8-neighbors of each other. That is, a region is a connected component. One of the most common tasks in image processing involves finding connected components in an image. In this context, a *component labeling* algorithm finds all connected components in an image and assigns a unique label to all pixels within the same connected component. In the following subsection we take a closer look at the area of image segmentation.

iv) **Parasite tracking**: As a video is a collection of still images, measurement of the phenotypic response of a specific parasite requires that we be able to identify it in each frame of the video. The process through which a correspondence can be established between specific parasites in different frames of a video is called tracking. In spite of the intuitive simplicity of this formulation, tracking is an exceedingly complex technical problem. Consider for instance the case illustrated in Figure 10.1d. In frame i, there are three identifiable regions labeled 1, 2, and 3 (corresponding to three parasites). In the next frame $i + 1$, three new regions can be identified (labeled 4, 5, and 6, respectively). An analysis of the two frames shows that region 4 in frame $i + 1$ is formed when the parasites denoted as 1 and 2 in frame i move and touch each other. By contrast, region 5 in frame $i + 1$ is due to a new parasite that has come into the field of view and region 6 in frame $i + 1$ corresponds to region 3 from frame i (the parasite having moved). These correspondences are shown as a bipartite graph in Figure 10.1d. As this example illustrates, a tracking method should be able to deal with possibly complex movement patterns, merging and splitting of regions, and objects appearing and disappearing from the field of view. A rich collection of tracking techniques can be found in the image processing literature. For a recent review of the area, we refer the reader to [27]. Later, we present an example of a tracking approach based on the mean-shift algorithm [28].

v) **Quantitative phenotyping**: Once all the parasites in a video are identified, their different characteristics can be measured. The simplest measurements for parasites include: (1) count or the number of parasites; (2) size, typically defined as the number of pixels inside each parasite or the area of each parasite; (3) intensity/color distribution, defined using the intensity and/or color histogram as well as the maximum, minimum, and total intensity of a parasite; (4) shape, which can be defined through a number of descriptors such as the medial axis of the parasite, ratio of the body thickness at different points, ratio of the length of the medial axis to the straight line joining the extremities, various descriptors of contour shape, and Zernike shape features; (5) texture descriptors that characterize spatial smoothness and regularity of the parasites (texture descriptors are obtained from the analysis of the intensity co-occurrence matrix and quantified using statistical properties such as energy, entropy, homogeneity, and contrast); and, finally, (6) motion descriptors, which include speed of movement along with descriptions of parasite movement patterns. An illustration of some of the shape descriptors can be found in Figure 10.1e.

Image Segmentation: A Closer Look

One of the conceptually simplest methods for region-based segmentation is based on the idea of *thresholding*. The idea lies in classifying a pixel as foreground if its intensity exceeds a certain threshold value. Global thresholding methods compute a single threshold for the entire image. This can be done, for instance, by fitting two probability distributions to the intensity data. The underlying assumption being that the foreground (parasites) and the background would have different intensity distributions. Local thresholding methods, by contrast, apply different thresholds to different parts of the image and have superior performance in case of nonuniform or variable image illumination.

An edge in an image is a significant local change in the intensity associated with a discontinuity in either the image intensity or the first derivative of the image intensity. Mathematically, the gradient is a measure of change in a function. Consequently, significant changes in the intensity of an image can be detected by assuming the image to be a sample of some continuous image intensity function and using a discrete approximation of the intensity gradient. Much of the work in this area is devoted to finding numerical approximations to the gradient that are suitable for use with real-world images. The Roberts operator, the Sobel operator, and the Prewitt operator are some of the techniques that provide different ways of approximating the image gradient (for details on these operators, see [21]). All these operators compute the first derivative and report an edge point if the derivative is above a threshold. This procedure can, however, report too many edge points. A more selective approach considers only those points that have local maxima in gradient values. Mathematically, this implies that at these points there is a peak in the first derivative and a zero crossing in the second derivative. The two-dimensional equivalent of the second derivative is called the Laplacian. However, the detection of zero crossings of the second derivative can be very sensitive to noise. The Laplacian of Gaussian edge detection operator combines Gaussian filtering with the Laplacian to deal with this problem. In this method the image is first convolved with a Gaussian filter to reduce noise. This is followed by the application of the Laplacian. The presence of a zero crossing in the second derivative with a corresponding (large) peak in the first derivative constitutes the edge detection criterion.

Another widely used approach to edge detection is the Canny operator [29] that approximates the product of signal-to-noise ratio and localization. This composite operator performs several operations to detect the edges of the original image. The first operation consists of filtering the original image, which is convolved with a Gaussian kernel to reduce noise. The next operation involves the detection of the intensity gradient of the image G and its direction angle Θ using an edge detection operator comprising four filters (vertical, horizontal, and diagonals). Depending on the edge direction angle Θ, the third operation called nonmaximum suppression detects if the gradient magnitude assumes a local maximum in the gradient direction. In such a case, the point is considered tentatively to belong to an edge. Finally, the tentatively selected edge points undergo thresholding with hysteresis to eliminate pixels with large magnitudes (essentially noise) and pixels with very low magnitudes.

Once the foreground/background distinction is achieved, additional processing is often required to separate touching parasites (e.g., see Figure 10.1c). Most of the algorithmic methods that have been designed for this problem can be placed in one of two categories: partitioning methods and methods based on morphological analysis. In partitioning methods, the first step is to approximate the centers of each parasite. This can be done either by identification of the local intensity extrema or by using a distance transformation. The former approach works well when the object is brighter/dimmer in the middle as compared to its edges. The later approach is suited for rounded shapes. In the second step, the partition lines between objects are established using techniques such as Voronoi tessellation or the watershed algorithm [30]. In the final step, an object model is applied to discard or merge existing objects. The object model represents a typical object in the domain. For instance, based on such a model, foreground entities that are smaller than a threshold size can be excluded to remove debris from the scene. It should be noted that the intensity/shape regularity that is critical for identifying approximate object centers does not apply for parasites like *S. mansoni* or *B. malayi*. In such cases morphological analysis can lead to better results. Later in this chapter, we describe three methods for separating touching parasites.

Segmentation and Automated Phenotype Analysis: A Brief Review

In biological imaging, phenotype analysis has primarily occurred either in the context of cell-based assays or for characterization of model organisms. We begin this section with a brief review of techniques for cell segmentation and analyze the applicability of such methods for segmentation of parasites. This is followed by a brief review of the state-of-the-art in terms of phenotypic analysis of whole organisms.

The problem of image segmentation has a long history in image processing research and many methods have been proposed. However, a direct application of traditional segmentation algorithms proposed in image processing literature on images of parasites (or cells) often leads to inadequate performance [31–33]. Consequently, a large number of techniques have been proposed, with the primary thrust on cell/nuclei segmentation [34]. Broadly, the following three classes of techniques can be distinguished in this context. (i) When only an image of a nuclear marker is available, Voronoi tessellation-based segmentation is used [35, 36]. However, the resulting segmentation masks have been observed to crop pieces off of individual cells [37] in cases where the cells clump together. (ii) When information about both cell centers and boundaries are available, the seeded watershed algorithm [38, 39] usually provides good segmentation. However, the performance of this algorithm is critically dependent on initial seeds. Furthermore, unless the background is seeded, the algorithm fails to produce tight contours. Owing to its popularity, a number of variations of the watershed algorithm have been proposed, such as the use of context information [32], and combinations of watershed and rule-based merging [40]. (iii) The final set of techniques involves parameterized models such as active contours [41–45] as well as level sets [46]. The computational costs of techniques based on both active contours and level sets can be significant, thereby making them difficult to apply in high-throughput settings. A few techniques fall outside the scope of the aforementioned three categories. Most of these involve the use of motion information for segmentation. For example, in [47], initial image-based region segmentation is followed by bipartite matching of the segmented regions across two consecutive frames of a video in order to topologically "align" them and obtain the final partition.

With respect to the state-of-the-art in bioimage analysis, it should be noted that a number of arguments underpin the need to develop novel algorithms for segmentation and analysis as applied to the pathogens such as *S. mansoni* or *B. malayi*. (i) The fact that no single method has been found that can produce satisfactory segmentation results for all organisms (see [48, 49] for studies on segmentation errors and comparison of different techniques as applied to cell-based assays). This is due, among others, to the fact that experimental conditions and instrumentation can significantly impact the nature of the segmentation task. (ii) Outside of the significant research in *C. elegans* [7, 8, 50–55] there is little research on algorithmic segmentation and analysis of complex phenotypes exhibited by helminths. (iii) The problem confronting us is also significantly distinct from that encountered by researchers in *C. elegans* phenotyping. Compared to the *C. elegans* mutants, the motion, morphology, and appearance of *S. mansoni* schistosomula are more complex and undergo a greater variety of changes when exposed to different compounds (e.g., clones of genotypically identical schistosomes do not exist). (iv) In the case of HTS against NTDs, the input data typically consists of images and video of multiple parasites residing in multiwell plates used in HTS. This leads to imaging conditions very different than those used for *C. elegans* (consisting of large Petri dishes with only few worms per dish). (v) Algorithms in an HTS setting have to be computationally efficient to ensure their usage – this is a constraint that is simply not critical in *C. elegans* phenotyping.

Efforts in algorithmic phenotyping, to date, have almost exclusively focused on model organisms like the nematode *C. elegans*. In [55], the shape of the *C. elegans* body was described through a curve that passes through the center of the body and positions along this curve were computed using the Frenet equations. Subsequently, the variation in the body shape was analyzed during small changes in the temperature; analysis of the covariance matrix of the angles along the body showed that the four largest eigenvectors accounted for 95% of the shape variance. In [51], the authors proposed a number of parameters for quantifying shape and movement of *C. elegans*. These were compared for a small set of mutant worms in which the signaling network controlling acetylcholine release at the neuromuscular junction had been altered.

The parameters included velocity of the worm centroid, worm velocity along its track, amplitude, and frequency of body bending. Finally, in [52], a number of numerical features were proposed for characterization of *C. elegans* motion, and the CART (classification and regression tree) algorithm was used for subsequent phenotype identification.

Although related to the above, phenotypic analysis of schistosomula involves greater complexity; unlike *C. elegans*, phenotypes in schistosomula are not just shape- and motion-based, but based on changes in color and appearance. Further, the motion patterns of schistosomula involve contractions and bending of the parasite body leading to greater shape perturbations when compared to those of *C. elegans*.

Automated Phenotype Analysis for Drug Screening Against Schistosomiasis and Filariasis

In this section, we present a review of our ongoing research efforts that target many of the problems described earlier with a goal of developing high-throughput whole-organism phenotypic screening methods for drug discovery against schistosomiasis and filariasis. We begin by describing some of the different technical directions we have taken to address the problem of segmenting parasites. Then we discuss parasite tracking, quantitative descriptor generation, and derivation of phenotypes using machine learning. The data used for method development and experiments comprise time-lapse videos of live schistosomula captured using a Zeiss Axiovert 40C inverted microscope outfitted with a Zeiss AxioCam MRc camera. Each video observation was of duration 25 s at 15 fps.

Algorithms for Schistosome Segmentation

In high-throughput settings, parasite segmentation is often the most significant technical challenge. This is because segmentation is the critical first step and variability in experimental conditions such as lighting characteristics or number of parasites in a well (even moderate number of parasites can cause them to lump together) can significantly impact the efficacy of automated processing. The problem of segmenting schistosomula is especially complex since a model "parasite shape" cannot be assumed *a priori*. This is in stark contrast to the problem of cellular segmentation, for instance, where a "rounded" shape is often assumed [32, 43, 56]. A stated above, the movement of schistosomula is based on extension and contraction of the musculature, in addition to bending. Therefore, the shape of the parasite's body changes within a single movement cycle. Additionally, parasites contain visible internal anatomical structures that complicate segmentation by creating edges that do not correspond to the boundaries of the body. Often, parasites can be touching over the course of the video recording. This can result in poor discrimination of individual parasites. Finally, the effects of different drugs are manifested in different ways through changes in the appearance, morphology (shape), and motion of the parasites. It is consequently impossible to assume a characteristic shape-appearance model.

Two key parts can therefore be identified within the segmentation problem. The first relates to the problem of distinguishing the parasites from the background. The second part involves identifying individual parasites. It has been our observation that efficacy of the segmentation process depends critically on solving the first of the above subproblems. Once accurate parasite/background separation is achieved, computational morphology-based methods can be used to separate and identify individual parasites with relatively high reliability. In the following, we review results from our ongoing research on this problem.

In [31], we proposed a multistep process for parasite segmentation. The initial step of this algorithm involves fitting a bimodal distribution to the intensity distribution of the frame and automatic intensity-based thresholding of the image into foreground and background regions. The threshold is selected at a point that maximizes the intensity variance between the foreground and background using the Otsu algorithm [57]. Even though the bimodality assumption is simplistic, it describes the intensity characteristics of most images we have encountered reasonably well. A critical advantage of this approach is that for most cases, the threshold value can be obtained automatically without any user intervention across a range of lighting conditions. Moreover, this step is used only as an initial estimate. Next, the foreground regions from this image are treated as the first approximation of the partition and used as object markers (in practice prior to use, the foreground regions are typically subjected to morphological closing followed by erosion). The background markers are also extracted from the binary image after determination of the SKIZ (skeleton of influence zones, which correspond to the generalized Voronoi regions) of the foreground objects followed by watershed transform of the distance transform of the image. Subsequently, the gradient magnitude of the grayscale image is modified to have regional minima at the foreground and background marker locations, and used as the segmentation function prior to application of the watershed transform. Finally, the parasite contours are extracted and touching parasites are separated by analyzing opposing concave/convex points. The separation is done under the constraint that each of the separated blobs contained a foreground region marker as determined in the previous step. The markers, object boundaries, and watershed ridge lines (in white) obtained using this method are shown superimposed on an original image in Figure 10.2a. Figure 10.2b illustrates the idea of concave/convex points based on which morphological thinning is performed to separate touching parasites.

In Figure 10.2c–f we illustrate a morphological approach to the problem of separating parasites from the background and from each other. We shall refer to this method in the following as the Mennillo–Singh method. The idea underlying this method forms the genesis of a more efficient approach proposed in [58], which is described later. The Mennillo–Singh method begins by using the mean-shift algorithm to identify regions by tessellating the image. The image on the left in Figure 10.1c constitutes an example of this step. A key insight of this approach lies in recognizing that in most images, the background pixels correspond to the largest mode. Consequently, all other modes correspond to foreground objects and are marked as such. The results from this step are shown in Figure 10.2c. As can be seen,

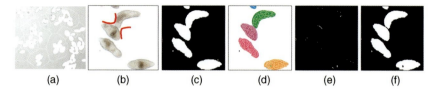

(a) (b) (c) (d) (e) (f)

Figure 10.2 Results from two methods for separating touching parasites. In the first method regional maxima obtained from automatic thresholding are superimposed on the original image and used as object markers prior to watershed segmentation. (a) markers, object boundaries, and watershed ridge lines are shown superimposed on the original image. (b) The idea of opposing concave/convex regions for two touching parasites. (c–f) Results from the Mennillo–Singh method: (c) results of foreground/background separation, (d) output of the Canny edge operator, (e) relevant edge pixels for this image, and (f) result of the method, showing separation of touching parasites.

the problem of separating touching parasites remains outstanding at this point. The next step involves detecting the edges of the original image. For this, the Canny edge operator [29] is used. The edges detected using the Canny operator are then subtracted from the foreground image identified using the mean-shift algorithm. The results of this step from the image in Figure 10.2c are shown in Figure 10.2d. The core idea of the Mennillo–Singh method is now implemented. This involves finding relevant edge pixels. The pixels lying on edges determined by the Canny operator are considered to be relevant if they are responsible of the separation of a connected component. In terms of image connectivity this means that every such edge pixel in the labeled image must have at least two different labels in its eight neighbors. The relevant pixels for the image in Figure 10.2c are shown in Figure 10.2e. The relevant edges are next subtracted from the foreground image. The reader may note that this results in separation of two different regions that are touching. The final step consists of filling holes of the image and removal of small connected components which are less than 200 pixels. The output of this method is shown in Figure 10.2f.

The Mennillo–Singh method has shown promise in experiments in terms of its accuracy. However, it is dependent on the computationally intensive mean-shift algorithm and can take approximately 26 s to process a single image. Recently, an alternate approach based on the core idea of the Mennillo–Singh method was proposed by Moody-Davis *et al.* [58]. This method shares with the Mennillo–Singh approach the idea of first identifying and separating the parasites from the background. However, it approaches this problem from a different computational perspective based on the idea of a region-based distribution function [56]. This formulation leads to significantly faster run times as compared to the mean-shift algorithm without compromising the quality of results. Once the parasite/background separation is achieved, morphological analysis similar to that in the Mennillo–Singh method is used to separate touching parasites. In the following, we briefly outline this method.

The purpose of a region-based distribution function is to rapidly identify the background by assigning a higher weight to background pixels. Initially, a low-pass filter is applied to remove noise and smooth the image. Next the average border intensity γ is subtracted and the image is multiplied by a term β called the harshness of the threshold. The term β is inversely proportional to the difference of the average background and foreground intensities; the smaller the difference, the higher the value assigned to β. The result is asymptotically bounded using a sigmoid function and finally a skewing factor α is applied. This results in pixel values below the average border intensity γ being skewed towards the background because they have a higher weight. The original formulation of the region-based distribution function is as follows [56]:

$$R_1(n) = \alpha \times \text{sig}\left(\beta \times \left((f * h)(n) - \gamma\right)\right) \tag{10.1}$$

where $\alpha \in (-1, 0)$ is the weight of the region-based distributing function, $\beta = 4/(H - L)$ is the harshness of the threshold, and $\gamma = (H + L)/2$ denotes the average border intensity. In the definition of the parameter β, H denotes the average region intensity and L denotes the average background intensity. Further, h denotes a low-pass filter which is used to remove high-frequency noise. Finally, the function sig(.) is defined as shown Equation 10.2 and is used to restrict the possible value range to the interval $[-1 +1]$:

$$\text{sig}(x) = \text{erf}(x) = \frac{2}{\sqrt{\pi}} \int_0^x e^{\frac{t^2}{2}} dt \tag{10.2}$$

In [58], the above method was modified to reduce the number of parameters in Equation 10.1 and a new version of the region-based distribution function was introduced as shown in Equation 10.3:

$$R_1(n) = -1 \times \text{sig}\left((f * h)(n) - \gamma\right) \tag{10.3}$$

Additionally, the parameter γ was reinterpreted to threshold the difference in the intensity between the background and foreground. The reader may note that as this threshold decreases (i.e., as the difference in the foreground and background intensities becomes smaller), the segmented results increasingly include regions with intensity values closer to the background intensity. This essentially increases the number of true-positive identification of parasites and beyond a point false-positives start to occur in the foreground. In the limit, the number of foreground objects decreases to one (as the entire image is treated as the foreground). Thus, the number of foreground objects is a function of the parameter γ. The method in [58] selects as the threshold that value of γ at which the slope of this function is maximum. It is important to note that at this point small regions representing debris from the medium constitute the false positives. These regions can be easily filtered.

After filtering, the remaining foreground regions are analyzed using the morphological processing approach used in the Mennillo–Singh method. In Figure 10.3, we present some of the segmentation results obtained using this approach. Figure 10.3a is the input image. The results after application of the region-based distribution function are shown in Figure 10.3b. The reader may observe the false positive regions of the foreground. The final results of the method are shown in

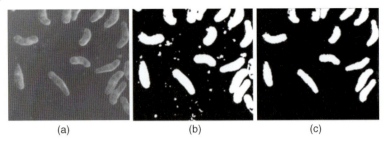

Figure 10.3 Results of the method from [58] combining a modified region-based distribution function with the morphological processing of the Mennillo—Singh method. (a) Original image. (b) Result from applying the region-based distribution function. (c) Final output of the method.

Figure 10.3c after filtering the false positives and morphological processing to separate touching parasites.

Segmentation of Filarial Parasites for HTS

In this section, we consider the problem of screening *B. malayi*, which is one of the three etiological agents of lymphatic filariasis (the others being *Wuchereria bancrofti* and *Brugia timori*). The morphology of this parasite is long and threadlike; consequently, the segmentation methods we have discussed earlier are inapplicable to this problem. In Figure 10.4a the reader can find two different images of this parasite, taken from two wells of a 24-well plate. A number of issues that pose technical challenges can be identified from these images. (i) Unlike schistosomula, the *B. malayi* parasite body can take complex configurations, such as self-intersections. (ii) The entire parasite body may not be in view, even if the assay is designed to have only one parasite per well. (iii) Different parts of the body of the parasite can lie in different planes of focus. This causes parts of the parasite body to be blurred due to being out of focus. (iv) Unlike schistosomula, *B. malayi* has a thrashing motion,

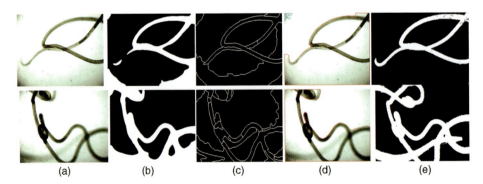

Figure 10.4 Segmentation of *B. malayi*. (a) Images of the parasites. (b) Results of segmentation using the Active Mask method of [56]. (c) Segmentation results using the JSEG method [60]. (d) Segmentation using the Mennillo–Singh method. (e) Segmentation using a variation of the codebook method.

which can be quite rapid under inducements by certain chemicals. While the speed of motion is in itself not a hindrance for segmentation, it can impact the effectiveness of tracking. (v) Due to the thrashing motion of the parasite, there can be significant displacement in the surrounding medium. Again, this does not directly affect segmentation, but can be problematic for tracking by introducing spurious motion in the background. It is interesting to note that conventional segmentation methods perform poorly for this parasite. Figure 10.4b–d show the results from applying some of the state-of-the-art segmentation techniques to the images in Figure 10.4a.

As part of our ongoing research in this area, we are experimenting with a novel approach to simultaneous segmentation and tracking that is inspired by prior research in the area of surveillance. Specifically, we are experimenting with a dictionary-based segmentation approach that was proposed by Kim *et al.* [59]. The basic idea of this approach lies in analyzing the joint intensity/frequency characteristics of each pixel in the video and identifying it as a foreground (parasite) pixel or a background pixel. For the kind of images shown in Figure 10.4a, the background will consist of high-intensity pixels that occur with high frequency. By contrast, low-intensity pixels that also change with lower frequency (as the body of the parasite moves in and out of this pixel) would belong to the parasite. The method works in a supervised setting, where in a "training phase" samples of the video are taken to identify characteristics of the foreground and the background pixels. These characteristics are then stored in a dictionary (or codebook). In the "test phase," pixels from a video are compared to the dictionary and identified as foreground (parasite) or background. In Figure 10.4e we show segmentation results from our work in progress based on this idea. The reader may note that the quality of segmentation far exceeds what is possible with other methods.

Tracking, Phenotype Quantification, and Phenotype Classification

In this section, we review the results from our research [31], which was applied to automated phenotyping of schistosomula. However, the algorithmic approach proposed in this work is sufficiently generic to be extended to other parasites. This method consists of the following four main steps: (i) delineation of the parasites from the medium (parasite/background segmentation), (ii) automatic tracking of individual parasites across the observation period, (iii) quantitative description of the phenotypes exhibited by the parasite in terms of its shape, appearance (texture and color), and movement patterns, and (iv) machine learning-based strategies for automatically analyzing and classifying the above (quantitative) characteristics into phenotype classes. Since we have already covered the problem of parasite segmentation in earlier sections, here we describe the other steps of the method and refer the reader to [31] for further details.

To determine the time-varying characteristics, including parasite motion, in [31] a tracking algorithm was designed based on the mean-shift algorithm [28], which has recently gained popularity in feature-based tracking [32, 61–63]. As stated earlier, the mean-shift algorithm clusters an n-dimensional dataset by associating each point

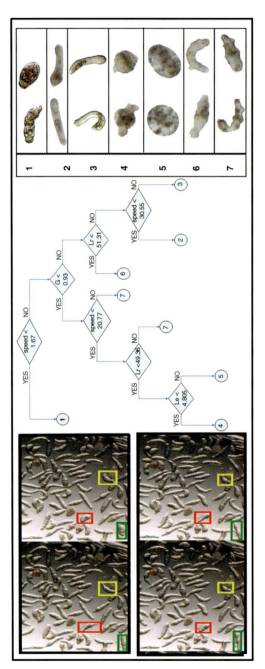

Figure 10.5 (Left) Example of parasite tracking from a video sequence using the method from [31]. Three parasites are tracked across the sequence. In the figure, the tracked positions are shown for the first frame (top-row left) and for every 25th frame thereafter (top-row right and bottom row). (Middle) The CART decision tree obtained after 10-fold cross-validation. Internal nodes represent decision boundaries. Terminal nodes represent a phenotype. (Right) Examples of the seven phenotypes obtained automatically from the data. Two parasites from each phenotype class are shown.

with a peak of the dataset's probability density. Based on this idea, the key steps of the tracking approach consisted of (i) representing the parasites through normalized histograms of their descriptors, (ii) defining a similarity function between parasites whose local maxima, when computed across frames, would imply similar parasites, and (iii) use of the mean-shift algorithm to determine the local maxima and establish the correspondences between the same parasite in different frames. In Figure 10.5, we present an example of parasite tracking with this approach, in which three parasites are tracked across a video.

After segmentation and tracking, each blob (corresponding to a parasite) was algorithmically characterized in terms of the following shape and appearance-based features: intensity/color distribution histogram, texture, area (defined as the number of pixels inside the blob), bounding box for each parasite, density (defined as the ratio of the area/bounding box area), centroid, and contour (defined by the set of coordinates of boundary pixels). All these descriptors were calculated for each parasite in each frame. To measure parasite activity, the displacement of the parasite extremities was measured across every 10 frames of a video recording.

We used the CART algorithm [64] to structure the numerical measurements into phenotypes. CART is a supervised learning strategy in which the training set is analyzed according to a splitting rule and a goodness-of-split criteria to create a binary classification tree. The internal nodes of this tree represent binary decisions with respect to the descriptor values and the leaves correspond to phenotype classes. The goal of CART is to perform a set of successive binary subdivisions of the training set such that data associated with the leaf nodes is as homogeneous as possible. A classifier obtained using data from four videos is shown in Figure 10.5 (middle). It is interesting to note that in the datasets analyzed by us, the algorithm found seven statistically stable phenotype classes, compared to the six classes identified by visual inspection [6]. These results underline (i) the importance of using algorithmic approaches to the problem, because the perceptual capabilities of humans (even trained experts) may not suffice to determine all statistically stable or nontrivial phenotypes, and (ii) the importance of developing systems that support human–machine synergy, whereby the computer/algorithms perform the labor- and attention-intensive tasks of phenotype identification while the domain experts focus on the questions of phenotype interpretability and importance. For instance, it is not yet known how many treatment-related phenotypes will predict *in vivo* efficacy and/or biological mechanism of action.

Conclusions

As complex multicellular organisms, the etiological agents of helminth NTDs display multiple and changing phenotypes in response to external insult. This multidimensional response provides a unique challenge and opportunity for developing novel types of HTS/HCS technologies that can measure the effect of a drug, even at the initial screening stage, in terms of the systemic response of the parasite. Decisions on which drug candidates to take further into lead optimization based on such comprehensive information can only increase the quality of molecules entering late-stage discovery and development. To realize this vision, HTS/HCS biology and computational sciences have to successfully address a rich set of questions. This chapter has highlighted many of these challenges. We have also provided the relevant background on image analysis to help the reader understand and evaluate potential solutions. Finally, we have described some of our own investigative efforts towards solving these technical challenges.

Acknowledgments

The author thanks his students Asher Moody-Davis, Laurent Mennillo, Utsab Saha, Dan Asarnaw, and Ai Sasho. The author would also like to thank his collaborators Jim McKerrow, Conor Caffrey, Judy Sakanari, and Michelle Arkin from the University of California San Francisco. This work was funded in part by the National Institutes of Health, National Institute of Allergy and Infectious Diseases through grant 1R01AI089896-01, the National Science Foundation through grant IIS-0644418 (CAREER), the Bill & Melinda Gates Foundation through grant OPP1017584, and a Joint Venture Grant from the California State University Program for Education and Research in Biotechnology. The findings and conclusions contained within are those of the author and do not necessarily reflect positions or policies of the funding agencies.

References

1 Caffrey, C.R. (2007) Chemotherapy of schistosomiasis: present and future. *Curr. Opin. Chem. Biol.*, **11**, 433–439.

2 Fenwick, A. and Webster, J.P. (2006) Schistosomiasis: challenges for control, treatment and drug resistance. *Curr. Opin. Infect. Dis.*, **19**, 577–582.

3 Lammie, P.J., Fenwick, A., and Utzinger, J. (2006) A blueprint for success: integration of neglected tropical disease control programmes. *Trends Parasitol.*, **22**, 313–321.

4 Steinmann, P., Keiser, J., Bos, R., Tanner, M., and Utzinger, J. (2006) Schistosomiasis and water resources development: systematic review, meta-analysis, and estimates of people at risk. *Lancet Infect. Dis.*, **6**, 411–425.

5 Michael, S., Auld, D., Klumpp, C., Jadhav, A., Zheng, W., Thorne, N., Austin, C.P., Inglese, J., and Simeonov, A. (2008) A robotic platform for quantitative high throughput screening. *Assay Drug Dev. Technol.*, **6**, 637–657.

6 Abdulla, M.H., Ruelas, D.S., Wolff, B., Snedecor, J., Lim, K.C., Xu, F., Renslo, A.R. et al. (2009) Drug discovery for schistosomiasis: hit and lead compounds identified in a library of known drugs by medium-throughput phenotypic screening. *PLoS Negl. Trop. Dis.*, **3**, e478.

7 Baek, J.-H., Cosman, P., Feng, Z., Silver, J., and Schafer, W.R. (2002) Using Machine Vision to analyze and classify *Caenorhabditis elegans* behavioral phenotypes quantitatively. *J. Neurosci. Methods*, **118**, 9–21.

8 Geng, W., Cosman, P., Berry, C.C., Feng, Z., and Schafer, W.R. (2004) Automatic tracking, feature extraction and classification of *C. elegans* phenotypes. *IEEE Trans. Biomed. Eng.*, **51**, 1811–1820.

9 Darland, T. and Dowling, J.E. (2001) Behavioral screening for cocaine sensitivity in mutagenized zebrafish. *Proc. Natl. Acad. Sci. USA*, **98**, 11691–11696.

10 Levin, E.D. and Cerutti, D.T. (2009) Behavioral neuroscience of zebrafish, in *Methods of Behavior Analysis in Neuroscience*, 2nd edn (ed. J.J. Buccafusco), CRC Press, Boca Raton, FL, pp. 291–308.

11 McNabb, S.L., Baker, J.D., Agapite, J., Steller, H., Riddiford, L.M., and Truman, J.W. (1997) Disruption of a behavioral sequence by targeted death of peptidergic neurons in *Drosophila*. *Neuron*, **19**, 813–823.

12 Dankert, H., Wang, L., Hoopfer, E.D., Anderson, D.J., and Perona, P. (2009) Automated monitoring and analysis of social behavior in drosophila. *Nat. Methods*, **6**, 297–303.

13 Halem, H.A., Cherry, J.A., and Baum, M.J. (1999) Vomeronasal neuroepithelium and forebrain Fos responses to male pheromones in male and female mice. *J. Neurobiol.*, **39**, 249–263.

14 Branson, K., Rabaud, W.R., and Belongie, S. (2003) Three brown mice: see how they run. IEEE International Workshop on Performance Evaluation of Tracking and Surveillance, Graz.

15 Mezoff, S., Papastathis, N., Takesian, A., and Trimmer, B.A. (2004) The biomechanical and neural control of hydrostatic limb movements in *Manduca sexta*. *J. Exp. Biol.*, **17**, 3043–3053.

16 Shimoide, A., Yoon, I., Fuse, M., Beale, H.C., and Singh, R. (2005) Automated behavioral phenotype detection and analysis using color-based motion tracking. Second Canadian Conference on Comput Robot Vision, Victoria, BC.

17 Vaughan, A., Singh, R., Shimoide, A., Yoon, I., and Fuse, M. (2005) EigenPhenotypes: towards an algorithmic framework for phenotype discovery. IEEE Computational Systems Bioinformatics Conference, Stanford, CA.

18 Caffrey, C.R. and Secor, W.E. (2011) Schistosomiasis: from drug deployment to drug development. *Curr. Opin. Infect. Dis.*, **24**, 410–417.

19 Geary, T.G., Woods, D.J., Williams, T., and Nwaka, S. (2009) Target identification and mechanism-based screening for anthelmintics: application of veterinary antiparasitic research programs to search for new antiparasitic drugs for human indications, in *Antiparasitic and Antibacterial Drug Discovery: From Molecular Targets to Drug Candidates* (ed. P.M. Selzer), Wiley-VCH Verlag GmbH, Weinheim, pp. 3–15.

20 Carpenter, A. (2007) Image based chemical screening. *Nat. Chem. Biol.*, **3**, 461–465.

21 Jain, R., Kasturi, R., and Schunck, B.G. (1995) *Machine Vision*, McGraw Hill, New York.

22 Ljosa, V. and Carpenter, A. (2009) Introduction to the quantitative analysis of two dimensional fluorescence microscopy images for cell-based screening. *PLoS Comp. Biol.*, **5**, e1000603.

23 Meijering, E. and Van Cappellen, G. (2007) Quantitative biological image analysis, in *Imaging Cellular and Molecular Biological Function* (eds S. Shorte and F. Frischknecht), Springer, Berlin, pp. 45–70.

24 Peng, H. (2008) Bioimage informatics: a new area of engineering biology. *Bioinformatics*, **24**, 1827–1836.

25 Chung, T.D. (2008) The management of chemical and biological information. *Curr. Opin. Drug Discov. Dev.*, **11**, 299–300.

26 Shannon, C.E. (1949) Communication in the presence of noise. *Proc. Inst. Radio Eng.*, **37**, 10–21.

27 Yilmaz, A., Javed, O., and Shah, M. (2006) Object tracking: a survey. *ACM Comput. Surv.*, **38**, article 13; doi: 10.1145/1177352.1177355

28 Comaniciu, D. and Meer, P. (2002) Mean shift: a robust approach towards feature space analysis. *IEEE Trans. Pattern Anal. Mach. Intell.*, **24**, 603–619.

29 Canny, J. (1986) A computational approach to edge detection. *IEEE Trans. Pattern Anal. Mach. Intell.*, **8**, 679–698.

30 Meyer, F. and Beucher, S. (1990) Morphological segmentation. *J. Visual Commun. Image Represent.*, **1**, 21–46.

31 Singh, R., Pittas, M., Heskia, I., Xu, F., McKerrow, J.H., and Caffrey, C.R. (2009) Automated image-based phenotypic screening for high-throughput drug discovery. IEEE Symposium on Computer-Based Medical Systems, Albuquerque, NM.

32 Yang, X., Li, H., and Zhou, X. (2006) Nuclei segmentation using marker-controlled watershed, tracking using mean-shift, and Kalman filter in time-lapse microscopy. *IEEE Trans. Circuits Syst.*, **53**, 2405–2414.

33 Wu, K., Gauthier, D., and Levine, M.D. (1995) Live cell image segmentation. *IEEE Trans. Biomed. Eng.*, **42**, 1–12.

34 Miura, K. (2005) Tracking movement in cell biology. *Adv. Biochem. Eng. Biotechnol.*, **95**, 267–295.

35 Rodenacker, K. and Bischoff, P. (1990) Quantification of tissue sections: graph theory and topology as modelling tools. *Pattern Recogn. Lett.*, **11**, 275–284.

36 Jones, T.R., Carpenter, A.E., and Golland, P. (2005) Voronoi-based segmentation of cells on image manifolds. ICCV Workshop on Computer Vision for Biomedical Image Applications, Beijing.

37 Chen, S.-C., Zhao, T., Gordon, G.J., and Murphy, R.F. (2006) A novel graphical model approach to segmenting cell images. IEEE Symposium on Computer Intelligence in Bioinformatics and Computational Biology, Toronto.

38 Meyer, F. (1994) Topographic distance and watershed lines. *Signal Process.*, **38**, 113–125.

39 Vincent, L. and Soille, P. (1991) Watersheds in digital spaces: an efficient algorithm based on immersion simulations. *IEEE Trans. Pattern Anal. and Mach. Intell.*, **13**, 583–598.

40 Adiga, P.S.U. and Chaudhuri, B.B. (2001) An efficient method based on watershed and rule-based merging for segmentation of 3-D histo-pathological images. *Pattern Recognit.*, **34**, 1449–1458.

41 Sacan, A., Ferhatosmanoglu, H., and Coskun, H. (2008) CellTrack: an open-source software for cell tracking and motility analysis. *Bioinformatics*, **24**, 1647–1649.

42 Meas-Yedid, V. and Olivo-Marin, J.-C. (2000) Active contours for the movement and motility analysis of biological objects. IEEE International Conference on Image Processing, Vancouver, BC.

43 Ray, N., Acton, S.T., and Ley, K. (2002) Tracking leukocytes *in vivo* with shape and size constrained active contours. *IEEE Trans. Med. Imaging*, **21**, 1222–1235.

44 Srinivasa, G., Fickus, M., Gonzales-Rivero, M.N., Hsieh, S.Y., Guo, Y., Linstedt, A.D., and Kovačević, J. (2008) Active mask segmentation for the cell-volume computation and Golgi-body segmentation of HeLa cell images. IEEE International Symposium on Biomedical Imaging, Paris.

45 Zimmer, C., Labruyère, E., Meas-Yedid, V., Guillén, N., and Olivo-Marin, J.C. (2002) Segmentation and tracking of migrating cells in videomicroscopy with parametric active contours: a tool for cell-based drug testing. *IEEE Trans. Med. Imaging*, **21**, 1212–1221.

46 Mukherjee, D.P., Ray, N., and Acton, S.T. (2004) Level set analysis for leukocyte detection and tracking. *IEEE Trans. Image Process.*, **13**, 562–572.

47 Mosig, A., Jager, S., Wang, C., Nath, S., Ersoy, I., Palaniappan, K.P., and Chen, S.S. (2009) Tracking cells in life cell imaging videos using topological alignments. *Algorithms Mol. Biol.*, **4**, 10.

48 Hill, A.A., LaPan, P., Li, Y., and Haney, S. (2007) Impact of image segmentation on high-content screening data quality for SK-BR-3 cells. *BMC Bioinformatics*, **8**, 340.

49 Coelho, L.P., Shariff, A., and Murphy, R.F. (2009) Nuclei segmentation in microscope cell images: a hand-segmented dataset and comparison of algorithms. IEEE International Symposium on Biomedical Imaging, Boston, MA.

50 Buckingham, S.D. and Sattelle, D.B. (2009) Fast automated measurement of nematode swimming (thrashing) without morphometry. *BMC Neurosci.*, **10**, 84.

51 Cronin, C.J., Mendel, J.E., Mukhtar, S., Kim, Y.M., Stirbl, R.C., Bruck, J., and Sternberg, P.W. (2005) An automated system for measuring parameters of nematode sinusoidal movement. *BMC Genet.*, **6**, 5.

52 Geng, W., Cosman, P., Baek, J.H., Berry, C.C., and Schafer, W.R. (2003) Quantitative classification and natural clustering of *Caenorhabditis elegans* behavioral phenotypes. *Genetics*, **165**, 1117–1126.

53 Huang, K., Cosman, P., and Schafer, W.R. (2009) Using articulated models for tracking multiple *C. elegans* in physical contact. *J. Signal Process. Syst.*, **55**, 113–126.

54 Roussel, N., Morton, C.A., Finger, F.P., and Roysam, B. (2007) A computational model for *C. elegans* locomotory behavior: application to multiworm tracking. *IEEE Trans. Biomed. Eng.*, **54**, 1786–1797.

55 Stephens, G.J., Johnson-Kerner, B., Bialek, W., and Ryu, W.S. (2008) Dimensionality and dynamics in the behavior of *C. elegans*. *PLoS Comput. Biol.*, **4**, e1000028.

56 Srinivasa, G., Fickus, M., Guo, Y., Linstedt, A.D., and Kovacevic, J. (2009) Active mask segmentation of fluorescence microscope images. *IEEE Trans. Image Process.*, **18**, 1817–1829.

57 Otsu, N. (1979) A threshold selection method from gray-level histograms. *IEEE Trans. Syst. Man. Cybernet.*, **9**, 62–66.

58 Moody-Davis, A., Mennillo, L., and Singh, R. (2011) Region-based segmentation of parasites for high-throughput screening. *Lect. Notes Comput. Sci.*, **6938**, 44–54.

59 Kim, K., Chalidabhongse, T.H., Harwood, D., and Davis, L. (2005) Real-time foreground-background segmentation using codebook model. *Real-Time Imaging*, **11**, 172–185.

60 Deng, Y. and Manjunath, B. (2001) Unsupervised segmentation of color-texture regions in images and video. *IEEE Trans. Pattern Anal. Mach. Intell.*, **23**, 800–810.

61 Collins, R. (2003) Mean-shift blob tracking through scale space. *IEEE Conf. Comput. Vision Pattern Recognit.*, **2**, 234–240.

62 Comaniciu, D., Ramesh, V., and Meer, P. (2003) Kernel-based object tracking. *IEEE Trans. Pattern Anal. Mach. Intell.*, **25**, 564–577.

63 Yang, C., Duraiswami, R., and Davis, L. (2005) Efficient mean-shift tracking via a new similarity measure. *IEEE Conf. Comput. Vision Pattern Recognit.*, **1**, 176–183.

64 Breiman, L., Friedman, J.H., Olshen, R.A., and Stone, C.J. (1984) *Classification and Regression Trees*, Wadsworth & Brooks/Cole, Pacific Grove, CA.

11
Use of Rodent Models in the Discovery of Novel Anthelmintics

Rebecca Fankhauser, Linsey R. Cozzie, Bakela Nare, Kerrie Powell, Ann E. Sluder, and Lance G. Hammerland*

Abstract

Successful drug development can be facilitated by the use of animal models to characterize the pharmacodynamic and pharmacokinetic properties of drug candidates. Rodent models have been described for several parasitic helminths, including gastrointestinal nematodes, filarids, and flatworms. In general, rodent models are employed during the lead optimization phase, and have the advantages, in most cases, of reduced compound requirements, shorter study duration, and lower costs when compared to studies in the target species. A primary assumption of rodent efficacy models is that the results generated should correlate with outcomes in humans or veterinary target species. Although false-positive results in screening models are an accepted risk in drug discovery, false-negative results can halt the progression of promising candidate compounds. In this chapter, we will examine and discuss several published rodent anthelmintic models, emphasizing their strengths and limitations to prioritize and select drug candidates for human and veterinary indications.

Introduction

Data-driven decisions in drug discovery ensure that the best candidates are advanced into the development pipeline. These decision steps illustrate why drug discovery is often described as an iterative process aimed at optimization of lead compounds into molecules that satisfy the rigorous requirements of a drug candidate [1]. The high throughput of *in vitro* or *ex vivo* screens enables the profiling of large numbers of compounds that may be generated during drug discovery's lead optimization phases. Animal models introduce further stringency and complexity to the screening process because multiple compound attributes can be assessed simultaneously. Rodent models offer advantages of reduced compound requirements, shorter study durations, and lower costs when compared to studies in veterinary target species or studies in humans. These model systems thus allow *in vitro* lead compounds to be profiled against the desired attributes of existing products or drug candidates, and

---

* Corresponding Author

Parasitic Helminths: Targets, Screens, Drugs and Vaccines, First Edition. Edited by Conor R. Caffrey.
© 2012 Wiley-VCH Verlag GmbH & Co. KGaA. Published 2012 by Wiley-VCH Verlag GmbH & Co. KGaA.

serve as an important translation step between *in vitro* systems and clinical or field settings.

Translational Science

In many disease areas the extent of unmet need remains great. In spite of the resources, time, and rigor applied to target validation and drug discovery processes, overall attrition rates of drug candidates exceed 80% [2]. Attrition most often results when the preclinically determined attributes of the drug candidate do not translate adequately to the clinical setting [3]. These failures in clinical development are explained by a number of factors, including poor efficacy or an unfavorable toxicological profile. Lack of efficacy may reflect an incomplete understanding of the disease and its accessibility to pharmaceutical intervention, while toxicity can result from target-mediated or off-target effects that are only manifest in the clinical setting.

All stages of drug discovery, including translational models, face the challenges of understanding the model systems in relation to the targeted disease. For drug discovery in virtually all disease areas, certain assumptions must be included in the design, development, and use of models. For example, rodent behavioral models have been used for decades to evaluate compounds for their potential to treat clinical depression. In this setting, the nature of the disorder is such that the efficacy endpoints require interpretation of specific behaviors. However, those behaviors are based on assumptions about psychological states that may not exist and that cannot be directly measured in rodents [4]. Hence, a candidate compound's effects in these models may not accurately forecast its potential to favorably translate in the clinical setting. In other therapeutic areas, access to and measurement of disease-related endpoints can increase confidence in the outputs of model systems. In endocrine and metabolic disease research, markers have been successfully employed to better understand various disease classes and to formulate treatment approaches [5]. These biomarkers have facilitated successful drug development because the marker-based model outcomes translated to the clinical setting [6]. Models of infectious disease, particularly those used to assess anthelmintic efficacy, should provide a sturdy translational bridge, because the infecting parasites are the end-point markers and their clearance is assumed to correlate with a positive treatment outcome [7]. The need to discover and screen new anthelmintic compounds in a rapid and cost-effective manner has motivated the continued development of rodent and other small-mammal models to profile and validate new anthelmintic compounds.

Nematode Infection Models

Nematode Infections in Livestock

The economic impact of helminth infections in ruminant livestock (e.g., goats, sheep, and cattle) is well documented, as is the potential for further losses related to treatment failure and the development of resistance [8–10]. Gastrointestinal nematode and heartworm infections in pets are also of ever-increasing concern, not only for the health and well-being of the pet, but also regarding the potential for zoonotic transmission [11, 12]. However, efforts in rodent model development and application for veterinary anthelmintic discovery have focused largely on parasites of ruminant livestock, where tractable small-animal laboratory models offer distinct advantages in terms of the cost and time required for compound screening compared to the larger target host species.

Haemonchus contortus, an abomasal parasite, and *Trichostrongylus colubriformis*, a nematode of the small intestine, are considered the most pathogenic and prolific parasitic nematodes affecting goats and sheep. *Ostertagia* spp., abomasal parasites, and *Cooperia* spp., which infest the small intestine, are the most prevalent nematodes found in cattle [13]. Nematode infections in ruminants may result in anemia, production losses of meat, milk, and fleece, and even death in severe cases [14].

Trichostrongylus Rodent Models
Induced infection of rodents with ruminant nematodes was first reported in 1931 when *Trichostrongylus axei* and *Trichostrongylus colubriformis* were recovered successfully from guinea pigs that had been fed infective larvae [15]. In subsequent studies, modifications of experimental design led to improved reproducibility in the model [16–19]. The validity of the model was supported later by a study profiling anthelmintic resistance in *T. colubriformis* strains [20].

Early attempts to develop a model of *T. colubriformis* or *T. axei* in mouse or rat yielded variable results [19, 21], but the reliability of the rat model was improved significantly when animals were immunosuppressed by treatment with a corticosteroid prior to infection with *T. colubriformis* [22]. In this study, several anthelmintics, including several benzimidazoles, levamisole, and morantel tartrate, showed efficacy at doses similar to their label-recommended doses in ruminants. One potential advantage of using rats or mice in an anthelmintic model is that they are used routinely in preclinical safety assessment and pharmacokinetic studies. By using a single species in the discovery and preclinical phases, a better overall profile may be obtained prior to more extensive and expensive studies in the target species.

The Mongolian gerbil (*Meriones unguiculatus*) has emerged as the most commonly used rodent species for *in vivo* anthelmintic screening against nematode parasites of ruminants. Leland first reported induced patent infections of *T. axei* in 1961 [23]. Since *T. axei* infections in gerbils can remain patent for at least 8 months, the parasite life cycle can be maintained. In 1967, Kates and Thompson established dual infections (*T. axei* and *T. colubriformis*) in gerbils and showed that two of three known anthelmintics administered at 24–36 days postinfection were efficacious against adult worms, consistent with the efficacy reported in ruminants at similar doses [24].

Haemonchus Rodent Models
H. contortus infection has been established in guinea pigs; however, the worms develop only to the L4 stage and are expelled 5–7 days after infection [25]. When mice are immunosuppressed, *H. contortus* is able to establish and maintain infection [26].

Induced infection of gerbils with *H. contortus* was first reported in 1990 using methods similar to those employed for the gerbil model of *Trichostrongylus* infection. Gerbils were immunosuppressed via a medicated diet containing 0.02% hydrocortisone starting 5 days prior to infection with 1000 exsheathed infective larvae. Animals were treated 10 days after infection and necropsied for worm recovery 3 days after treatment [27]. Several anthelmintics were evaluated in this study, including the benzimidazoles, febantel, ivermectin, levamisole, and milbemycin; each was efficacious in the gerbil at doses comparable to those used in the treatment of sheep and cattle. The model also has been used to screen for anthelmintic activity from extracts of *Prosopis laevigata* (smooth mesquite) plants [28], orange oil emulsion [29], extracts of artemisinin, and *Artemisia* species plant extracts [30].

In 1991, Conder *et al.* reported the successful dual infection of the gerbil with *H. contortus* and *T. colubriformis*, and validated use of the model as an anthelmintic screen [31]. Several anthelmintics, including the benzimidazoles, febantel, ivermectin, levamisole, and milbemycin, were effective against both parasites in gerbils at doses similar to those effective in sheep and cattle [31]. More recently, the gerbil dual-infection model was used to profile and validate the anthelmintic activity of novel amino-acetonitrile derivatives, including monepantel [32, 33].

Other Nematode Species
Experimental infections of gerbils with other ruminant nematode species also have been reported. Court *et al.* established infections of *Ostertagia circumcincta* in gerbils, but infection rates were low, patent infections could not be established, and most worms were expelled by 21 days postinfection [34]. Conder *et al.* infected gerbils with *Ostertagia ostertagi* and used this model to profile the anthelmintic activity of the cyclodepsipeptide PF1022A [35]. A triple infection model was used to profile the spectrum and efficacy of paraherquamide against *H. contortus*, *T. colubriformis* and *Trichostrongylus sigmodontis* [36].

The dual-infection model in gerbils (*T. colubriformis* and *H. contortus*) has been used extensively for compound screening and characterization of anthelmintic sensitivity of numerous nematode strains. The validity of the model is reinforced further by its ability to distinguish between compounds known to possess anthelmintic efficacy and those that lack it. By infecting with two species, a preliminary assessment of spectrum can be determined. Given the broad-spectrum requirements of new anthelmintics, the gerbil model can support the selection or removal of compounds from the preclinical pipeline. Results from several studies in which this model has been used for anthelmintic profiling are summarized in Table 11.1, along with reference data from sheep.

Gastrointestinal Nematode Parasites of Humans

Disease and Impact
The most common parasites infecting the gastrointestinal tract in humans are the soil-transmitted helminth (STHs), which include *Ascaris lumbricoides*, *Strongyloides stercoralis*, *Trichuris trichiura*, and the hookworms, *Ancylostoma duodenale* and *Necator*

Table 11.1 Efficacious doses of selected compounds against parasites of sheep when tested in gerbils and sheep.

Parasite	Compound	Gerbils (mg/kg)	Reference	Sheep (mg/kg)	Reference
Trichostrongylus axei	cambendazole	NE	[107]	NA	
	fenbendazole	NE	[107]	5	[108]
	levamisole	16	[107]	7.5	[108]
	morantel–HCl	NE	[107]	NE	[108]
	phenothiazine	NE	[24]	550–600	[24, 106, 108]
	ruelene	NE	[24]	NA	
	thiabendazole	200	[24]	44–100	[24, 106]
Trichostrongylus colubriformis	albendazole	3.1–12.5	[31, 36]	5.0	[108]
	bithionol	NE	[31]	NA	
	cambendazole	40	[107]	NA	
	closantel	NE	[31]	NE	[108]
	diethylcarbamazine	NE	[31]	NA	
	febantel	37.5	[31]	5.0	[108]
	fenbendazole	3.1–10	[31, 107]	5.0	[108]
	ivermectin	0.0625	[31, 36]	0.2	[108]
	levamisole	1.875–16	[31, 107]	7.5	[108]
	milbemycin D	1.25	[31]	NA	
	morantel–HCl	12.5–20	[36, 107]	10	[108]
	oxfendazole	3.1–25	[31, 36]	5.0	[108]
	oxibendazole	125	[31]	10.0	[108]
	paraherquamide	0.781	[36]	NA	
	PF1022A	2.75	[35]	NA	
	phenothiazine	NE	[24]	600	[24]
	piperazine	NE	[31]	NA	
	pyrantel tartrate	12.5	[31]	25.0	[108]
	ruelene	400	[24]	100–200	[24]
	thiabendazole	100–200	[24, 36]	44–100	[24, 106]
Haemonchus contortus	albendazole	1.875–3.125	[27, 36]	5.0	[108]
	bithionol	NE	[27]	NA	
	closantel	7.5	[27]	5.0	[108]
	diethylcarbamazine	NE	[27]	NA	
	febantel	187.5	[31]	5.0	[108]
	fenbendazole	1.875	[27]	5.0	[108]
	ivermectin	0.125	[31, 36]	0.2	[108]
	levamisole	10–12.5	[27, 36]	7.5	[108]
	milbemycin D	0.469	[31]	NA	
	morantel–HCl	200	[36]	10	[108]
	oxfendazole	1.875–3.125	[27, 36]	5.0	[108]
	oxibendazole	187.5	[27]	10.0	[108]
	paraherquamide	12.5	[36]	NA	
	PF1022A	2.75	[35]	NA	

(*Continued*)

Table 11.1 (Continued)

Parasite	Compound	Gerbils (mg/kg)	Reference	Sheep (mg/kg)	Reference
	piperazine	NE	[27]	NA	
	pyrantel tartrate	187.5	[31]	25	[108]
	thiabendazole	187.5–400	[27, 36]	75.0	[108]

NE, no dose that clears greater than 90% reported; NA, not available.

americanus [37–40]. An estimated 2–3 billion people suffer from STH infections and over 4 billion people are at risk, with the highest rates of infection occurring in sub-Saharan Africa, Asia, and South America [41, 42]. Adult worms of these species inhabit the small intestine and their eggs are passed in the feces. The eggs embryonate in soil and, when ingested, hatch in the duodenum. Larvae penetrate the intestine, enter the lymphatic system, and are carried to the liver, heart, and lungs. Once the larvae migrate through the trachea, coughing can lead to ingestion of larvae. STH infection is rarely fatal, but high parasite load is associated with anemia and poor nutritional absorption, which, in children, may result in delayed physical and cognitive development [41]. In infected communities, mebendazole is distributed typically through mass drug administration (MDA) programs [40]. Mebendazole is the current primary treatment for STH infections, but recent reports of lack of efficacy have raised concerns about the potential for the development of resistance [37].

T. trichiura, commonly known as human whipworm, manifests infection symptoms that are directly related to worm burden, with low-level infections often being asymptomatic and heavy infections causing gastrointestinal issues and cognitive delay in children [41, 43].

T. muris, a natural intestinal parasite of mice, has been used extensively as a model for *T. trichiura* infection and is the model considered most equivalent to human infection [44, 45]. Mice ingest eggs that hatch and develop into larvae in the small intestine, and then migrate into the cecum and colon [45]. One of the advantages of this model, in addition to the ease of laboratory maintenance, is that infections of selected mice strains mimic much of the pathology observed in humans.

Hookworm Infection and Rodent Models

The majority of human hookworm infections are caused by *N. americanus* and *A. duodenale*, with an estimated prevalence rate of 10% globally. *Anyclostoma ceylanicum* also infects humans, but is found in limited locations [46]. Like other STH, the intensity of clinical effects correlates with the extent of worm burden [43].

The Syrian Golden hamster, *Mesocricetus auratus*, has been used as a model for hookworm disease for over 30 years. Experimental infection by oral gavage with infective larvae in the hamster model mimics the route of infection in human [47–51]. The hamster [52] can be infected experimentally with *N. americanus*, but although this model offers a potential for evaluating drugs on one of the major human STH species, it is better suited for profiling single candidates because of logistical and biological limitations restricting its throughput capabilities. Hamsters also are permissive hosts for *A. ceylanicum* infection and this model shares key clinical pathologies seen in human infections, such as anemia and stunted growth [50]. As the *A. ceylanicum* life cycle can be maintained readily in hamsters, this model offers logistical advantages for lead optimization and compound screening. Efficacy of emerging preclinical candidates on a major human STH parasite then can be confirmed in the *N. americanus* model, in a manner similar to its use in evaluating the efficacy of tribendimidine and its metabolites [53].

Strongyloides Stercoralis
Like the other STHs, *S. stercoralis* larvae are able to infect their host through penetration of the skin by L3 larvae. *S. stercoralis* is unique among human helminths in that it is able to reproduce in a free-living reproductive cycle as well as within the human host. Autoinfection, in which the first stage larvae develop while in the intestine of the host, can account for the persistence of infection in individuals who no longer live in endemic areas [38, 43, 54].

Rodent Models
S. stercoralis will establish patent infections in the gerbil, but not in the mouse, rat, or guinea pig. Infections in the gerbil remain for over 130 days and autoinfection can be induced with the treatment of steroids or by infecting with larger numbers of L3 larvae [55–57]. The model, therefore, allows for the screening of compounds against various parasitic stages. An infection model with a surrogate rodent parasite, *Strongyloides ratti*, has also been used for compound profiling, but this model is limited in that the parasites cannot reproduce in the rodent by autoinfection [55, 58].

Rodent Models of Other STH Infections
Although *A. lumbricoides* is a very common intestinal nematode in humans, it is not well-suited for use in rodent models. *Ascaris suum*, a common swine parasite that also can infect humans, was used to develop models of induced infection in the guinea pig and mouse [44, 59]. *A. suum* can migrate and establish in rodents, but its larvae will not reach the adult stage. However, because larval migration is responsible for morbidity, the efficacy of compounds in this model correlates well with clinical outcomes in the treatment of human infections [51, 60].

Filarial Parasite Models

Filarial Parasites of Humans

Lymphatic Filariasis
More than 100 million people in the tropics and subtropics suffer from lymphatic filariasis, and over 1 billion in are at risk of infection by the causative nematodes [61]. Although many infected individuals are asymptomatic, the more

severe manifestations of the disease result in a chronic obstruction of the lymphatic system that can be disabling and disfiguring. *Wuchereria bancrofti*, *Brugia malayi*, and *Brugia timori* infections account for virtually all lymphatic filariasis, with *W. bancrofti* being responsible for over 90% of filarial parasite infections world-wide [62]. Infection occurs via the bite of the mosquito that carries L3 infective larvae. Those larvae then migrate through the skin and enter the lymphatic vessels, where they develop into adults over a period of a few months. As adult females may release thousands of microfilariae per day into the bloodstream of the host, the life cycle readily continues, as long as the vector is present and feeding.

Current treatments rely on annual MDA of single-dose combination treatments of ivermectin or diethylcarbamazine with albendazole. Significant unmet need remains because current drug options are limited in that they control only the microfilarial stage. In addition, concerns over resistance have increased the need for new therapies [63].

Rodent Models of Lymphatic Filarial Infection
Early development of filarial rodent models used native rodent parasites, because these life cycles were experimentally accessible. In 1944, Hewitt *et al.* reported the microfilaricidal activity of diethylcarbamazine in cotton rats (*Sigmodon hispidus*) naturally infected with *Litomosoides carinii* (now *L. sigmodontis*). However, this model system had limited value because infection levels varied greatly between individual animals [64]. This limitation was addressed when mice were infected via pleural or subcutaneous injection of L3 larvae. Using these modified methods, more consistent worm recoveries were achieved [65–67].

W. bancrofti is the leading cause of lymphatic filariasis in humans, but because this species does not survive in rodents, models for lymphatic filariasis have been developed in gerbils and mice with induced infections of *B. malayi*. These model systems are favored particularly because the entire life cycle can be readily maintained [68]. In subperiodic filariasis, microfilariae counts in host blood do not change significantly from day to night, whereas in periodic forms the microfilariae levels in blood are higher at night when the mosquitoes are active. The periodic form of *B. malayi* is specific to human, but the subperiodic form readily infects other mammals [69].

Ash and Riley first reported the successful infection of the gerbil with subperiodic forms of *B. pahangi* and *B. malayi* by subcutaneous injection of infective larvae [70]. McCall *et al.* demonstrated that intraperitoneal infection of larvae resulted in higher recovery. As the larvae are restricted to the peritoneal cavity, they are accessed easily for efficacy counts. However, their tissue distribution is not representative of the human infections, as would be expected following subcutaneous infection in gerbils [71].

Onchoceriasis
Onchocerciasis, resulting from infection with the filarial nematode *Onchocerca volvulus*, affects up to 20 million people, the majority of those in West and Central

Africa [72, 73]. Infected individuals may develop severe skin lesions, musculoskeletal pain, and are at risk of blindness. Ivermectin is the only treatment available through MDA programs and it must be dosed over the course of an individual's lifetime because the drug is not efficacious against adult worms [69, 74].

Rodent Models of Onchocerciasis
As induced infections of *O. volvulus* cannot be generated in rodents, surrogate parasites have been used to develop rodent models of infection [72]. The *L. sigmodontis* model is preferred over the *Brugia* rodent models because patent infections of circulating microfilaria are achieved [51]. In another model, gerbils are infected by subcutaneous delivery of *Acanthocheilonema vitae* to enable efficacy testing on worms residing in the skin [51, 61–69]. Table 11.2 summarizes results from a variety of rodent studies of filiarial parasite and STH infection models.

Trematode and Cestode Infection Models

Trematode Infections in Humans and Livestock

Trematode species cause several types of infections in human and ruminants. Common parasitic trematodes include *Schistosoma* species (blood flukes), *Paragonimus westermani* (lung fluke), *Clonorchis sinensis* and *Fasciola hepatica* (liver flukes), and *Echinostoma caproni* (intestinal fluke). Trematode (primarily *F. hepatica*) infection in ruminants results in decreased milk production and liver condemnation [75, 76]. In humans, inflammatory lesions and damage to tissues and target organs can occur, and symptoms vary depending on the tissue distribution of the parasite. Therefore, clinical manifestations may include fever, loss of appetite, jaundice, pain, fatigue, cough, and vomiting [37].

Schistosomiasis
Schistosomiasis is prevalent in tropical and subtropical regions where over 200 million people are infected and another 700 million are at risk of the disease. The disease is caused by any of three major species: *Schistosoma mansoni* (Africa and South America), *Schistosoma heamatobium* (Africa and the Middle East), and *Schistosoma japonicum* (Philippines and China). Treatment with praziquantel through MDA programs is the primary pharmaceutical means of disease control [39]. Although praziquantel has been effective in the control of schistosomiasis [77, 78], the potential for drug resistance [79] and its markedly decreased efficacy against juvenile stages [80, 81] motivate continued efforts in discovery and development of antischistosomal drugs [82, 83] (see also Chapter 20).

Rodent Models
Among rodent species evaluated, the mouse model has emerged as the most suitable for schistosome infection, largely because activity in this model appears predictive of

Table 11.2 Activity of selected compounds in rodent models of infection for STHs and filarial parasites.

Parasite	Compound	Host	Dose (mg/kg)	Route	Efficacy (%)	Reference
Brugia malayi	ivermectin	mice	0.75 × 5 days	p.o.	90	[109]
	diethylcarbamazine	mice	250 × 5 days	p.o.	90	[109]
	mebendazole	mice	6.25 × 5 days	s.c.	74 (adult)	[109]
		mice	200 × 5 days	p.o.	73 (adult)	[109]
Litomosoides sigmodontis	ivermectin	mice	0.2	s.c.	100	[109]
	diethylcarbamazine	mice	0.03 × 5 days	s.c.	100	[109]
Onchocerca lienalis	diethylcarbamazine	mice	50 × 5 days	s.c.	62–76	[110]
	moxidectin	mice	0.15 × 5 days	s.c.	100	[111]
		mice	0.015 × 5 days	s.c.	100	[111]
		mice	0.0015 × 5 days	s.c.	90–98	[111]
	ivermectin	mice	0.15 × 5 days	s.c.	100	[111]
		mice	0.015 × 5 days	s.c.	98	[111]
Trichuris muris	imidacloprid + moxidectin	mice	128 mg/kg (I) + 32 mg/kg (M)	topical	95	[112]
	emodepside + praziquantel	mice	3 mg/kg (E) + 12 mg/kg (P)	topical	93	[113]
Necator americanus	tribendimidine	hamsters	16	p.o.	94, 72 (larvae)	[114, 115]
	pyrantel pamoate	hamsters	100	p.o.	100 (larvae)	[115]
	albendazole	hamsters	100	p.o.	99.3 (larvae)	[115]
	tribendimidine	hamsters	100	p.o.	98.8 (larvae)	[115]
	ivermectin	hamsters	0.1–0.5	s.c.	100 (larvae)	[116]
Ancylostoma ceylanicum	ivermectin	hamsters	10	p.o.	93	[114, 116]
Strongyloides ratti	cambendazole	mice	50 × 7 days	p.o.	100 (larvae)	[117]
	thiabendazole	mice	50 × 7 days	p.o.	91 (larvae)	[117]
	mebendazole	mice	50 × 7 days	p.o.	100 (larvae)	[117]
	tribendimidine	mice	25	p.o.	91.4 (larvae) 100 (adult)	[117]
	ivermectin	mice	2.5	p.o.	90 (larvae) 100 (adult)	[117]

human clinical outcomes [84–87]. The mouse *S. mansoni* model is the most widely used for both basic research and drug screening. This model provides relevant pathogenesis of the disease, including the chronic aspects that are primarily due to granulomatous inflammatory response to parasite eggs that become trapped in host tissues [88, 89]. Further, *S. mansoni* is the human-infective schistosome species with the widest geographic distribution [90]. For compound testing, mice are treated at different points during the development of the parasite up to and including maturity and egg laying at about 40 days postinfection. This is with a view to identifying compounds with broader schistosomicidal activity given praziquantels predominant bioactivity against adult parasites. The primary efficacy end-point is determined by worm burdens recovered from the hepatic portal and mesenteric venous systems of treated versus untreated mice. Egg counts and morphological assessment of parasites in the drug-treated groups are also common end-points [91, 92].

Fascioliasis
Fascioliasis is caused by the trematodes *F. hepatica* or *Fasciola gigantica*. Human infection results from ingestion of metacercariae in contaminated food or water. Although *F. hepatica* can infect and reach maturity in a variety of laboratory animals, the rat has emerged as the model system of choice for compound screening [93].

Following ingestion, metacercariae excyst and juvenile flukes penetrate the intestinal wall to enter the abdominal cavity. Once in the abdominal cavity, juveniles migrate to the liver and then to the bile duct where they develop to adults. For compound testing, rats are treated either 3–5 or 8–12 weeks after experimental infection in order to test efficacy against juveniles or adult flukes, respectively [94, 95]. The primary efficacy end-point is determined by worm burdens in livers and bile ducts of treated versus untreated rats. Egg counts and morphological assessment of parasites in the drug-treated groups are also common end-points [96, 97].

In a mouse model developed for the intestinal fluke, *Echinostoma caproni*, orally delivered metacercariae reach the adult stage within 2 weeks. One of the advantages of this model is that cycle times (around 2 weeks) for compound evaluation are decreased dramatically compared to life cycles in the *Schistosoma* or *Fasciola* models. Validity of the *E. caproni* model has been demonstrated by the activity of several anthelmintics [98–100].

Cestode Infection in Humans and Livestock

Tapeworms are parasitic cestodes found in the intestine or other tissues, and may cause symptoms such as nausea, vomiting, and diarrhea in infected individuals. Cystic echinococcosis is also responsible for production losses in ruminants [101]. Owing to low host specificity during the metacestode stage, several rodent species have been evaluated as potential hosts, including mouse, gerbil, vole, and rat [102]. Induced infection by *Echinococcus granulosus* or *Echinococcus multilocularis* in animal models has been accomplished by oral delivery of eggs or intraperitoneally infection with metacestodes or protoscolices [103].

Several compounds have been profiled in the echinoccocal metacestode model, including albendazole, ivermectin, praziquantel, mitomycin, cyclosporin A, and oltipraz [104]. An alternative is the gerbil model of induced infection using *Hymenolepis diminuta*. In this model, parasites can be reared and recovered in the intermediate host, *Tenebrio molitor* (beetle). Infected gerbils may be treated 4–6 days postinfection and efficacy determined 3–4 days later by worm counts at necropsy. Praziquantel, albendazole, and niclosamide are among the anthelmintics profiled in this model [105]. Table 11.3 summarizes results from trematode and cestode models in rodent species.

Table 11.3 Activity of selected compounds in rodent models of trematode and cestode infection.

Parasite	Compound	Host	Dose (mg/kg)	Route	Worm reduction (%)	Reference
Schistosoma mansoni	oxamniquine	mice	40–50	i.m.	36	[118]
	oxamniquine	hamsters	12	i.m.	82	[118]
	praziquantel	humans	40	p.o.	80	[118]
	praziquantel	mice	500	p.o.	93	[119]
	niridazole	mice	35 × 5 days	p.o.	30–70	[118]
	artemether	mice	200 × 6 days	p.o.	99	[120]
	mefloquine	mice	400	p.o.	77	[121]
	triclabendazole	mice	120	p.o.	36	[119]
	OZ78	mice	200	p.o.	82	[122]
	OZ78	hamsters	200	p.o.	80	[122]
Schistosoma japonicum	oxamniquine	mice	4–50	i.m.	0	[120]
	praziquantel	humans	60	p.o.	80–90	[120]
	oltipraz	mice	25–35	p.o.	0	[120]
	niridazole	mice	35 × 5 days	p.o.	50	[120]
	mefloquine	mice	400	p.o.	95	[121]
Schistosoma haematobium	oxamniquine	mice	40–50	i.m.	0	[120]
	praziquantel	humans	40	p.o.	75–85	[120]
	niridazole	mice	35 × 5 days	p.o.	80–100	[120]
Fasciola hepatica	artemether	rats	200	p.o.	100	[97]
	artesunate	rats	400	p.o.	100	[123]
	OZ78	rats	100	p.o.	100	[99]
Echinostoma caproni	praziquantel	mice	50	p.o.	100	[100]
	artemisinin	mice	1500	p.o.	99	[100]
	OZ78	mice	1000	p.o.	100	[100]
Hymenolepis dimunuta	praziquantel	gerbils	10 × 3 days	p.o.	100	[105]
	albendazole	gerbils	90 × 3 days	p.o.	95	[105]
	niclosamide	gerbils	350 × 3 days	p.o.	80	[105]

Conclusions

Successful discovery, development, and marketing of a new chemical entity are rare, and anthelmintic drugs are no exception. Limited funding for anthelmintic discovery and development likely has contributed to the paucity of new anthelmintics to reach the market over the past few decades. Other factors include the inherent challenges related to the treatment of helmintic diseases, particularly the requirement for a sufficiently broad activity spectrum of potential drug candidates and concerns regarding anthelmintic resistance. Given the stringent requirements for new anthelmintic products, the strategies and workflows associated with discovery of novel drug candidates should be developed to maximize efforts on the most promising candidates. It is in this context that the effective use of rodent efficacy models can make a substantial impact.

References

1 Woods, D.J. and Williams, T.M. (2007) The challenges of developing novel antiparasitic drugs. *Invert. Neurosci.*, **7**, 245–250.
2 Booth, B. and Zemmel, R. (2004) Prospects for productivity. *Nat. Rev. Drug Discov.*, **2**, 451–456.
3 Hutchinson, L. and Kirk, R. (2011) High drug attrition rates – where are we going wrong? *Nat. Rev. Clin. Oncol.*, **8**, 189–190.
4 Holmes, P. (2003) Rodent models of depression: reexamining validity without anthropomorphic inference. *Crit. Rev. Neurobiol.*, **15**, 143–174.
5 Nemeth, E.F., Heaton, W.H., Miller, M., Fox, J., Balandrin, M.F., Van Wagenen, B.C., Colloton, M. et al. (2004) Pharmacodynamics of the type II calcimimetic compound cinacalcet HCl. *J. Pharmacol. Exp. Ther.*, **308**, 627–635.
6 Shahapuni, I., Monge, M., Oprisiu, R., Mazouz, H., Westeel, P.F., Morinière, P., Massy, Z. et al. (2006) Drug insight: renal indications of calcimimetics. *Nat. Clin. Pract. Nephrol.*, **6**, 316–325.
7 Rothwell, J.T., Sangster, N.C., Conder, G.A., Dobson, R.J., and Johnson, S.S. (1993) Kinetics of expulsion of *Haemonchus contortus* from sheep and jirds after treatment with closantel. *Int. J. Parasitol.*, **23**, 885–889.
8 Sutherland, I.A., Bailey, J., and Shaw, R.J. (2010) The production costs of anthelmintic resistance in sheep managed within a monthly preventive drench program. *Vet. Parasitol.*, **171**, 300–304.
9 Sutherland, I.A. and Leathwick, D.M. (2011) Anthelmintic resistance in nematode parasites of cattle: a global issue? *Trends Parasitol.*, **27**, 176–181.
10 Corwin, R.M. (1997) Economics of gastrointestinal parasitism of cattle. *Vet. Parasitol.*, **72**, 451–457.
11 Mohamed, A.S., Moore, G.E., and Glickman, L.T. (2009) Prevalence of intestinal nematode parasitism among pet dogs in the United States (2003–2006). *J. Am. Vet. Med. Assoc.*, **234**, 631–637.
12 McCall, J.W., Gench, C., Kramer, L.H., Guerrero, J., and Venco, L. (2008) Heartworm disease in animals and humans. *Adv. Parasitol.*, **66**, 193–285.
13 Scott, I. and Sutherland, I. (2010) *Gastrointestinal Nematodes of Sheep and Cattle: Biology and Control*, Wiley-Blackwell, Ames, IA.
14 Radostits, O.M., Gay, C.C., Blood, D.C. and Hinchcliff, K.W. (eds) (1999) Diseases caused by helminth parasites: nematode diseases of the alimentary tract, in *Veterinary Medicine: A Textbook of the Diseases of Cattle, Sheep, Pigs, Goats and Horses*, 9th edn, Saunders, St Louis, MO, pp. 1339–1350.

15 Zavadovskii, M.M. and Zakharova, M. (1931) Artificial infection of guinea-pigs with *Trichostrongylus extenuatus* and *Trichostrongylus instabilis*. *Trudy Dinamike Razvit.*, **6**, 303–305.

16 Herlich, H., Douvres, F.W., and Isenstein, R.S. (1956) Experimental infections of guinea pigs with *Trichostrongylus colubriformis*, a parasite of ruminants. *Proc. Helm. Soc. Wash.*, **23**, 104–105.

17 Herlich, H. (1958) Further observations on the experimental host–parasite relations of the guinea pig and the ruminant parasite, *Trichostrongylus colubriformis*. *J. Parasitol.*, **44**, 602.

18 Sturrock, R.F. (1963) Observations on the use of *Trichostrongylus colubriformis* (Nematoda) infections of guinea-pigs for laboratory experiments. *Parasitology*, **53**, 189–199.

19 Williams, G.A.H. and Palmer, B.H. (1964) *Trichostrongylus colubriformis* (a nematode parasite of sheep and other ruminants) as a test organism in screening for sheep anthelmintics in the laboratory. *Nature*, **203**, 1399–1400.

20 Kelly, J.D., Sangster, N.C., Porter, C.J., Martin, I.C.A., and Gunawan, M. (1981) Use of guinea pigs to assay anthelmintic resistance in ovine isolates of *Trichostrongylus colubriformis*. *Res. Vet. Sci.*, **30**, 131–137.

21 Kates, K.C. and Thompson, D.E. (1968) Susceptibility of gerbils and young white rats to simultaneous infection with *Trichostrongylus axei* and *Trichostrongylus colubriformis*. *Proc. Helm. Soc. Wash.*, **35**, 102–106.

22 Gration, K.A.F., Bishop, B.F., Martin-Short, M.R., and Herbert, A. (1992) A new anthelmintic assay using rats infected with *Trichostrongylus colubriformis*. *Vet. Parasitol.*, **42**, 273–279.

23 LeLand, S.E. Jr (1961) Studies on *Trichostrongylus axei* (Cobbold, 1879). VII. Some quantitative aspects of experimental infection of the Mongolian gerbil (*Meriones unguiculatus*). *J. Parasitol.*, **49**, 617–622.

24 Kates, K.C. and Thompson, D.E. (1967) Activity of three anthelmintics against mixed infections of two *Trichostrongylus* species in gerbils, sheep and goats. *Proc. Helm. Soc. Wash.*, **34**, 228–236.

25 Wagland, B.M., Abeydeera, L.R., Rothwell, T.L.W., and Ouwerkerk, D. (1989) Experimental *Haemonchus contortus* infections in guinea pigs. *Int. J. Parasitol.*, **19**, 301–305.

26 Adams, D.B. (1990) Infection of immunosuppressed mice with the abomasal nematode parasite of ruminants, *Haemonchus contortus*. *Int. J. Parasitol.*, **20**, 631–636.

27 Conder, G.A., Jen, L.W., Marbury, K.S., Johnson, S.S., Guimond, P.M., Thomas, E.M., and Lee, B.L. (1990) A novel anthelmintic model utilizing jirds, *Meriones unguiculatus*, infected with *Haemonchus contortus*. *J. Parasitol.*, **76**, 168–170.

28 De Jesús-Gabino, A.F., Mendoza-de Gives, P., Salinas-Sánchez, D.O., López-Arellano, M.E., Liébano-Hernández, E., Hernández-Velázquez, V.M., and Valladares-Cisneros, G. (2010) Anthelmintic effects of *Prosopis laevigata* n-hexanic extract against *Haemonchus contortus* in artificially infected gerbils (*Meriones unguiculatus*). *J. Helminthol.*, **84**, 71–75.

29 Squires, J.M., Foster, J.G., Lindsay, D.S., Caudell, D.L., and Zajac, A.M. (2010) Efficacy of an orange oil emulsion as an anthelmintic against *Haemonchus contortus* in gerbils (*Meriones unguiculatus*) and in sheep. *Vet. Parasitol.*, **172**, 95–99.

30 Squires, J.M., Ferreira, J.F., Lindsay, D.S., and Zajac, A.M. (2011) Effects of artemisinin and *Artemisia* extracts on *Haemonchus contortus* in gerbils (*Meriones unguiculatus*). *Vet. Parasitol.*, **175**, 103–108.

31 Conder, G.A., Johnson, S.S., Guimond, P.M., Cox, D.L., and Lee, B.L. (1991) Concurrent infections with the ruminant nematodes *Haemonchus contortus* and *Trichostrongylus colubriformis* in jirds, *Meriones unguiculatus*, and use of this model for anthelmintic studies. *J. Parasitol.*, **77**, 621–623.

32. Kaminsky, R., Ducray, P., Jung, M., Clover, R., Rufener, L., Bouvier, J., Weber, S.S. et al. (2008) A new class of anthelmintics effective against drug-resistant nematodes. *Nature*, **452**, 176–180.

33. Kaminsky, R., Gauvry, N., Schorderet Weber, S., Skripsky, T., Bouvier, J., Wenger, A., Shroeder, F. et al. (2008) Identification of the amino-acetonitrile derivative monepantel (AAD 1566) as a new anthelmintic drug development candidate. *Parasitol. Res.*, **103**, 931–939.

34. Court, J.P., Lees, G.M., Coop, R.L., Angus, K.W., and Beesley, J.E. (1988) An attempt to produce *Ostertagia circumcincta* infections in Mongolian gerbils. *Vet. Parasitol.*, **28**, 79–91.

35. Conder, G.A., Johnson, S.S., Nowakowski, D.S., Blake, T.E., Dutton, F.E., Nelson, S.J., Thomas, E.M. et al. (1995) Anthelmintic profile of the cyclodepsipeptide PF1022A in *in vitro* and *in vivo* models. *J. Antibiot.*, **48**, 820–823.

36. Ostlind, D.A., Cifelli, S., Mickle, W.G., Smith, S.K., Ewanciw, D.V., Rafalko, B., Felcetto, T., and Misura, A. (2006) Evaluation of broad-spectrum anthelmintics activity in a novel assay against *Haemonchus contortus, Trichostrongylus colubriformis*, and *T. sigmodontis* in the gerbil *Meriones unguiculatus*. *J. Helminthol.*, **80**, 393–396.

37. Keiser, J. and Utzinger, J. (2008) Efficacy of current drugs against soil-transmitted helminth infections: systematic review and meta-analysis. *J. Am. Med. Assoc.*, **299**, 1937–1948.

38. Mahmoud, A.A. (1996) Strongyloidiasis. *Clin. Infect. Dis.*, **23**, 949–952.

39. Hotez, P.J. and Kamath, A. (2009) Neglected tropical diseases in sub-Saharan Africa: review of their prevalence, distribution, and disease burden. *PLoS Negl. Trop. Dis.*, **3**, e412.

40. Harhay, M.O., Horton, J., and Olliaro, P.L. (2010) Epidemiology and control of human gastrointestinal parasites in children. *Expert Rev. Anti Infect. Ther.*, **8**, 219–234.

41. Hotez, P.J., Bundy, D.A.P., Beegle, K., Brooker, S., Drake, L., de Silva, N., Montresor, A. et al. (2006) Helminth infections: soil-transmitted helminth infections and schistosomiasis, in *Disease Control Priorities in Developing Countries*, 2nd edn (eds D.T. Jamison, J.G. Breman, A.R. Measham, G. Alleyne, M. Claeson, D.B. Evans, P. Jha, A. Mills, and P. Musgrove), World Bank Publications, Washington, DC, pp. 467–482.

42. Olliaro, P., Seiler, J., Kuesel, A., Horton, J., Clark, J.N., Don, R., and Keiser, J. (2011) Potential drug development candidates for human soil-transmitted helminthiases. *PLoS Negl. Trop. Dis.*, **5**, e1138.

43. Cross, J.H. (1996) Enteric nematodes of humans, in *Medical Microbiology*, 4th edn (ed. S. Baron), University of Texas Medical Branch, Galveston, TX, pp. 1065–1177.

44. Boes, J. and Helwigh, A.B. (2000) Animal models of intestinal nematode infections of humans. *Parasitology*, **121** (Suppl.), S97–S111.

45. Cliffe, L.J. and Grencis, R.K. (2004) The *Trichuris muris* system: a paradigm of resistance and susceptibility to intestinal nematode infection. *Adv. Parasitol.*, **57**, 255–307.

46. Bungiro, R. and Cappello, M. (2011) Twenty-first century progress toward the global control of human hookworm infection. *Curr. Infect. Dis. Rep.*, **13**, 210–217.

47. Sen, H.G. and Seth, D. (1970) Development of *Necator americanus* in golden hamsters *Mesocricetus auratus*. *Indian J. Med. Res.*, **58**, 1356–1360.

48. Sen, H.G. (1972) *Necator americanus*: behaviour in hamsters. *Exp. Parasitol.*, **32**, 26–32.

49. Sen, H.G. and Deb, B.N. (1973) Effect of cortisone upon serial passage with the human hookworm, *Necator americanus* in golden hamsters, *Mesocricetus auratus*. *Indian J. Med. Res.*, **61**, 486–494.

50. Bungiro, R.D., Anderson, B.R., and Cappello, M. (2003) Oral transfer of adult *Ancylostoma ceylanicum* hookworms into permissive and nonpermissive host species. *Infect. Immun.*, **71**, 1880–1886.

51 Murthy, P.K., Joseph, S.K., and Murthy, P.S. (2011) Plant products in the treatment and control of filariasis and other helminth infections and assay systems for antifilarial/anthelmintic activity. *Planta Med.*, **77**, 647–661.

52 Behnke, J.M., Paul, V., and Rajasekariah, G.R. (1986) The growth and migration of *Necator americanus* following infection of neonatal hamsters. *Trans. R. Soc. Trop. Med. Hyg.*, **80**, 146–149.

53 Xue, J., Xiao, S.H., Xu, L.L., and Qiang, H.Q. (2010) The effect of tribendimidine and its metabolites against *Necator americanus* in golden hamsters and *Nippostrongylus braziliensis* in rats. *Parasitol. Res.*, **106**, 775–781.

54 Siddiqui, A.A. and Berk, S.L. (2001) Diagnosis of *Strongyloides stercoralis* infection. *Clin. Infect. Dis.*, **33**, 1040–1047.

55 Nolan, T.J., Megyeri, Z., Bhopale, V.M., and Schad, G.A. (1993) *Strongyloides stercoralis*: the first rodent model for uncomplicated and hyperinfective strongyloidiasis, the Mongolian gerbil (*Meriones unguiculatus*). *J. Infect. Dis.*, **168**, 1479–1484.

56 Nolan, T.J., Bhopale, V.M., Rotman, H.L., Abraham, D., and Schad, G.A. (2002) *Strongyloides stercoralis*: high worm population density leads to autoinfection in the jird (*Meriones unguiculatus*). *Exp. Parasitol.*, **100**, 173–178.

57 Lok, J.B. (2007) *Strongyloides stercoralis*: a model for translational research on parasitic nematode biology, in *WormBook* (ed. The *C. elegans* Research Community), doi: 10.1895/wormbook.1.134.1.

58 Steinmann, P., Zhou, X.N., Du, Z.W., Jiang, J.Y., Xiao, S.H., Wu, Z.X., Zhou, H., and Utzinger, J. (2008) Tribendimidine and albendazole for treating soil-transmitted helminths, *Strongyloides stercoralis* and *Taenia* spp: open-label randomized trial. *PLoS Negl. Trop. Dis.*, **2**, e322.

59 Pawlowski, Z.S. (1982) Ascariasis: host–pathogen biology. *Rev. Infect. Dis.*, **4**, 806–814.

60 Katiyar, J.C., Gupta, S., and Sharma, S. (1989) Experimental models in drug development for helminthic diseases. *Rev. Infect. Dis.*, **11**, 638–654.

61 Addiss, D. (2010) The Global Alliance to Eliminate Lymphatic Filariasis. The 6th Meeting of the Global Alliance to Eliminate Lymphatic Filariasis: a half-time review of lymphatic filariasis elimination and its integration with the control of other neglected tropical diseases. *Parasit. Vectors*, **3**, 100.

62 Gupta, R., Tyagi, K., Jain, S.K., and Misra-Bhattacharya, S. (2003) *Brugia malayi*: establishment in inbred and outbred strains of mice. *Exp. Parasitol.*, **103**, 57–60.

63 Bockarie, M.J. and Deb, R.M. (2010) Elimination of lymphatic filariasis: do we have the drugs to complete the job? *Curr. Opin. Infect. Dis.*, **23**, 617–620.

64 Hewitt, R.I. and Wallace, W.S. (1947) Experimental chemotherapy of filariasis; experimental methods for testing drugs against naturally acquired filarial infections in cotton rats and dogs. *J. Lab. Clin. Med.*, **32**, 1293–1303.

65 Taubert, A. and Zahner, H. (2001) Cellular immune responses of filaria (*Litomosoides sigmodontis*) infected BALB/c mice detected on the level of cytokine transcription. *Parasite Immunol.*, **23**, 453–462.

66 Babayan, S., Ungeheuer, M.N., Martin, C., Attout, T., Belnoue, E., Snounou, G., Rénia, L. et al. (2003) Resistance and susceptibility to filarial infection with *Litomosoides sigmodontis* are associated with early differences in parasite development and in localized immune reactions. *Infect. Immun.*, **71**, 6820–6829.

67 Taylor, M.D., LeGoff, L., Harris, A., Malone, E., Allen, J.E., and Maizels, R.M. (2005) Removal of regulatory T cell activity reverses hyporesponsiveness and leads to filarial parasite clearance *in vivo*. *J. Immunol.*, **174**, 4924–4933.

68 Lawrence, R.A. (1996) Lymphatic filariasis: what mice can tell us. *Parasitol. Today*, **12**, 267–271.

69 Singh, P.K., Ajay, A., Kushwaha, S., Tripathi, R.P., and Misra-Bhattacharya, S.

(2010) Towards novel antifilarial drugs: challenges and recent developments. *Future Med. Chem.*, **2**, 251–283.

70 Ash, L.R. and Riley, J.M. (1970) Development of *Brugia pahangi* in the jird, *Meriones unguiculatus*, with notes on infections in other rodents. *J. Parasitol.*, **56**, 962–968.

71 McCall, J.W., Malone, J.B., Hyong-Sun, A., and Thompson, P.E. (1973) Mongolian jirds (*Meriones unguiculatus*) infected with *Brugia pahangi* by the intraperitoneal route: a rich source of developing larvae, adult filariae, and microfilariae. *J. Parasitol.*, **59**, 436.

72 Allen, J.E., Adjei, O., Bain, O., Hoerauf, A., Hoffmann, W.H., Makepeace, B.L., Schulz-Key, H. *et al.* (2008) Of mice, cattle, and humans: the immunology and treatment of river blindness. *PLoS Negl. Trop. Dis.*, **2**, e217.

73 Gloeckner, C., Garner, A.L., Mersha, F., Oksov, Y., Tricoche, N., Eubanks, L.M., Lustigman, S. *et al.* (2010) Repositioning of an existing drug for the neglected tropical disease Onchocerciasis. *Proc. Natl. Acad. Sci. USA*, **107**, 3424–3429.

74 Müllner, A., Helfer, A., Kotlyar, D., Oswald, J., and Efferth, T. (2011) Chemistry and pharmacology of neglected helminthic diseases. *Curr. Med. Chem.*, **18**, 767–789.

75 Schweizer, G., Braun, U., Deplazes, P., and Torgerson, P.R. (2005) Estimating the financial losses due to bovine fasciolosis in Switzerland. *Vet. Rec.*, **157**, 188–193.

76 Sargison, N.D. and Scott, P.R. (2011) Diagnosis and economic consequences of triclabendazole resistance in *Fasciola hepatica* in a sheep flock in south-east Scotland. *Vet. Rec.*, **168**, 159.

77 Cioli, D. and Pica-Mattoccia, L. (2003) Praziquantel. *Parasitol. Res.*, **90**, S3–S9.

78 Utzinger., J., Raso, G., Brooker, S., De Savigny, D., Tanner, M., Ornbjerg, N., Singer, B.H., and N'goran, E.K. (2009) Schistosomiasis and neglected tropical diseases: towards integrated and sustainable control and a word of caution. *Parasitology*, **136**, 1859–1874.

79 Lamberton, P.H., Hogan, S.C., Kabatereine, N.B., Fenwick, A., and Webster, J.P. (2010) *In vitro* praziquantel test capable of detecting reduced *in vivo* efficacy in *Schistosoma mansoni* human infections. *Am. J. Trop. Med. Hyg.*, **83**, 1340–1347.

80 Sabah, A.A., Fletcher, C., Webbe, G., and Doenhoff, M.J. (1986) *Schistosoma mansoni*: chemotherapy of infections of different ages. *Exp. Parasitol.*, **61**, 294–303.

81 Xiao, S.H., Yue, W.J., Yang, Y.Q., and You, J.Q. (1987) Susceptibility of *Schistosoma japonicum* to different developmental stages to praziquantel. *Chin. Med. J.*, **100**, 759–768.

82 Xiao, S.H., Mei, J.Y., and Jiao, P.Y. (2009) The *in vitro* effect of mefloquine and praziquantel against juvenile and adult *Schistosoma japonicum*. *Parasitol. Res.*, **106**, 237–246.

83 Dong, Y., Chollet, J., Vargas, M., Mansour, N.R., Bickle, Q., Alnouti, Y., Huang, J., Keiser, J., and Vennerstrom, J.L. (2010) Praziquantel analogs with activity against juvenile *Schistosoma mansoni*. *Bioorg. Med. Chem. Lett.*, **20**, 2481–2484.

84 Coles, G.C. (1999) Schistosomosis, in *Handbook of Animal Models of Infection* (eds O. Zak and M.A. Sande), Academic Press, London, pp. 873–884.

85 el Kouni, M.H. (1991) Efficacy of combination therapy with tubercidin and nitrobenzylthioinosine 5′-monophosphate against chronic and advanced stages of schistosomiasis. *Biochem. Pharmacol.*, **41**, 815–820.

86 Penido, M.L., Nelson, D.L., Vieira, L.Q., Watson, D.G., and Kusel, J.R. (1995) Metabolism by *Schistosoma mansoni* of a new schistosomicide: 2-[(1-methylpropyl)amino]-1-octanethiosulphuric acid. *Parasitology*, **111**, 177–185.

87 Manivannan, B., Rawson, P., Jordan, T.W., Secor, W.E., and La Flamme1, A.C. (2010) Differential patterns of liver proteins in experimental murine hepatosplenic schistosomiasis. *Infect. Immun.*, **78**, 618–628.

88 Pearce, E.J. and MacDonald, A.S. (2002) The immunobiology of schistosomiasis. *Nat. Rev. Immunol.*, **2**, 499–511.

89 Cheever, A.W., Lenzi, J.A., Lenzi, H.L., and Andrade, Z.A. (2002) Experimental models of *Schistosoma mansoni* infection. *Mem. Inst. Oswaldo Cruz*, **97**, 917–940.

90 Lewis, F.A., Liang, Y.S., Raghavan, N., and Knight, M. (2008) The NIH-NIAID schistosomiasis resource center. *PLoS Negl. Trop. Dis.*, **2**, e267.

91 Sayed, A.A., Simeonov, A., Thomas, C.J., Inglese, J., Austin, C.P. *et al.* (2008) Identification of oxadiazoles as new drug leads for the control of schistosomiasis. *Nat. Med.*, **14**, 407–412.

92 Abdulla, M.H., Lim, K.C., Sajid, M., McKerrow, J.H., and Caffrey, C.R. (2007) Schistosomiasis mansoni: novel chemotherapy using a cysteine protease inhibitor. *PLoS Med.*, **4**, e14.

93 Keiser, J. (2010) *In vitro* and *in vivo* trematode models for chemotherapeutic studies. *Parasitology*, **137**, 589–603.

94 Keiser, J., Shu-Hua, X., Tanner, M., and Utzinger, J. (2006) Artesunate and artemether are effective fasciolicides in the rat model and *in vitro*. *J. Antimicrob. Chemother.*, **57**, 1139–1145.

95 McConville, M., Brennan, G.P., Flanagan, A., Edgar, H.W., Hanna, R.E., McCoy, M., Gordon, A.W. *et al.* (2009) An evaluation of the efficacy of compound alpha and triclabendazole against two isolates of *Fasciola hepatica*. *Vet. Parasitol.*, **162**, 75–88.

96 McKinstry, B., Fairweather, I., Brennan, G.P., and Forbes, A.B. (2003) *Fasciola hepatica*: tegumental surface alterations following treatment *in vivo* and *in vitro* with nitroxynil (Trodax). *Parasitol. Res.*, **91**, 251–263.

97 Keiser, J. and Morson, G. (2008) *Fasciola hepatica*: tegumental alterations in adult flukes following *in vitro* and *in vivo* administration of artesunate and artemether. *Exp. Parasitol.*, **118**, 228–237.

98 Saric, J., Li, J.V., Wang, Y., Keiser, J., Veselkov, K., Dirnhofer, S., Yap, I.K., Nicholson, J.K., Holmes, E., and Utzinger, J. (2009) Panorganismal metabolic response modeling of an experimental *Echinostoma caproni* infection in the mouse. *J. Proteome Res.*, **8**, 3899–3911.

99 Keiser, J., Utzinger, J., Tanner, M., Dong, Y., and Vennerstrom, J.L. (2006) The synthetic peroxide OZ78 is effective against *Echinostoma caproni* and *Fasciola hepatica*. *J. Antimicrob. Chemother.*, **58**, 1193–1197.

100 Keiser, J., Brun, R., Fried, B., and Utzinger, J. (2006) Trematocidal activity of praziquantel and artemisinin derivatives: *in vitro* and *in vivo* investigations with adult *Echinostoma caproni*. *Antimicrob. Agents Chemother.*, **50**, 803–805.

101 Sariözkan, S. and Yalçin, C. (2009) Estimating the production losses due to cystic echinococcosis in ruminants in Turkey. *Vet. Parasitol.*, **163**, 330–334.

102 Kamiya, M. and Sato, H. (1990) Complete life cycle of the canid tapeworm, *Echinococcus multilocularis*, in laboratory rodents. *FASEB J.*, **4**, 3334–3339.

103 Romig, T. and Bilger, B. (1999) Animal models for echinococcosis, in *Handbook of Animal Models of Infection* (eds O. Zak and M.A. Sande), Academic Press, London, pp. 877–884.

104 Taylor, D.H., Morris, D.L., Reffin, D., and Richards, K.S. (1989) Comparison of albendazole mebendazole and praziquantel chemotherapy of *Echinoccocus multilocularis* in a gerbil model. *Gut.*, **30**, 1401–1405.

105 Johnson, S.S., Thomas, E.M., and Geary, T.G. (1999) Cestode model: *Hymenolepis diminuta* in the jird, in *Handbook of Animal Models of Infection* (eds O. Zak and M.A. Sande), Academic Press, London, pp. 892–896.

106 Drudge, J.H., Leland, S.E. Jr, Wyant, Z.N., and Elam, G.W. (1955) Studies on *Trichostrongylus axei* (Cobbold, 1879) I. Some experimental host relationships. *J. Parasitol.*, **41**, 505–511.

107 Panitz, E. and Shum, K.L. (1981) Efficacy of four anthelmintics in *Trichostrongylus axei* or *T. colubriformis* infections in the gerbil, *Meriones unguiculatus*. *J. Parasitol.*, **67**, 135–136.

108 Boersema, J.H. (1985) Chemotherapy of gastrointestinal nematodiasis in ruminants, in *Chemotherapy of*

Gastrointestinal Helminths (eds H. Vanden Bossche, D. Thienpont, and P.G. Janssens), Springer, New York, pp. 407–442.

109 Zahner, H. and Schares, G. (1993) Experimental chemotherapy of filariasis: comparative evaluation of the efficacy of filaricidal compounds in *Mastomys coucha* infected with *Litomosoides carinii, Acanthocheilonema viteae, Brugia malayi* and *B. pahangi. Acta Trop.*, **52**, 221–266.

110 Townson, S., Connelly, C., Dobinson, A., and Muller, R. (1987) Drug activity against *Onchocerca gutturosa* males *in vitro*: a model for chemotherapeutic research on onchocerciasis. *J. Helminthol.*, **61**, 271–281.

111 Tagboto, S.K. and Townson, S. (1996) *Onchocerca volvulus* and *O. lienalis*: the microfilaricidal activity of moxidectin compared with that of ivermectin *in vitro* and *in vivo. Ann. Trop. Med. Parasitol.*, **90**, 497–505.

112 Mehlhorn, H., Schmahl, G., and Mevissen, I. (2005) Efficacy of a combination of imidacloprid and moxidectin against parasites of reptiles and rodents: case reports. *Parasitol. Res.*, **97**, S97–S101.

113 Mehlhorn, H., Schmahl, G., Frese, M., Mevissen, I., Harder, A., and Krieger, K. (2005) Effects of a combinations of emodepside and praziquantel on parasites of reptiles and rodents. *Parasitol. Res.*, **97**, S65–S69.

114 Rajasekariah, G.R., Dhage, K.R., Deb, B.N., and Bose, S. (1985) *Necator americanus* and *Ancylostoma ceylanicum*: development of protocols for dual infection in hamsters. *Acta Trop.*, **42**, 45–54.

115 Xue, J., Qiang, H.Q., Yao, J.M., Fujiwara, R., Zhan, B., Hotez, P., and Xiao, S.H. (2005) *Necator americanus*: optimization of the golden hamster model for testing anthelmintic drugs. *Exp. Parasitol.*, **111**, 219–223.

116 Behnke, J.M., Tose, R., and Garside, P. (1993) Sensitivity to ivermectin and pyrantel of *Ancylostoma ceylanicum* and *Necator americanus. Int. J. Parasitol.*, **23**, 945–952.

117 Grove, D. (1982) *Strongyloides ratti* and *S. stercoralis*: the effects of thiabendazole, mebendazole, and cambendazole in infected mice. *Am. J. Trop. Med. Hyg.*, **31**, 469–476.

118 Cioli, D., Pica-Mattoccia, L., and Archerm, S. (1995) Antischistosomal drugs: past, present and future. *Clin. Pharmacol. Ther.*, **68**, 35–85.

119 Keiser, J., El Ela, N.A., El Komy, E., El Lakkany, N., Diab, T., Chollet, J., Utzinger, J., and Barakat, R. (2006) Triclabendazole and its two main metabolites lack activity against *Schistosoma mansoni* in the mouse model. *Am. J. Trop. Med. Hyg.*, **75**, 287–291.

120 Xiao, S.H. and Catto, B.A. (1989) *In vitro* and *in vivo* studies of the effect of artemether on *Schistosoma mansoni. Antimicrob Agents Chemother.*, **33**, 1557–1562.

121 Keiser, J., Chollet, J., Xiao, S.H., Mei, J.Y., Jiao, P.Y., Utzinger, J., and Tanner, M. (2009) 2009 Mefloquine – an aminoalcohol with promising antischistosomal properties in mice. *PLoS Negl. Trop. Dis.*, **3**, e350.

122 Xiao, S.H., Keiser, J., Chollet, J., Utzinger, J., Dong, Y., Endriss, Y., Vennerstrom, J.L., and Tanner, M. (2007) *In vitro* and *in vivo* activities of synthetic trioxolanes against major human Schistosome species. *Antimicrob. Agents Chemother.*, **51**, 1440–1445.

123 Keiser, J. and Utzinger, J. (2007) Artemisinins and synthetic trioxolanes in the treatment of helminth infections. *Curr. Opin. Infect. Dis.*, **20**, 605–612.

12
To Kill a Mocking Worm: Strategies to Improve *Caenorhabditis elegans* as a Model System for use in Anthelmintic Discovery

*Andrew R. Burns and Peter J. Roy**

Abstract

The nematode *Caenorhabditis elegans* can be a powerful model system for the discovery and characterization of new anthelmintics. *C. elegans* is free-living and its use therefore circumvents the complications of culturing parasitic nematodes that are invariably dependent on a host to complete their life cycle. *C. elegans* is also small (1 mm in length), hermaphroditic, and has a 3-day life cycle. These features make *C. elegans* a seemingly ideal high-throughput platform with which to discover novel anthelmintics. However, *C. elegans* has formidable xenobiotic defenses that have likely evolved to protect it from a plethora of chemical insults in its native environment. In this chapter, we will discuss the extent of *C. elegans* xenobiotic resistance and review strategies to circumvent this resistance in order to take full advantage of one of the most powerful animal models available.

Introduction

The impact of parasitic nematodes on human productivity and well-being cannot be overstated. Parasitic nematodes infect over 1 billion people worldwide [1], and impose significant agricultural losses through infected livestock and crops [2, 3]. Resistance to commonly used anthelmintics among animals is escalating and the recent increase in the use of mass drug administration for the treatment of human helminth infections raises the risk that clinically relevant resistance will soon develop [2, 4]. Despite the obvious need for new anthelmintic drugs, the last 30 years has seen only three new anthelmintic classes marketed for veterinary use (monepantel and derquantel for sheep [5–7], and emodepside for cats and dogs [1]) and only one new drug approved for use in humans (tribendimidine in China [1, 8]). Clearly, there is a pressing need to discover new anthelmintic drug classes.

The relatively large size and complex life cycles of many parasitic nematode species present significant challenges for their manipulation in a laboratory setting, particularly when considering their use in high-throughput chemical screens.

---

* Corresponding Author

Parasitic Helminths: Targets, Screens, Drugs and Vaccines, First Edition. Edited by Conor R. Caffrey
© 2012 Wiley-VCH Verlag GmbH & Co. KGaA. Published 2012 by Wiley-VCH Verlag GmbH & Co. KGaA.

The free-living nematode Caenorhabditis elegans provides an experimentally tractable alternative to parasitic worms for the discovery and characterization of novel anthelmintic drugs. C. elegans is small (around 1 mm fully grown), hermaphroditic, easy to culture, and has only a 3-day life cycle [9]. These attributes enable the high-throughput screening of small molecules for bioactivity in the context of the whole animal over its entire life cycle (Figure 12.1a). Indeed, a number of compounds with novel bioactivities have been identified from C. elegans chemical screens [10–13]. Furthermore, genetic analyses of C. elegans have revealed the mechanism of action for many bioactive molecules, including anthelmintics [5, 10, 14, 15].

In this chapter, we briefly discuss the important role C. elegans has played in the describing the mechanism of action of anthelmintics. We describe the historical and biological reasons of why C. elegans has not played a pre-eminent role in the discovery of novel anthelmintics in the past, and discuss new methodologies that now allow researchers to use C. elegans as an effective platform in large-scale screens for novel anthelmintics.

C. elegans as a Platform for Anthelmintic Characterization

The power of C. elegans as an animal model system lies in the relative simplicity of its biology and genetics, which can be taken advantage of to define the mode of action of bioactive molecules. Tens of thousands of mutagenized C. elegans worms can be screened for mutants that are resistant to the effects of a given bioactive molecule in a relatively short timeframe (Figure 12.1b). Depending on the design, these forward genetic screens may yield mutations in the target's biochemical pathway, the target itself, or even residues within the target that comprise the small molecule's binding site [16]. Forward genetic screens in C. elegans have been used successfully to characterize the modes of action for a number of bioactive molecules, including many anthelmintics [10, 14, 17]. For example, the protein targets of the novel class of anthelmintics, called amino-acetonitrile derivatives (AADs), were discovered through a screen for resistant C. elegans mutants [5, 18]. Kaminsky et al. obtained 44 AAD-resistant mutants from a screen of C. elegans mutant F2s, of which 36 fell into a single complementation group. Genetic mapping and subsequent DNA sequencing revealed 27 independent mutations in the C. elegans acr-23 gene. acr-23 encodes a nicotinic acetylcholine receptor (nAChR) of the DEG-3 group. The authors found that isolates of Haemonchus contortus that are resistant to AADs had lost at least part of the acr-23 gene homolog and at least part of the des-2 gene homolog (another member of the DEG-3 group of nAChRs). These results suggest that the AADs function by activating nAChRs of the DEG-3 subfamily. Indeed, subsequent electrophysiological analysis has shown that the AADs act as positive allosteric modulators of H. contortus DEG-3/DES-2 channels [18]. One of the AADs, monepantel, is currently marketed as an anthelmintic therapy for sheep [6]. The use of C. elegans in defining the mode of action of the AADs is a clear example of the utility of this simple nematode for anthelmintic target identification.

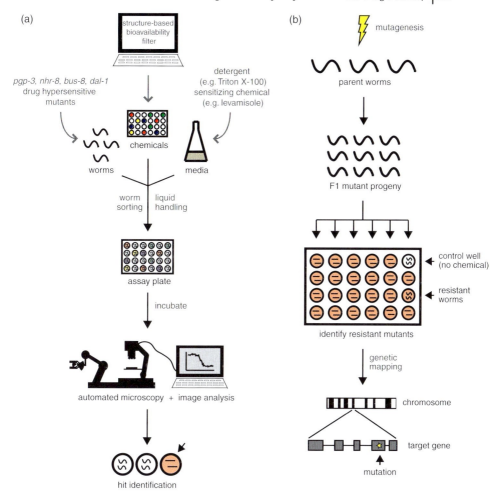

Figure 12.1 High-throughput chemical screening and target identification in *C. elegans*. (a) Workflow for a high-throughput chemical screen in *C. elegans*. Liquid handling, worm sorting, and imaging can be fully automated with the use of robots and automated imaging platforms. The worm strains, media, and chemicals used for screening can be optimized to maximize the bioavailability of the compounds being screened. (b) Upon identifying a compound that is bioactive in *C. elegans*, forward genetic screens can be performed to identify candidate pathways, targets, and docking sites of the molecule of interest (see [16] for more details). In the diagram, pink represents a solution of the compound of interest.

C. elegans as a Platform for Anthelmintic Drug Discovery

Several lines of evidence support the idea that *C. elegans* is also a suitable model for anthelmintic drug discovery. (i) Comparative genomic analyses of *C. elegans* and parasitic nematodes suggest that *C. elegans* is no more distinct from any parasitic nematode than any two parasitic nematodes are from each other [17, 19]. (ii) The majority of anthelmintic drugs used to treat parasitic worm infections of humans and livestock are effective against *C. elegans*, and most have conserved modes of action [5, 17]. (iii) Both established and putative anthelmintic drug targets are conserved in *C. elegans* [17, 20–24]. (iv) It has recently been shown that the long-lived nonreproductive *C. elegans* dauer stage is analogous to the infective larval stage (iL3) of parasitic nematodes, and that a conserved endocrine signaling mechanism controls entry into and recovery from both dauer and iL3 [22, 24]. It therefore follows that anthelmintics developed against *C. elegans* might be equally effective against parasitic nematodes based on the genomic and biological relationships between the nematodes.

The potential utility of *C. elegans* for anthelmintic drug screens was recognized early in the development of this animal model system [25]. In the 1980s and 1990s, industrial anthelmintic discovery efforts employed *C. elegans* as a primary screening tool for the identification of novel anthelmintic lead molecules [26]. Many positive hits were obtained from these initial screens, but few exhibited adequate activity in infection models to warrant testing in target animals. To date, no new anthelmintic class has resulted from a *C. elegans* primary screen. Due to the low-throughput nature of previous *C. elegans* screening protocols, the predominance of unviable leads, and a paradigm shift from broad whole-organism-based screens to more rational high-throughput approaches to drug discovery, *C. elegans* was essentially abandoned as a screening platform for novel anthelmintics [26].

Despite the pharmaceutical industry's current focus on target-based approaches to drug discovery, there are advantages to whole organism-based screens [27, 28]. (i) *A priori* knowledge of the protein target is not required for a phenotype-based screen. (ii) Mode-of-action studies of bioactive compounds obtained from whole-organism screens can reveal several components that act in the same pathway as the targeted compound and consequently yield potentially novel targets for further drug development. (iii) Bioactive hits obtained from whole-organism screens are active *in vivo*, which is a property that typically requires significant additional investment with lead compounds identified with targeted-based *in vitro* screens. Furthermore, all of the currently available anthelmintic therapies were discovered through whole-organism screens. Hence, reviving *C. elegans* as an anthelmintic discovery tool may be warranted. However, the issues that plagued the initial *C. elegans*-based screens first need to be addressed. Future screens using *C. elegans* will have to be of higher throughput, the workload needs to be lessened, and the number of viable leads must increase.

Several technological advances over the past decade have enabled the development of high-throughput screens with *C. elegans* [16, 27, 29, 30]. (i) There are a number of commercially available automated liquid-handling systems that can be used to standardize the addition of media and chemicals to screening plates, and our group has made use of such technologies for genetic screens in *C. elegans* [31]. (ii) Worm deposition in *C. elegans*-based screens can be automated using the COPAS Biosort (Union Biometrica) [32]. This machine sorts worms based on user-defined selection criteria, such as size and fluorescence, and then precisely dispenses defined numbers of worms into the wells of multiwell assay plates in a high-throughput fashion.

The COPAS Biosort has been used by a number of groups to automate worm handling for both chemical and genetic screens in C. elegans [16, 29, 31, 33]. (iii) Methods for automated image acquisition and analyses of C. elegans samples cultured in multiwell plates have been developed [16, 29, 34, 35]. Our lab uses a high-throughput digital imager (HiDI 2100; Elegenics) to automate plate handling and image acquisition of worms on top of solid media in multiwell plates [16]. Combined, these technologies facilitate a throughput that might be considered high even by industrial standards (i.e., tens of thousands of chemicals per day [29]) and transforms C. elegans into a viable platform for industrial anthelmintic discovery.

Initial C. elegans-based anthelmintic screens were performed by inspecting 96-well screening plates for chemical-induced changes in behavior, viability, or reproduction [26]. These gross phenotypes can result from the perturbation of a plethora of target proteins, which may or may not be conserved in pathogenic worm species. Thus, the use of such holistic phenotypes fails to enrich the target space of the screen with proteins that are conserved in parasitic worms and could account for the high rate of nonviable leads obtained from these early C. elegans-based screens. One way to increase viable leads in C. elegans anthelmintic screens is to develop high-content assays that provide immediate insight into a potential mechanism of action of candidate hits.

One paradigm that holds promise for yielding specific modulators of an infective state is to screen for compounds that alter C. elegans dauer development. As mentioned previously, a conserved endocrine signaling pathway regulates the development of both the dauer stage of C. elegans and the infective larval stage of parasitic nematodes (iL3) [22, 24]. In C. elegans, the dafachronic acid steroid hormones control dauer entry through their interaction with the nuclear receptor DAF-12 [36]. The orthologous dafachronic acid–DAF-12 signaling system also regulates iL3 development. Reduced dafachronic acid induces the dauer/iL3 state and increased dafachronic acid promotes dauer recovery or iL3 escape. It has been proposed that the dafachronic acid–DAF-12 signaling system may be a pertinent drug target for disseminated strongyloides infection, which is characterized by an auto-infection cycle in which Strongyloides stercoralis never leaves its host [24]. Given that dauers are a readily distinguishable developmental state of C. elegans, a straightforward screening paradigm for novel anthelmintics is to screen for molecules that modulate the dauer state. Such focused phenotype-based assays would hopefully reduce the number of unviable leads obtained from C. elegans primary screens.

With our improving ability to screen chemical libraries in a high-throughput fashion against whole worms and the development of more focused phenotypic assays, C. elegans-based chemical screens have the potential to resurge as a powerful complementary approach to rational mechanism-based methods for anthelmintic drug discovery.

Xenobiotic Resistance of C. elegans

A potential drawback to the use of C. elegans for anthelmintic discovery is its general resistance to xenobiotic perturbation, despite the conservation of many known and well-characterized pharmacological targets [10, 37]. Given its extensive xenobiotic defenses [37, 38], which include a four-layered cuticle and a genome replete with putative detoxification proteins, a reasonable explanation for this resistance is that exogenous molecules have limited bioavailability in *C. elegans* tissues. Indeed, molecules having no effect on whole worms can perturb their target proteins if they are provided direct access [10, 39, 40]. For example, the anthelmintic nAChR antagonist derquantel has little to no activity on intact *C. elegans* at concentrations as high as 100 µM, but shows clear effects on motility in cut worms at concentrations as low as 10 µM [41]. The anthelmintic nAChR agonist amidantel has similar properties [42]. Both derquantel and amidantel are potent anthelmintics in animal models of nematode infection. Moreover, in a high-performance liquid chromatography-based survey of the accumulation of more than 1000 drug-like molecules, our group found that fewer than 10% of the molecules accumulate to concentrations greater than half of the concentration in the environment and that accumulation is generally required for bioactivity [37]. Thus, target access is likely a major limiting factor for drug efficacy in *C. elegans*. The obvious concern is that *C. elegans* high-throughput chemical screens will miss potential anthelmintic lead structures, simply because the molecules screened do not achieve effective concentrations at the target site.

It is not surprising that a free-living worm such as *C. elegans* has evolved strategies to resist the accumulation of exogenous compounds in its tissues, given the diverse and potentially harmful nature of the dissolved substances in the soil and associated niches. Conversely, the tissue stages of parasitic worms may require less extensive xenobiotic defenses to survive the relatively homogeneous and predictable chemistry of their host niche. The observation that the free-living L3 stage of *H. contortus* is less sensitive to anthelmintics than its adult stage supports this idea [41, 43] and suggests that free-living worms may be, in general, more resistant to xenobiotic insult than their host-dwelling counterparts.

It has been proposed that previous *C. elegans*-based anthelmintic discovery efforts failed, in part, because the worms were insensitive to potentially useful anthelmintic lead compounds [41]. Our previous small-molecule screens of *C. elegans* that included a number of known anthelmintics [10] provide a test case for this hypothesis. Our screens were performed on solid substrate, over the course of one generation (4 days), and at a small-molecule concentration of 25 µM. Common nematicidal anthelmintics included in the screens were piperazine, levamisole, pyrantel, morantel, selamectin, ivermectin, avermectin B1, thiabendazole, albendazole, mebendazole, fenbendazole, and oxybendazole. All three avermectins had nematicidal activity against *C. elegans*. Levamisole, albendazole, mebendazole, fenbendazole, and oxybendazole induced obvious motility defects. Piperazine, pyrantel, morantel, and thiabendazole had no effect on the growth or behavior of *C. elegans*. Therefore, although established anthelmintics can be identified from large-scale chemical screens in *C. elegans*, some compounds will be missed at typical screening concentrations.

If *C. elegans* is to be used as a screening tool for anthelmintic lead discovery, it is important to consider sensitizing the worm to a broader range of chemical structures and to include "worm-bioavailable" structures in screening collections. Below, we describe modifications to screening parameters that serve to improve *C. elegans* drug sensitivity and increase the rate at which bioactives are identified from *C. elegans* chemical screens. These modifications, alone or in combination, should help bolster the utility of *C. elegans* as a platform for anthelmintic discovery and drug discovery in general.

Circumventing Xenobiotic Resistance

Modifying the Screening Paradigm
C. elegans can be cultured in both liquid media and on solid substrate, and chemical screens performed in both media types have been described [10, 12]. We have observed relatively higher hit rates for liquid-based versus solid-based screens (unpublished observations), likely because the worms are bathing in the chemical solution, which provides greater opportunity for the chemicals to penetrate the animals and access target proteins. Aside from bioavailability considerations, liquid-based screens are more amenable to miniaturization and high-throughput screening using, for example, 384-well microtiter plates and microfluidic chips. Thus, for maximal throughput and bioavailability, liquid media is likely the best choice for *C. elegans* anthelmintic discovery screens.

The simplest method to achieve higher internal xenobiotic concentrations in the worm is to increase the compound's external concentration. However, increasing the screening concentration can be cost-prohibitive, and result in the precipitation of the xenobiotic and consequently reduce its bioavailability. Also, the screening concentration is limited by the concentration of the stock solution and by the amount of solvent that the organism can reasonably tolerate. Chemicals in purchasable libraries are typically dissolved in dimethylsulfoxide (DMSO) at a concentration of 10 mM. DMSO concentrations greater than 1% can adversely affect the development and behavior of *C. elegans* (unpublished observations). Thus, the upper concentration limit for a screen of purchasable chemicals in *C. elegans* is fixed at 100 μM and published chemical screens employing *C. elegans* have typically used concentrations equivalent to or lower than this value [10–13, 29, 44].

A second method to increase target accessibility in the worm is to spike the screening media with a small amount of mild detergent such as Triton X-100 or Tween-20. For example, wild-type *C. elegans* treated with 0.1% Triton X-100 arrests at the first larval stage when exposed to 200 μg/ml of the mushroom toxin α-amanitin, whereas detergent-free worms are resistant to α-amanitin at concentrations as high as 800 μg/ml [45]. Furthermore, Semple *et al.* found that wild-type worms treated with 0.1% Triton X-100 showed more than 100-fold greater sensitivity to 0.5 mg/ml puromycin after 2 days of exposure, relative to detergent-free animals [46]. Triton X-100 also sensitized worms to two other antibiotics, G418 and phleomycin. Presumably the detergent permeabilizes the cuticle and/or the intestine; however, the mechanism of sensitization is unclear. In addition to serving as permeability agents, mild detergents could also solubilize lipophilic molecules in the screening media that would otherwise precipitate out of solution, thereby enhancing compound availability to the worm. To our knowledge, mild detergents have never been used as permeability agents in *C. elegans* high-throughput chemical screens, but they could easily be incorporated into the media preparation for this type of screening platform. Before universally adopting "detergent-spiked" media for anthelmintic discovery screens, it is critical to assess how general the detergent-sensitizing effects are for a broad range of pharmacologically active molecules, including established anthelmintics. Purchasable collections of pharmacologically active compounds are available that can be used for this purpose.

A third approach to sensitize worms to xenobiotics is to screen them in the background of a low dose of a characterized compound that elicits the desired phenotype at higher concentrations. For example, spiking the screening media with an EC_{10} of the anthelmintic nAChR agonist levamisole could sensitize *C. elegans* to novel nAChR agonists that may not elicit obvious motility defects in *C. elegans* when administered alone. Earlier, we discussed a screen for compounds that antagonize *C. elegans* dauer formation as a means to identify novel DAF-12 activators that could be developed into therapies to treat parasitic nematode infections. This screen might benefit from the incorporation of a low dose of dafachronic acid (the dauer antagonizing hormone) in the screening media in order to sensitize the worms to chemicals that promote reproductive development. In addition to sensitizing worms to anthelmintic lead compounds, "combination chemical screens" also have the potential to uncover therapeutically useful synergistic chemical combinations that would be missed in a "single-chemical screen." A caveat to combination chemical screens is that chemical combinations can act antagonistically (i.e., one compound can reduce the efficacy of another) [47]. However, this limitation is easily circumvented by screening single molecules in parallel to any combinatorial screen. Also, we have found that pooling large numbers of chemicals generally reduces hit rates. In previous chemical screens we found that pooling eight small molecules per well, as opposed to screening the same chemicals one molecule per well, resulted in the identification of 10-fold fewer actives ([10, 16] and unpublished observations). The reason for the reduction in hit rate is not clear. One possibility may be that the worm's xenobiotic defenses are upregulated in response to the large number of different structures and that the upregulated defenses limit the accessibility of what would otherwise be a genuine hit. Regardless, combination chemical screens have the potential to sensitize worms to new anthelmintic lead compounds and could uncover therapeutically useful chemical combinations.

Modifying the Chemistry
In 1991, the main cause for clinical attrition of pharmaceutical drug candidates was adverse pharmacokinetic and bioavailability properties, accounting for 40% of all attrition [48]. By 2000, the percentage of clinical failures attributed to adverse pharmacokinetics decreased 4-fold and poor bioavailability was no longer the root cause for attrition. Efforts to define property-based rules of small-molecule drug absorption and permeation likely contributed to the observed decrease. A particularly influential example is Lipinski's "Rule-of-Five," whereby small molecules will generally have unfavorable absorption and permeation properties if they have a $\log P > 5$, a molecular weight above 500, and more than five hydrogen bond donors or more than 10 hydrogen bond acceptors [49]. The Rule-of-Five serves as a useful

computational tool to exclude molecules from high-throughput screens that are likely to have poor oral bioavailability in humans. As a result of its established utility, the majority of chemicals in purchasable libraries are "Lipinski-like" [50]. Lipinski's Rule-of-Five describes a chemical space with good oral absorption properties for humans, but it likely does not define an optimal chemical space for worms, free-living or otherwise. As discussed above, our analysis of the accumulation of more than 1000 drug-like (also Lipinski-like) molecules in *C. elegans* revealed that less than 10% of the molecules accumulate to concentrations greater than half of the assay concentration and that accumulation is generally required for bioactivity [37]. Indeed, *C. elegans* is resistant to many pharmacologically active compounds, despite most of these molecules being Rule-of-Five compliant.

We reasoned that higher hit rates could be achieved for *C. elegans* chemical screens if the molecules were selected from a "worm-bioavailable" chemical space. To define a worm-focused chemistry, we used our *C. elegans* drug-like molecule accumulation data as a training set to model the structural signatures of accumulating compounds using computer-based chemical fingerprinting and machine-learning techniques (see [37] for a more detailed description of the method). The resultant structure-based accumulation model (SAM) scores substructural features positively if they have a high likelihood of being found in accumulating molecules, whereas features unlikely to be found in accumulating compounds are scored negatively. The five top- and bottom-scoring substructural features derived from the SAM are shown in Figure 12.2a and b, respectively. The structural scaffolds from which the top-scoring features are derived are shown in Figure 12.2c. Of the 74 molecules in our dataset that accumulate to concentrations greater than half the external concentration, 30 contain at least one of these structural scaffolds. Interestingly, of the 12 accumulating molecules that contain the "unfused" biaryl scaffold (Figure 12.2c), 11 induce penetrant lethality in *C. elegans* at a concentration of 25 µM. Thus, the "unfused" biaryl scaffold may serve as a useful building block in the construction of novel nematicides. The bottom-scoring features B1, B2, and B4 are derived from molecules that contain carboxylic acid, aliphatic hydroxyl, and sulfonyl groups, respectively. It is not unexpected that these features are found primarily in nonaccumulating molecules given that the hydrogen and oxygen atoms they contain can make hydrogen bond contacts with water molecules, thereby promoting aqueous solubility and preventing cell membrane permeability. Consistent with these data, an analysis of the molecular properties used to define Lipinski's Rule-of-Five (log P, molecular weight, number of hydrogen bond donors, and number of hydrogen bond acceptors) reveals that the accumulating molecules in our dataset generally have fewer hydrogen bond donors and acceptors compared to the nonaccumulating compounds, and molecules that accumulate in worms are generally more hydrophobic than those that fail to accumulate (Figure 12.2d). We hope that the molecular features and structural scaffolds we have identified will guide the design of novel "worm-bioavailable" chemical matter targeted for nematode screens.

Aside from determining structural features that promote or antagonize accumulation, the SAM can also be used to determine the likelihood that a given molecule, or a collection of molecules, will accumulate in worm tissue [37]. A molecule's

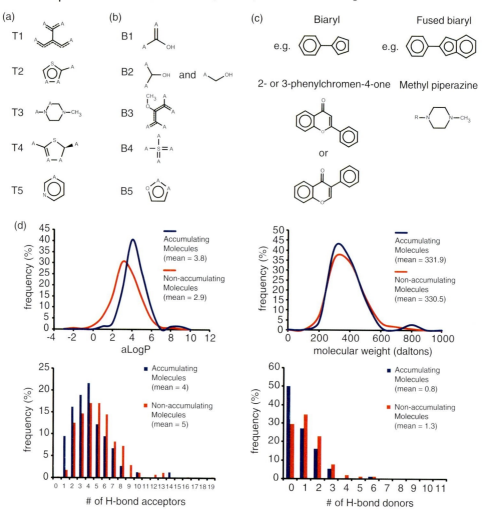

Figure 12.2 Molecular properties that influence exogenous drug-like molecule accumulation in C. elegans. (a) Top-scoring substructural features derived from our C. elegans SAM; these features are found predominantly in molecules that accumulate in worms. Where appropriate A = C, N, O, or S. (b) Bottom-scoring substructural features derived from the SAM; these features are found predominantly in molecules that fail to accumulate in worms. (c) Molecular scaffolds of molecules enriched for accumulators. (d) Distributions of the Lipinski parameters (log P, molecular weight, number of hydrogen bond acceptors, and number of hydrogen bond donors) for the compounds in the accumulation dataset. The term alog P is a computationally derived estimate of the log P of an organic compound, which is a measure of hydrophobicity.

"accumulation score" is simply the sum of the scores of the substructural features present in the molecule. Compounds with higher accumulation scores are more likely to accumulate in worms than molecules with lower scores. A key utility of the SAM is that it can be used to generate accumulation scores for the molecules in available compound collections. The SAM-scored molecules can then be prioritized based on their likelihood of accumulating in worms and hence their likelihood of accessing a biologically relevant target. Indeed, when we analyzed the accumulation of SAM-ranked molecules from the DIVERSet™ chemical library (ChemBridge), we found that 60% of the compounds selected from the top-scoring 5% accumulate to concentrations greater than half of the assay concentration [37]. This accumulation rate represents a 5.5-fold enrichment relative to randomly selected compounds and a 15-fold enrichment relative to compounds selected from the bottom-scoring 5%. Furthermore, when we used our SAM to rank 9740 molecules of the same DIVERSet library that we had previously screened for the induction of gross phenotypes in wild-type *C. elegans*, we found that the top-scoring 5% are 6-fold enriched for bioactives relative to an equivalent number of molecules chosen at random from the same library [37]. We envision our SAM as a structure-based bioavailability filter that will be used to preselect "worm-bioavailable" molecules for inclusion in *C. elegans* high-throughput screening assays. Applying our SAM to other Lipinski-like small-molecule libraries will increase the likelihood that any hit found using *C. elegans* will also be bioavailable in humans and facilitate its development as a human anthelmintic drug lead.

Similar "worm-bioavailable" chemical spaces could be defined for parasitic worms as well, although the generation of analogous accumulation datasets would likely be technically more difficult for these species. Encouragingly, the molecular properties that influence bioavailability in *C. elegans* are similar to those for parasitic worms [37, 51], suggesting that our model may have some utility in predicting drug bioavailability for parasitic worm species as well. For example, lipophilicity is a major determinant of drug entry into parasitic worms [51] and we find that molecules that accumulate in *C. elegans* are generally more hydrophobic than those that fail to accumulate (Figure 12.2d). In addition, two of the lowest scoring features defined by our SAM are sulfoxide and sulfonyl groups, and these features have been shown to reduce anthelmintic bioavailability in parasitic worms ([51] and references therein). For instance, the sulfoxide metabolite of albendazole has poorer bioavailability in *Ascaris suum*, *Moniezia* spp., and *Fasciola hepatica* compared to the unmodified structure. Furthermore, *F. hepatica* can sulfoxidate and sulfonate the anthelmintic triclabendazole (TCBZ), and it has been shown that the rate of TCBZ sulfoxidation is significantly higher in TCBZ-resistant isolates of *F. hepatica* relative to susceptible worms, suggesting that sulfoxidation plays a role in TCBZ detoxification. Of the 34 compounds in our accumulation dataset that contain a sulfonyl or sulfoxide group, zero accumulate in *C. elegans* to concentrations greater than half the external concentration. Despite these similarities, there are documented differences in the pharmacokinetics of established anthelmintics between *C. elegans* and parasitic worms. For example, amidantel and derquantel are potent anthelmintics in animal models of nematode infection, but have minimum effective concentrations in *C. elegans* at or above 350 and 100 µM, respectively [41, 42]. Nevertheless, as most established anthelmintics are effective against *C. elegans*, the "bioavailability spaces" of parasitic worms and *C. elegans* certainly overlap, even if they are not identical.

We have made our SAM freely available to the scientific community [37] and we hope that it will serve as a useful tool for *C. elegans* chemical biologists, as well as researchers interested in using C. elegans for the discovery of novel anthelmintic drugs.

Modifying C. elegans

Unlike parasitic nematodes, C. elegans is free-living for its entire life cycle and has adapted to survive the dynamic stresses of a soil environment. As a consequence, C. elegans has evolved extensive physical and enzymatic defenses to resist the uptake and accumulation of xenobiotics in its tissues. The physical barriers comprise an intestine through which solutes are rapidly pumped [52] and a four-layered collagenous cuticle that lines its exterior, as well as its oral and rectal cavities [53]. In addition, the C. elegans genome encodes a number of putative xenobiotic detoxification genes including 86 cytochrome P450 (CYP) and 72 UDP-glucuronosyltransferase (UGT) enzymes [38], as well as 15 P-glycoprotein (PGP) and nine multidrug resistance protein (MRP) pumps, many of which are implicated in xenobiotic efflux [54]. The expression of detoxifying genes can be induced by xenobiotics in C. elegans [55, 56] and this induction is likely mediated by one or more of the 284 C. elegans nuclear hormone receptor (*nhr*) genes [38]. Indeed, it has been shown that C. elegans glucosylates the broad-spectrum anthelmintic albendazole, and that albendazole can induce the expression of both CYP and UGT detoxification enzymes [55]. Furthermore, increased expression of PGP and MRP proteins in C. elegans is associated with resistance to the anthelmintic ivermectin [57].

Mutant worms that are defective in xenobiotic defense have the potential to exhibit multidrug sensitivity, and mutants of this class would be invaluable for anthelmintic screens and drug screens in general. For example, C. elegans *pgp-3* mutants are hypersensitive to the growth defects induced by colchicine and chloroquine – two structurally distinct molecules with differing modes of action [58]. The C. elegans PGP-3 protein is expressed in the apical membranes of the intestinal cells and the excretory cell, consistent with a role in xenobiotic efflux. A C. elegans *nhr-8* deletion mutant is also sensitive to colchicine and chloroquine [59]. The *nhr-8* promoter drives expression in the intestine, consistent with a role in xenobiotic defense in this tissue. Both the *pgp-3* and *nhr-8* mutants develop normally and are morphologically indistinguishable from wild-type worms.

Mutations in a number of genes required for C. elegans cuticle integrity also result in drug hypersensitivity [60–62]. Partial loss-of-function mutants of one of these genes, *bus-8*, are hypersensitive to nicotine, 1-phenoxypropan-2-ol, and the anthelmintic ivermectin [62]. These molecules are structurally disparate and have distinct modes of action. *bus-8* mutants also show increased uptake of Hoechst 33258 dye, suggesting that these mutants are generally more permeable to exogenous molecules. Finally, a C. elegans mutant called *dal-1*, which was identified from a forward genetic screen for mutant worms with abnormal intestinal morphologies, exhibits multidrug sensitivity (Paulson and Waddle, personal communication). Despite having altered gut morphology, characterized by membrane invaginations that span the length of the intestine, *dal-1* worms develop normally and are grossly indistinguishable from wild-type worms. *dal-1* mutants are hypersensitive to the effects of colchicine and chloroquine, the neurotransmitters serotonin and octopamine, as well as the L-type calcium channel antagonists nemadipine A, felodipine, and verapamil. Presumably the altered intestinal morphology of *dal-1* mutants improves the absorption of solutes dissolved in the intestinal lumen; however, the mechanism of *dal-1* drug hypersensitivity has not been determined.

The use of multidrug-sensitive mutants in high-throughput chemical screens will likely uncover novel bioactives that would otherwise elicit no phenotype in wild-type worms. However, the utility of the above-mentioned mutants in large-scale screening ventures has, to our knowledge, not been demonstrated. Before employing these mutants in screens for novel anthelmintics, it will be necessary to determine if they are generally sensitive to a broad range of pharmacologically active molecules, including established anthelmintics, and to assess the well-to-well variability in their growth and behavior. Nonetheless, multidrug-sensitive mutants have great potential to improve the hit rates of *C. elegans* chemical screens.

Conclusions

Over the past four decades, the study of *C. elegans* has made innumerable and invaluable contributions to our understanding of animal development. Consequently, it is one of the best understood animals and, correspondingly, is one of the best animal model systems with which to characterize the mechanism by which small bioactive molecules exert their effects. Recent technological advances now allow us to extend the utility of *C. elegans* beyond target identification to high-throughput screens for novel anthelmintics. Given the pressing need for novel structural classes of nematicides, we anticipate that *C. elegans* will play an ever-increasing role in anthelmintic discovery in the future.

Acknowledgments

This work was supported by a Canadian Institutes of Health Research operating grants to P.J.R. (68813) and a Natural Sciences and Engineering Research Council of Canada Graduate Scholarship doctoral award to A.R.B. P.J.R. is a Canadian Research Chair in Molecular Neurobiology.

References

1 Keiser, J. and Utzinger, J. (2010) The drugs we have and the drugs we need against major helminth infections. *Adv. Parasitol.*, **73**, 197–230.

2 Besier, B. (2007) New anthelmintics for livestock: the time is right. *Trends Parasitol.*, **23**, 21–24.

3 Fuller, V.L., Lilley, C.J., and Urwin, P.E. (2008) Nematode resistance. *New Phytol.*, **180**, 27–44.

4 Sutherland, I.A. and Leathwick, D.M. (2011) Anthelmintic resistance in nematode parasites of cattle: a global issue? *Trends Parasitol.*, **27**, 176–181.

5 Kaminsky, R., Ducray, P., Jung, M., Clover, R., Rufener, L., Bouvier, J. et al. (2008) A new class of anthelmintics effective against drug-resistant nematodes. *Nature*, **452**, 176–180.

6 Kaminsky, R., Mosimann, D., Sager, H., Stein, P., and Hosking, B. (2009) Determination of the effective dose rate for monepantel (AAD 1566) against adult gastro-intestinal nematodes in sheep. *Int. J. Parasitol.*, **39**, 443–446.

7 Little, P.R., Hodges, A., Watson, T.G., Seed, J.A., and Maeder, S.J. (2010) Field efficacy and safety of an oral formulation of the novel combination anthelmintic, derquantel–abamectin, in sheep in New Zealand. *NZ Vet. J.*, **58**, 121–129.

8 Hu, Y., Xiao, S.H., and Aroian, R.V. (2009) The new anthelmintic tribendimidine is an L-type (levamisole and pyrantel) nicotinic acetylcholine receptor agonist. *PLoS Negl. Trop. Dis.*, **3**, e499.

9 Brenner, S. (1974) The genetics of *Caenorhabditis elegans*. *Genetics*, **77**, 71–94.

10 Kwok, T.C., Ricker, N., Fraser, R., Chan, A.W., Burns, A., Stanley, E.F. et al. (2006) A small-molecule screen in *C. elegans* yields a new calcium channel antagonist. *Nature*, **441**, 91–95.

11 Lemieux, G.A., Liu, J., Mayer, N., Bainton, R.J., Ashrafi, K., and Werb, Z. (2011) A whole-organism screen identifies new regulators of fat storage. *Nat. Chem. Biol.*, **7**, 206–213.

12 Petrascheck, M., Ye, X., and Buck, L.B. (2007) An antidepressant that extends lifespan in adult *Caenorhabditis elegans*. *Nature*, **450**, 553–556.

13 Samara, C., Rohde, C.B., Gilleland, C.L., Norton, S., Haggarty, S.J., and Yanik, M.F. (2010) Large-scale *in vivo* femtosecond laser neurosurgery screen reveals small-molecule enhancer of regeneration. *Proc. Natl. Acad. Sci. USA*, **107**, 18342–18347.

14 Jones, A.K., Buckingham, S.D., and Sattelle, D.B. (2005) Chemistry-to-gene screens in *Caenorhabditis elegans*. *Nat. Rev. Drug Discov.*, **4**, 321–330.

15 Kokel, D., Li, Y., Qin, J., and Xue, D. (2006) The nongenotoxic carcinogens naphthalene and *para*-dichlorobenzene suppress apoptosis in *Caenorhabditis elegans*. *Nat. Chem. Biol.*, **2**, 338–345.

16 Burns, A.R., Kwok, T.C., Howard, A., Houston, E., Johanson, K., Chan, A. et al. (2006) High-throughput screening of small molecules for bioactivity and target identification in *Caenorhabditis elegans*. *Nat. Protoc.*, **1**, 1906–1914.

17 Holden-Dye, L. and Walker, R.J. (2007) Anthelmintic drugs, in *WormBook* (ed. The *C. elegans* Research Community), doi: 10.1895/wormbook.1.143.1.

18 Rufener, L., Baur, R., Kaminsky, R., Maser, P., and Sigel, E. (2010) Monepantel allosterically activates DEG-3/DES-2 channels of the gastrointestinal nematode *Haemonchus contortus*. *Mol. Pharmacol.*, **78**, 895–902.

19 Mitreva, M., Blaxter, M.L., Bird, D.M., and McCarter, J.P. (2005) Comparative genomics of nematodes. *Trends Genet.*, **21**, 573–581.

20 Hetherington, S., Gally, C., Fritz, J.A., Polanowska, J., Reboul, J., Schwab, Y. et al. (2011) PAT-12, a potential anti-nematode target, is a new spectraplakin partner essential for *Caenorhabditis elegans* hemidesmosome integrity and embryonic morphogenesis. *Dev. Biol.*, **350**, 267–278.

21 McVeigh, P., Leech, S., Mair, G.R., Marks, N.J., Geary, T.G., and Maule, A.G. (2005) Analysis of FMRFamide-like peptide (FLP) diversity in phylum Nematoda. *Int. J. Parasitol.*, **35**, 1043–1060.

22 Ogawa, A., Streit, A., Antebi, A., and Sommer, R.J. (2009) A conserved endocrine mechanism controls the formation of dauer and infective larvae in nematodes. *Curr. Biol.*, **19**, 67–71.

23 Stepek, G., McCormack, G., and Page, A.P. (2010) Collagen processing and cuticle formation is catalysed by the astacin metalloprotease DPY-31 in free-living and parasitic nematodes. *Int. J. Parasitol.*, **40**, 533–542.

24 Wang, Z., Zhou, X.E., Motola, D.L., Gao, X., Suino-Powell, K., Conneely, A. et al. (2009) Identification of the nuclear receptor DAF-12 as a therapeutic target in parasitic nematodes. *Proc. Natl. Acad. Sci. USA*, **106**, 9138–9143.

25 Simpkin, K.G. and Coles, G.C. (1981) The use of *Caenorhabditis elegans* for anthelmintic screening. *J. Chem. Technol. Biotechnol.*, **31**, 66–69.

26 Geary, T.G., Thompson, D.P., and Klein, R.D. (1999) Mechanism-based screening: discovery of the next generation of anthelmintics depends upon more basic research. *Int. J. Parasitol.*, **29**, 105–112, discussion 113–114.

27 Giacomotto, J. and Segalat, L. (2010) High-throughput screening and small animal models, where are we? *Br. J. Pharmacol.*, **160**, 204–216.

28 Segalat, L. (2007) Invertebrate animal models of diseases as screening tools in drug discovery. *ACS Chem. Biol.*, **2**, 231–236.

29 Gosai, S.J., Kwak, J.H., Luke, C.J., Long, O.S., King, D.E., Kovatch, K.J. et al. (2010) Automated high-content live animal drug screening using *C. elegans* expressing the aggregation prone serpin alpha1-antitrypsin Z. *PLoS One*, **5**, e15460.

30 O'Rourke, E.J., Conery, A.L., and Moy, T.I. (2009) Whole-animal high-throughput screens: the *C. elegans* model. *Methods Mol. Biol.*, **486**, 57–75.

31 Byrne, A.B., Weirauch, M.T., Wong, V., Koeva, M., Dixon, S.J., Stuart, J.M. et al. (2007) A global analysis of genetic interactions in *Caenorhabditis elegans*. *J. Biol.*, **6**, 8.

32 Pulak, R. (2006) Techniques for analysis, sorting, and dispensing of *C. elegans* on the COPAS flow-sorting system. *Methods Mol. Biol.*, **351**, 275–286.

33 Okoli, I., Coleman, J.J., Tampakakis, E., An, W.F., Holson, E., Wagner, F. et al. (2009) Identification of antifungal compounds active against Candida albicans using an improved high-throughput *Caenorhabditis elegans* assay. *PLoS One*, **4**, e7025.

34 Buckingham, S.D. and Sattelle, D.B. (2008) Strategies for automated analysis of *C. elegans* locomotion. *Invert. Neurosci.*, **8**, 121–131.

35 Buckingham, S.D. and Sattelle, D.B. (2009) Fast, automated measurement of nematode swimming (thrashing) without morphometry. *BMC Neurosci.*, **10**, 84.

36 Motola, D.L., Cummins, C.L., Rottiers, V., Sharma, K.K., Li, T., Li, Y. et al. (2006) Identification of ligands for DAF-12 that govern dauer formation and reproduction in *C. elegans*. *Cell*, **124**, 1209–1223.

37 Burns, A.R., Wallace, I.M., Wildenhain, J., Tyers, M., Giaever, G., Bader, G.D. et al. (2010) A predictive model for drug bioaccumulation and bioactivity in *Caenorhabditis elegans*. *Nat. Chem. Biol.*, **6**, 549–557.

38 Lindblom, T.H. and Dodd, A.K. (2006) Xenobiotic detoxification in the nematode *Caenorhabditis elegans*. *J. Exp. Zool. A*, **305**, 720–730.

39 Franks, C.J., Pemberton, D., Vinogradova, I., Cook, A., Walker, R.J., and Holden-Dye, L. (2002) Ionic basis of the resting membrane potential and action potential in the pharyngeal muscle of *Caenorhabditis elegans*. *J. Neurophysiol.*, **87**, 954–961.

40 Jospin, M., Jacquemond, V., Mariol, M.C., Segalat, L., and Allard, B. (2002) The L-type voltage-dependent Ca^{2+} channel EGL-19 controls body wall muscle function in *Caenorhabditis elegans*. *J. Cell Biol.*, **159**, 337–348.

41 Ruiz-Lancheros, E., Viau, C., Walter, T.N., Francis, A., and Geary, T.G. (2011) Activity of novel nicotinic anthelmintics in cut preparations of *Caenorhabditis elegans*. *Int. J. Parasitol.*, **41**, 455–461.

42 Tomlinson, G., Albuquerque, C.A., and Woods, R.A. (1985) The effects of amidantel (BAY d 8815) and its deacylated derivative (BAY d 9216) on *Caenorhabditis elegans*. *Eur. J. Pharmacol.*, **113**, 255–262.

43 Folz, S.D., Pax, R.A., Thomas, E.M., Bennett, J.L., Lee, B.L., and Conder, G.A. (1987) Detecting *in vitro* anthelmintic effects with a micromotility meter. *Vet. Parasitol.*, **24**, 241–250.

44 Min, J., Kyung Kim, Y., Cipriani, P.G., Kang, M., Khersonsky, S.M., Walsh, D.P. et al. (2007) Forward chemical genetic approach identifies new role for GAPDH in insulin signaling. *Nat. Chem. Biol.*, **3**, 55–59.

45 Rogalski, T.M., Golomb, M., and Riddle, D.L. (1990) Mutant *Caenorhabditis*

elegans RNA polymerase II with a 20,000-fold reduced sensitivity to alpha-amanitin. *Genetics*, **126**, 889–898.

46 Semple, J.I., Garcia-Verdugo, R., and Lehner, B. (2010) Rapid selection of transgenic *C. elegans* using antibiotic resistance. *Nat. Methods*, **7**, 725–727.

47 Lehar, J., Stockwell, B.R., Giaever, G., and Nislow, C. (2008) Combination chemical genetics. *Nat. Chem. Biol.*, **4**, 674–681.

48 Kola, I. and Landis, J. (2004) Can the pharmaceutical industry reduce attrition rates? *Nat. Rev. Drug Discov.*, **3**, 711–715.

49 Lipinski, C.A., Lombardo, F., Dominy, B.W., and Feeney, P.J. (1997) Experimental and computational approaches to estimate solubility and permeability in drug discovery and development settings. *Adv. Drug. Deliv. Rev.*, **23**, 3–25.

50 Irwin, J.J. and Shoichet, B.K. (2005) ZINC – a free database of commercially available compounds for virtual screening. *J. Chem. Inf. Model.*, **45**, 177–182.

51 Alvarez, L.I., Mottier, M.L., and Lanusse, C.E. (2007) Drug transfer into target helminth parasites. *Trends Parasitol.*, **23**, 97–104.

52 Avery, L. and Shtonda, B.B. (2003) Food transport in the *C. elegans* pharynx. *J. Exp. Biol.*, **206**, 2441–2457.

53 Cox, G.N., Kusch, M., and Edgar, R.S. (1981) Cuticle of *Caenorhabditis elegans*: its isolation and partial characterization. *J. Cell Biol.*, **90**, 7–17.

54 Sheps, J.A., Ralph, S., Zhao, Z., Baillie, D.L., and Ling, V. (2004) The ABC transporter gene family of *Caenorhabditis elegans* has implications for the evolutionary dynamics of multidrug resistance in eukaryotes. *Genome Biol.*, **5**, R15.

55 Laing, S.T., Ivens, A., Laing, R., Ravikumar, S., Butler, V., Woods, D.J. et al. (2010) Characterization of the xenobiotic response of *Caenorhabditis elegans* to the anthelmintic drug albendazole and the identification of novel drug glucoside metabolites. *Biochem. J.*, **432**, 505–514.

56 Menzel, R., Rodel, M., Kulas, J., and Steinberg, C.E. (2005) CYP35: xenobiotically induced gene expression in the nematode *Caenorhabditis elegans*. *Arch. Biochem. Biophys.*, **438**, 93–102.

57 James, C.E. and Davey, M.W. (2009) Increased expression of ABC transport proteins is associated with ivermectin resistance in the model nematode *Caenorhabditis elegans*. *Int. J. Parasitol.*, **39**, 213–220.

58 Broeks, A., Janssen, H.W., Calafat, J., and Plasterk, R.H. (1995) A P-glycoprotein protects *Caenorhabditis elegans* against natural toxins. *EMBO J.*, **14**, 1858–1866.

59 Lindblom, T.H., Pierce, G.J., and Sluder, A.E. (2001) A *C. elegans* orphan nuclear receptor contributes to xenobiotic resistance. *Curr. Biol.*, **11**, 864–868.

60 Bounoutas, A., O'Hagan, R., and Chalfie, M. (2009) The multipurpose 15-protofilament microtubules in *C. elegans* have specific roles in mechanosensation. *Curr. Biol.*, **19**, 1362–1367.

61 Gravato-Nobre, M.J., Nicholas, H.R., Nijland, R., O'Rourke, D., Whittington, D.E., Yook, K.J. et al. (2005) Multiple genes affect sensitivity of *Caenorhabditis elegans* to the bacterial pathogen *Microbacterium nematophilum*. *Genetics*, **171**, 1033–1045.

62 Partridge, F.A., Tearle, A.W., Gravato-Nobre, M.J., Schafer, W.R., and Hodgkin, J. (2008) The *C. elegans* glycosyltransferase BUS-8 has two distinct and essential roles in epidermal morphogenesis. *Dev. Biol.*, **317**, 549–559.

Part Three
Drugs

13
Anthelmintic Drugs: Tools and Shortcuts for the Long Road from Discovery to Product

Eugenio L. de Hostos[*] and Tue Nguyen

Abstract

The development of new drugs is a complex and expensive process, but a convergence of scientific, business, and social trends is generating new opportunities to fill in gaps in the treatment of neglected tropical diseases (NTDs) that still affect billions of lives. Globalization has led to a raised awareness of the medical needs of the poor in the developing world, and at the same time has brought to bear new philanthropic, industrial, and governmental resources on those needs. Although the resources available for NTD drug development pale in comparison to those available for profitable indications, drug development programs can be cobbled together by product development partnerships (PDPs) that harness material and technical support from a variety of sources. In particular, PDPs can help bridge the "valley of death" between the increasingly easier and automated discovery associated with new drug leads and clinical trials. With the fact that NTDs are becoming less neglected, and that the drug development process is becoming more routine, affordable, and accessible, we are likely to see a more robust pipeline of products in this field in the years ahead. Veterinary anthelmintics offer a good opportunity to fill in gaps in the treatment of human helminth infections by shortcutting the standard drug development process. The regulatory standards for veterinary drugs in the United States and in Europe are compatible with those for human drugs, making cross-over development a relatively straightforward and cost-effective alternative to starting a human drug development program from scratch. In addition to a potentially complete preclinical dossier, a veterinary anthelmintic candidate is also likely to have a robust chemical process for its production on a large scale and a valuable record of its use in animals. Currently, a number veterinary anthelmintics are attractive candidates for cross-over development for the treatment for human soil-transmitted helminth infections.

[*] Corresponding Author

Parasitic Helminths: Targets, Screens, Drugs and Vaccines, First Edition. Edited by Conor R. Caffrey
© 2012 Wiley-VCH Verlag GmbH & Co. KGaA. Published 2012 by Wiley-VCH Verlag GmbH & Co. KGaA.

Introduction

The drug development process has evolved over the years to guarantee that new drugs are relatively safe and efficacious. It involves extensive testing, and it is therefore long and costly. This paradigm represents a huge challenge for the development of drugs against neglected tropical diseases (NTDs), which have received little attention by the pharmaceutical industry because of their small or nonprofitable markets [1, 2]. NTDs are at the wrong end of the often-quoted statistic that globally 90% of the research and development (R&D) funds are spent on diseases that afflict only 10% of the world's population (www.globalforumhealth.org/About/10-90-gap). Fortunately, many investigators and organizations such as nonprofit product development partnerships (PDPs) are busy trying to compensate for this imbalance, with the support of government agencies, philanthropic foundations, and pharmaceutical companies.

Here, we provide investigators in the helminth field with an overview of the drug development process, and share our insight into the particular challenges and opportunities for the development of new drugs to treat NTDs. We will base much of our discussion on our own efforts to develop new treatments for soil-transmitted helminth (STH) infections and highlight the "cross-over" potential of veterinary anthelmintics.

STHs colonize the intestines of billions and have been called the "great burden of mankind" [3]. The insidious effects on general health, the physical and mental development of children, and the overall socioeconomic development of communities [4] by these "leeches in your intestine" [5] have been recognized at least since the establishment in 1909 of the Rockefeller Sanitary Commission for the Eradication of Hookworm Disease to help the rural southern United States escape poverty and underdevelopment [6, 7]. As stated by the World Health Organization (WHO), "deworming school-aged children is probably the most economically efficient public health activity that can be implemented in any low-income country where soil-transmitted helminths are endemic" (http://www.who.int/intestinal_worms/strategy/en/).

Yet, in terms of R&D, helminth infections in humans are a particularly neglected, even in comparison to diseases such as malaria or tuberculosis [8]. This is because they are, for the most part, debilitating rather than lethal diseases and because they tend to diminish on their own with the improved sanitation that comes with economic development [8, 9]. The most important tools of the Rockefeller Sanitary Commission were latrines and shoes, not drugs. Human helminth infections are neglected, but fortunately agricultural and small companion animals represent a profitable market for anthelmintics, and this drives the development of a small stream of new drugs. The availability of veterinary anthelmintics that can be repurposed for human use not only has the potential to partially compensate for the lack of R&D into human anthelmintics, but also to provide a shortcut in the long and costly development process [10, 11].

The road between veterinary and human anthelmintics has been traveled before, but not in a long time. There are currently only four drugs listed on the WHO Model List of Essential Medicines (http://www.who.int/medicines/publications/essentialmedicines/en) for the treatment of STH infections (albendazole, mebendazole, pyrantel pamoate, and levamisole), and only albendazole and mebendazole are widely used in mass drug administration (MDA) campaigns that treat a whole school or village at a time. All four entered the human pharmacopeia from veterinary R&D over 30 years ago [4]. Fortunately, the path that can allow veterinary medicines to cross-over into human use is now shorter than ever.

Target Product Profile: First Know Where You Want to Go

The starting point for most drug development projects is the target product profile (TPP). The TPP is an essential tool of designers, be they drug developers or the designers of consumer gadgets. As the name suggests, the TPP is a description of the desired product and serves as a detailed articulation of what the project is aiming to achieve. Ideally, this profile has been developed in consultation with "stakeholders" who, in the case of a new NTD drug, should include clinicians, public health professionals, nongovernmental organizations, regulatory consultants, and patients. The consultation process should identify what are the shortcomings of existing treatments (e.g., efficacy, safety, dosing regimen) and what characteristics the desired product should have in order to fill in those gaps. The TPP becomes the document that guides development and by which progress is measured.

The TPPs for new NTD medicines are highly constrained by the special requirements for drugs of this kind (low cost, in particular), but they are also constrained by the limited resources available for these projects in general. Although the pharmaceutical industry may have the resources necessary for multiple "shots on goal" and be able to develop, for example, several new anticholesterol drugs in a few years, the collective global resources available for new anthelmintics (including the support of organizations like the Bill & Melinda Gates Foundation, Wellcome Trust, WHO, as well as major pharmaceuticals and governments) may only be sufficient to develop a single new drug in a decade or more. What this means is that the TPP for such a new drug has to be spot-on in correcting the shortcomings of existing drugs. In the NTD space there is no room for "me too" drugs; new drugs have to have the potential to provide a very significant improvement over existing treatments.

The TPP consists of a list of parameters and their minimal criteria. The parameters include efficacy spectrum, safety, formulation, and dosing, as well as cost. In the case of a drug to treat STH infections, for example, the TPP needs to be very specific about defining efficacy. For example, not all STH species can be expected to respond equally to a drug and the TPP should specify the acceptable efficacy parameter for each. A new STH drug would ideally be effective against all four major species of intestinal nematodes [10–12], but a new drug could be acceptable, for example, if it was highly efficacious against roundworms (*Ascaris*) and hookworms (*Necator* and *Ancylostoma*), but not necessarily superior to existing drugs that treat whipworms (*Trichuris*). In the case of parasites with complex life cycles, there may need to be an additional level of detail. For example, the TPP for a new drug to treat lymphatic filariasis may require efficacy against macrofilaria (adult parasites), which is a shortcoming of existing treatments [13].

The formulation and dosing regimen expected for the new drug product is of particular importance for deployment in the developing world. For example, a drug that requires intramuscular injection may be acceptable in a first-world situation, but would be impractical for use in a rural clinic where access to and disposal of hypodermic needles presents challenges and dangers of its own. For the treatment of STH infections, drugs have to be compatible with MDA campaigns, which is the preferred access model. MDA campaigns are employed because the cost of drug delivery in general exceeds the cost of the drugs and because they reduce the reinfection rate by suppressing the presence of infectious larvae in the environment. To fit this access model, a treatment that requires only a single tablet is ideal [10], whereas drugs that require multiple doses or doses that need to be adjusted according to size (such as pyrantel), while useful, are not optimal for a new generation drug.

Another parameter of particular relevance to NTD drugs is the cost of the drug product [14]. For public health organizations working in developing countries, choosing between a new drug and an alternative intervention (e.g., a new STH drug versus shoes and latrines) may be a zero-sum game. Thus, the parameters for the cost of a new drug may be very narrow. Current single-dose treatments for STH infections cost less than US$0.03 (http://www.who.int/intestinal_worms/strategy/en), therefore the TPP of a new STH drug might specify an ideal cost no higher than this, while a highly efficacious drug costing US$0.10 might be acceptable. Higher prices may put the drug out of reach of those who need it unless the drug is donated (as is regularly the case for albendazole and mebendazole) or otherwise subsidized.

In general, albendazole sets a high bar for the next-generation of STH drug: it is very cheap and reasonably effective against the major STH species, with the exception of whipworm [10]. As a drug on the WHO's List of Essential Medicines, it is currently administered to school-age children in MDA campaigns in endemic regions around the world and has a good safety record. However, there is room for improvement [10]. To start with, albendazole and other benzimidazole anthelmintics are microtubule poisons that have the potential to disrupt cell division in the mammalian hosts. While this may seem risky, millions of doses of these compounds have been administered to children and adults, and are generally regarded as safe [15]. That said, a new drug with a spotless toxicological profile would be welcome, as it would allow the inclusion of women in their first trimester of pregnancy, which is counterindicated for benzimidazoles [10]. This is a significant gap in current treatments that leaves an important population at risk. The first trimester is a critical period in fetal development and being able to treat women without fear of affecting fetal development would be a welcome improvement over the current therapy.

Arguably the major driving force behind the development of new veterinary anthelmintics has been the emergence of resistance. Resistance to anthelmintics in veterinary use is well-documented and widespread [16, 17]. The evidence for drug resistance in human STH infections is more fragmentary, as efficacy data is rarely collected even in endemic areas where the drugs are in common use. However, it is clear that levamisole and pyrantel are inferior to the benzimidazole stalwarts [12], and even the efficacy of mebendazole has waned in areas where it has been used extensively for years [18–20].

Although drug resistance does not seem to be an immediate problem in the treatment of STH infections, there is general agreement in the public health community that there should be more drugs in the development pipeline to be prepared for the time when resistance does become a major issue [4, 10, 21, 22]. It is worth pointing out that in the case of lymphatic filariasis the issue is not the emergence of resistance, but the fact there has never been a single drug or drug combination that can deal decisively with both macro- and microfilaria [13]. New chemistries, targets, and mechanisms of action will be required to overcome the problem of resistance or poor efficacy [10, 22, 23]. For example, the veterinary anthelmintics, monepantel [24], which belongs to a new chemical class and has a unique nicotinic receptor target distinct from that targeted by pyrantel and levamisole, and emodepside [25], which involves a new target class and mechanism of action, are of great interest, and represent good candidates for cross-over development to treat human STH infections [10]. Similarly, flubendazole, an alternative benzimidazole in veterinary use, is being investigated as a macrofilaricide [26].

Drug Development Stages

The drug development process can be divided into three broad and sequential stages: discovery, preclinical development, and clinical development. Discovery and the preclinical development stages can overlap in an intermediate phase when animal efficacy and toxicity studies inform chemical lead selection and optimization in an iterative process. These days, discovery is usually viewed as the high-attrition and relatively low-cost phase, whereas for drug candidates in clinical development, attrition is proportionately low but the stakes and cost are high [27]. Clinical development culminates in marketing approval by a regulatory agency such as the US Food and Drug Administration (FDA) or the European Medicines Agency (EMA). These three phases are followed by a range of postapproval activities aimed at monitoring safety (Phase IV, pharmacovigilance), marketing, and further development to expand and extend the utility of the drug in new formulations, dosing regimes, or combinations. For NTD drugs, approval may be followed by an advocacy phase that promotes the adoption of the drug and facilitates its access to those in need.

Table 13.1 shows a rough outline of the drug development phases, approximate durations, and costs. The duration and costs of the clinical phases are derived from a project planning exercise for the development of a new STH drug.

Discovery

The process leading to the discovery of a "hit" molecule with promising antiparasitic activity has become much faster and cheaper with the advent of automation and high-throughput screening (HTS) technologies. HTS campaigns are no longer the realm of biotech and pharmaceutical companies. Chemical biology is booming – many

Table 13.1 Stages of drug development.

Phase	Duration (years)	Cost (US$ millions)
Discovery	2–3	2–5
Preclinical development		
Exploratory (non-GLP)	0.5–1	1
IND-enabling (GLP)	0.75	0.75
CMC	preclinical through clinical	1
Clinical development		
Phase I (focus on safety)	0.5–1	1
Reproductive toxicology, metabolism, and distribution studies in animals and humans	1	1.5
Phase II (identify doses and efficacy end-points; adults and children)	0.75–1 each for adult and pediatric trials	1 each for adult and pediatric trials
Phase III (confirm efficacy and safety)	1.5–3	4–7
Totals	8–12	13–20

research universities have central screening facilities and even individual investigators may have their own screening operations. Compound libraries are now routinely screened against protozoan [28, 29] and helminth [30] parasites, and image-based methods have been developed for screening against whole helminths (e.g., [31]; see also Chapter 10).

The free-living nematode *Caenorhabditis elegans* has become a productive workhorse for compound screening and mechanism of action studies (see also Chapters 1, 2 and 12). However, despite the proliferation of reports of new biochemical and biological screens aimed at NTD pathogens maintained by academia, the "valley of death" remains a serious and demanding challenge between hit identification and eventual candidates that enter clinical trials (http://www.xconomy.com/sanfrancisco/2010/08/19/nonprofits-and-the-valley-of-death-in-drug-discovery). Major funding and the support of contracted services in medicinal chemistry and pharmacology are usually required to make it through the "valley." Even if these are obtained, animal models for NTDs can be rate-limiting. These "boutique" animal models (as opposed to commercially available models for diseases such as cancer, inflammation, and heart disease) may be complicated, intrinsically slow, and only available in academic laboratories that often do not have the capacity to process large numbers of compounds. Animal models of helminth infection, especially those with complex life cycles and multiple hosts, can be particularly challenging (see also Chapter 11 for a relevant discussion).

Preclinical Studies

Once efficacy has been established, preclinical studies focus on selected compounds to establish their pharmacokinetic/pharmacodynamic properties, effective dose range, and safety profile. The major transition point in preclinical development is that between the exploratory and relatively inexpensive studies and those conducted under the much more costly Good Laboratory Practice (GLP) that is required for filing an FDA Investigational New Drug (IND) application or the EMA Investigational Medicinal Product Dossier. Whereas non-GLP toxicology studies may be conducted on a number of compounds, the field is usually narrowed down to a single lead compound and a backup compound for the GLP phase. The IND-enabling studies are specified by regulatory standards and therefore most of the GLP studies are the same for all drug candidates. However, the toxicology studies may be customized based on factors such as the expected dosing regimen (i.e., single, multiple, or chronic). After the drug candidate has entered clinical trials there is usually a second set of prescribed and costly animal studies focused on reproductive toxicology, as well as drug metabolism and distribution studies with radiolabeled compound.

The repurposing of an approved veterinary drug eliminates the need for discovery and can greatly facilitate the preclinical development of the drug for human use. For the approval of an FDA New Animal Drug Application (NADA), veterinary products must be shown to be safe and effective in the target animal(s), and to meet stringent human safety standards if the animals treated will be used in a human food product. The veterinary dossier may also include animal reproductive toxicology data that for human drugs is normally not collected until after clinical trials have been initiated. The good news for the NTD community is that these studies now need to be conducted under GLP guidelines and may support an IND application for human use. However, in order to meet IND regulations it is possible that additional "bridging" studies may be required to complement and fill gaps in a NADA dossier. It is important to note that the veterinary dossier is the proprietary information of the company that developed the veterinary drug. Thus any agreement negotiated between the owner and a third party seeking to develop the drug for human use (such as a PDP) must include not just freedom to operate, but access to this information as well.

Chemistry, Manufacturing, and Controls

Running in parallel to the biology and pharmacology, the chemistry, manufacturing, and controls (CMC) aspect of the project aims to provide an adequate supply of active pharmaceutical ingredient (API) at the required purity and in the correct formulation. In the course of the project, the process for making API will be scaled-up from perhaps a 100-mg scale (sufficient for *in vitro* or *in vivo* efficacy studies) to the more than 100-g scale required for GLP toxicology. A further 100 times scale-up (to 10 kg) may be required for clinical trials followed by an additional 100–1000 times scale-up (from 1000 to 10 000 kg) for commercialization. A critical and expensive transition in the CMC process is manufacturing the API under Good Manufacturing Practice (GMP) standards. GMP ensures that only product of the highest purity is used in clinical trials, and requires rigorous control, tracking, and documentation of the ingredients, processes and equipment used during manufacture. Only a subset of chemical contract research organizations (CROs) and manufacturers have GMP manufacturing capability.

In the case of a veterinary product, it is likely that an industrial-scale manufacturing process has already been developed and that GMP API is available. Thus, in addition to being nearly IND-ready, a commercial veterinary product can bring a well-established manufacturing process into the bargain as well as enough GMP material for preclinical and clinical studies. Together these represent substantial savings in the development time and costs. As with the preclinical dossier, a licensing agreement for clinical development should ideally include access to the CMC dossier and GMP API if available. It is important to note that, ironically, the manufacturing process for a veterinary drug (especially one used for companion animals) may need further optimization to bring the cost down to meet the TPP for human use. The formulation for human use may also require additional work and investment, both in the formulation itself and how it affects the pharmacokinetics/pharmacodynamics and toxicology. For example, an anthelmintic formulated for drenching (e.g., monepantel) or transdermal application (emodepside) would have to be reformulated for human use. In the case of some veterinary drugs, developing the human formulation is the key and greatest challenge of the repurposing process [26].

Clinical Trials

Repurposing a veterinary anthelmintic can eliminate the need for much of the preclinical phase and chemical process development at a savings of years and millions of dollars. Although this can allow resources to be focused on clinical trials, it does not allow for cutting corners. One consolation is that, for example, an anthelmintic that has been in widespread veterinary use is likely to have a well-documented safety, toxicology, and efficacy record that can be both reassuring to the clinician as well as provide critical dosing information. Clinical study design and execution is a vast field, but three issues are of particular relevance to anthelmintic drug development.

A key consideration for clinical efficacy studies is the end-point. The term "clinical end-point" originally defined the point at which a clinical study was designed to stop, but it now refers to, as somewhat of a misnomer, measures of success (i.e., the levels of specific parameters that must be achieved in order to allow a trial to continue or to consider the trial successful). Selection of clinical efficacy end-points can be complex and should reflect the desired TPP. In the case of clinical trials dealing with STH infections, two end-points have been used traditionally – the cure rate (the elimination of parasites as determined by the absence of helminth eggs in the feces) and the egg reduction rate (a before and after comparison of the number of eggs per gram of feces). With the shift in thinking in the public health community away from the goal of curing and reducing the number of people with STH infections to the more achievable goal of reducing the intensity of infection or worm load (http://www.who.int/intestinal_worms/strategy/en), an egg reduction rate end-point is now favored. It is important to point out, however, that an end-point based on egg reduction rate, although quickly measured and adequate for veterinary purposes, may not be an adequate surrogate for the impact on a community. The success of any deworming campaign is now more frequently measured in terms of reducing disability-adjusted life years, which may require multiple MDA interventions over many years. This metric is more difficult to establish, but it more accurately reflects the current mission of the WHO, as well as the mission of the Rockefeller Sanitary Commission more than a century ago.

The very low prevalence of NTDs such as helminth infections in developed regions makes clinical testing in resource-poor and sometimes remote locations necessary. This is expensive, time-consuming, and logistically challenging [32]. Extensive capacity building may be necessary before trials can be conducted in such locations. For example, to support its hookworm and schistosome vaccine development program, the Sabin Vaccine Institute, in collaboration with the Fundação Oswaldo Cruz (FIOCRUZ), has built and operates its own field laboratory and clinical site capable of conducting Phase I trials in Americaninhas – a remote community in the Brazilian state of Minas Gerais (http://www.sabin.org/vaccine-development/vaccines/hookworm). Similarly, OneWorld Health, with help from Quintiles, the Swiss TPH (Tropical and Public health Institute), and financial support from a Swiss philanthropic organization, has been involved in training and laboratory capacity building in Vietnam and India, specifically to support helminth studies. Fortunately, clinical CROs are expanding operations in developing countries. This is primarily to conduct trials on new treatments for developed world diseases, but they are eager to become involved in NTD trials, both to capture a share of that market and as a way of recruiting and building resources in developing countries that can be used for their more standard trials.

Regulatory Considerations

For a drug that is expected to be used in many developing countries, including in MDA deworming campaigns, approval by the FDA or EMA is a big advantage in obtaining widespread approval for use. Some developing countries lack sufficient clinical trial guidelines or regulatory requirements of their own, and therefore require clinical trials and drug distribution programs to be run according to FDA or EMA regulatory guidelines [33]. However, many developing countries have their own regulations that must be adhered to when designing studies and projecting the development timeline and budget. These are often aimed at providing greater confidence in the safety of the drug in the indigenous population and its efficacy against local strains of a pathogen. For example, the Drug Controller General of India requires foreign drug developers to carry out the initial Phase I studies in another country and then to conduct additional Phase I trials in India before going into Phase II.

For NTD drugs, an important step in enabling their widespread adoption is their incorporation into the WHO's model List of Essential Medicines. The List of Essential Medicines is the WHO's recommended medicine cabinet. In addition, it identifies the medicines that developing countries can request in the form of medical aid. Unfortunately, inclusion in the List of Essential Medicines is not always sufficient to guarantee widespread adoption and this sometimes requires significant advocacy at the local level, engaging both local authorities and healthcare providers.

Getting the Job Done

Regardless of how cleverly or efficiently it is conducted, or what shortcuts are taken, drug development remains an expensive proposition as the funds available for NTD drug development are highly constrained. However, this is a good time for NTD drug development. The multifaceted phenomenon that we call "globalization" has made the world smaller in many ways, helping to mobilize resources and raise the consciousness in developed countries of the health needs of the developing world. In this era, CROs distributed around the world offer the entire range of drug development services and compete aggressively with each other to offer lower costs.

PDPs

In the past decade, nonprofit organizations called PDPs have become engaged in the development of drugs for NTDs [34, 35]. PDPs such as PATH (www.path.org), DNDi (www.dndi.org), and OneWorld Health (www.oneworldhealth.org) have brought the rigor and cohesion characteristic of large pharmaceutical companies to bear on NTD vaccine and drug development. The impact of PDPs is impressive and one study [35] suggests that approximately 75% of NTD drug development is now conducted by organizations of this kind. In recent years, the drug development pipeline of PDPs has brought to clinical trials treatments for a number of NTDs, including, for example, Human African Trypanosomiasis (DNDi), rotavirus (PATH), and cholera (OneWorld Health).

A multimillion dollar grant from a large philanthropic organization such as the Bill & Melinda Gates Foundation or the Wellcome Trust can be a decisive enabler for a PDP, but this does not eliminate their need to harness other resources available for NTD R&D and bring them to bear on specific projects. Some PDPs, like OneWorld Health and DNDi, are "virtual," meaning they have no laboratories of their own, but rely entirely on contract services and collaborations with industry and academia for the laboratory work [36]. PDPs can help academic investigators translate their basic research findings into products, such as by shepherding promising compounds through the "valley of death" discussed earlier. Academic researchers in turn can advise PDPs on the best approaches to achieving a desired therapeutic outcome and the design of clinical trials. Experts from the pharmaceutical industry can provide advice on medicinal chemistry, pharmacology, and the selection of drug candidates.

Government Resources and Incentives

In addition to drawing down funding from philanthropic sources, PDPs can also benefit from a range of government resources and incentives such as those offered in the United States by the National Institutes of Health (NIH) and the FDA. One problem with these resources is that they are spread over a number of agencies and that no single program is likely to support a single development phase in its entirety, let alone a complete drug development program. However, with a bit of time and patience can be found at the NIH that can greatly aid an NTD drug development program. The National Institute of Allergy and Infectious Diseases (NIAID) is the nexus for many of these resources and has in recent years gone to great lengths to expand its offerings and make these more accessible. The NIAID's Division of Microbiology and Infectious Diseases (www.niaid.nih.gov/labsandresources/resources/dmid/pages/default.aspx) offers drug development services ranging from discovery to Phase II trials through government contractors. Also, the NIH recently launched a program called Therapeutics for Rare and Neglected Diseases (TRND, trnd.nih.gov) that can make available the expertise and resources of institutes such as NIAID through a partnership with the applicant. For example, TRND serves as a portal for resources at NIAID earmarked for work on schistosomiasis (see also Chapter 20) and hookworm disease. Services offered through the TRND umbrella are available to applicants from outside the United States.

On the regulatory side, the FDA has established several programs to encourage development of treatments for diseases neglected by the pharmaceutical industry. Two are particularly relevant to NTD R&D. The Orphan Drug Act is aimed at reducing the cost of developing drugs for diseases that affect less that 200 000 patients per year in the United States or that are not expected to recoup their unaided development costs (both categories include drugs for NTDs). The Office of Orphan Products Development (OOPD, http://www.fda.gov/ForIndustry/DevelopingProductsfor-RareDiseasesConditions/default.htm) at the FDA has the responsibility of facilitating orphan drug development. One of the mechanisms that the OOPD promotes is the repurposing of existing drugs for the treatment of orphan diseases and it has drawn attention to the potential of veterinary anthelmintics to meet the gaps in the current human pharmacopeia.

In 2007 the US Congress enacted an amendment of the FDA charter (bill HR 3580, Section 1102) to include a new mechanism that is hoped will encourage drug development for NTDs. This mechanism will grant a Priority Review Voucher (PRV) to an organization that obtains a New Drug Application (NDA) for a New Chemical Entity (NCE) to move into clinical trials for a disease on their list of NTDs (which include STHs). The PRV in turn gives the bearer the right to an expedited review of another NDA application for a drug that need not be for the treatment of an NTD. The PRV can be sold to a third party that is seeking to shorten the time-to-market of its own drug candidate. A PRV generated by a PDP with a new anthelmintic, for example, could be sold to a pharmaceutical company to shorten its time-to-market for a new blockbuster cardiovascular medicine. Accordingly, a pharmaceutical company may be willing to pay a significant amount of money to a PDP for a PRV generated by the approval of an NTD drug. The PRV mechanism may attract the private capital into NTD drug development that would otherwise be absent due to the weak profit margins at stake (http://www.bvgh.org/What-We-Do/Incentives/Priority-Review-Vouchers.aspx). However, the value of a PRV remains unproven, both in financial terms and in terms of the actual regulatory time saved. Thus far, only one PRV has been issued (to Novartis for Coartem®) and it has not been used or sold. PDPs, pharmaceutical companies, and philanthropic organizations still await the day that a market for PRVs develops and a new stimulus is created in the NTD field.

Conclusions

The development of new drugs is a complex and expensive process,, but a convergence of scientific, business, and social trends is generating new opportunities to fill in gaps in the treatment of NTDs that affect billions of people. In this resource-constrained corner of the pharmaceutical world, PDPs will continue to take a leading role in harnessing the public, industrial, academic, and philanthropic resources available in order to build development programs for NTDs. Until the development of new drugs for NTDs becomes a profitable business, it will remain a cottage industry. Yet, progress is being made due to the increasing availability of human and technical expertise from the pharmaceutical industry and the provision of resources and incentives from government agencies. Although it is regrettable that research into new human anthelmintics is particularly neglected, it is fortunate that the animal health industry provides opportunities for cross-over development that is faster and less expensive than designing drugs from scratch, and this should facilitate the development of new anthelmintics in the near future.

Acknowledgments

The authors would like to thank Deborah Tranowski for conducting much of the research for this manuscript and Robert Choy for critical reading of the manuscript. This work was supported by the UK Department for International Development, the Bill & Melinda Gates Foundation, and a Swiss philanthropic foundation.

References

1 Trouiller, P., Olliaro, P., Torreele, E., Orbinski, J., Laing, R., and Ford, N. (2002) Drug development for neglected diseases: a deficient market and a public-health policy failure. *Lancet*, **359**, 2188–2194.

2 Pink, R., Hudson, A., Mouriès, M.-A., and Bendig, M. (2005) Opportunities and challenges in antiparasitic drug discovery. *Nat. Rev. Drug. Discov.*, **4**, 727–740.

3 Stoll, N.R. (1962) On endemic hookworm, where do we stand today? *Exp. Parasitol.*, **12**, 241–252.

4 Bethony, J., Brooker, S., Albonico, M., Geiger, S.M., Loukas, A., Diemert, D., and Hotez, P.J. (2006) Soil-transmitted helminth infections: ascariasis, trichuriasis, and hookworm. *Lancet*, **367**, 1521–1532.

5 Hotez, P.J. (2010) How to cure 1 billion people? Defeat neglected tropical diseases. *Sci. Am.*, **302**, 90–94.

6 Bleakly, H. (2007) Disease and development: evidence from hookworm eradication in the American South. *Q. J. Econ.*, **122**, 73–117.

7. Boccaccio, M. (1972) Ground Itch and Dew poison the Rockefeller Sanitary Commission 1909–14. *J. Hist. Med. Allied Sci.*, **XXVII**, 30–53.
8. Hotez, P.J., Brindley, P.J., Bethony, J.M., King, C.H., Pearce, E.J., and Jacobson, J. (2008) Helminth infections: the great neglected tropical diseases. *J. Clin. Invest.*, **118**, 1311–1321.
9. Hotez, P.J., Bundy, D.A.P., Beegle, K., Brooker, S., Drake, L., de Silva, N., Montresor, A. *et al.* (2006) Helminth infections: soil-transmitted helminth infections and schistosomiasis, in *Disease Control Priorities in Developing Countries* (eds D.T. Jamison, J.G. Breman, A.R. Measham, and G. Alleyne), World Bank Publications, Washington, DC, pp. 467–482.
10. Keiser, J. and Utzinger, J. (2010) The drugs we have and the drugs we need against major helminth infections. *Adv. Parasitol.*, **73**, 197–230.
11. Olliaro, P., Seiler, J., Kuesel, A., Horton, J., Clark, J.N., Don, R., and Keiser, J. (2011) Potential drug development candidates for human soil-transmitted helminthiases. *PLoS Negl. Trop. Dis.*, **5**, e1138.
12. Keiser, J. and Utzinger, J. (2008) Efficacy of current drugs against soil-transmitted helminth infections: systematic review and meta-analysis. *J. Am. Med. Assoc.*, **299**, 1937–1948.
13. Katiyar, D. and Singh, L.K. (2011) Filariasis: current status, treatment and recent advances in drug development. *Curr. Med. Chem.*, **18**, 2174–2185.
14. Boutayeb, A. (2007) Developing countries and neglected diseases: challenges and perspectives. *Int. J. Equity Health*, **6**, 20.
15. Keiser, J., Ingram, K., and Utzinger, J. (2011) Antiparasitic drugs for paediatrics: systematic review, formulations, pharmacokinetics, safety, efficacy and implications for control. *Parasitology*, **138**, 1620–1632.
16. Sangster, N. (1999) Pharmacology of anthelmintic resistance. *Parasitol. Today*, **15**, 141–146.
17. Kaplan, R.M. (2004) Drug resistance in nematodes of veterinary importance: a status report. *Trends Parasitol.*, **20**, 477–481.
18. Albonico, M., Bickle, Q., Ramsan, M., Montresor, A., Savioli, L., and Taylor, M. (2003) Efficacy of mebendazole and levamisole alone or in combination against intestinal nematode infections after repeated targeted mebendazole treatment in Zanzibar. *Bull. World Health Organ.*, **81**, 343–352.
19. Flohr, C., Tuyen, L.N., Lewis, S., Minh, T.T., Campbell, J., Britton, J., Williams, H. *et al.* (2007) Low efficacy of mebendazole against hookworm in Vietnam: two randomized controlled trials. *Am. J. Trop. Med. Hyg.*, **76**, 732–736.
20. De Clercq, D., Sacko, M., Behnke, J., Gilbert, F., Dorny, P., and Vercruysse, J. (1997) Failure of mebendazole in treatment of human hookworm infections in the southern region of Mali. *Am. J. Trop. Med. Hyg.*, **57**, 25–30.
21. Geerts, S. and Gryseels, B. (2000) Drug resistance in human helminths: current situation and lessons from livestock. *Clin. Microbiol. Rev.*, **13**, 207–222.
22. Kaminsky, R. (2003) Drug resistance in nematodes: a paper tiger or a real problem? *Curr. Opin. Infect. Dis.*, **16**, 559–564.
23. Prichard, R.K. and Geary, T.G. (2008) Drug discovery: fresh hope to can the worms. *Nature*, **452**, 157–158.
24. Kaminsky, R., Ducray, P., Jung, M., Clover, R., Rufener, L., Bouvier, J., Weber, S.S. *et al.* (2008) A new class of anthelmintics effective against drug-resistant nematodes. *Nature*, **452**, 176–180.
25. Welz, C., Krüger, N., Schniederjans, M., Miltsch, S.M., Krücken, J., Guest, M., Holden-Dye, L. *et al.* (2011) SLO-1 channels of parasitic nematodes reconstitute locomotor behaviour and emodepside sensitivity in *Caenorhabditis elegans slo-1* loss of function mutants. *PLoS Pathog.*, **7**, e1001330.
26. Mackenzie, C.D. and Geary, T.G. (2011) Flubendazole: a candidate macrofilaricide for lymphatic filariasis and onchocerciasis field programs. *Expert Rev. Anti Infect. Ther.*, **9**, 497–501.

27 Brown, D. and Superti-Furga, G. (2003) Rediscovering the sweet spot in drug discovery. *Drug Discov. Today*, **8**, 1067–1077.

28 Gut, J., Ang, K.K.H., Legac, J., Arkin, M.R., Rosenthal, P.J., and McKerrow, J.H. (2011) An image-based assay for high throughput screening of *Giardia lamblia*. *J. Microbiol. Methods*, **84**, 398–405.

29 Caffrey, C.R., Steverding, D., Swenerton, R.K., Kelly, B., Walshe, D., Debnath, A., Zhou, Y.-M. *et al.* (2007) Bis-acridines as lead antiparasitic agents: structure-activity analysis of a discrete compound library *in vitro*. *Antimicrob. Agents Chemother.*, **51**, 2164–2172.

30 Abdulla, M.H., Ruelas, D.S., Wolff, B., Snedecor, J., Lim, K.C., Xu, F., Renslo, A.R. *et al.* (2009) Drug discovery for schistosomiasis: hit and lead compounds identified in a library of known drugs by medium-throughput phenotypic screening. *PLoS Negl. Trop. Dis.*, **3**, e478.

31 Mansour, N.R. and Bickle, Q.D. (2010) Comparison of microscopy and Alamar blue reduction in a larval based assay for schistosome drug screening. *PLoS Negl. Trop. Dis.*, **4**, e795.

32 Hotez, P.J., Bethony, J.M., Diemert, D.J., Pearson, M., and Loukas, A. (2010) Developing vaccines to combat hookworm infection and intestinal schistosomiasis. *Nat. Rev. Microbiol.*, **8**, 814–826.

33 Moran, M., Strub-Wourgaft, N., Guzman, J., Boulet, P., Wu, L., and Pecoul, B. (2011) Registering new drugs for low-income countries: the African challenge. *PLoS Med.*, **8**, e1000411.

34 Nwaka, S., Ramirez, B., Brun, R., Maes, L., Douglas, F., and Ridley, R. (2009) Advancing drug innovation for neglected diseases – criteria for lead progression. *PLoS Negl. Trop. Dis.*, **3**, e440.

35 Moran, M. (2005) A breakthrough in R&D for neglected diseases: new ways to get the drugs we need. *PLoS Med.*, **2**, e302.

36 Nwaka, S. and Ridley, R.G. (2003) Virtual drug discovery and development for neglected diseases through public–private partnerships. *Nat. Rev. Drug Discov.*, **2**, 919–928.

14
Antinematodal Drugs – Modes of Action and Resistance: And Worms Will Not Come to Thee (Shakespeare: *Cymbeline*: IV, ii)

Alan P. Robertson, Samuel K. Buxton, Sreekanth Puttachary, Sally M. Williamson, Adrian J. Wolstenholme, Cedric Neveu, Jacques Cabaret, Claude L. Charvet, and Richard J. Martin*

Abstract

There are two main types of anthelmintics: those that act more rapidly on membrane ion channels, and those that act biochemically and more slowly. The modes of action of 11 classes of antinematodal drugs are summarized: the first five act on membrane ion channels, the remaining six act biochemically. The 11 classes are: (i) cholinergic agonists, imidazothiazole (levamisole), tetrahydropyrimidines (pyrantel, morantel, and oxantel), quaternary/tertiary amines (bephenium and tribendimidine), pyridines (methyridine), and amino-acetonitrile derivatives (monepantel); (ii) cholinergic antagonists (derquantel and phenothiazine); (iii) allosteric modulators of glutamate-gated chloride channels (GluCls): avermectins (ivermectin, doramectin, eprinomectin, and abamectin) and milbemycins (moxidectin and milbemycin); (iv) γ-aminobutyric acid agonist (piperazine); (v) SLO-1 potassium channel activator (emodepside); (vi) β-tubulin ligands (thiabendazole, mebendazole, flubendazole, oxibendazole, and albendazole); (vii) chitinase inhibitor/ionophore (closantel); (viii) lipooxygenase inhibitor (diethylcarbamazine); (ix) SH ligand (melarsomine); (x) pyruvate: ferredoxin oxidoreductase inhibitor (nitazoxanide); and (xi) isothiocyanate-ATP and cholinesterase inhibition (nitroscanate and amoscanate). The current knowledge of the mechanisms of resistance to the nicotinic cholinergic agonists (reduced receptor expression and truncated receptor subunit expression), GluCl allosteric modulators (increased expression of P-glycoproteins and multidrug resistance proteins), and β-tubulin ligands (single nucleotide polymorphisms) is summarized.

Introduction

Parasitic worms have been recognized since ancient times and we assume that treatments developed early on after their recognition. The ancient Romans described *Ascaris lumbricoides* as an earthworm that could live in humans [1]. Early cures included santonica from the Levant wormseed (*Artemisia cina*) that was used by the

* Corresponding Author

ancient Greeks and chenopod oil (from *Chenopodium ambrosioides*) used by the Aztecs (referred to in the Sahagun Florentine code written by Aztec physicians in the sixteenth century [2]). Originally, treatments were referred to as "vermifuges," but this has now been replaced by "anthelmintic" (antihelminthic). Following the introduction of piperazine in 1949 by Fayard [3], safer, more effective synthetic or semisynthetic drugs have been introduced, replacing the older vermifuges. We summarize the mode of action of 11 classes of these newer anthelmintics. The first five act on membrane ion channels of the nematode and produce a rapid effect (around 3 h); the remaining six act biochemically, killing the parasite more slowly (1–4 days). We then summarize the known mechanisms of resistance to levamisole, monepantel, macrocyclic lactones, and benzimidazoles.

Modes of Action of Anthelmintics

Cholinergic Agonists

Imidazothiazoles (Levamisole and Butamisole), Tetrahydropyrimidines (Pyrantel, Morantel, and Oxantel), Quaternary/Tertiary Amines (Bephenium and Tribendimidine), Pyridines (Methyridine), and Amino-Acetonitrile Derivatives (AADs) (Monepantel)

The earliest of these anthelmintics (bephenium and methyridine) were introduced soon after 1958, although the most recent of this group (monepantel) appeared in 2008. These drugs act selectively as agonists to open acetylcholine-gated ion channels (Figures 14.1 and 14.2) of nematode body muscle. This type of ion channel receptor is known as a nicotinic acetylcholine ion channel receptor (nAChR) for historical reasons since early known vertebrate receptors were activated by nicotine. We use this convention of nAChRs for nematode ligand-gated acetylcholine receptors, even if nicotine and sometimes acetylcholine is for them a low potency agonist. They are not G-protein-coupled acetylcholine receptors. Activation of nematode nAChRs on body muscle produces depolarization, contraction, and spastic paralysis of the parasites, so they are swept away from their normal location. The chemical structure of the cholinergic anthelmintics is very heterogeneous. As a result, these drugs have different selectivities for the different subtypes of acetylcholine ion channel receptors that are present in each of the parasitic nematodes. In the large nematode of the pig, *Ascaris suum*, three subtypes of receptor have been characterized (Figure 14.1a): the L-subtype (preferentially sensitive to levamisole), the B-subtype (preferentially sensitive to bephenium), and the N-subtype (preferentially activated by oxantel and methyridine and nicotine). It turns out that there are potentially a very large number of nematode nAChRs subtypes that are separate and discrete drug targets within a single worm. Those subtypes that have a sufficiently distinctive pharmacology from the host nAChRs are major drug targets to be exploited for therapeutic purposes [4].

We have most knowledge of the nAChRs of the model nematode, *Caenorhabditis elegans*, but know less about this class of receptors in parasitic nematodes. The nAChRs are made up of five subunits (Figures 14.2 and 14.3) and each is about 500 amino acids

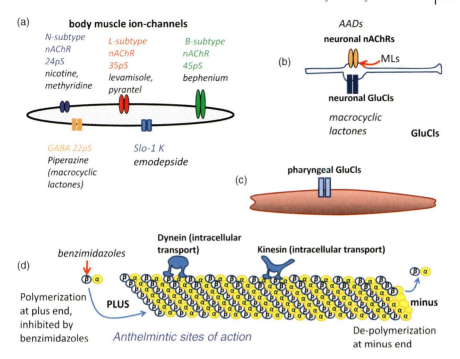

Figure 14.1 Sites of action of different classes of anthelmintic. (a) Ion channel targets of anthelmintics on somatic muscle of nematodes. Cholinergic agonists: nicotine, methyridine, and oxantel have a selective effect on the N-subtype of nAChR; levamisole has a selective effect on the L-subtype of nAChR; bephenium has a selective effect on the B-subtype of nAChR. Piperazine acts as an agonist on the GABA receptors, which are also affected by macrocyclic lactones. Emodepside leads to opening of the SLO-1 potassium channel. (b) On neurons there are different subtypes of nAChR, some of which are activated by monepantel. Also present on some neurons are GluCls, on which macrocyclic lactones act as allosteric modulators. (c) Macrocyclic lactones are allosteric modulators that potentiate and activate opening of pharyngeal GluCls. (d) Benzimidazole anthelmintics bind to β-tubulin and αβ-tubulin dimers, and prevent the formation of microtubules at the positive pole. Microtubules are involved in a number of intracellular tasks including mitosis and intracellular transport with the motor molecules dynein and kinesin.

in length. Each acetylcholine receptor subunit possesses typical sequence features including a signal peptide, an extracellular N-terminal region containing a dicysteine loop (two cysteines separated by 13 amino acids), four transmembrane domains (TM1–TM4), and a highly variable intracellular loop between TM3 and TM4. Acetylcholine receptor subunits are defined as α or non-α depending on the presence of adjacent cysteine residues in the acetylcholine binding site. Homopentameric nAChRs are made of five identical α-subunits, whereas heteropentameric comprise at least two non-α-subunits in combination with α-subunits. The agonist binding site is at the interface of two adjacent α-subunits or between an α-subunit and a non-α-subunit depending upon the receptor subtype (hetero- or homopentamer). In *C. elegans*, there are at least 27 subunit genes, encoding different α- or non-α-subunits

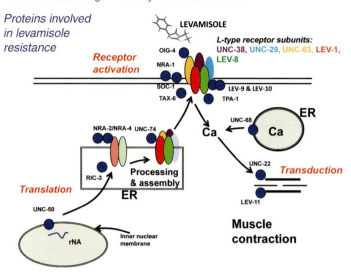

Figure 14.2 Summary diagram of the proteins (and genes) associated with levamisole resistance and receptor regulation based on C. elegans. LEV-8 has been replaced by ACR-8 for clade V parasitic nematodes. The proteins are involved in the signal transduction process, and regulation and expression of levamisole receptors on the muscle membrane surface.

that are assembled into different combinations leading to expression of many different nAChR subtypes that have specific pharmacologies [4]. Alternative splicing of some of the subunit genes can also occur, increasing the possible number of subtypes of nAChR.

A well-characterized cholinergic receptor of *C. elegans* is the levamisole receptor (usually abbreviated to L-AChR rather than L-nAChR) which is found at neuromuscular junctions in somatic muscle. Characteristics of the levamisole receptor and associated proteins are illustrated in Figure 14.2. The molecular composition of this receptor was deciphered using the powerful genetic tools available in this model organism [4, 9–11]. Forward genetic screens for levamisole-resistant mutants in *C. elegans* identified the five genes encoding the five subunits of L-AChRs. They include three α-subunits (UNC-63, UNC-38, and LEV-8) and two non-α-subunits (UNC-29 and LEV-1). Boulin *et al.* demonstrated that the subunits encoded by these five genes associate to reconstitute a functional L-AChR when coexpressed with ancillary proteins in *Xenopus* oocytes [9].

unc-38, unc-63, unc-29, lev-1, and *lev-8* are subunit genes required for full sensitivity to levamisole (Figure 14.2). In addition, there is a second group of genes, *nra-1, soc-1, tax-6,* and *tpa-1,* the products of which modify the channel opening in response to levamisole with null mutants showing less channel opening to levamisole. Next, the products of a third set of genes, *unc-68* (ryanodine receptor), *unc-22,* and *lev-11,* are involved in the calcium signaling cascade and the contraction response to levamisole.

A fourth set of gene products, *unc-50*, *ric-3*, *unc-74*, and *nra-2/nra-4*, are involved in processing and assembly of the levamisole receptor in the endoplasmic reticulum. *unc-50*, *ric-3*, and *unc-74* are essential for expression of levamisole receptors [9]. *nra-2* and *nra-4* are thought to be involved in the selection of the subunit combinations, the subtype of levamisole receptor, and its sensitivity to levamisole [10, 11]. Finally, a fifth set of genes, *lev-10*, *lev-9*, and *oig-4*, encodes proteins involved in the synaptic clustering of the nAChRs at the neuromuscular junctions, especially the levamisole receptors (L-AChRs) [12].

It has been suggested that in parasitic nematodes there are fewer nAChR subunit genes than in *C. elegans* [13], although recent transcriptomic and genetic studies show a wider range of subunit genes in nematode parasites of clade V. *lev-8* appears to be missing in parasitic nematodes of clade V, but four copies of *unc-29* have been identified in *Haemonchus contortus* and *Teladordagia circumcincta* [5, 14, 15]. For the clade III nematode, *A. suum*, however, expression of *Asu-unc-38* and *Asu-unc-29* subunits in the *Xenopus* oocyte system was sufficient to produce a functional levamisole receptor [16]. Also, changing the expression ratio (stoichiometry) of the two subunits altered the pharmacology of the receptor from an N-subtype to an L-subtype. The L-subtype was more sensitive to levamisole and pyrantel; the N-subtype was more sensitive to oxantel and nicotine. The function of *Asu-unc-63* and *Asu-unc-8* remains to be investigated. Recently, the expression of the *H. contortus* subunits, *Hco-unc-38*, *Hco-unc-29.1*, *Hco-unc-63a*, and *Hco-acr-8*, together with the addition of the ancillary proteins, *Hco-ric-3*, *Hco-unc-74*, and *Hco-unc-50*, led to a functional L-AChR [15] (Figure 14.3a). Interestingly, ACR-8 is critical for the expression of an *H. contortus* levamisole receptor and, if omitted, produces a receptor (L-AChR2; Figure 14.3b) that is more sensitive to pyrantel than levamisole. The pharmacology of this expressed receptor is strikingly different from the *C. elegans* prototype.

AADs (Monepantel)
Monepantel is a recently introduced (2008) anthelmintic belonging to the AAD chemical class. The compound has effects against levamisole-resistant and multi-resistant parasites. It produces contraction of *H. contortus* body muscle leaving the head and tail regions motile, suggesting that it is a cholinomimetic that has a different site of action to levamisole and pyrantel. Use of null mutants in *C. elegans* showed that monepantel is selective for a subtype of nAChR (Figure 14.1b) that is made up of subunits from the DEG-3 family including ACR-23 [17]. In the absence of homologs of *acr-23* in *H. contortus*, other genes associated with monepantel resistance include *Hco-des-2* and *Hco-mptl-1* [18]. So far, expression of *Hco-mptl-1* subunits have failed to produce receptors sensitive to monepantel [19]. However, *Xenopus* oocyte expression of *Hco-deg-3/Hco-deg-2* subunits with *Hco-ric-3* has produced a subtype of nAChRs that is more sensitive to choline than acetylcholine and with which monepantel acts allosterically to reverse receptor desensitization (a type II positive allosteric modulator). Further studies are required to decipher the subunit structure of the monepantel receptor in parasitic nematodes.

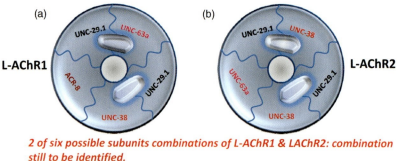

2 of six possible subunits combinations of L-AChR1 & LAChR2: combination still to be identified.

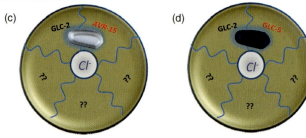

GluCl subunits in C. elegans pharynx

GluCl subunits in H. contortus motor neuron commissures

Figure 14.3 Diagram of subunits that contribute to the formation of the L-AChR1 and LAChR2 of strongylid nematode parasites, and GluCl subunits of *C. elegans*. The red triangle denotes the presence of a putative agonist binding site. (a) Putative arrangements of the L-AChR1 receptor subunits [5], which are more sensitive to levamisole. (b) Putative arrangements of the L-AChR2 receptor subunits [5], which are more sensitive to pyrantel. Expression requires RIC-3, UNC-74, and UNC-50. (c and d) Subunits that contribute to the formation of GluCls in nematodes. (c) *C. elegans* pharyngeal receptor that has AVR-15 and GLC-2. (d) GluCls present on the motoneuron commissures of *H. contortus* possess GLC-2, GLC-5, and possibly other subunits [6]. The drug-binding site lies in the outer membrane-spanning region of the channel [7], with binding sites to the M1, M2, and M3 transmembrane regions at the interface [8].

Cholinergic Antagonists (Derquantel and Phenothiazine)

Derquantel

Derquantel is a spiroindole (2-desoxyparaherquamide) that began to be marketed in 2010 for animal use. To enhance its effect, derquantel is mixed with the macrocyclic lactone, abamectin (Startect®; Pfizer). Derquantel is a selective and competitive antagonist of nematode muscle nicotinic receptors, but has effects against levamisole-resistant and macrocyclic-resistant parasitic worms. It selectively inhibits the B-subtype of nAChR [20]. The combination with abamectin is predicted to have synergistic effects.

Phenothiazine

Phenothiazine was introduced in 1940 and has modest nAChR inhibitory effects in nematodes [21].

Glutamate-gated chloride ion channels (GluCls) and γ-Aminobutyric Acid (GABA) Allosteric Modulators

Avermectins (Ivermectin, Doramectin, Eprinomectin, and Abamectin) and Milbemycins (Moxidectin and Milbemycin)

The avermectins were first characterized and assayed for anthelmintic activity by Merck Sharp & Dohme in 1979 following their isolation from a soil sample near a golf course at Kawana, Ito City in Japan. The macrocyclic lactones (the avermectins and milbemycins) are effective and potent drugs against roundworms and biting insects, but not tapeworms or flatworms. They are good substrates for P-glycoproteins in vertebrates and do not accumulate in the vertebrate central nervous system, which may permit their selective action on the parasites. They exert their anthelmintic effect by acting in the outer membrane layer in the lipophilic region of thus GluCls [7, 8, 22] of the nematode parasite (Figure 14.1c). They act as allosteric modulators, increasing the probability of opening of GluCls that are found in the pharynx and neurons of nematodes. The increased opening of the chloride channels results in hyperpolarization and inhibition of body movement and pharyngeal pumping. Molecular and genetic studies of macrocyclic lactone sensitivity in *C. elegans* and parasitic nematodes, including *H. contortus* [23], have identified multiple subtypes (isoforms) of GluCls and other ligand-gated chloride channels (dopamine- and serotonin-gated chloride channels [24–28]) that are sensitive to macrocyclic lactones.

The macrocyclic lactones have little effect, however, on adult filariae of *Brugia*, *Dirofilaria*, and *Onchocerca*, which survive treatment, perhaps because they do not need feed by pharyngeal pumping. In these species, the main effect is on the larval stages. For the canine heartworm, *Dirofilaria immitis*, it is the infective L3 and L4 larvae that are exquisitely sensitive to the drugs and regular monthly dosing is required for their effective action as a preventative. In human filarial infections, lymphatic filariasis and onchocerciasis, the major effects are on the microfilariae, which are rapidly cleared by treatment. Very recently, Moreno et al. [29] have shown that the macrocyclic lactones inhibit protein secretion by *Brugia malayi* microfilariae and suggest that this may be responsible for the rapid clearance of this life stage following drug treatment.

Again, like the cholinomimetic drugs, the genes required for macrocyclic lactone sensitivity were initially identified in *C. elegans*. The genes include: (i) *glc-1* (a GluClα1 subunit that forms a homo-oligomer gated by ivermectin, but not glutamate, and that forms hetero-oligomers with GluClβ to form channels gated by glutamate and ivermectin) [22], (ii) *glc-3* (a GluClα4 subunit that forms glutamate-gated channels) [30–32], (iii) *avr-14* (that encodes the subunits GluClα3A and GluClα3B splicing variants) [33, 34], and (iv) *avr-15* (that encodes the subunits GluClα2A and GluClα2B) [35, 36]. Resistance to ivermectin in *C. elegans* occurs at different concentrations and is also affected by a large number of genes associated with amphid structures (*dyf* genes), transporter genes (P-glycoproteins and multidrug resistance proteins, multiple drug resistance transporters) as well as the GluCl subunits. For the highest level of resistance, null mutants of *glc-1*, *avr-14*, and avr-15 [34] have to be present simultaneously. Innexins also affect electrical coupling between neurons [34].

In parasitic nematodes, some of the *C. elegans* GluCl genes are missing and some additional genes are present. In *H. contortus*, glc-1 appears to be missing, Hco-glc-2, Hco-glc-3, and Hco-glc-4 are present, but there are two additional subunit genes, Hco-glc-5 and Hco-glc-6. There are even fewer GluCl subunit sequences in the clade III parasite, *B. malayi*, and in the clade I parasite, *Trichinella spiralis*. *B. malayi* has avr-14, glc-2, and glc-4; glc-2 is not present in *T. spiralis* [13]. We can predict that the multiple subunits come together in different pentameric arrangements to give rise to a range of GluCl subtypes with differing sensitivities to the macrocyclic lactones.

GABA Agonist

Piperazine

Piperazine is a saturated heterocyclic ring and was introduced by Faynard in 1949 as an anthelmintic. It acts as a GABA agonist and hyperpolarizes muscle by opening chloride channels to induce flaccid paralysis [37]. Its potency may be increased in high CO_2 environments. Siddiqui et al. [28] identified and expressed two genes from *H. contortus*, Hco-unc-49B and Hco-unc-49C, that encode two GABA-gated chloride channel subunits.

SLO-1 Potassium Channel Activator

Emodepside

Emodepside was introduced in 2001 by Bayer. It has an inhibitory effect on nematode movements. It does not act as a GABA agonist or as a nicotinic antagonist [38]. Guest et al. [39] described a *C. elegans* mutagenesis screen to generate alleles of slo-1 that encode a calcium-activated potassium channel in *C. elegans* (Figure 14.1a). They observed that (i) slo-1 but not slo-2 null mutants are more resistant to the inhibitory effects of emodepside than lat-1 and lat-2 (latrophilin receptor) double-null mutants, and (ii) inhibition of feeding by emodepside is facilitated by the presence of lat-1 [40]. The effects of emodepside on heterologously expressed slo-1 in *C. elegans* [41] predicted that SLO-1 is a direct target for emodepside, whereas the human ortholog of SLO-1, KCNMA1, is less sensitive to emodepside. In *A. suum*, a slo-1 homolog gene is expressed in *A. suum* muscle flaps where it is presumed to produce the Ca^{2+}-dependent voltage-activated potassium currents in *A. suum* muscle [41–43]. In *A. suum*, emodepside produces a slow (minutes) hyperpolarization of the muscle membrane potential [42, 43], and potentiates voltage- and calcium-dependent, SLO-1-like channel currents that are affected by modulators of the nitric oxide and protein kinase C (PKC) signaling pathways. Emodepside has no effect on voltage-activated calcium currents. These latter effects are consistent with a model in which nitric oxide, PKC, and emodepside signaling pathways are separate and converge on the SLO-1 potassium channels, and/or in which emodepside activates one or more of these signaling pathways [43].

β-Tubulin Ligands

Thiabendazole, Mebendazole, Flubendazole, Oxibendazole, and Albendazole
The first benzimidazole to be introduced was thiabendazole in 1961 by Merck Sharpe & Dohme. Benzimidazoles produce degenerative changes in the cuticle and cells of the intestine of nematode parasites by binding to colchicine-binding sites of tubulin (β-tubulin and αβ-tubulin dimers), and inhibiting polymerization and assembly of tubulin [44] into microtubules (Figure 14.1d). Loss of cytoplasmic microtubules reduces intracellular transport, glucose uptake by larvae and adults, and drains their glycogen stores. Degeneration of the endoplasmic reticulum and mitochondria in the underlying germinal layer facilitates the release of lysosome enzymes that further damages the cell. There is decreased ATP production. As the energy is depleted, the parasite becomes immobilized and dies. The benzimidazoles have also been reported to inhibit the parasite fumarate reductase, but this may be a secondary effect related to the decreased absorption of glucose. Albendazole is larvicidal against *Necator* hookworm and also has ovicidal activity against the *Ancylostoma* hookworm, *Ascaris*, and *Trichuris*. Binding studies [45] show that the affinity series is: albendazole > fenbendazole > mebendazole > oxibendazole > parbendazole > thiabendazole for β-tubulin and αβ-heterodimers, but the affinities are lower for binding to α-tubulin. The incorporation of benzimidazole-bound αβ-heterodimers into assembling microtubules arrests polymerization. These findings indicate that a benzimidazole-β-tubulin cap was formed at the growing end of the microtubule and that this cap prevented elongation of the microtubule.

The *C. elegans* genome encodes nine α- and six β-tubulin genes [46, 47]. Some of these, particularly *tba-1, tba-2, tbb-1*, and *tbb-2*, are expressed broadly during embryogenesis, and function redundantly in spindle assembly and positioning [48–50]. *tba-1* and *tbb-2* have also been recently shown to be important for axon outgrowth and synaptogenesis [51]. Others, including *mec-7* and *mec-12*, were identified through genetic screens for touch insensitivity, but only mutants of *ben-1* are associated with benzimidazole resistance [52–54]. In parasitic nematodes there are two and sometimes three isotypes (genes) coding for β-tubulin [54], but it is isotype I that is recognized as being relevant for the action of benzimidazoles [55].

Chitinase Inhibitor/Ionophore

Closantel
Closantel was developed by Janssen Pharmaceuticals in 1979; it is a broad-spectrum anthelmintic used against trematodes, nematodes, and some arthropods. It is a salicylanilide, which can be protonated such that it abolishes the pH gradients found across mitochondria, thus inhibiting oxidative phosphorylation. *In vitro* studies have shown that closantel is an uncoupler of oxidative phosphorylation in rat liver, and an inhibitor of mitochondrial phosphorylation in *Fasciola hepatica* and *H. contortus* [56, 57]. Recently, it has also been shown to be a potent and specific inhibitor of filarial chitinases [58]. It completely inhibits molting of *Onchocerca volvulus* infective L3 stage larvae. It may therefore act by targeting two important biochemical

processes in filarial parasites. Structure–activity studies found that closantel has a dual proton ionophore and chitinase activity; simple chemical modification of the salicylanilide scaffold structure could produce compounds that acted only as protonophores or chitinase inhibitors [59]. These studies found that there is a synergistic effect between the chitinase inhibitor effect and the proton ionophore effect [59] consistent with a dual mode of action for closantel.

Innate Immune Response Inhibitor

Diethylcarbamazine
Diethylcarbamazine was discovered in 1947. It is a piperazine derivative and has been used for many years to treat human lymphatic filariasis [60]. It has been reported to have direct inhibitory effects at low concentrations (below 100 µM) on adult parasites and excitatory effects at higher concentrations (above 100 µM) [61], although direct effects on microfilaria are not seen. Whilst it is a piperazine derivative, unchanged diethylcarbamazine does not mimic the action of piperazine [37]. It inhibits the metabolism of arachidonic acid and, therefore, alters the inflammatory response of the host. Within 5 min, microfilaria are cleared from the circulation and this effect is inhibited by dexamethasone or indomethacin [62]. Arachidonic acid is metabolized through two pathways: the cyclooxygenase pathway to different prostaglandins or via the lipooxygenase to produce leukotrienes. Diethylcarbamazine affects (inhibits) both pathways, and because it has little direct action on microfilaria (in contrast to effects on adult preparations) it is suggested that the microfilaricidal activity is due to modulation of the host innate immune system pathways involving cyclooxygenase-1 and cyclooxygenase-2 and inducible nitric oxide synthase [62, 63].

SH Ligand

Melarsamine
Melarsamine (also spelt melarsomine and also known as MelCy or melaminylthioarsenate) was introduced as an antitrypanosomal drug in 1991 following development of a series of organic arsenic compounds. Its action as a heartworm macrofilaricide was reported in 1992. The mode of action of this trivalent organo-arsenic compound has not been completely defined, but its actions include binding to SH groups of enzymes, including glutathione reductase, and their inactivation through denaturation. Melarsamine inhibits the uptake of glucose by the parasite and disrupts the structure of the parasites' intestine. It is used to treat adult heartworm in dogs, but is relatively toxic to the host.

Pyruvate: Ferredoxin Oxidoreductase Inhibitor

Nitazoxanide
Nitazoxanide is a synthetic nitrothizolyl-salicylamide. Originally used as an antiprotozoal drug (*Cryptosporidium* and *Giardia*), it interferes with pyruvate: ferredoxin oxidoreductase, which is required to maintain redox potential (electron transfer)

during anaerobic energy metabolism [64]. It is also an effective anthelmintic against roundworms [65].

Isothiocyanate-ATP Inhibition

Nitroscanate, Amoscanate, and Sulfoscanate
Nitroscanate and amoscanate have antinematodal, anticestodal, and antischistosomal actions [66, 67]. These drugs are 4-isothiocyanate-4-nitrodiphenyl derivatives. The thiourea group appears to be responsible for an anticholinesterase action, and the nitrophenyl group appears to be responsible for the oxidative uncoupling that damages the mitochondria of the parasite and reduces ATP levels in the parasites [68].

Resistance

Cholinergic Agonists

Levamisole and Pyrantel Resistance
In *H. contortus*, the first levamisole-binding experiments performed on wild-type and levamisole-resistant isolates identified changes in the binding characteristics or in the expression level of levamisole-sensitive receptors rather than the complete loss of levamisole receptors, as was the case in *C. elegans* null mutants [69]. This resistance mechanism involving the downregulation of the receptors is compatible with the need of the parasite to maintain its mobility to complete its life cycle. The nAChRs are a family of heterogeneic pentameric receptors resulting from different combinations of subunits. Examination of the gene sequences of *unc-29*, *unc-38*, and *unc-63* from *Ancylostoma caninum* found no evidence of specific amino acid substitutions associated with pyrantel resistance [70]. However, a pyrantel-resistant isolate was found to have decreased expression of *Aca-unc-38*, *Aca-unc-29*, and *Aca-unc-63* [70]. This is predicted to reduce the number of nAChRs, suggesting that these genes may be part of a functional pyrantel receptor that has not yet been described. This is consistent with studies with *Oesophagostomum dentatum* that found fewer L-subtype channels present in a levamisole resistant isolate [71]. In *H. contortus*, *T. circumcincta*, and *Trichostrongylus colubriformis*, a truncated form of *unc-63* (*unc-63b*) is associated with levamisole resistance [5, 14, 15]. A truncated form of *acr-8* (*Hco-acr-8b*) was also described as a levamisole resistance marker in several *H. contortus* isolates [14]. These truncated transcripts may give rise to truncated subunits that inhibit the formation of normal receptors [72]. Accordingly, when coexpressed with the Hco-L-AChR1 in *Xenopus* oocytes, the truncated Hco-unc-63b subunit had a strong dominant-negative effect on receptor expression, thus providing mechanistic insight into levamisole resistance [5]. Figure 14.2 illustrates the signaling cascade (based on *C. elegans*) following the opening of a levamisole-activated channel. In addition to null mutants of the channel protein subunits that produce levamisole resistance, other genes associated with the levamisole receptor (*lev-10*, *oig-4*, *nra-1*, *soc-1*, *tax-6*, and *tpa-1*), the calcium signaling cascade producing contraction (*unc-68*, *unc-22*, and *lev-11*), and

processing and assembly of the receptor protein in the endoplasmic reticulum (*unc-50*, *ric-3*, *nra-2/nra-4*, and *unc-74*) may be involved as well [73].

Monepantel Resistance (AADs)
AADs (monepantel) target the nAChRs composed of DEG-3-like subunits [17]. In *C. elegans*, resistance to monepantel is associated with mutations in the genes *acr-23*, *acr-29*, *des-2*, or *deg-3*. In *H. contortus*, experimentally induced monepantel resistance is associated with truncation of *Hco-mptl-1 (acr-23H)*, *Hco-des-2H*, and *Hco-deg-3H*, and reduced expression of the subunit RNA [19]. Resistance appears to be associated with changes to the subunit encoded by the *mptl-1* gene, but physiological evidence for it has not been demonstrated yet. Specific single nucleotide polymorphisms (SNPs) associated with monepantel resistance remain to be identified.

GluCl Modulators (Changed Receptor Subunit SNPs, and Increased Expression of P-Glycoproteins and Multidrug Resistance Proteins)
The macrocyclic lactones are allosteric modulators of nematode GluCl channels, and other ligand-gated chloride channels including those gated by GABA, dopamine, and tyramine. A number of genes and SNPs ([74] and Table 14.1) have been associated

Table 14.1 Summary of genes and the molecular changes described in the text that are associated with resistance to the different anthelmintics.

Anthelmintic	Site of action	Gene carrying resistance	Molecular change
Benzimidazoles	β-tubulin	*ben-1* (isotype I)	F200Y
			E198A
			F167Y
Levamisole	body muscle nAChR	*unc-38*	decreased expression
		unc-29	decreased expression
		unc-63	truncated transcript
		acr-8	truncated transcript
Monepantel	neuronal nAChR	*mpt-1*	decreased expression and truncated transcript
		des-2	decreased expression and truncated transcript
		deg-3	decreased expression and truncated transcript
Macrocyclic lactones	GluCl channel (+ GABA, dopamine, tyramine Cl channel?)	*avr-14*	L256F
		glc-5	A169V
		ggr-3	decreased expression
		lgc-37	K169R
	transporter	*pgp*	increased expression

with expressed receptors that have reduced responses to the macrocyclic lactones. A clear link between field resistance and these SNPs remains to be demonstrated.

In C. elegans, loss of macrocyclic lactone sensitivity requires the deletion of all three GluCl genes (i.e., *avr-14*, *avr-15*, and *glc-1*) [33]. Moxidectin is less potent on pharyngeal pumping in C. elegans [74, 75] and this difference in sensitivity disappears when the *glc-2* is deleted, suggesting that moxidectin and ivermectin have different selectivities for receptor subtypes. Reduced macrocyclic lactone sensitivity is also produced by P-glycoprotein transporters (*pgp-1* and *pgp-2*) and molecules associated with ABC transporter family (*mrp* genes) [74, 75]. Also, in parasitic nematodes, resistance has been associated with increased expression of P-glycoprotein multidrug transporters. We already have good evidence that different alleles of the mammalian ABCG2 transporter, S581Y, have different affinities to selamectin and ivermectin [76]. In addition to resistance associated with ligand-gated chloride channels and transporter molecules, there may also be a genetic relationship between macrocyclic lactone and benzimidazole resistance [77].

β-Tubulin Ligands – Benzimidazole Resistance
Since 1964, resistance to benzimidazoles has been observed in parasitic nematodes of livestock. A null mutant of *ben-1* [51] confers benomyl resistance in C. elegans. In parasitic nematodes, SNPs found on isotype I β-tubulin are associated with resistance (F167Y, E198A, and F200Y) [74]. In addition, using transformation of a C. elegans ben-1 mutant with parasite wild-type and F200Y mutated *β-tubulin*, Kwa et al. [78] clearly demonstrated that the F200Y mutation in the *β-tubulin* isotype I is the molecular mechanism for benzimidazole resistance in H. contortus. This change has been found in different veterinary parasites and each time the affinity of β-tubulin for benzimidazoles is decreased [74]. Given the many isotypes of β-tubulin that are present and the presence of P-glycoprotein transporters that might exclude benzimidazoles, we anticipate that there are still unrecognized molecular mechanisms for resistance to benzimidazoles. A role for other genes affecting the activity of tubulin-binding genes in mammals has been reviewed [79].

Acknowledgments

The project was supported by grant **2R56AI047194-11** from the National Institute of Allergy and Infectious Diseases to R.J.M. and A.P.R., and by the French National Institute for Agricultural Research to C.L.C., C.N., and J.C. S.K.B. is the grateful recipient of a scientific Chateaubriand doctoral fellowship granted by the Office for Science and Technology of the Embassy of France in the USA and from the "Santé, Sciences, Technologies" doctoral school Tours University. C.L.C. held a 2011 Fellowship award from the OECD's Cooperative Research Program "Biological Resource Management for Sustainable Agricultural Systems." The content is solely the responsibility of the authors and does not necessarily represent the official views of the National Institute of Allergy and Infectious Diseases of the National Institutes of Health.

References

1 Bowman, W.C. and Rand, J. (eds) (1980) *Textbook of Pharmacology*, Blackwell Scientific, Oxford.

2 Kliks, M.M. (1990) Helminths as heirlooms and souvenirs: a review of new world paleoparasitology. *Parasitol. Today*, **6**, 93–100.

3 Fayard, G. (1949) Ascaridiose et piperazine, These de Doctorat, University of Paris.

4 Jones, A.K. and Sattelle, D.B. (2004) Functional genomics of the nicotinic acetylcholine receptor gene family of the nematode, *Caenorhabditis elegans*. *Bioessays*, **26**, 39–49.

5 Boulin, T., Fauvin, A., Charvet, C., Cortet, J., Cabaret, J., Bessereau, J.-L., and Neveu, C. (2001) Functional reconstitution of *Haemonchus contortus* acetylcholine receptors in *Xenopus* oocytes provides mechanistic insights into levamisole resistance. *Br. J. Pharmacol.*, **164**, 1421–1432.

6 Portillo, V., Jagannathan, S., and Wolstenholme, A.J. (2003) Distribution of glutamate-gated chloride channel subunits in the parasitic nematodes *Haemonchus contortus*. *J. Comp. Neurol.*, **462**, 213–222.

7 Martin, R.J. and Kusel, J.R. (1991) On the distribution of a fluorescent ivermectin probe (4″,5,7 dimethyl-bodipy proprionylivermectin) in *Ascaris* membranes. *Parasitology*, **104**, 549–555.

8 Hibbs, R.E. and Gouaux, E. (2011) Princicples of activation and permeation in an anion-selective Cys-loop receptor. *Nature*, **474**, 54–60.

9 Boulin, T. et al. (2008) Eight genes are required for functional reconstitution of the *Caenorhabditis elegans* levamisole-sensitive acetylcholine receptor. *Proc. Natl. Acad. Sci. USA*, **105**, 18590–18595.

10 Gottschalk, A. et al. (2005) Identification and characterization of novel nicotinic receptor-associated proteins in *Caenorhabditis elegans*. *EMBO J.*, **24**, 2566–2578.

11 Almedom, R.B. et al. (2009) An ER-resident membrane protein complex regulates nicotinic acetylcholine receptor subunit composition at the synapse. *EMBO J.*, **28**, 2636–2649.

12 Rapti, G., Richmond, J., and Bessereau, J.L. (2011) A single-imunoglobulin-domain protein for clustering acetylcholine receptors in *C. elegans*. *EMBO J.*, **30**, 706–718.

13 Williamson, S.M., Walsh, T.K., and Wolstenholme, A.J. (2007) The cys-loop ligand-gated ion channel gene family of *Brugia malayi* and *Trichinella spiralis*: a comparison with *Caenorhabditis elegans*. *Invert. Neurosci.*, **7**, 219–226.

14 Fauvin, A. et al. (2010) cDNA-AFLP analysis in levamisole-resistant *Haemonchus contortus* reveals alternative splicing in a nicotinic acetylcholine receptor subunit. *Mol. Biochem. Parasitol.*, **170**, 105–107.

15 Neveu, C. et al. (2010) Genetic diversity of levamisole receptor subunits in parasitic nematode species and abbreviated transcripts associated with resistance. *Pharmacogenet. Genomics*, **20**, 414–425.

16 Williamson, S.M. et al. (2009) The nicotinic acetylcholine receptors of the parasitic nematode *Ascaris suum*: formation of two distinct drug targets by varying the relative expression levels of two subunits. *PLoS Pathog.*, **5**, e1000517.

17 Kaminsky, R. et al. (2008) A new class of anthelmintics effective against drug-resistant nematodes. *Nature*, **452**, 176–180.

18 Rufener, L. et al. (2009) *Haemonchus contortus* acetylcholine receptors of the DEG-3 subfamily and their role in sensitivity to monepantel. *PLoS Pathog.*, **5**, e1000380.

19 Rufener, L. et al. (2010) Monepantel allosterically activates DEG-3/DES-2 channels of the gastrointestinal nematode *Haemonchus contortus*. *Mol. Pharmacol.*, **78**, 895–902.

20 Qian, H., Martin, R.J., and Robertson, A.P. (2006) Pharmacology of N-, L- and B-subtypes of nematode nAChR resolved at

the single-channel level in *Ascaris suum*. *FASEB J.*, **20**, 2606–2608.
21. Zinser, E.W. et al. (2002) Anthelmintic paraherquamides are cholinergic antagonists in gastrointestinal nematodes and mammals. *J. Vet. Pharmacol. Ther.*, **25**, 241–250.
22. Cully, D.F. et al. (1994) Cloning of an avermectin-sensitive glutamate-gated chloride channel from *Caenorhabditis elegans*. *Nature*, **371**, 707–711.
23. Forrester, S.G. et al. (2003) *Haemonchus contortus*: HcGluCla expressed in Xenopus oocytes forms a glutamate-gated ion channel that is activated by ibotenate and the antiparasitic drug ivermectin. *Mol. Biochem. Parasitol.*, **129**, 115–121.
24. Forrester, S.G. and Siddiqui, S.Z. (2008) A novel member of the ligand-gated chloride channel gene family from *Haemonchus contortus*. *Parasitology*, **135**, 539–545.
25. Rao, V.T. et al (2010) Characterization of a novel tyramine-gated chloride channel from *Haemonchus contortus*. *Mol. Biochem. Parasitol.*, **173**, 64–68.
26. Rao, V.T. et al. (2011) Localisation of serotonin and dopamine in *Haemonchus contortus*. *Int. J. Parasitol.*, **41**, 249–254.
27. Rao, V.T. et al. (2009) A dopamine-gated ion channel (HcGGR3*) from *Haemonchus contortus* is expressed in the cervical papillae and is associated with macrocyclic lactone resistance. *Mol. Biochem. Parasitol.*, **166**, 54–61.
28. Siddiqui, S.Z. et al. (2010) An UNC-49 GABA receptor subunit from the parasitic nematode *Haemonchus contortus* is associated with enhanced GABA sensitivity in nematode heteromeric channels. *J. Neurochem.*, **113**, 1113–1122.
29. Mareno, Y. et al. (2010) Ivermectin disrupts the function of the excretory-secretory apparatus in microfilariae of *Brugia malayi*. *Proc. Natl. Acad. Sci. USA*, **46**, 20120–20125.
30. Horoszok, L. et al. (2001) GLC-3: a novel fipronil and BIDN-sensitive, but picrotoxinin-insensitive, L-glutamate-gated chloride channel subunit from *Caenorhabditis elegans*. *Br. J. Pharmacol.*, **132**, 1247–1254.
31. Jagannathan, S. et al. (1999) Ligand-gated chloride channel subunits encoded by the *Haemonchus contortus* and *Ascaris suum* orthologues of the *Caenorhabditis elegans gbr-2 (avr-14)* gene. *Mol. Biochem. Parasitol.*, **103**, 129–140.
32. Cully, D.F. et al. (1996) Identification of a *Drosophila melanogaster* glutamate-gated chloride channel sensitive to the antiparasitic agent avermectin. *J. Biol. Chem.*, **271**, 20187–20191.
33. Laughton, D.L., Lunt, G.G., and Wolstenholme, A.J. (1997) Alternative splicing of a *Caenorhabditis elegans* gene produces two novel inhibitory amino acid receptor subunits with identical ligand binding domains but different ion channels. *Gene*, **201**, 119–125.
34. Dent, J.A. et al. (2000) The genetics of ivermectin resistance in *Caenorhabditis elegans*. *Proc. Natl. Acad. Sci. USA*, **97**, 2674–2679.
35. Barnes, T.M. and Hekimi, S. (1997) The *Caenorhabditis elegans* avermectin resistance and anesthetic response gene *unc-9* encodes a member of a protein family implicated in electrical coupling of excitable cells. *J. Neurochem.*, **69**, 2251–2260.
36. Vassilatis, D.K. et al. (1997) Evolutionary relationship of the ligand-gated ion channels and the avermectin-sensitive, glutamate-gated chloride channels. *J. Mol. Evol.*, **44**, 501–508.
37. Martin, R.J. (1982) Electrophysiological effects of piperazine and diethylcarbamazine on *Ascaris suum* somatic muscle. *Br. J. Pharmacol.*, **77**, 255–265.
38. Martin, R.J. et al. (1996) Anthelmintic actions of the cyclicdepsipeptide PF1022A and its electrophysiological effects on muscle cells of *Ascaris suum*. *Pesticide Sci.*, **38**, 343–349.
39. Guest, M. et al. (2007) The calcium-activated potassium channel, SLO-1, is required for the action of the novel cyclo-octadepsipeptide anthelmintic, emodepside, in *Caenorhabditis elegans*. *Int. J. Parasitol.*, **37**, 1577–1588.

40 Crisford, A. et al. (2011) Selective toxicity of the anthelmintic emodepside revealed by heterologous expression of human KCNMA1 in *Caenorhabditis elegans*. *Mol. Pharmacol.*, **79**, 1031–1043.

41 Verma, S., Robertson, A.P., and Martin, R.J. (2009) Effects of SDPNFLRF-amide (PF1) on voltage-activated currents in *Ascaris suum* muscle. *Int. J. Parasitol.*, **39**, 315–326.

42 Willson, J. et al. (2003) The effect of the anthelmintic emodepside at the neuromuscular junction of the parasitic nematode *Ascaris suum*. *Parasitology*, **126**, 79–86.

43 Buxton, S.K., Neveu, C., Charvet, C.L., Robertson, A.P., and Martin, R.J. (2011) On the mode of action of emodepside: effects on membrane potential and voltage-activated currents in *Ascaris suum*. *Br. J. Pharmacol.*, **164**, 453–470.

44 Lacey, E. and Prichard, R.K. (1986) Interactions of benzimidazoles (BZ) with tubulin from BZ-sensitive and BZ-resistant isolates of *Haemonchus contortus*. *Mol. Biochem. Parasitol.*, **19**, 171–181.

45 MacDonald, L.M. et al. (2004) Characterisation of benzimidazole binding with recombinant tubulin from *Giardia duodenalis*, *Encephalitozoon intestinalis*, and *Cryptosporidium parvum*. *Mol. Biochem. Parasitol.*, **138**, 89–96.

46 Fukushige, T. et al. (1999) MEC-12, an alpha-tubulin required for touch sensitivity in *C. elegans*. *J. Cell Sci.*, **112**, 395–403.

47 Gogonea, C.B. et al. (1999) Computational prediction of the three-dimensional structures for the *Caenorhabditis elegans* tubulin family. *J. Mol. Graph. Model.*, **17**, 90–100. 126–130.

48 Phillips, J.B. et al. (2004) Roles for two partially redundant alpha-tubulins during mitosis in early *Caenorhabditis elegans* embryos. *Cell Motil. Cytoskeleton*, **58**, 112–126.

49 Lu, C. and Mains, P.E. (2005) Mutations of a redundant alpha-tubulin gene affect *Caenorhabditis elegans* early embryonic cleavage via MEI-1/katanin-dependent and -independent pathways. *Genetics*, **170**, 115–126.

50 Lu, C., Srayko, M., and Mains, P.E. (2004) The *Caenorhabditis elegans* microtubule-severing complex MEI-1/MEI-2 katanin interacts differently with two superficially redundant beta-tubulin isotypes. *Mol. Biol. Cell*, **15**, 142–150.

51 Baran, R. et al. (2010) Motor neuron synapse and axon defects in a *C. elegans* alpha-tubulin mutant. *PLoS One*, **5**, e9655.

52 Driscoll, M. et al. (1989) Genetic and molecular analysis of a *Caenorhabditis elegans* beta-tubulin that conveys benzimidazole sensitivity. *J. Cell Biol.*, **109**, 2993–3003.

53 Savage, C. et al. (1989) *mec-7* is a beta-tubulin gene required for the production of 15-protofilament microtubules in *Caenorhabditis elegans*. *Genes Dev.*, **3**, 870–881.

54 Luduena, R.F. (1993) Are tubulin isotypes functionally significant. *Mol. Biol. Cell*, **4**, 445–457.

55 Geary, T.G. et al. (1992) Three beta-tubulin cDNAs from the parasitic nematode *Haemonchus contortus*. *Mol. Biochem. Parasitol.*, **50**, 295–306.

56 Van den Bossche, H. et al. (1983) Alterations in rat liver mitochondria caused by *Fasciola hepatica*. *Contrib. Microbiol. Immunol.*, **7**, 30–38.

57 Rothwell, J.T. and Sangster, N.C. (1996) The effects of closantel treatment on the ultrastructure of *Haemonchus contortus*. *Int. J. Parasitol.*, **26**, 49–57.

58 Gloeckner, C. et al. (2010) Repositioning of an existing drug for the neglected tropical disease Onchocerciasis. *Proc. Natl. Acad. Sci. USA*, **107**, 3424–3429.

59 Garner, A.L. et al. (2011) Design, synthesis, and biological activities of closantel analogues: structural promiscuity and its impact on *Onchocerca volvulus*. *J. Med. Chem.*, **54**, 3963–3972.

60 Hawking, F., Sewell, P., and Thurston, J.P. (1948) Mode of action of hetrazan in filariasis. *Lancet*, **ii**, 730.

61 Terada, M. and Sano, M. (1986) Effects of diethylcarbamazine on the motility of *Angiostrongylus cantonensis* and *Dirofilaria immitis*. *Z. Parasitenkd.*, **72**, 375–385.

62 McGarry, H.F., Plant, L.D., and Taylor, M.J. (2005) Diethylcarbamazine activity against *Brugia malayi* microfilariae is dependent on inducible nitric-oxide synthase and the cyclooxygenase pathway. *Filaria J.*, **4**, 4.

63 Queto, T. *et al.* (2010) Inducible nitric oxide synthase/CD95L-dependent suppression of pulmonary and bone marrow eosinophilia by diethylcarbamazine. *Am. J. Respir. Crit. Care Med.*, **181**, 429–437.

64 Anderson, V.R. and Curran, M.P. (2007) Nitazoxanide: a review of its use in the treatment of gastrointestinal infections. *Drugs*, **67**, 1947–1047.

65 Hoffman, P.S. *et al.* (2007) Antiparasitic drug nitazoxanide inhibits the pyruvate oxidoreductases of *Helicobacter pylori*, selected anaerobic bacteria and parasites, and *Campylobacter jejuni*. *Antimicrob. Agents Chemother.*, **51**, 868–76.

66 Boray, J.C. *et al.* (1997) Nitroscanate a new broad-spectrum anthelmintic against nematodes and cestodes of dogs and cats. *Aust. Vet. J.*, **55**, 45–53.

67 Voge., E. and Bueding, E. (1980) *Schistosoma mansoni*: tegmental surface alterations induced by sub-curative does of the schistosmocide, amoscanate. *Exp. Parasitol.*, **50**, 251–259.

68 Kohler, P., Davies, K.P., and Zahner, H. (1992) Activity, mechanism of action and pharmacokinetics of 2-tert-butylbenzothiazole and CGP 6140 (amocarzine) antifilarial drugs. *Acta Trop.*, **51**, 195–211.

69 Sangster, N.C. *et al.* (1989) Binding of [^{3}H] *m*-aminolevamisole to receptors in levamisole-susceptible and -resistant *Haemonchus contortus*. *Int. J. Parasitol.*, **28**, 707–717.

70 Kopp, S.R. *et al.* (2006) High-level pyrantel resistance in the hookworm *Ancylsotoma caninum*. *Vet. Parasitol.*, **143**, 299–304.

71 Robertson, A.P., Bjorn, H.E., and Martin, R.J. (1999) Resistance to levamisole resolved at the single-channel level. *FASEB J.*, **13**, 749–760.

72 Saragoza, P.A. *et al.* (2003) Identification of an alternatively processed nicotinic receptor alpha7 subunit RNA in mouse brain. *Brain Res. Mol. Brain Res.*, **117**, 15–26.

73 Martin, R.J. and Robertson, A.P. (2007) Mode of action of levamisole and pyrantel, anthelmintic resistance, E153 and Q57. *Parasitology*, **134**, 1093–1104.

74 Beech, R.N. *et al.* (2010) Anthelmintic resistance: markers for resistance, or susceptibility? *Parasitology*, **138**, 160–74.

75 Ardelli, B.F. *et al.* (2009) A comparison of the effects of ivermectin and moxidectin on the nematode *Caenorhabditis elegans*. *Vet. Parasitol.*, **165**, 96–108.

76 Merino, G. *et al.* (2009) Natural allelic variants of bovine ATP-binding cassette transporter ABCG2: increased activity of the Ser581 variant and development of tools for the discovery of new ABCG2 inhibitors. *Drug Metab. Dispos.*, **37**, 5–9.

77 Mottier, MD. and Prichard, R.K. (2008) Genetic analysis of a relationship between macrocyclic lactone and benzimidazole anthelmintic selection on *Haemonchus contortus*. *Pharmacogenet. Genomics*, **18**, 129–140.

78 Kwa, M.S.G. *et al.* (1995) Beta-tubulin genes from the parasitic nematode *Haemonchus contortus* modulate drug-resistance in *Caenorhabditis elegans*. *J. Mol. Biol.*, **246**, 500–510.

79 Kavallaris, M. (2010) Microtubules and resistance to tubulin-binding agents. *Nat. Rev. Cancer*, **10**, 194–204.

15
Drugs and Targets to Perturb the Symbiosis of *Wolbachia* and Filarial Nematodes

Mark J. Taylor[*], *Louise Ford, Achim Hoerauf, Ken Pfarr, Jeremy M. Foster, Sanjay Kumar, and Barton E. Slatko*

Abstract

A novel approach to the treatment of filarial nematodes has been to target the *Wolbachia* bacterial endosymbionts, which are essential for nematode development, embryogenesis, and survival. A 4- to 6-week course of doxycycline (200 mg/kg/day) results in the long-term sterility and ultimate death of the adult parasite. In addition to its potent antiparasitic effects, doxycycline therapy reduces the severity of clinical disease (hydrocele and lymphedema). The therapeutic effect of targeting *Wolbachia* on microfilariae and adult worms is slow and prolonged, delivering a good safety profile while both avoiding parasite- or *Wolbachia*-mediated inflammatory adverse reactions, and producing a sustained interruption of transmission. The use of doxycycline in widespread community-based control is compromised by the logistics of lengthy courses of treatment, and contraindications in children and pregnant women. To overcome these barriers, the Anti-*Wolbachia* Consortium (A·WOL), was established to optimize current regimens, and discover and develop new anti-*Wolbachia* drugs to deliver therapy compatible with mass drug administration (MDA) approaches. The potent sterilizing and macrofilaricidal activity of antiwolbachial therapy would greatly reduce MDA program timeframes, which may be required in regions where sustained delivery is problematic or in the event of reduced efficacy of currently used drugs. A·WOL has established screening approaches to exploit focused anti-infective and diversity-based libraries of existing and novel drugs and natural products. Target discovery has ranked essential genes to guide library selection and selected key pathways and enzymes thought to be involved in the symbiotic relationship for small-molecule library screening. Antiwolbachial therapy has become the most effective way to treat individuals with onchocerciasis and lymphatic filariasis, and the hope is that A·WOL can deliver a new generation of drugs and regimens needed to ensure the elimination of onchocerciasis and lymphatic filariasis.

[*] Corresponding Author

Introduction

Diseases due to filarial nematodes inflict serious public health problems throughout tropical communities [1]. The major disease-causing species include those responsible for lymphatic filariasis, *Wuchereria bancrofti* and *Brugia malayi*, and onchocerciasis, *Onchocerca volvulus*, which together infect more than 150 million people – ranking filariasis as one of the leading causes of global morbidity.

The search for a safe macrofilaricidal drug for filarial nematodes has been a sought-after goal for the past 35 years, but without the successful delivery of a drug suitable for large-scale use in endemic countries [2]. Existing drugs principally target the larval microfilarial stage of the parasites and so require sustained delivery with high treatment coverage to endemic communities in order to break the transmission cycle of the long-lived (10–14 years) adult worms (Table 15.1). The growing evidence for resistance to ivermectin [3–5] has refocused the need and urgency for new and alternative drugs, particularly for onchocerciasis, which is solely reliant on ivermectin.

In the past 10 years, a promising alternative approach has been to target the bacterial symbiont, *Wolbachia*, which is essential for larval and embryonic growth and development, and the fertility and survival of adult worms [6]. Anti-*Wolbachia* therapy delivers superior therapeutic outcomes compared to all standard antifilarial treatments for individual patients. These outcomes can be achieved with existing registered drugs (e.g., doxycycline) that are cheap, available in endemic communities, and have well-known safety profiles. Anti-*Wolbachia* treatment is safe because it is slowly microfilaricidal or macrofilaricidal, thus avoiding the risk of severe adverse events due to coinfections with *Loa loa* (a filarial species that is free of *Wolbachia*).

The use of doxycycline in widespread community-based control is compromised by the logistics of a relatively lengthy course of treatment, and contraindications in children under 8 years and pregnancy. These barriers have stimulated the formation of the "Anti-*Wolbachia* Consortium" (A·WOL, www.a-wol.com), which aims to search for new drugs active against *Wolbachia* that are suitable for community-directed mass drug administration (MDA). A secondary goal is to optimize regimens of existing drugs and repurposed registered drugs for use in more restricted populations: (i) communities that are not covered by existing control strategies or for which sustained MDA is compromised, (ii) communities in which current drugs demonstrate reduced efficacy, and (iii) communities in which the risk of severe adverse events to ivermectin treatment due to *L. loa* coinfections restricts existing strategies. Finally, optimized regimens of existing drugs would facilitate programmatic endgame "mop-up" phases, where elimination is the goal.

Anti-*Wolbachia* Treatment as an Effective Antifilarial Therapy

In their initial description of intracellular bacteria within *O. volvulus*, Kozek and Marroquin [7] speculated on whether these endosymbionts could serve as a chemotherapeutic target with macrofilaricidal potential. The prophecy took more than two

Table 15.1 Current recommended treatment strategies for MDA, IDA, and morbidity control and treatment [1].

	MDA		IDA	Morbidity control and treatment
	Africa	Rest of world		
Lymphatic filariasis, *Wuchereria bancrofti*, *Brugia malayi*, and *Brugia timori*	Ivermectin and albendazole for at least 5 years	Diethylcarbamazine and albendazole for at least 5 years	Diethylcarbamazine (with or without albendazole) single dose treatment[a] or 12-day course of 6 mg/kg/day; or doxycycline 200 mg/day for 4 weeks plus ivermectin (or without ivermectin if risk of serious adverse events with *L. loa*)	Lymphedema: hygiene physiotherapy, doxycycline 200 mg/day for 6 weeks; hydrocoele: surgical hydrocelectomy, doxycycline 200 mg/day for 6 weeks; tropical pulmonary eosinophilia: doxycycline 200 mg/day for 4 weeks plus ivermectin
Onchocerciasis	Ivermectin every year for at least 15–17 years	Ivermectin twice every year until transmission has been interrupted	Ivermectin;[a] doxycycline 200 mg/day for 4 weeks or 100 mg/day for 6 weeks[b] followed by one ivermectin single dose after 4–6 months; or doxycycline 200 mg/day for 6 weeks[c] followed by ivermectin single dose after 4–6 months (or without ivermectin if risk of serious adverse events with *L. loa*)	Same as individual drug administration for onchocerciasis

a) If patient continues to live in endemic area or is less than 9 years of age (contraindication of doxycycline).
b) If interruption in embryogenesis and cessation of microfilariae production is desired.
c) If a strong macrofilaricidal effect is desired.

decades to reach fruition when animals treated with tetracycline led to the depletion of *Wolbachia* from *B. pahangi* and *Dirofilaria immitis* (dog heart worm), and subsequently resulted in embryonic defects in the parasites [8]. The effect of tetracycline is specific to the endobacteria as filarial species that do not contain *Wolbachia* are unaffected after tetracycline treatment [9] and the observed detrimental effects are always preceded by the loss of *Wolbachia* [10, 11]. Several studies with animal filariae and infections of human filariae in animals have shown *in vitro* and *in vivo* the antifilarial effects of a short list of antirickettsial drugs, with the most effective being the tetracyclines and rifampicin (reviewed in [6]).

The effects of depleting *Wolbachia* are not limited to one stage of the life cycle. As noted above, embryogenesis is blocked and embryos degenerate when filarial-infected animals are treated with tetracycline. Oogenesis is also affected, resulting in infertile worms [9–12]. As the worms become infertile and residual microfilaria are cleared from the blood or skin either naturally or with microfilaricidal drugs, the infected person presents with a sustained amicrofilarial state [12–14] and transmission is interrupted over the longer term. Although the first-stage larvae of filarial nematodes can survive without *Wolbachia*, their ability to develop within their arthropod vector is severely limited [15, 16], with female worms being more sensitive to the loss of the endosymbionts [17]. Larval development within the mammalian host is also impaired, resulting in stunted worms that fail to develop into adults [9]. The most dramatic outcome is the killing of adult worms after the depletion of *Wolbachia*. Unlike the effects on larval and embryonic development, which occur soon after *Wolbachia* depletion, macrofilaricidal activity observed in human trials occurs after 12 months for lymphatic filariasis and 18–27 months for onchocerciasis. This outcome was first seen in cattle infected with *O. ochengi* that had received a protracted course of tetracycline for an unrelated infection [11]. A comprehensive series of phase II field trials have confirmed the macrofilaricidal effects of *Wolbachia* depletion in *W. bancrofti* [13, 18–20] and *O. volvulus* [21–23].

The preceding studies established anti-*Wolbachia* therapy as a valid treatment for the major filarial infections causing human disease. Additionally, the life stages responsible for pathogenesis of onchocerciasis (microfilariae) and lymphatic filariasis (adults) are successfully targeted by doxycycline. *Wolbachia* endosymbionts are unique drug targets for filarial disease control and doxycycline offers the best macrofilaricidal treatment to date, thus adding to the limited arsenal of antifilarial therapeutics.

Indications for Doxycycline as an Antifilarial Treatment

The phase II trials stated above [13, 18–23] provided anti-*Wolbachia* therapy with or without the addition of the classical antifilarial drugs (diethylcarbamazine and ivermectin with or without albendazole). They also demonstrated that addition of doxycycline leads to higher antifilarial efficacy against lymphatic filariasis, onchocerciasis, and *Mansonella perstans* [24]. Treatment of lymphatic filariasis with 200 mg/day doxycycline for 3 weeks plus a single dose of 6 mg/kg diethylcarbamazine (in India) or for 4 weeks plus a single-dose of 200 μg/kg ivermectin plus 400 mg albendazole (in Ghana) achieved more than 90% macrofilaricidal effects scored as the proportion of male patients who lost worm nests in the scrotum as monitored by ultrasound [19, 20]. For onchocerciasis, treatment with 200 mg/day doxycycline for 4 weeks or with 100 mg/day for 5 weeks led to sterile female worms, effectively clearing the patients of microfilariae [21, 22]. The macrofilaricidal effect is dose- and time-dependent with 200 mg/day doxycycline for 6 weeks showing the greatest macrofilaricidal rate of 60% [21, 23]. By subtracting newly acquired worms that had infected the participants between the long follow-up periods, the macrofilaricidal effect of doxycycline treatment increased to 70% [25].

Such an effective treatment would warrant that doctors, who are obliged to provide the best possible treatment to their patients, include doxycycline in antifilarial treatment of lymphatic filariasis, onchocerciasis, and mansonellosis patients who privately seek out treatment in clinics because of disease symptoms. This "individual drug administration" (IDA) concept has been introduced to underpin the requirements of individuals (whose number will rise as both incomes and health care systems improve in endemic countries) as compared to MDA programs that aim to reduce or eliminate disease transmission (rather than cure patients) at the best possible cost-to-benefit ratio. Of particular note is the fact that doxycycline has so far been the only lymphatic filariasis treatment to reduce the dilation of lymph vessels, and lead to amelioration of lymphedema [18] and a reduction in hydroceles [26].

Doxycycline is contraindicated in children and pregnant/lactating women, restricting coverage of the target population in filaria-endemic areas. Rifampicin has equivalent activity in *Wolbachia* depletion and inhibition of maturation of L3 to adult worms as doxycycline in the *Litomosoides sigmodontis* mouse model (Specht *et al.*, unpublished). Pilot studies with rifampicin have demonstrated the loss of *Wolbachia* and infertility of adult worms in onchocerciasis patients [27] – an observation that a larger, randomized, placebo controlled noninferiority trial will test. As rifampicin can be administered to children, it may be possible to include children in anti-*Wolbachia* treatment schemes to eliminate filariasis.

Although very successful, a 6-week regimen with doxycycline has been viewed as being impractical given the poor health resources in endemic communities. This position has been elegantly countered by a study in Cameroon where the feasibility of large-scale distribution of doxycycline for the treatment of onchocerciasis was tested [28]. In this study, a community-directed delivery of a 6-week course of 100 mg/day doxycycline in five health areas co-endemic for *O. volvulus* and *L. loa* was introduced. In total, 21 355 individuals were recruited, of which 17 519 were eligible for treatment and 12 936 received doxycycline – a therapeutic coverage of 73.8% of the eligible population. At the end of the 6 weeks, 97.5% of the 12 936 who had started treatment had complied with the full course of treatment as assessed by directly observed intake of doxycycline by community health implementers and staff of the front-line health facilities. The study demonstrated that with the necessary empowerment of the target population, advocacy at the national, regional, and health district levels, and the engagement of community health implementers and front-line health facilities, a multiweek regimen is not an impediment to doxycycline mass distribution.

Search for Second-Generation Anti-*Wolbachia* Drugs

The therapeutic success of doxycycline stimulated the search for alternative drugs with anti-*Wolbachia* activity, and which could be used in MDA control programs by overcoming the contraindications of doxycycline and reducing the timeframe of drug delivery. These goals formed the basis of the A·WOL consortium – a group of academic laboratories and pharmaceutical company partners established to discover and develop new and existing anti-*Wolbachia* drugs.

A·WOL Drug Regimen Refinement

The first objective was to refine regimens of drugs with known anti-*Wolbachia* efficacy (doxycycline and rifampicin) to provide alternative treatment for use within the timeframes of existing MDA programs. Trials on both lymphatic filariasis and onchocerciasis were designed to test combinations of doxycycline and rifampicin delivered in shorter timeframes (3 weeks, 2 weeks, and 10 days) and lower doses of doxycycline (100 versus 200 mg/day) to provide an optimized regimen. These can then be deployed in restricted populations, for which current program strategies are compromised (e.g., in *L. loa* coendemic areas) or where existing drugs show evidence of reduced efficacy (e.g., Ghana). These regimens could also be deployed in the MDA program end-game that would treat the remaining cases of infection prior to elimination of the disease. Follow-up sampling has been completed and analyses of the trial's outcomes are currently underway (www.controlled-trials.com; ISRCTN15216778 and ISRCTN68861628).

A·WOL Assay Development and Screening Strategy

The A·WOL screening strategy uses a pipeline of approaches (Figure 15.1) optimized to identify and validate anti-*Wolbachia* compounds by screening of both focused anti-infective and diversity-based libraries of existing and novel drugs and natural products.

In order to screen these large compound libraries a *Wolbachia* cell-based assay was developed as the primary *in vitro* drug-screening tool. This validated assay, which has been adapted to automated high-throughput screening, and represents a rapid, sensitive, and efficient assay for screening chemical libraries, utilizes a *Wolbachia*-containing *Aedes albopictus* cell line (C6/36 Wp) [29], in a 96-well format, with a quantitative polymerase chain reaction (qPCR) readout to quantify the *Wolbachia* 16S rRNA gene copy number following treatment [30]. Hits from this primary *in vitro* cell-based screening assay are selected based on their log drop depletion of *Wolbachia*, reproducibility, and, if using known drugs, the target product profile as defined by A·WOL to include oral formulation, and the safe use in children and pregnancy. These selected hits are then moved down the screening pipeline into both *in vitro* and *in vivo* nematode screening. *In vitro* nematode screening, using either adult male

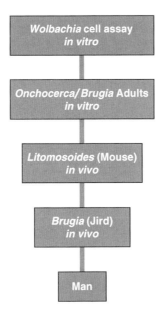

Figure 15.1 A·WOL screening strategy.

O. gutturosa [31] or both male and female *B. malayi* [30], is performed to verify that hits are effective against nematode *Wolbachia*. These *in vitro* screens also provide a valuable tool to identify compounds that have no direct antinematode activity yet show significant reductions in *Wolbachia* load. For *in vivo* nematode screening, established animal models of filarial infection are utilized, and include *L. sigmodontis* in mice [9] and *B. malayi* in Mongolian jirds [32]. For all *in vivo* models, the reduction of *Wolbachia* load following treatment is measured by qPCR. The primary *in vivo* screening model with *L. sigmodontis* allows for rapid screening of compounds, and yields a visible and quantifiable phenotype of larvae with retarded growth (Figure 15.2). The secondary *in vivo* model with *B. malayi* uses a human filarial nematode, and evaluates macrofilaricidal activity, effects on female fertility, and reductions in *Wolbachia* load.

A·WOL Library Screening

Registered Drug Library Screening

Following the validation of the primary cell-based screen the first priority was to screen approved human drug pharmacopeia for potential repurposing for anti-*Wolbachia* activity. Repurposing or repositioning of drugs provides a less risky route to drug discovery given that candidates will already have well-known safety and pharmacokinetic profiles [33, 34], and could provide a cost- and time-effective strategy to identify a novel A·WOL therapeutic. By screening 2664 compounds from the

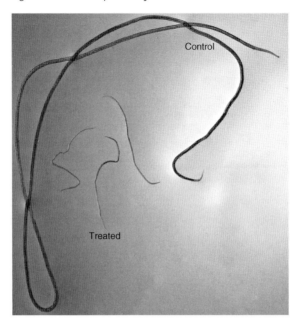

Figure 15.2 Stunted *L. sigmodontis* larvae following anti-*Wolbachia* treatment with a 14-day course of doxycycline compared to untreated control worms.

human drug pharmacopeia, this strategy identified 121 hits that had anti-*Wolbachia* activity; 69 of these were orally available from different diverse drug categories (Table 15.2), with nine compounds being more effective than doxycycline. Several drugs have progressed further along the screening pipeline into *in vitro* nematode assays and *in vivo* screening models. The most advanced lead has shown an increase in potency of 50% compared to doxycycline in the secondary *in vivo* screen. As many of these hits are drugs already in human use for other diseases, they represent an opportunity to quickly develop alternative chemotherapy for filarial diseases.

Table 15.2 Hits from the human drug pharmacopeia screen grouped into different drug classes.

Drug class	Number of hits	Percent of hits (%)
Anti-infectives	24	35
Antipsychotics/anticonvulsants	8	12
Natural products/nutraceuticals	7	10
Receptor antagonists	6	9
Antihypertensives	6	9
Others	6	6
Muscle relaxants	5	7
Nonsteroidal anti-inflammatory drugs	4	6
Antineoplastic agents	4	6

Focused Anti-Infective Library Screening

Focused anti-infective libraries have been sourced from several pharmaceutical companies and include near-to-market lead candidate drugs or drug class derivatives, which are selected from known and bioinformatically predicted essential gene targets. Focused anti-infective library screening has, thus far, involved A·WOL *in vitro* screening of 3062 novel compounds from five chemical libraries. To date this has generated 184 diverse hit compounds, a number of which have progressed further into the screening funnel. Encouragingly, there is a good agreement between the reduction in *Wolbachia* load in the cell-based and *O. gutturosa in vitro* assays with no effect on worm motility. This suggests that the hits do not directly effect the nematode (and are, therefore, predicted to avoid direct parasite-mediated adverse events). Notably, the ability to identify hit compounds from these focused libraries, which are effective at reducing *Wolbachia* load and have improved efficacy over doxycycline, is highly supportive of the long-term goal to identify A·WOL new chemical entities (NCEs).

Diversity-Based Library Screening

In order to expand the capacity of novel NCE screening and to explore novel anti-*Wolbachia* chemical space, A·WOL screening has included large diversity-based libraries. Two diversity-based chemical libraries consisting in total of more than 60 000 compounds have entered the primary cell-based assay screen. Hits from these libraries will be tested for narrow-spectrum activity against *Wolbachia* in order to produce targeted treatments that do not overlap with other antibacterial treatment domains.

A·WOL Target Discovery

A final objective of the A·WOL consortium is the identification and validation of new *Wolbachia*-specific targets for entry into the drug discovery pipeline. In the absence of any tools for the genetic analysis of *Wolbachia*, researchers have devised bioinformatic and comparative genomic approaches that take advantage of the completed genome sequences of *Wolbachia* from *B. malayi* (*w*Bm) [35], *B. malayi* [36], and humans [37] to predict the essential gene repertoire of *w*Bm and to uncover candidate drug targets.

An essentiality score for each predicted gene of *w*Bm was determined by two separate approaches [38]. The first method compared each gene to entries in the Database of Essential Genes (DEG) [39], a collection of around 5000 experimentally identified essential genes from 15 different bacterial species, to predict essential genes that are mostly conserved across the bacterial domain. The second approach used phyletic conservation across members of the order Rickettsiales, to which *Wolbachia* belongs, in order to highlight genes that are well conserved and, thus, likely to be essential. Conservation of genes in these rickettsial genomes that are undergoing reductive evolution underscores their importance. A ranked essentiality list was produced by each method, and showed complementary and partially overlapping sets of wBm genes. A gene identified by both methods has a particularly high likelihood of being essential. A gene predicted essential by comparison to DEG would offer the potential to develop a broad-spectrum antibiotic, whereas a gene identified only by phyletic conservation could lead to an inhibitor with a more restricted activity profile. Many of the top-ranking genes fall into classes of genes targeted by current antibiotics and are in functional categories predicted to be essential for bacterial growth [38]. For example, DNA gyrase and topoisomerase family proteins were well represented and are known targets of quinolones [40], and DNA-directed RNA polymerase is the target of rifampicin [41]. Certain tRNA synthetases also ranked highly and are the targets of a variety of compounds [42]. The high essentiality prediction of such known targets validates the computational approach. The ranked lists can be further curated to prioritize candidate drug targets by filtering for genes with no similarity to human proteins, for example. The druggability of the wBm proteins was addressed by comparing them to known protein targets contained within the DrugBank database, a collection of around 5000 US Food and Drug Administration-approved small-molecule drugs and compounds with details of their protein-binding partners and relevant chemical and pharmacological data [43]. This analysis correlated well with the essential gene predictions, and revealed classes of wBm proteins that appear to be essential and druggable [38]. The ranked essential gene list and druggability data have been used by A·WOL to guide selection of focused library compounds supplied by several leading pharmaceutical companies.

Analysis of the wBm genome suggested *Wolbachia* might provide heme, flavin adenine dinucleotide, riboflavin, and nucleotides to the *B. malayi* host, which cannot synthesize these molecules *de novo* [35, 36]. Disruption of the symbiotic association through targeting *Wolbachia* enzymes involved in the biosynthesis of these molecules could offer new avenues towards filarial control. For example, two enzymes of the wBm heme biosynthetic pathway, aminolevulinic acid dehydratase (ALAD) and ferrochelatase, have been evaluated as candidate targets based on their low conservation to the corresponding human proteins, their distinct biochemical properties, and their sensitivities to inhibitors relative to the human enzymes [44]. As ALAD is not found in the genome of *B. malayi* and is significantly different from the human ortholog [44], it was subjected to both aptamer and chemical library screening as part of the A·WOL program. Screening of aptamers uses short nucleic acid ligands, most often RNA, that fold into three-dimensional structures and specifically bind to proteins with a high probability of inhibition of function (reviewed in [45]). By screening a small-molecule library, displacement of the aptamer can identify drugs or compounds that mimic the inhibitory action of the aptamer without performing an enzymatic assay [46, 47].

Comparative genomic analyses and examination of metabolic pathway maps can indicate key differences between processes that are otherwise conserved between *Wolbachia* and humans, leading to the identification of additional potential drug targets in *Wolbachia*. For example, despite the ubiquity of glycolysis/gluconeogensis in almost all prokaryotes and eukaryotes, the pathway contains several nonhomologous isofunctional enzymes (NISEs), alternative enzymes, and highly variant forms. The interconversion of 3-phosphoglycerate and 2-phosphoglycerate is catalyzed by cofactor-dependent phosphoglycerate mutase (dPGM) in mammals, whereas in *Wolbachia*, a cofactor-independent PGM (iPGM) is used. These PGM NISEs have no similarity in primary sequence, three-dimensional structure, or catalytic mechanism, making the *Wolbachia* iPGM enzyme an attractive drug target [48]. Similarly, the final step in glycolysis is catalyzed by pyruvate kinase in humans, but by a distinct alternative enzyme, pyruvate phosphate dikinase (PPDK), in *Wolbachia* [49]. PPDK is not found in mammals. The *Wolbachia* PPDK enzyme has also been included in both aptamer-based and conventional library screening as part of A·WOL.

To date, there has been no biochemical evidence for a cell wall in *Wolbachia*, yet the *w*Bm genome predicts all the genes required for biosynthesis of lipid II – the monomer that is polymerized into peptidoglycan [35]. This pathway is active and sensitive to at least one antibiotic, fosfomycin, that blocks synthesis of lipid II [50]. Akin to *Chlamydia*, lipid II biosynthesis appears to be important despite the apparent lack of a cell wall. At best, *Wolbachia* has a rudimentary or very atypical cell wall structure. This structure may provide an anchor point between the inner and outer membranes for outer membrane proteins. Alternatively, the machineries of cell division and cell wall biosynthesis have components in common, and it has been proposed that lipid II may be involved in cell division [50]. The *Wolbachia* lipid II pathway is being pursued as an antifilarial target as it has been shown to be both functional and sensitive to specific inhibition [50].

Lipoproteins are essential structural and functional components of bacteria, and those from *Wolbachia* are potent stimulators of the innate and adaptive inflammatory pathogenesis of filarial disease [51]. Analysis of the *w*Bm genome indicates that the *Wolbachia* lipoproteins are only diacylated because the necessary *lgt* and *lspA* genes are predicted, whereas the third gene responsible for triacylation, *lnt*, appears to be absent. This is consistent with recognition by the diacyl-lipoprotein receptor complex Toll-like receptor 2 and 6 [51]. The *Wolbachia* prolipoprotein signal peptidase II (LspA) was shown to be functional, and both an arthropod cell line containing *Wolbachia* from *A. albopictus* and adult *B. malayi* were sensitive to inhibition with a known LspA inhibitor, globomycin [30]. As a result, drugs targeting the *Wolbachia* lipoprotein biosynthetic pathway are being evaluated within the A·WOL framework. The *Wolbachia* chaperone protein DnaK is also considered as a target within A·WOL as it shows differential sensitivity to inhibitors of the *Escherichia coli* ortholog, suggesting that the identification of inhibitors with selected specificity for the *Wolbachia* protein is feasible.

Further studies that address the biological basis of the mutualistic association between *Wolbachia* and its filarial nematode hosts are underway, and are expected to unravel the mechanisms that sustain the relationship, revealing additional opportunities for disrupting the symbiosis and, as a consequence, producing antifilarial activity. Many of these genes are expected to be critical for *Wolbachia* and maintenance of its symbiotic status, and will also include those filarial gene products that interact with *Wolbachia* proteins. Their identification will increase the number of candidate *Wolbachia* targets that can be evaluated for development of antifilarial therapies.

Conclusions

Since its inception in 2007 the A·WOL consortium has made significant progress towards its goals of identifying new and improved drugs with activity against *Wolbachia* that could potentially be used in widespread MDA programs. The program has included field trials to optimize regimes of existing drugs, assay development of an anti-*Wolbachia* screening strategy, registered drug, focused anti-infective, and diversity-based library screening, and a target discovery program. The A·WOL program has (i) identified registered drug combinations that can reduce treatment times from weeks to a few days *in vivo*, (ii) discovered 69 registered drug hits, the most advanced of which displays an increase in potency of 50% over doxycycline, and (iii) identified a further 138 hits for advancement. In addition, A·WOL is completing a screen of a further more than 60 000 compounds and has validated essential *Wolbachia* gene targets.

The next steps will require a period of hit-to-lead optimization to focus A·WOL hits to a small number of credible candidates that we can pursue through the screening pathway.

The hope is that this process will deliver new and improved drugs active against *Wolbachia*, which will provide the tools needed to ensure that the goal of eliminating onchocerciasis and lymphatic filariasis can be ultimately achieved.

Acknowledgments

We thank the Bill & Melinda Gates Foundation for their support of the A·WOL consortium, the EU, Volkswagen Foundation, and DFG (German Research Foundation) for financial support, and Dr Donald Comb, Dr Clotilde Carlow, and New England Biolabs for continued interest and support.

References

1 Taylor, M.J., Hoerauf, A., and Bockarie, M. (2010) Lymphatic filariasis and onchocerciasis. *Lancet*, **376**, 1175–1185.

2 Duke, B.O. (2002) A plea to continue the search for an *Onchocerca volvulus* macrofilaricide. *Trans. R. Soc. Trop. Med. Hyg.*, **96**, 575–576.

3 Awadzi, K., Boakye, D.A., Edwards, G., Opoku, N.O., Attah, S.K., Osei-Atweneboana, M.Y., Lazdins-Helds, J.K. *et al.* (2004) An investigation of persistent microfilaridermias despite multiple treatments with ivermectin, in two onchocerciasis-endemic foci in Ghana. *Ann. Trop. Med. Parasitol.*, **98**, 231–249.

4 Osei-Atweneboana, M.Y., Eng, J.K., Boakye, D.A., Gyapong, J.O., and

Prichard, R.K. (2007) Prevalence and intensity of *Onchocerca volvulus* infection and efficacy of ivermectin in endemic communities in Ghana: a two-phase epidemiological study. *Lancet*, **369**, 2021–2029.

5 Osei-Atweneboana, M.Y., Awadzi, K., Attah, S.K., Boakye, D.A., Gyapong, J.O., and Prichard, R.K. (2011) Phenotypic evidence of emerging ivermectin resistance in *Onchocerca volvulus*. *PLoS Negl. Trop. Dis.*, **5**, e998.

6 Taylor, M.J., Bandi, C., and Hoerauf, A. (2005) *Wolbachia* bacterial endosymbionts of filarial nematodes. *Adv. Parasitol.*, **60**, 245–284.

7 Kozek, W.J. and Marroquin, H.F. (1977) Intracytoplasmic bacteria in *Onchocerca volvulus*. *Am. J. Trop. Med. Hyg.*, **26**, 663–678.

8 Bandi, C., McCall, J.W., Genchi, C., Corona, S., Venco, L., and Sacchi, L. (1999) Effects of tetracycline on the filarial worms *Brugia pahangi* and *Dirofilaria immitis* and their bacterial endosymbionts *Wolbachia*. *Int. J. Parasitol.*, **29**, 357–364.

9 Hoerauf, A., Nissen-Pahle, K., Schmetz, C., Henkle-Duhrsen, K., Blaxter, M.L., Buttner, D.W., Gallin, M.Y. *et al.* (1999) Tetracycline therapy targets intracellular bacteria in the filarial nematode *Litomosoides sigmodontis* and results in filarial infertility. *J. Clin. Invest.*, **103**, 11–18.

10 Hoerauf, A., Mand, S., Volkmann, L., Buttner, M., Marfo-Debrekyei, Y., Taylor, M., Adjei, O. *et al.* (2003) Doxycycline in the treatment of human onchocerciasis: kinetics of *Wolbachia* endobacteria reduction and of inhibition of embryogenesis in female *Onchocerca* worms. *Microbes Infect.*, **5**, 261–273.

11 Langworthy, N.G., Renz, A., Mackenstedt, U., Henkle-Duhrsen, K., de Bronsvoort, M.B., Tanya, V.N., Donnelly, M.J. *et al.* (2000) Macrofilaricidal activity of tetracycline against the filarial nematode *Onchocerca ochengi*: elimination of *Wolbachia* precedes worm death and suggests a dependent relationship. *Proc. Biol. Sci.*, **267**, 1063–1069.

12 Hoerauf, A., Mand, S., Adjei, O., Fleischer, B., and Buttner, D.W. (2001) Depletion of *Wolbachia* endobacteria in *Onchocerca volvulus* by doxycycline and microfilaridermia after ivermectin treatment. *Lancet*, **357**, 1415–1416.

13 Taylor, M.J., Makunde, W.H., McGarry, H.F., Turner, J.D., Mand, S., and Hoerauf, A. (2005) Macrofilaricidal activity after doxycycline treatment of *Wuchereria bancrofti*: a double-blind, randomised placebo-controlled trial. *Lancet*, **365**, 2116–2121.

14 Supali, T., Djuardi, Y., Pfarr, K.M., Wibowo, H., Taylor, M.J., Hoerauf, A., Houwing-Duistermaat, J.J. *et al.* (2008) Doxycycline treatment of *Brugia malayi*-infected persons reduces microfilaremia and adverse reactions after diethylcarbamazine and albendazole treatment. *Clin. Infect. Dis.*, **46**, 1385–1393.

15 Srivastava, K. and Misra-Bhattacharya, S. (2003) Tetracycline, a tool for transmission blocking of *Brugia malayi* in *Mastomys coucha*. *Curr. Sci.*, **85**, 588–589.

16 Arumugam, S., Pfarr, K.M., and Hoerauf, A. (2008) Infection of the intermediate mite host with *Wolbachia*-depleted *Litomosoides sigmodontis* microfilariae: impaired L1 to L3 development and subsequent sex-ratio distortion in adult worms. *Int. J. Parasitol.*, **38**, 981–987.

17 Casiraghi, M., McCall, J.W., Simoncini, L., Kramer, L.H., Sacchi, L., Genchi, C., Werren, J.H. *et al.* (2002) Tetracycline treatment and sex-ratio distortion: a role for *Wolbachia* in the moulting of filarial nematodes? *Int. J. Parasitol.*, **32**, 1457–1468.

18 Debrah, A.Y., Mand, S., Specht, S., Marfo-Debrekyei, Y., Batsa, L., Pfarr, K., Larbi, J. *et al.* (2006) Doxycycline reduces plasma VEGF-C/sVEGFR-3 and improves pathology in lymphatic filariasis. *PLoS Pathog.*, **2**, e92.

19 Debrah, A.Y., Mand, S., Marfo-Debrekyei, Y., Batsa, L., Pfarr, K., Buttner, M., Adjei, O. *et al.* (2007)

Macrofilaricidal effect of 4 weeks of treatment with doxycycline on *Wuchereria bancrofti. Trop. Med. Int. Health*, **12**, 1433–1441.

20 Mand, S., Pfarr, K., Sahoo, P.K., Satapathy, A.K., Specht, S., Klarmann, U., Debrah, A.Y. et al. (2009) Macrofilaricidal activity and amelioration of lymphatic pathology in bancroftian filariasis after 3 weeks of doxycycline followed by single-dose diethylcarbamazine. *Am. J. Trop. Med. Hyg.*, **81**, 702–711.

21 Hoerauf, A., Specht, S., Buttner, M., Pfarr, K., Mand, S., Fimmers, R., Marfo-Debrekyei, Y. et al. (2008) *Wolbachia* endobacteria depletion by doxycycline as anti-filarial therapy has macrofilaricidal activity in onchocerciasis: a randomized placebo-controlled study. *Med. Microbiol. Immunol.*, **197**, 295–311.

22 Hoerauf, A., Specht, S., Marfo-Debrekyei, Y., Buttner, M., Debrah, A.Y., Mand, S., Batsa, L. et al. (2009) Efficacy of 5-week doxycycline treatment on adult *Onchocerca volvulus*. *Parasitol. Res.*, **104**, 437–447.

23 Turner, J.D., Tendongfor, N., Esum, M., Johnston, K.L., Langley, R.S., Ford, L., Faragher, B. et al. (2010) Macrofilaricidal activity after doxycycline only treatment of *Onchocerca volvulus* in an area of *Loa loa* co-endemicity: a randomized controlled trial. *PLoS Negl. Trop. Dis.*, **4**, e660.

24 Coulibaly, Y.I., Dembele, B., Diallo, A.A., Lipner, E.M., Doumbia, S.S., Coulibaly, S.Y., Konate, S. et al. (2009) A randomized trial of doxycycline for *Mansonella perstans* infection. *N. Engl. J. Med.*, **361**, 1448–1458.

25 Specht, S., Hoerauf, A., Adjei, O., Debrah, A., and Buttner, D.W., (2009) Newly acquired *Onchocerca volvulus* filariae after doxycycline treatment. *Parasitol. Res.*, **106**, 23–31.

26 Debrah, A.Y., Mand, S., Marfo-Debrekyei, Y., Batsa, L., Pfarr, K., Lawson, B., Taylor, M. et al. (2009) Reduction in levels of plasma vascular endothelial growth factor-A and improvement in hydrocele patients by targeting endosymbiotic *Wolbachia* sp. in *Wuchereria bancrofti* with doxycycline. *Am. J. Trop. Med. Hyg.*, **80**, 956–963.

27 Specht, S., Mand, S., Marfo-Debrekyei, Y., Debrah, A.Y., Konadu, P., Adjei, O., Buttner, D.W. et al. (2008) Efficacy of 2- and 4-week rifampicin treatment on the *Wolbachia* of *Onchocerca volvulus*. *Parasitol. Res.*, **103**, 1303–1309.

28 Wanji, S., Tendongfor, N., Nji, T., Esum, M., Che, J.N., Nkweschu, A., Alassa, F. et al. (2009) Community-directed delivery of doxycycline for the treatment of onchocerciasis in areas of co-endemicity with loiasis in Cameroon. *Parasite Vectors*, **2**, 39.

29 Turner, J.D., Langley, R.S., Johnston, K.L., Egerton, G., Wanji, S., and Taylor, M.J. (2006) *Wolbachia* endosymbiotic bacteria of *Brugia malayi* mediate macrophage tolerance to TLR- and CD40-specific stimuli in a MyD88/TLR2-dependent manner. *J. Immunol.*, **177**, 1240–1249.

30 Johnston, K.L., Wu, B., Guimaraes, A., Ford, L., Slatko, B.E., and Taylor, M.J. (2010) Lipoprotein biosynthesis as a target for anti-*Wolbachia* treatment of filarial nematodes. *Parasite Vectors*, **3**, 99.

31 Townson, S., Tagboto, S., McGarry, H.F., Egerton, G.L., and Taylor, M.J. (2006) *Onchocerca* parasites and *Wolbachia* endosymbionts: evaluation of a spectrum of antibiotic types for activity against *Onchocerca* gutturosa *in vitro*. *Filaria J.*, **5**, 4.

32 Ash, L.R. and Riley, J.M. (1970) Development of subperiodic *Brugia malayi* in the jird, *Meriones unguiculatus*, with notes on infections in other rodents. *J. Parasitol.*, **56**, 969–973.

33 Ashburn, T.T. and Thor, K.B. (2004) Drug repositioning: identifying and developing new uses for existing drugs. *Nat. Rev. Drug Discov.*, **3**, 673–683.

34 Tobinick, E.L. (2009) The value of drug repositioning in the current pharmaceutical market. *Drug News Perspect.*, **22**, 119–125.

35 Foster, J., Ganatra, M., Kamal, I., Ware, J., Makarova, K., Ivanova, N., Bhattacharyya, A. et al. (2005) The *Wolbachia* genome of *Brugia malayi*: endosymbiont evolution within a

human pathogenic nematode. *PLoS Biol.*, **3**, e121.

36 Ghedin, E., Wang, S., Spiro, D., Caler, E., Zhao, Q., Crabtree, J., Allen, J.E. *et al.* (2007) Draft genome of the filarial nematode parasite *Brugia malayi*. *Science*, **317**, 1756–1760.

37 Lander, E.S., Linton, L.M., Birren, B., Nusbaum, C., Zody, M.C., Baldwin, J., Devon, K. *et al.* (2001) Initial sequencing and analysis of the human genome. *Nature*, **409**, 860–921.

38 Holman, A.G., Davis, P.J., Foster, J.M., Carlow, C.K., and Kumar, S. (2009) Computational prediction of essential genes in an uncultureable endosymbiotic bacterium, *Wolbachia* of *Brugia malayi*. *BMC Microbiol.*, **9**, 243.

39 Zhang, R. and Lin, Y. (2009) DEG 5.0, a database of essential genes in both prokaryotes and eukaryotes. *Nucleic Acids Res.*, **37**, D455–458.

40 Drlica, K. and Zhao, X. (1997) DNA gyrase, topoisomerase IV, and the 4-quinolones. *Microbiol. Mol. Biol. Rev.*, **61**, 377–392.

41 Floss, H.G. and Yu, T.W. (2005) Rifamycin – mode of action, resistance, and biosynthesis. *Chem. Rev.*, **105**, 621–632.

42 Kim, S., Lee, S.W., Choi, E.C., and Choi, S.Y. (2003) Aminoacyl-tRNA synthetases and their inhibitors as a novel family of antibiotics. *Appl. Microbiol. Biotechnol.*, **61**, 278–288.

43 Wishart, D.S., Knox, C., Guo, A.C., Cheng, D., Shrivastava, S., Tzur, D., Gautam, B. *et al.* (2008) DrugBank: a knowledgebase for drugs, drug actions and drug targets. *Nucleic Acids Res.*, **36**, D901–906.

44 Wu, B., Novelli, J., Foster, J., Vaisvila, R., Conway, L., Ingram, J., Ganatra, M. *et al.* (2009) The heme biosynthetic pathway of the obligate *Wolbachia* endosymbiont of *Brugia malayi* as a potential anti-filarial drug target. *PLoS Negl. Trop. Dis.*, **3**, e475.

45 Famulok, M. and Mayer, G. (2005) Intramers and aptamers: applications in protein-function analyses and potential for drug screening. *ChemBioChem*, **6**, 19–26.

46 Niebel, B., Lentz, C., Pofahl, M., Mayer, G., Hoerauf, A., Pfarr, K.M., and Famulok, M. (2010) ADLOC: an aptamer-displacement assay based on luminescent oxygen channeling. *Chemistry*, **16**, 11100–11107.

47 Hafner, M., Vianini, E., Albertoni, B., Marchetti, L., Grune, I., Gloeckner, C., and Famulok, M. (2008) Displacement of protein-bound aptamers with small molecules screened by fluorescence polarization. *Nat. Protoc.*, **3**, 579–587.

48 Foster, J.M., Raverdy, S., Ganatra, M.B., Colussi, P.A., Taron, C.H., and Carlow, C.K. (2009) The *Wolbachia* endosymbiont of *Brugia malayi* has an active phosphoglycerate mutase: a candidate target for anti-filarial therapies. *Parasitol. Res.*, **104**, 1047–1052.

49 Raverdy, S., Foster, J.M., Roopenian, E., and Carlow, C.K. (2008) The *Wolbachia* endosymbiont of *Brugia malayi* has an active pyruvate phosphate dikinase. *Mol. Biochem. Parasitol.*, **160**, 163–166.

50 Henrichfreise, B., Schiefer, A., Schneider, T., Nzukou, E., Poellinger, C., Hoffmann, T.J., Johnston, K.L. *et al.* (2009) Functional conservation of the lipid II biosynthesis pathway in the cell wall-less bacteria *Chlamydia* and *Wolbachia*: why is lipid II needed? *Mol. Microbiol.*, **73**, 913–923.

51 Turner, J.D., Langley, R.S., Johnston, K.L., Gentil, K., Ford, L., Wu, B., Graham, M. *et al.* (2009) *Wolbachia* lipoprotein stimulates innate and adaptive immunity through Toll-like receptors 2 and 6 to induce disease manifestations of filariasis. *J. Biol. Chem.*, **284**, 22364–22378.

16
Promise of *Bacillus thuringiensis* Crystal Proteins as Anthelmintics

*Yan Hu and Raffi V. Aroian**

Abstract

Bacillus thuringiensis crystal (Cry) proteins are the most widely used biological insecticides in the world. Their value in safely controlling insects that destroy crops and transmit human diseases is well established. Here, we review B. *thuringiensis* Cry proteins as novel anthelmintics with a unique mode of action. In laboratory studies, Cry proteins are highly effective against a broad range of free-living roundworms and parasitic roundworms that infect plants and animals. Cry5B is therapeutic for two different intestinal roundworm parasitic infections – one in mice and the other in hamsters. The latter infection involves a minor hookworm parasite of humans, *Ancylostoma ceylanicum*, which is closely related to the more prevalent *Ancylostoma duodenale*. Therapy is observed despite the fact that much of the protein is likely degraded in the stomach prior to reaching the parasites. Cry21A is also therapeutic in mice infected with the roundworm parasite, *Heligmosomoides bakeri*. Cry proteins offer excellent combinatorial therapeutic properties with nicotinic acetylcholine receptor agonists – one of two classes of compounds approved by the World Health Organization for treatment of intestinal roundworms in humans. Given their nontoxicity to humans and their broad spectrum of nematicidal action, Cry proteins show great potential as next-generation anthelmintics.

Introduction

Soil-transmitted helminths (STHs) are nematodes that parasitize the human intestine, and include hookworms, the whipworm (*Trichuris trichuria*), and the giant roundworm (*Ascaris lumbricoides*). They cause significant disease burden in the world's poorest, infecting one in three people in the world and causing morbidity comparable to that of malaria [1–5]. STH infections in children result in growth and cognitive stunting, and severely impact learning, school attendance, and future income potential [1–3, 5, 6]. Over 44 million hookworm-infected pregnant women, including 7.5 million women in sub-Saharan Africa, are at an increased risk for premature delivery, low birth weight, maternal ill health, and maternal death [7].

*Corresponding Author

In general, intestinal roundworms impair workers' productivity and contribute to keeping large populations entrapped in poverty [8, 9]. Furthermore, intestinal roundworm infections modulate the immune system, and are correlated with increased HIV severity, susceptibility to malaria, and probability of having active tuberculosis [10–12]. In addition, those infected have generally poorer responses to tuberculosis and cholera vaccines [13–15]. Clearly, STHs are one of the great causes of disease in our time.

Four anthelmintics are currently approved by the World Health Organization for treatment of STHs – two benzimidazoles (mebendazole and albendazole) and two nicotinic acetylcholine receptor (nAChR) agonists (pyrantel and levamisole) [16]. Albendazole is considered best and is preferred for STH mass drug administration [17]. The problem with having so few anthelmintic classes is the emergence of parasite resistance. Reduction of efficacy or failure of current anthelmintics, including increasingly to albendazole, has been seen in Australia, Tanzania, Vietnam, Mali, Ethiopia, Sri Lanka, and Ghana [18–23]. These reports have evoked urgent and repeated appeals for the development of new anthelmintics [2, 5, 16, 22].

Since albendazole's introduction in 1983 [24], only one new single-dose drug targeting human parasitic roundworms has reached clinical development – tribendimidine (TBD). TBD was developed by the Chinese Centers for Disease Control and Prevention [25]. It was approved for clinical use in 2004. In clinical trials in China, TBD offered single-dose efficacy against all parasites comparable to albendazole [25, 26]. The mechanism of action of TBD is the same as the levamisole/pyrantel class nAChR agonists [27], to which resistance in human populations has already been documented [22]. Another drug, nitazoxanide, shows efficacy against *Ascaris*, hookworm, and *Trichuris trichiura* when delivered as six doses over 3 days [28]. New anthelmintics continue to be developed for veterinary applications as roundworm resistance to all of the classes currently available is now widespread in farm animals [29]. These new anthelmintics include monepantel (see Chapter 17), the cyclooxadepsipeptides, and the paraherquamides [30–32] (see Chapter 18). When these drugs will be available for human clinical trials, how safe they will be for humans and how effective they will be against STHs that infect humans are outstanding questions.

Our laboratory is pioneering work on a novel class of anthelmintics, crystal (Cry) proteins made by the soil bacterium *Bacillus thuringiensis* [33, 34, 43, 46, 57, 61, 70, 71, 79]. *B. thuringiensis* is a Gram-positive, spore-forming bacterium characterized by parasporal crystalline protein inclusions (Figure 16.1). These inclusions often appear microscopically as distinctively shaped crystals and therefore are referred to as "Cry proteins." Cry proteins are pore-forming toxins that bind to receptors on the intestines of invertebrates, intoxicating and killing their targets [33, 35].

Safety of *B. thuringiensis* Cry Proteins

Five decades of intense use of Cry proteins as insecticides, including major aerial spraying over populated areas [36, 37], mosquito and black fly control programs, transgenic food crops, and in the organic farming industry (*B. thuringiensis* Cry proteins are the insecticide of choice by organic farmers), has proven that

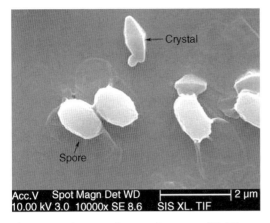

Figure 16.1 Scanning electron microscope of Cry5B spores and crystals.

B. thuringiensis and its crystal proteins are nontoxic to vertebrates [38, 39]. Over a dozen studies with spores and crystals have been performed in small mammals and humans, and all have showed no evidence of toxicity [38]. These data indicating nontoxicity of Cry proteins towards mammals include acute oral toxicity studies in which rodents were given greater than 4000 mg/kg/day [38]. Cry proteins are expressed in a number of food crops. For example, they are approved by the US Environmental Protection Agency for expression in corn and around 60% of all the corn grown in the United States currently expresses Cry protein [40].

Much of our pioneering work on Cry protein anthelmintics has focused on Cry5B – a three-domain Cry protein related by primary sequence and predicted secondary structures to the Cry proteins used to kill insects [33, 34, 41]. In terms of phylogeny, Cry5B is located between families of Cry proteins known to be safe to vertebrates, such as Cry1A and Cry2A [42]. To understand how Cry5B interacts with its invertebrate hosts, our laboratory carried out forward genetics screens for Cry5B-resistant animals in the common free-living laboratory roundworm, *Caenorhabditis elegans* [43]. Identification of various *C. elegans* genes that mutate to Cry protein resistance revealed four glycosyltransferases [44, 45]. Further research demonstrated that Cry5B binds to the carbohydrate moiety of *C. elegans* glycolipids and this binding is essential for toxin action *in vivo* [46]. These carbohydrates contain the arthroseries core conserved in insects and roundworms, but lacking in vertebrates. These data provide a molecular basis for the mammalian safety of Cry5B and perhaps other Cry proteins such as Cry1A family proteins, because vertebrates lack at least two of the enzymes required for biosynthesis of the carbohydrate moiety [46].

Mechanism of Action

B. thuringiensis Cry proteins are ingestible toxins. Once ingested by target invertebrates, they are solubilized into monomers and proteolytically activated in the invertebrate intestinal lumen. Protein monomers bind to receptors on intestinal cells, then oligomerize and insert into the plasma membrane to form pores [33, 35, 47]. Cry proteins are pore-forming toxins (PFTs) and as such are part of the single largest group of bacterial protein virulence factors [48]. Cry5B itself has been demonstrated to form pores in planar lipid bilayers [49]. PFTs poke holes in the plasma membrane in the cells, breaching cellular integrity, and disrupting ion balances and membrane potential [50, 51]. The net result is death or severe dysregulation of target cells. There has been a little discussion as to whether the mode of lethality of Cry proteins involves osmotic lysis or signal transduction events [47]. Both are consistent with the effects of PFTs. PFTs trigger a multitude of signal transduction effects in cells [50, 52]. Studies in *C. elegans* have demonstrated that numerous signal transduction and cellular effects of Cry5B are conserved with those of mammalian-acting PFTs [49, 53–56]. Thus, the mechanism of action of Cry5B is an invertebrate-specific acting PFT.

Cry Proteins Have a Broad-Spectrum of Activity Against Free-Living and Parasitic Roundworms *Ex Vivo*

Cry Proteins Intoxicate a Wide Range of Free-Living Roundworms

We exposed five phylogenetically diverse free-living roundworms (*C. elegans* strain N2, *Pristionchus pacificus* strain PS312, *Panagrellus redivivus* strain PS1163, *Acrobeloides* spp. strain PS1146, and *Distolabrellus veechi* strain LKC10) to *Escherichia coli*-expressed Cry proteins from the Cry5 and Cry6 subfamilies. We found that three Cry5 subfamily proteins (Cry5B, Cry14A, and Cry21A) and one Cry6 subfamily protein (Cry6A) are generally toxic to the free-living roundworms [57]. The Cry5 subfamily proteins Cry5A and Cry12A, as well as the Cry6 subfamily protein, Cry6B, are generally not toxic to roundworms [57]. To date, every roundworm tested, be it free-living, plant-parasitic (see below), or animal-parasitic (see below), is susceptible to Cry5B.

Cry Proteins Intoxicate Plant-Parasitic Roundworms

Plant-parasitic nematodes feed, live, and reproduce inside plant roots, and cause significant damage to commercially important crops world-wide [58, 59]. To test the efficacy of Cry proteins it is therefore essential that plants be engineered to express the Cry proteins so that the parasites have access to the protein. Our laboratory has demonstrated that Cry6A and Cry5B proteins transgenically expressed in tomato roots intoxicate the endoparasitic root-knot nematode, *Meloidogyne incognita*, resulting, for example, in significant inhibition of endoparasite reproduction [60, 61]. Cry proteins represent potentially powerful tools in the control of plant-parasitic nematodes.

Cry proteins Intoxicate Animal-Parasitic Roundworms *Ex Vivo*

Early studies suggested that *B. thuringiensis* might have effects on animal parasitic roundworms, although these involved the use of the entire bacterium (not purified Cry proteins) and the use of uncharacterized *B. thuringiensis* strains (reviewed in [62]).

The role of Cry proteins in the intoxication of the parasites was unclear from these studies. More definitive indication that Cry protein could act against animal-parasitic roundworms came from our study demonstrating that Cry5B, Cry14A, and Cry21A expressed in nonpathogenic *E. coli* are toxic to the free-living larval stages of the rodent-parasitic roundworm, *Nippostrongylus brasiliensis* [57]. Subsequently, a research group from Australia screened a collection of *B. thuringiensis* strains for nematicidal activity [62]. They found two *B. thuringiensis* strains that intoxicated *in vitro* larval and adult stages of three economically important roundworm parasites of livestock (i.e., *Haemonchus contortus*, *Trichostrongylus colubriformis*, and *Ostertagia circumcincta*). One *B. thuringiensis* strain expressed Cry5A and Cry5B proteins, and the other expressing the Cry5 family member Cry13A [62].

B. thuringiensis as a Natural Pathogen of Roundworms

That *B. thuringiensis* Cry proteins have widespread and potent activity against roundworms suggests that the bacterium *B. thuringiensis* evolved these proteins specifically to target roundworms. This suggestion is not surprising given that *B. thuringiensis* and many free-living roundworms (nematodes) coexist in the soil [57]. Studies on the interaction, evolution, and ecology of *B. thuringiensis* and *B. thuringiensis* Cry proteins in association with free-living nematodes are all consistent with the hypothesis that the intoxication/killing of roundworms with *B. thuringiensis* Cry proteins is part of a natural host–pathogen interaction [57, 63–66].

Therapeutic Activity of Cry Proteins (Cry5B and Cry21A) Against Two Mammalian Intestinal Roundworm Parasites *In Vitro* and *In Vivo*

Cry5B is Active Against Hookworms *In Vitro* and *In Vivo*

Hamsters are permissive hosts for the hookworm parasite, *Ancylostoma ceylanicum*, which is a minor human hookworm parasite most commonly found in Asia and which is closely related to the prevalent human hookworm parasite *Ancylostoma duodenale* [2]. Like human hookworm infection, *A. ceylanicum* infection in hamsters causes weight loss and anemia, and, accordingly, is considered a good model [67–69]. *A. ceylanicum* hookworm adults and larvae show dose-dependent intoxication by purified Cry5B when cultured *in vitro* [70]. Cry5B is very intoxicating to early-stage hookworm larvae – the percentage of motile larvae after 48 h of incubation was reduced from 90% (no Cry5B) to 6% in 5 µg/ml Cry5B [70]. Incubation with Cry5B also resulted in significant morphological changes to *A. ceylanicum* larvae (i.e., stunted growth and loss of integrity of most internal structures) [70]. Exposure of adult *A. ceylanicum* to Cry5B was also associated with significant toxicity, including a substantial reduction in egg excretion by adult female worms [70]. Females exposed to 0.1 µg/ml Cry5B demonstrated a 95% reduction in the number of eggs compared with control worms [70].

Most significantly, Cry5B shows excellent anthelmintic activity against hookworms *in vivo*. Purified Cry5B administered in three doses on 3 consecutive days (15 mg/kg/

dose) to *A. ceylanicum*-infected hamsters decreased fecal egg counts and worm burdens by 81 and 89%, respectively [70] (Figure 16.2a and b). These data demonstrated for the first time that a Cry protein can act as an anthelmintic *in vivo*.

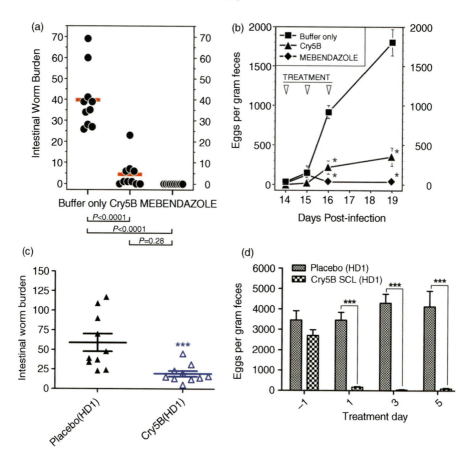

Figure 16.2 Cry5B treatment reduces intestinal worm burden (a and c) and fecal egg excretion (b and d) in roundworm-infected mammals. (a and b) *A. ceylanicum* (hookworm)-infected hamster experiments; (c and d) *H. bakeri*-infected mouse experiments. (a) Worm burdens in individual hamsters are indicated by closed circles and the means of each group are shown by red horizontal bars. Square brackets underneath indicate statistical comparisons between groups by analysis of variance (ANOVA). (b) Fecal samples from infected animals were collected at the times indicated and hookworm eggs quantified. All values are the means ± standard error (SE). Asterisks indicate statistical significance ($P < 0.05$) versus the infected control group (ANOVA). (c) Intestinal worm burdens in placebo (HD1)- and Cry5B (HD1)-treated mice. Worm burdens in individual mice are indicated by triangles. Long horizontal bars represent mean worm burdens; smaller bars indicate SE. ***$P < 0.001$ Mann–Whitney. (d) Shown are the average eggs/gram of feces/mouse for both placebo ($n = 10$)- and Cry5B HD1 ($n = 10$)-treated groups the day before treatment, (-1) and then every other day thereafter until the animals were euthanized on day 5 post-treatment. Error bars = SE. Two-way ANOVA. (Modified from [70] © (2006) National academy of Sciences, USA, and [71]).

Statistically similar, although more complete, curative results were obtained for three 15 mg/kg/dose treatments with mebendazole [70]. It is interesting to note that on a molar basis, the dose of mebendazole used was 475 times that of Cry5B.

Cry5B has Superior Single-Dose Anthelmintic Activity Against *Heligmosomoides bakeri* Intestinal Roundworm Infections in Mice

H. bakeri (also known as *H. polygyrus* and *Nematospiroides dubius* [72]) in the mouse is a commonly employed rodent model for infection by an intestinal roundworm [72–74]. *H. bakeri* infection in mice was the model that led to the discovery of ivermectin [75]. We tested whether Cry5B could provide significant single-dose therapy of *H. bakeri* and found that one dose of Cry5B at 715 nmol/kg (100 mg/kg) clears approximately 70% of the parasites relative to placebo in two different experiments (one of which is shown in Figure 16.2c) [71]. Cry5B-treated animals showed more than 98% reduction in fecal egg counts (Figure 16.2d) [71]. That the percent egg reduction was greater than the percent worm burden reduction suggested that the female parasites remaining in the intestine were severely intoxicated (the difference could not be attested to by preferential elimination of female over male parasites [71]).

To understand the potency of Cry5B relative to known anthelmintics, we performed an identical set of experiments (same mouse strain, *H. bakeri* culture, timing of infection, and treatment) using the latest anthelmintic developed for human use, TBD [71]. As noted above, TBD, along with albendazole, has the best single-dose efficacy in humans among any of the current anthelmintics. We found that a 3-fold higher dose of TBD is required to achieve the same level of parasite clearing (70%) as Cry5B [71]. A search through the literature confirmed that, relative to known anthelmintics tested against *H. bakeri* infections in mice, Cry5B has excellent efficacy (Table 16.1) [71, 76–78].

As Cry5B is a large protein (around 140 kDa), we hypothesized that it might fair poorly in the mammalian stomach in transit to the mammalian intestine. To test this hypothesis, we incubated Cry5B in simulated gastric fluids. Within 4 min, virtually all of the protein is degraded [71]. Given that the transit time through the stomach is of the order of a few hours, it is likely that the amount of protein reaching the parasites in our gavage experiments is miniscule, which makes the strong therapeutic effects seen with Cry5B even more remarkable. These data suggest that formulation of Cry5B protein to protect it against gastric juices should result in significantly higher anthelmintic effects superior to current anthelmintics.

Effect of Cry21A on *H. bakeri* Infections in Mice

H. bakeri-infected Swiss Webster mice were treated with three doses of Cry21A protein (13 mg/kg or 99 nM/kg per dose) or with three doses of placebo orally. Five days after treatment, the mice were euthanized and the number of intestinal adult parasites counted. Cry21A treatment resulted in a 40% reduction in parasite burden relative to placebo, demonstrating *in vivo* anthelmintic activity [79].

Table 16.1 The efficacy of different anthelmintics against *H. bakeri* as compared to Cry5B *in vivo*.

Anthelmintic	Dose given (μmol/kg)	Dose relative to Cry5B (-fold)	Day(s) treatment was given (days postinfection)	Reduction in intestinal worm burden (%)	Reference
Cry5B	0.7	1	15	70	[71]
Levamisole	49	70	12	90	[76]
Ivermectin	5.7	8	18	87	[77]
Pyrantel	84	120	18	99	[77]
Piperazine	6224	8891	18	34	[77]
Mebendazole	75	107	9–15	84	[78]
Tribendimidine	2.2	3	15	70	[71]

Powerful Combinatorial Antiroundworm Activity Between Cry Proteins and nAChR Agonists

Combination drug therapies are the best and standard of treatment for infectious diseases like HIV/AIDS, malaria, and tuberculosis [80–82]. Although anthelmintics have been used in combination [83], detailed studies regarding design of combination therapies have generally been lacking. We therefore set out to measure the combinatorial characteristics of nematicidal Cry proteins with approved human anthelmintics, namely the nAChR agonist class. Using the roundworm *C. elegans*, we find that nAChR agonists and nematicidal Cry proteins, namely Cry5B and Cry21A, display what is known as mutual hypersusceptibility (from the antivirus field [84–86]); that is, when the roundworms become resistant to one class, they become hypersensitive (relative to wild-type roundworms) to the other class. Furthermore, we find that when Cry5B and nAChR agonists are combined, their activities are strongly synergistic, producing combination index values as good or better than seen with antitumor, anti-HIV, and insecticide combinations.

Hypersusceptibility Studies Between nAChR Agonists and Cry Proteins

In order to determine hypersusceptibility characteristics, roundworms resistant to one anthelmintic are needed for testing with another anthelmintic. As we have been working on both *B. thuringiensis* Cry proteins (like Cry5B and Cry21A) and nAChR agonists (like TBD), we set out to study hypersusceptibility characteristics for these two classes of compounds. We treated *C. elegans* roundworms resistant to Cry proteins with TBD and reciprocally treated *C. elegans* roundworms resistant to nAChR agonists with Cry5B [79]. The response of these roundworms was compared to the response of wild-type roundworms to both drugs using dose-dependence assays to measure mortality and the inhibition of larval development [79]. We found that roundworms resistant to Cry5B protein are hypersusceptible to nAChR agonists, and that roundworms resistant to nAChR agonists are reciprocally hypersusceptible to Cry5B and Cry21A [79]. In other words, if *C. elegans* becomes resistant to L-subtype nAChR agonists, it is more susceptible to Cry proteins than wild-type *C. elegans*. Reciprocally, if *C. elegans* becomes resistant to Cry proteins, it is more susceptible to nAChR agonists than wild-type *C. elegans*. Given that hypersusceptibility is associated with excellent clinical efficacy with anti-HIV therapy, these results suggest that the combination of Cry proteins and nAChR agonists might also have excellent clinical utility against STHs.

Synergy Between Cry Proteins and nAChR Agonists

In addition to hypersusceptibility, another characteristic of combination therapies that is important to measure is synergy – the ability of two drugs to show a stronger effect in combination than predicted from their individual efficacies. Wild-type *C. elegans* were subjected to various doses of Cry5B, TBD, and a 1:1 ratio mixture of the two based either on mass (μg/ml : μg/ml) or efficacy ($LC_{50} : LC_{50}$, where LC_{50} is the dose of drug required to kill 50% of the animals), essentially following the algorithm and experimental design of Chou and Talalay [87]. We used the data from these experiments (proportion of animals killed at each dose of drugs individually and in combination) to calculate combination index (CI) values at different dose effect levels [79]. We found CI values for the Cry5B–TBD combination ranging from between 0.1 and 0.5, indicating strong synergy between the drugs that was comparable or superior to those found in combinations used for HIV or cancer chemotherapy or insecticides [79]. Similar results were obtained using Cry5B and levamisole [79]. We also calculated the dose-reduction index (DRI) values [79]. DRI is a measure of how many fold the dose of each drug in a combination may be reduced relative to the dose of each drug alone in order to achieve the same effect [87]. We found, for example, at the ED_{90} (effective dose for 90% lethality) in the Cry5B and levamisole *combination*, Cry5B can be reduced 6-fold and levamisole 39-fold relative to what it would take for each of these drugs to achieve the same effect on their own [79]. These data indicate that Cry proteins can potentiate the effects of nAChR agonists, like TBD, and their use in combination could significantly reduce drug doses and delay parasite resistance.

Cry Proteins are More Difficult for *C. elegans* to Resist

In the same hypersusceptibility and synergy study, we undertook a mutagenic forward genetic screen for *C. elegans* resistant to anthelmintics, comparing the frequencies to which *C. elegans* develops resistance to Cry5B, Cry21A, levamisole, albendazole, and ivermectin (Table 16.2) [79]. We found that *C. elegans* developed resistance to Cry5B more rarely than to levamisole or albendazole and at a frequency similar to that of ivermectin [79]. Resistance to Cry21A was more rare than any of the others, including Cry5B, and in fact was not seen in this screen. These data suggest that, under the laboratory conditions used here, Cry proteins have superior anti-resistance properties relative to the currently approved anthelmintics for STH chemotherapy.

Table 16.2 Results of a forward genetic screen to generate C. elegans mutants resistant to different classes of anthelmintics [79].

Anthelmintic screened	No. of mutagenized F2 C. elegans screened	No. of F2 resistant worms found
Cry5B	10000	8
Cry21A	10000	0
Albendazole	10000	22
Levamisole	10000	31
Ivermectin	10000	8

Conclusions

This chapter has highlighted the potential of B. thuringiensis Cry proteins to control intestinal roundworm parasites of humans and potentially livestock. Such a biological control strategy that would target both late-larval and adult roundworms resident in the intestine, in addition to free-living larvae, would provide a safe, powerful, attractive, and mechanistically distinct alternative to chemically based STH control. This chapter has also highlighted quantitative approaches to studying anthelmintic drug combinations, demonstrating the potential power of combining Cry proteins with nAChR agonists. As with the other major infectious diseases of humankind, most notably HIV, malaria, and tuberculosis, it is combination drug therapies that hold the greatest long-term potential for treatment and elimination of these parasites.

We are currently developing Cry5B as an anthelmintic for use in humans. In collaboration with others, we are testing Cry5B against additional intestinal roundworms of humans and animals, and are studying different formulations to protect Cry5B from the rapid digestion in the mammalian digestive tract while releasing it intact in the small intestine. These formulations are predicted to produce efficacies superior to the current anthelmintics. Finally, Cry proteins may also have excellent resistance characteristics relative to current anthelmintics.

Acknowledgments

This work was funded by a National Institutes of Health grant to R.V.A. (National Institute of Allergy and Infectious Diseases 2R01AI056189-06A1).

References

1 Albonico, M., Allen, H., Chitsulo, L., Engels, D., Gabrielli, A.F., and Savioli, L. (2008) Controlling soil-transmitted helminthiasis in pre-school-age children through preventive chemotherapy. *PLoS Negl. Trop. Dis.*, **2**, e126.

2 Bethony, J., Brooker, S., Albonico, M., Geiger, S.M., Loukas, A., Diemert, D., and

Hotez, P.J. (2006) Soil-transmitted helminth infections: ascariasis, trichuriasis, and hookworm. *Lancet*, **367**, 1521–1532.

3 Hall, A., Hewitt, G., Tuffrey, V., and de Silva, N. (2008) A review and meta-analysis of the impact of intestinal worms on child growth and nutrition. *Matern. Child Nutr.*, **4** (Suppl. 1), 118–236.

4 Hotez, P.J., Molyneux, D.H., Fenwick, A., Kumaresan, J., Sachs, S.E., Sachs, J.D., and Savioli, L. (2007) Control of neglected tropical diseases. *N. Engl. J. Med.*, **357**, 1018–1027.

5 Tchuente, L.A. (2011) Control of soil-transmitted helminths in sub-Saharan Africa: diagnosis, drug efficacy concerns and challenge. *Acta Trop.*, **20** (Suppl. 1), S4–S11.

6 Bundy, D.A., Kremer, M., Bleakley, H., Jukes, M.C., and Miguel, E. (2009) Deworming and development: asking the right questions, asking the questions right. *PLoS Negl. Trop. Dis.*, **3**, e362.

7 Hotez, P. (2008) Hookworm and poverty. *Ann. NY Acad. Sci.*, **1136**, 38–44.

8 Hotez, P.J. (2008) *Forgotten People, Forgotten Diseases: The Neglected Tropical Diseases and their Impact on Global Health and Development*, ASM Press, Washington, DC.

9 Martin, M.G. and Humphreys, M.E. (2006) Social consequence of disease in the American South, 1900–World War II. *South Med. J.*, **99**, 862–864.

10 Alexander, P.E. and De, P. (2009) HIV-1 and intestinal helminth review update: updating a Cochrane Review and building the case for treatment and has the time come to test and treat? *Parasite Immunol.*, **31**, 283–286.

11 Brooker, S., Akhwale, W., Pullan, R., Estambale, B., Clarke, S.E., Snow, R.W., and Hotez, P.J. (2007) Epidemiology of *Plasmodium*–helminth co-infection in Africa: populations at risk, potential impact on anemia, and prospects for combining control. *Am. J. Trop. Med. Hyg.*, **77**, 88–98.

12 Walson, J.L., Otieno, P.A., Mbuchi, M., Richardson, B.A., Lohman-Payne, B., Macharia, S.W., Overbaugh, J., Berkley, J., Sanders, E.J., Chung, M.H., and John-Stewart, G.C. (2008) Albendazole treatment of HIV-1 and helminth co-infection: a randomized, double-blind, placebo-controlled trial. *AIDS*, **22**, 1601–1609.

13 Cooper, P.J., Chico, M., Sandoval, C., Espinel, I., Guevara, A., Levine, M.M., Griffin, G.E., and Nutman, T.B. (2001) Human infection with *Ascaris lumbricoides* is associated with suppression of the interleukin-2 response to recombinant cholera toxin B subunit following vaccination with the live oral cholera vaccine CVD 103-HgR. *Infect. Immun.*, **69**, 1574–1580.

14 Cooper, P.J., Chico, M.E., Losonsky, G., Sandoval, C., Espinel, I., Sridhara, R., Aguilar, M., Guevara, A., Guderian, R.H., Levine, M.M., Griffin, G.E., and Nutman, T.B. (2000) Albendazole treatment of children with ascariasis enhances the vibriocidal antibody response to the live attenuated oral cholera vaccine CVD 103-HgR. *J. Infect. Dis.*, **182**, 1199–1206.

15 Elias, D., Britton, S., Kassu, A., and Akuffo, H. (2007) Chronic helminth infections may negatively influence immunity against tuberculosis and other diseases of public health importance. *Expert Rev. Anti Infect. Ther.*, **5**, 475–484.

16 Keiser, J. and Utzinger, J. (2008) Efficacy of current drugs against soil-transmitted helminth infections: systematic review and meta-analysis. *J. Am. Med. Assoc.*, **299**, 1937–1948.

17 Smits, H.L. (2009) Prospects for the control of neglected tropical diseases by mass drug administration. *Expert Rev. Anti Infect. Ther.*, **7**, 37–56.

18 Adugna, S., Kebede, Y., Moges, F., and Tiruneh, M. (2007) Efficacy of mebendazole and albendazole for *Ascaris lumbricoides* and hookworm infections in an area with long time exposure for antihelminthes, Northwest Ethiopia. *Ethiop. Med. J.*, **45**, 301–306.

19 Flohr, C., Tuyen, L.N., Lewis, S., Minh, T.T., Campbell, J., Britton, J., Williams, H., Hien, T.T., Farrar, J., and Quinnell, R.J. (2007) Low efficacy of

mebendazole against hookworm in Vietnam: two randomized controlled trials. *Am. J. Trop. Med. Hyg.*, **76**, 732–736.

20 Gunawardena, N.K., Amarasekera, N.D., Pathmeswaran, A., and de Silva, N.R. (2008) Effect of repeated mass chemotherapy for filariasis control on soil-transmitted helminth infections in Sri Lanka. *Ceylon. Med. J.*, **53**, 13–16.

21 Humphries, D., Mosites, E., Otchere, J., Twum, W.A., Woo, L., Jones-Sanpei, H., Harrison, L.M., Bungiro, R.D., Benham-Pyle, B., Bimi, L., Edoh, D., Bosompem, K., Wilson, M., and Cappello, M. (2011) Epidemiology of hookworm infection in Kintampo north municipality, Ghana: patterns of malaria coinfection, anemia, and albendazole treatment failure. *Am. J. Trop. Med. Hyg.*, **84**, 792–800.

22 Stepek, G., Buttle, D.J., Duce, I.R., and Behnke, J.M. (2006) Human gastrointestinal nematode infections: are new control methods required? *Int. J. Exp. Pathol.*, **87**, 325–341.

23 Stothard, J.R., Rollinson, D., Imison, E., and Khamis, I.S. (2009) A spot-check of the efficacies of albendazole or levamisole, against soil-transmitted helminthiases in young Ungujan children, reveals low frequencies of cure. *Ann. Trop. Med. Parasitol.*, **103**, 357–360.

24 Cowden, J. and Hotez, P. (2000) Mebendazole and albendazole treatment of geohelminth infections in children and pregnant women. *Pediatr. Infect. Dis. J.*, **19**, 659–660.

25 Xiao, S.H., Hui-Ming, W., Tanner, M., Utzinger, J., and Chong, W. (2005) Tribendimidine: a promising, safe and broad-spectrum anthelmintic agent from China. *Acta Trop.*, **94**, 1–14.

26 Steinmann, P., Zhou, X.N., Du, Z.W., Jiang, J.Y., Xiao, S.H., Wu, Z.X., Zhou, H., and Utzinger, J. (2008) Tribendimidine and albendazole for treating soil-transmitted helminths, *Strongyloides stercoralis* and *Taenia* spp.: open-label randomized trial. *PLoS Negl. Trop. Dis.*, **2**, e322.

27 Hu, Y., Xiao, S.H., and Aroian, R.V. (2009) The new anthelmintic tribendimidine is an L-type (levamisole and pyrantel) nicotinic acetylcholine receptor agonist. *PLoS Negl. Trop. Dis.*, **3**, e499.

28 Abaza, H., El-Zayadi, A.R., Kabil, S.M., and Rizk, H. (1998) Nitazoxanide in the treatment of patients with intestinal protozoan and helminthic infections: a report on 546 patients in Egypt. *Curr. Ther. Res. Clin. E*, **59**, 116–121.

29 Kaplan, R.M. (2004) Drug resistance in nematodes of veterinary importance: a status report. *Trends Parasitol.*, **20**, 477–481.

30 Jeschke, P., Harder, A., Schindler, M., and Etzel, W. (2005) Cyclohexadepsipeptides (CHDPs) with improved anthelmintical efficacy against the gastrointestinal nematode (*Haemonchus contortus*) in sheep. *Parasitol. Res.* **97** (Suppl. 1), S17–S21.

31 Kaminsky, R., Ducray, P., Jung, M., Clover, R., Rufener, L., Bouvier, J., Weber, S.S., Wenger, A., Wieland-Berghausen, S., Goebel, T., Gauvry, N., Pautrat, F., Skripsky, T., Froelich, O., Komoin-Oka, C., Westlund, B., Sluder, A., and Maser, P. (2008) A new class of anthelmintics effective against drug-resistant nematodes. *Nature*, **452**, 176–180.

32 Zinser, E.W., Wolf, M.L., Alexander-Bowman, S.J., Thomas, E.M., Davis, J.P., Groppi, V.E., Lee, B.H., Thompson, D.P., and Geary, T.G. (2002) Anthelmintic paraherquamides are cholinergic antagonists in gastrointestinal nematodes and mammals. *J. Vet. Pharmacol. Ther.*, **25**, 241–250.

33 de Maagd, R.A., Bravo, A., and Crickmore, N. (2001) How *Bacillus thuringiensis* has evolved specific toxins to colonize the insect world. *Trends Genet.*, **17**, 193–199.

34 Schnepf, E., Crickmore, N., Van Rie, J., Lereclus, D., Baum, J., Feitelson, J., Zeigler, D.R., and Dean, D.H. (1998) *Bacillus thuringiensis* and its pesticidal crystal proteins. *Microbiol. Mol. Biol. Rev.*, **62**, 775–806.

35 Bravo, A., Gill, S.S., and Soberon, M. (2007) Mode of action of *Bacillus*

thuringiensis Cry and Cyt toxins and their potential for insect control. *Toxicon*, **49**, 423–435.

36 Siegel, J.P. (2001) The mammalian safety of *Bacillus thuringiensis*-based insecticides. *J. Invertebr. Pathol.*, **77**, 13–21.

37 Stephen, C., Pearce, M., and Bender, C. (2001) Human health effects of aerial spraying of *Bacillus thuringiensis kurstaki*-based biological pesticides – a review of observational data and overview of surveillance conducted in Victoria, British Columbia, Canada 1999. *Environ. Health Rev.*, **Fall**, 73–81.

38 Betz, F.S., Hammond, B.G., and Fuchs, R.L. (2000) Safety and advantages of *Bacillus thuringiensis*-protected plants to control insect pests. *Regul. Toxicol. Pharmacol.*, **32**, 156–173.

39 Roh, J.Y., Choi, J.Y., Li, M.S., Jin, B.R., and Je, Y.H. (2007) *Bacillus thuringiensis* as a specific, safe, and effective tool for insect pest control. *J. Microbiol. Biotechnol.*, **17**, 547–559.

40 US Department of Agriculture Economic Research Service (2010) *Adoption of Genetically Engineered Crops in the US*. Department of Agriculture Economic Research Service, Washington, DC.

41 Xia, L.Q., Zhao, X.M., Ding, X.Z., Wang, F.X., and Sun, Y.J. (2008) The theoretical 3D structure of *Bacillus thuringiensis* Cry5Ba. *J. Mol. Model.*, **14**, 843–848.

42 Griffitts, J.S. and Aroian, R.V. (2005) Many roads to resistance: how invertebrates adapt to Bt toxins. *Bioessays*, **27**, 614–624.

43 Marroquin, L.D., Elyassnia, D., Griffitts, J.S., Feitelson, J.S., and Aroian, R.V. (2000) *Bacillus thuringiensis* (Bt) toxin susceptibility and isolation of resistance mutants in the nematode *Caenorhabditis elegans*. *Genetics*, **155**, 1693–1699.

44 Griffitts, J.S., Whitacre, J.L., Stevens, D.E., and Aroian, R.V. (2001) Bt toxin resistance from loss of a putative carbohydrate-modifying enzyme. *Science*, **293**, 860–864.

45 Griffitts, J.S., Huffman, D.L., Whitacre, J.L., Barrows, B.D., Marroquin, L.D., Muller, R., Brown, J.R., Hennet, T., Esko, J.D., and Aroian, R.V. (2003) Resistance to a bacterial toxin is mediated by removal of a conserved glycosylation pathway required for toxin-host interactions. *J. Biol. Chem.*, **278**, 45594–45602.

46 Griffitts, J.S., Haslam, S.M., Yang, T., Garczynski, S.F., Mulloy, B., Morris, H., Cremer, P.S., Dell, A., Adang, M.J., and Aroian, R.V. (2005) Glycolipids as receptors for *Bacillus thuringiensis* crystal toxin. *Science*, **307**, 922–925.

47 Pigott, C.R. and Ellar, D.J. (2007) Role of receptors in *Bacillus thuringiensis* crystal toxin activity. *Microbiol. Mol. Biol. Rev.*, **71**, 255–281.

48 Alouf, J.E. (2003) Molecular features of the cytolytic pore-forming bacterial protein toxins. *Folia Microbiol.*, **48**, 5–16.

49 Kao, C.Y., Los, F.C., Huffman, D.L., Wachi, S., Kloft, N., Husmann, M., Karabrahimi, V., Schwartz, J.L., Bellier, A., Ha, C., Sagong, Y., Fan, H., Ghosh, P., Hsieh, M., Hsu, C.S., Chen, L., and Aroian, R.V. (2011) Global functional analyses of cellular responses to pore-forming toxins. *PLoS Pathog.*, **7**, e1001314.

50 Aroian, R. and van der Goot, F.G. (2007) Pore-forming toxins and cellular non-immune defenses (CNIDs). *Curr. Opin. Microbiol.*, **10**, 57–61.

51 Bischofberger, M., Gonzalez, M.R., and van der Goot, F.G. (2009) Membrane injury by pore-forming proteins. *Curr. Opin. Cell Biol.*, **21**, 589–595.

52 Gonzalez, M.R., Bischofberger, M., Pernot, L., van der Goot, F.G., and Freche, B. (2008) Bacterial pore-forming toxins: the (w)hole story? *Cell Mol. Life Sci.*, **65**, 493–507.

53 Huffman, D.L., Abrami, L., Sasik, R., Corbeil, J., van der Goot, F.G., and Aroian, R.V. (2004) Mitogen-activated protein kinase pathways defend against bacterial pore-forming toxins. *Proc. Natl. Acad. Sci. USA*, **101**, 10995–11000.

54 Bischof, L.J., Kao, C.Y., Los, F.C., Gonzalez, M.R., Shen, Z., Briggs, S.P., van der Goot, F.G., and Aroian, R.V. (2008) Activation of the unfolded protein response is required for defenses against bacterial pore-forming toxin *in vivo*. *PLoS Pathog.*, **4**, e1000176.

55 Bellier, A., Chen, C.S., Kao, C.Y., Cinar, H.N., and Aroian, R.V. (2009) Hypoxia and the hypoxic response pathway protect against pore-forming toxins in C. elegans. PLoS Pathog., 5, e1000689.

56 Los, F.C., Kao, C.Y., Smitham, J., McDonald, K.L., Ha, C., Peixoto, C.A., and Aroian, R.V. (2011) RAB-5- and RAB-11-dependent vesicle-trafficking pathways are required for plasma membrane repair after attack by bacterial pore-forming toxin. Cell Host Microbe, 9, 147–157.

57 Wei, J.Z., Hale, K., Carta, L., Platzer, E., Wong, C., Fang, S.C., and Aroian, R.V. (2003) Bacillus thuringiensis crystal proteins that target nematodes. Proc. Natl. Acad. Sci. USA, 100, 2760–2765.

58 Sasser, J.N. and Freckman, D.W. (1987) A world perspective on nematology: the role of the society, in Vistas on Nematology (eds J.A. Veech and D.W. Dickerson), Society of Nematologists, Hyattsville, MD, pp. 7–14.

59 Williamson, V.M. and Gleason, C.A. (2003) Plant–nematode interactions. Curr. Opin. Plant. Biol., 6, 327–333.

60 Li, X.Q., Tan, A., Voegtline, M., Bekele, S., Chen, C.S., and Aroian, R.V. (2008) Expression of Cry5B protein from Bacillus thuringiensis in plant roots confers resistance to root-knot nematode. Biol. Control, 47, 97–102.

61 Li, X.Q., Wei, J.Z., Tan, A., and Aroian, R.V. (2007) Resistance to root-knot nematode in tomato roots expressing a nematicidal Bacillus thuringiensis crystal protein. Plant Biotechnol. J., 5, 455–464.

62 Kotze, A.C., O'Grady, J., Gough, J.M., Pearson, R., Bagnall, N.H., Kemp, D.H., and Akhurst, R.J. (2005) Toxicity of Bacillus thuringiensis to parasitic and free-living life-stages of nematode parasites of livestock. Int. J. Parasitol., 35, 1013–1022.

63 Rae, R., Riebesell, M., Dinkelacker, I., Wang, Q., Herrmann, M., Weller, A.M., Dieterich, C., and Sommer, R.J. (2008) Isolation of naturally associated bacteria of necromenic Pristionchus nematodes and fitness consequences. J. Exp. Biol., 211, 1927–1936.

64 Schulenburg, H. and Ewbank, J.J. (2004) Diversity and specificity in the interaction between Caenorhabditis elegans and the pathogen Serratia marcescens. BMC Evol. Biol., 4, 49.

65 Schulte, R.D., Makus, C., Hasert, B., Michiels, N.K., and Schulenburg, H. (2010) Multiple reciprocal adaptations and rapid genetic change upon experimental coevolution of an animal host and its microbial parasite. Proc. Natl. Acad. Sci. USA, 107, 7359–7364.

66 Schulte, R.D., Makus, C., Hasert, B., Michiels, N.K., and Schulenburg, H. (2011) Host-parasite local adaptation after experimental coevolution of Caenorhabditis elegans and its microparasite Bacillus thuringiensis. Proc. Biol. Sci., 78, 2832–2839.

67 Behnke, I.M., Guest, J., and Rose, R. (1997) Expression of acquired immunity to the hookworm Ancylostoma ceylanicum in hamsters. Parasite Immunol., 19, 309–318.

68 Bungiro, R.D. Jr, Sun, T., Harrison, L.M., Shoemaker, C.B., and Cappello, M. (2008) Mucosal antibody responses in experimental hookworm infection. Parasite Immunol., 30, 293–303.

69 Fujiwara, R.T., Geiger, S.M., Bethony, J., and Mendez, S. (2006) Comparative immunology of human and animal models of hookworm infection. Parasite Immunol., 28, 285–293.

70 Cappello, M., Bungiro, R.D., Harrison, L.M., Bischof, L.J., Griffitts, J.S., Barrows, B.D., and Aroian, R.V. (2006) A purified Bacillus thuringiensis crystal protein with therapeutic activity against the hookworm parasite Ancylostoma ceylanicum. Proc. Natl. Acad. Sci. USA, 103, 15154–15159.

71 Hu, Y., Georghiou, S.B., Kelleher, A.J., and Aroian, R.V. (2010) Bacillus thuringiensis Cry5B protein is highly efficacious as a single-dose therapy against an intestinal roundworm infection in mice. PLoS Negl. Trop. Dis., 4, e614.

72 Behnke, J.M. and Harris, P. (2009) Heligmosomoides bakeri or Heligmosomoides polygyrus? Am. J. Trop. Med. Hyg., 804, 684.

73 Behnke, J.M., Menge, D.M., and Noyes, H. (2009) *Heligmosomoides bakeri*: a model for exploring the biology and genetics of resistance to chronic gastrointestinal nematode infections. *Parasitology*, **136**, 1565–1580.

74 Monroy, F.G. and Enriquez, F.J. (1992) *Heligmosomoides polygyrus*: a model for chronic gastrointestinal helminthiasis. *Parasitol. Today*, **8**, 49–54.

75 Omura, S. (2008) Ivermectin: 25 years and still going strong. *Int. J. Antimicrob. Agents*, **31**, 91–98.

76 Fonseca-Salamanca, F., Martinez-Grueiro, M.M., and Martinez-Fernandez, A.R. (2003) Nematocidal activity of nitazoxanide in laboratory models. *Parasitol Res.*, **91**, 321–324.

77 Githiori, J.B., Hoglund, J., Waller, P.J., and Leyden Baker, R. (2003) Evaluation of anthelmintic properties of extracts from some plants used as livestock dewormers by pastoralist and smallholder farmers in Kenya against *Heligmosomoides polygyrus* infections in mice. *Vet. Parasitol.*, **118**, 215–226.

78 Wabo Pone, J., Mbida, M., and Bilong Bilong, C.F. (2009) *In vivo* evaluation of potential nematicidal properties of ethanol extract of *Canthium mannii* (Rubiaceae) on *Heligmosomoides polygyrus* parasite of rodents. *Vet. Parasitol.*, **166**, 103–107.

79 Hu, Y., Platzer, E.G., Bellier, A., and Aroian, R.V. (2010) Discovery of a highly synergistic anthelmintic combination that shows mutual hypersusceptibility. *Proc. Natl. Acad. Sci. USA*, **107**, 5955–5960.

80 Gleeson, T.D. and Decker, C.F. (2006) Treatment of tuberculosis. *Dis. Mon.*, **52**, 428–434.

81 Lin, J.T., Juliano, J.J., and Wongsrichanalai, C. (2010) Drug-resistant malaria: the era of ACT. *Curr. Infect. Dis. Rep.*, **12**, 165–173.

82 Mocroft, A., Ledergerber, B., Katlama, C., Kirk, O., Reiss, P., d'Arminio Monforte, A., Knysz, B., Dietrich, M., Phillips, A.N., and Lundgren, J.D. (2003) Decline in the AIDS and death rates in the EuroSIDA study: an observational study. *Lancet*, **362**, 22–29.

83 Keiser, J. and Utzinger, J. (2010) The drugs we have and the drugs we need against major helminth infections. *Adv. Parasitol.*, **73**, 197–230.

84 Tozzi, V., Zaccarelli, M., Narciso, P., Trotta, M.P., Ceccherini-Silberstein, F., De Longis, P., D'Offizi, G., Forbici, F., D'Arrigo, R., Boumis, E., Bellagamba, R., Bonfigli, S., Carvelli, C., Antinori, A., and Perno, C.F. (2004) Mutations in HIV-1 reverse transcriptase potentially associated with hypersusceptibility to nonnucleoside reverse-transcriptase inhibitors: effect on response to efavirenz-based therapy in an urban observational cohort. *J. Infect. Dis.*, **189**, 1688–1695.

85 Kim, R. and Baxter, J.D. (2008) Protease inhibitor resistance update: where are we now? *AIDS Patient Care STDS*, **22**, 267–277.

86 Haubrich, R.H. (2004) Resistance and replication capacity assays: clinical utility and interpretation. *Top. HIV Med.*, **12**, 52–56.

87 Chou, T.C. (2006) Theoretical basis, experimental design, and computerized simulation of synergism and antagonism in drug combination studies. *Pharmacol. Rev.*, **58**, 621–681.

17
Monepantel: From Discovery to Mode of Action

*Ronald Kaminsky** and Lucien Rufener*

Abstract

Until recently, only three broad-spectrum classes of anthelmintics for the control of gastrointestinal nematodes of livestock were available: the benzimidazoles, the imidazothiazoles, and the macrocyclic lactones. In 2008, Novartis Animal Health reported the discovery of the amino-acetonitrile derivatives (AADs) as a potential new class of broad-spectrum anthelmintics for livestock. The objectives of the present chapter are to introduce the AADs, their discovery, their safety and efficacy profiles, the selection of monepantel as the first candidate for commercial use, and, finally, the investigation of the mode of action of this active ingredient.

Discovery of the Amino-Acetonitrile Derivatives

In mid-2000, the first active compound from the amino-acetonitrile derivatives (AADs) class was detected in a high-throughput screening program, using a larval development assay (LDA) for *Haemonchus contortus* and *Trichostrongylus colubriformis*. Optimization of the lead molecule (AAD-450) was then pursued using a rodent model (*Meriones unguiculatus*) in which marked decreases in *H. contortus* burdens but no activity against *T. colubriformis* was observed. In these initial tests, a dose of 10 mg racemate/kg was used. (A racemate is an equimolar mixture of a pair of enantiomers. This is the case when a chiral center is present in a synthetic molecule.) It was then shown that only the *S*- and not the *R*-enantiomer had antiparasitic activity [1].

The *N*-acyl amino-acetonitriles were previously described in the literature as fungicides, antibacterials, and insecticides, but never as potential anthelmintics [1]. The AADs are low-molecular-mass compounds bearing different aryloxy and aroyl moieties on an amino-acetonitrile core (Figure 17.1) [1]. Based on the initial results with AAD-450, more than 700 different AAD molecules were generated and their potential anthelmintic activity was assessed. Promising candidates were selected using a LDA *in vitro* test on *H. contortus* and *T. colubriformis*, and then tested *in vivo* in the rodent model. It was observed that substitutions with OCF_3 and CF_3 on residues R3 or R4 tended to provide the best anthelmintic activity.

* Corresponding Author

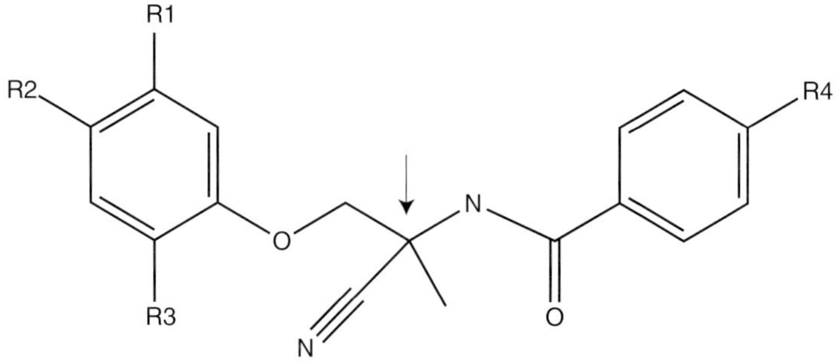

Figure 17.1 Chemical structure of the AADs. The arrow points out the chiral center. R stands for sites for various residues and are substitution points on the backbone structure.

Out of this screening, the better molecules were selected for further testing in sheep and cattle. Various studies using AAD analogs have been performed and confirmed as active against levamisole- and benzimidazole-resistant populations of *H. contortus* and levamisole/benzimidazole-multiresistant *T. colubriformis*. One of the selected compounds, AAD-1470, cured sheep (treated with 5 mg racemate/kg) infected with the "Howick" isolate from South Africa that is resistant to the three older broad-spectrum anthelmintic classes including the macrocyclic lactones [2]. This was a substantial hint that the AADs were acting through a completely novel mode of action because no cross-resistance was observed.

Selection of AAD-1566 (Monepantel)

At the end of the lead optimization program, that included efficacy and tolerability testing in sheep and cattle, one compound in particular emerged as the first drug development candidate. When tested in the rodent models at a dose of 0.32 mg racemate/kg, it was active against *H. contortus* and *T. colubriformis* [3]. The enantiomers of that compound were separated and both molecules (including the racemic mixture) were then tested in the gerbil against drug-resistant nematode isolates. The racemic mixture showed 84–100% activity at 1 mg/kg, the active enantiomer (AAD-1566) showed a higher efficacy of 99–100%, whereas the inactive enantiomer (AAD-1566i) possessed no activity. After a full battery of tests, AAD-1566 was selected for entering the industrial development phase as an oral anthelmintic for sheep. AAD-1566 was given the nonproprietary name monepantel by the World Health Organization and was approved as an oral anthelmintic for sheep in New Zealand in January 2009. Monepantel is now commercially available in many countries (France, United Kingdom, Australia, New Zealand, Germany, Switzerland, Uruguay, Argentina, and South Africa) under the tradename of Zolvix®.

The efficacy of monepantel in its commercial formulation against nematodes in sheep was evaluated in numerous pen studies and field trials [4–7]. When applied at the recommended dose of 2.5 mg/kg, monepantel is effective against all major gastrointestinal nematodes, including those that are resistant to benzimidazoles,

Table 17.1 Efficacy (%) of monepantel against various nematodes in sheep.

	H. contortus Howick	H. contortus Haecon 51	T. colubriformis	T. circumcincta
Fenbendazole	0	—	0	25
Levamisole	0	—	80	21
Ivermectin	3	1	100	24
Moxidectin	—	28	—	—
Oxfendazole + levamisole + abamectin	—	5	—	—
Monepantel	99.7	99.7	99.8	99.9

Sheep were treated with the commercially recommended doses of products containing the active compounds indicated in the table. Efficacy was determined as reductions in worm counts.

imidazothiazole, and macrocyclic lactones, and a recent commercialized combination of derquantel and abamectin [8]. An example of the efficacy of monepantel is presented in Table 17.1.

Tolerability of the AADs

A high level of efficacy and safety (for people, animals, and the environment) is desirable for new products. In most cases, new compounds that do not fulfill all of these target requirements are dropped from research and development programs. Preliminary toxicology testing (Ames test, micronucleus test, and acute toxic dosing) was performed with the racemate of AAD-450 and both enantiomers of AAD-1470. No evidence of clastogenic (i.e., giving rise to or inducing disruption or breakages, as of chromosomes), aneugenic (i.e., promoting aneuploidy in cells by affecting normal cell division and migration of chromosomes during mitosis (or meiosis)), or mutagenic potentials of these compounds was identified. The oral toxic dose in rats was determined to be greater than 2000 mg/kg. Tolerability and safety of monepantel were demonstrated in numerous studies [9–11]. In sheep, oral doses up to 200 mg/kg were tested and no adverse effects were noted. This safety profile is proposed to be due to the nematode-specific target of the AADs as described below.

Investigation of the Mode of Action of Monepantel

The mode of action of AAD-1566 was investigated using a forward genetics approach with the nonparasitic model organism, *Caenorhabditis elegans* (Figure 17.2). There are numerous examples of forward genetic screens to select *C. elegans* mutants that resist anthelmintics. This is the starting point to understand their mode of action and potential resistance mechanisms. Examples include screens for resistance to levamisole [12], benzimidazoles [13], aldicarb [14], and ivermectin [15, 16]. The complete genome sequence of *C. elegans* is known and the worms are easily amenable to

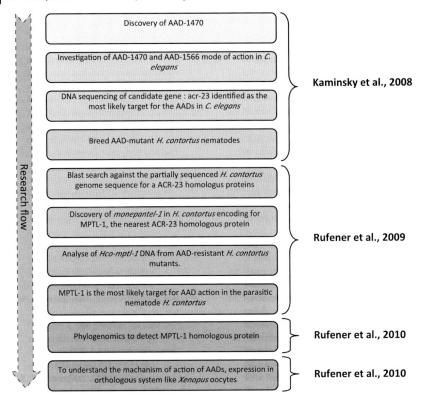

Figure 17.2 Outline of the approach and sequence of main discoveries to identify the biological target of the AADs using C. elegans and H. contortus mutant nematodes.

genetic manipulation. Fortunately, AAD-1566 interfered with the movement, growth, and viability of C. elegans as well. This manifests as a hypercontraction of the body wall muscles leading to paralysis, spasmodic contractions of the anterior portion of the pharynx, and, ultimately, death.

A screen was performed on C. elegans worms that had been exposed to the mutagenic agent ethane methyl sulfonate and approximately 40 mutants with different levels of resistance to AAD-1566 were selected. Gene mapping was then performed using a genetic recombination approach [17] where most of the resistant alleles isolated mapped to a 5-map-unit interval on chromosome V. Further DNA sequencing in this region revealed 27 independent mutations in *acr-23*, a gene coding for a putative nicotinic acetylcholine receptor (nAChR) subunit, designating it as the major candidate contributor to the AAD response in C. elegans.

Neurotransmitter-gated ion channels provide the molecular basis for rapid signal transmission at chemical synapses. They can transiently form a channel upon binding of a specific neurotransmitter and allow small cations (Na^+ and K^+ in the case of an excitatory channel or Cl^- if its an inhibitory channel) to pass through the central pore. The movement of the ions through the open pore lasts for several

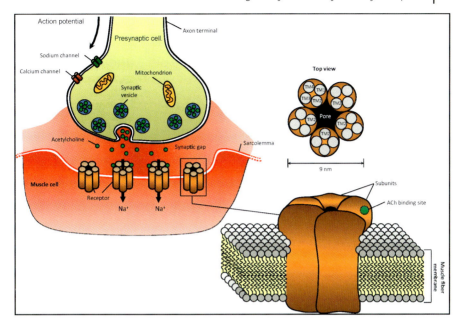

Figure 17.3 Schematic representation of a synaptic region with the axon terminal and the muscle cell (left part of the picture). On the right, the pentameric channel is represented in two different views (transversal and lateral). The five subunits that make up the receptor are arranged around a central pore formed by TM2.

milliseconds and results in a current pulse of several picoamps that flows across the membrane. An nAChR consists of five subunits, which assemble to form a channel through the cell membrane (Figure 17.3). This cholinergic receptor can be homomeric (five α-subunits) or heteromeric (both α- and non-α-subunits; see Chapter 1 for an extensive discussion on ligand-gated ion channels).

All known sequences of subunits from neurotransmitter-gated ion channels are structurally related. They are composed of a large extracellular glycosylated N-terminal domain, followed by three hydrophobic transmembrane regions, which form the ionic channel, followed by an intracellular region of variable length. A fourth transmembrane region is found at the C-terminal part of the sequence. The second transmembrane domain is the main contributor of the channel pore. The extracellular domain is composed of different loops (A–F), which are involved in the ligand binding [18]. Subunits possessing two adjacent cysteines in loop C are defined as nAChR α-subunits. A Cys-loop, consisting of two cysteines separated by 13 conserved amino acids, is used to classify subunits possessing the motif in the "Cys-loop superfamily" of ligand-gated ion channels.

It is remarkable that the *C. elegans* genome is extraordinarily rich in genes encoding nAChR subunits [18, 19]. For comparison, the human genome contains 17 genes encoding nAChR subunits, whereas as many as 27 nAChR genes are found in *C. elegans* [20]. Five subfamilies of nAChR subunits have been identified based on

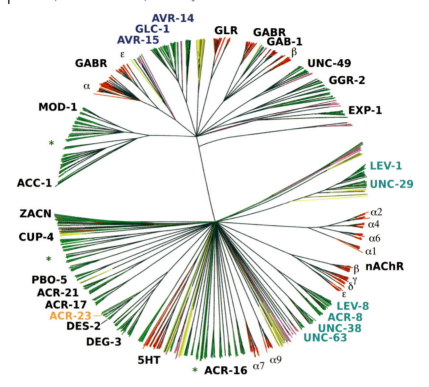

Figure 17.4 Phylogenetic tree based on the ligand-binding domain region of putative ligand-gated ion channel genes. A neighbor-joining tree (ClustalW) of the ligand-binding domain region of conceptually translated putative ligand-gated ion channel genes as detected with GeneWise after an initial BLAST screen with the 210 seeds (1426 sequences in total). A thousand bootstrap iterations were performed and branches below 50% bootstrap support were collapsed. Nematode sequences are shown in shades of green, platyhelminthes in yellow, insects in purple, and vertebrates in red. Some *C. elegans* and human subunits are labeled, and the labels for proteins involved in drug susceptibility are colored as follows; levamisole, cyan; monepantel, orange; and ivermectin, blue. Green asterisks indicate branches that are similar to these latter, and appear broad and nematode-specific. These could be attractive for further investigation as targets for other compounds. (Adapted from [20].)

sequence similarity: UNC-29, UNC-38, ACR-8, ACR-16, and DEG-3 [18, 19, 21], with ACR-8 and DEG-3 being nematode-specific classes [22]. The ACR-23 protein belongs to the DEG-3 subfamily of nAChR subunits and is, therefore, nematode-specific (Figure 17.4). This means that ACR-23 orthologs are not found in vertebrates (e.g., mammals, birds), providing the first explanation for the safety profile of AAD-1566. The nAChR subunits involved in AAD action are different from those targeted by levamisole [20, 23, 24] and there is no cross-resistance between the two chemical classes [25]. Levamisole targets subunits belonging to the UNC-38 and UNC-29 subfamily (Figure 17.4).

Elucidating the Molecular Mode of Action of Monepantel

Use of *C. elegans* as a Model

The genetic screening performed with *C. elegans* allowed the identification of one major molecular target for monepantel action – the nAChR subunit ACR-23. Further research (Rufener *et al.*, manuscript in preparation) showed that the mutant *acr-23* (*cb27*) can be fully rescued (i.e., AAD sensitivity is restored) by expressing the wild-type *acr-23* gene. For this, a wild-type copy of *acr-23*, including the promoter region (4 kb) and the 3′-untranslated region (UTR), was amplified by polymerase chain reaction (PCR) from genomic DNA extracted from the N2 strain and injected into *acr-23* (*cb27*) adults. The resulting rescue was complete with worms becoming as sensitive as the wild-type. This is the first direct evidence of the involvement of ACR-23 in the sensitivity phenotype. To gain knowledge about the function of ACR-23, its *in vivo* expression in *C. elegans* was localized using a Green Fluorescent Protein (GFP) fused in frame with *acr-23*. Wild-type or mutant *acr-23* (*cb27*) adults were injected with roller DNA plus two PCR-generated fragments coding for *acr-23* (promoter region and complete coding region) and GFP. In the case of *acr-23* (cb27), the transgenic animals were rescued and completely sensitive to the AADs (30 μg/ml). The presence of the fused transgene was verified by PCR. Integrated lines expressed GFP in various tissues, including body wall muscles (Figure 17.5), and head and tail neurons; no GFP expression was observed in eggs or first-stage larvae. This expression pattern (muscles and neurons) is in agreement with the paralysis phenotype observed on nematodes exposed to monepantel. Head and tail neurons have not yet been identified, and more work will be necessary to characterize them with the help of neuron-specific antibodies for instance.

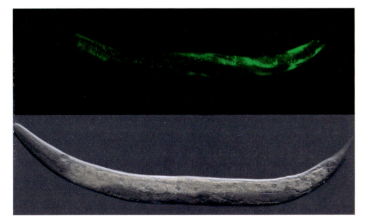

Figure 17.5 Expression of *acr-23*(+):GFP, L$_2$ larvae, ×100. Expression is detected in the body wall muscles. (Courtesy of Samantha Rey, University of Fribourg, Switzerland.)

Functional Characterization of the Cel-ACR-23 Receptor

To functionally characterize the receptor, *Xenopus* oocytes (Rufener *et al.*, manuscript in preparation) were injected with *Cel-acr-23* cRNA and current was recorded using a two-electrode voltage clamp after addition of the agonist. The *Cel-acr-23* gene was cloned in a vector containing the 5'- and 3'-UTR of β-globulin from *X. laevis*, reverse-transcribed *in vitro*, 5'-capped, and injected into *X. laevis* oocytes. After 24 h, currents were elicited by the addition of acetylcholine, choline, or nicotine. Choline proved to be a more potent agonist of the *C. elegans* ACR-23 channels than acetylcholine or nicotine. Currents measured with choline were characterized by a fast channel opening followed by a slow desensitization. The oocytes rapidly recovered to the initial resting membrane potential once the agonist was washed away. Interestingly, no saturation of the channel could be observed even when very high choline chloride concentrations were used (Figure 17.6).

The potential of monepantel to act as an allosteric modulator on the ACR-23 receptor was tested when coupled with choline chloride. Figure 17.7 shows current traces of a concentration–response curve with monepantel combined with 1 mM choline. When used alone, 1 mM choline elicited 350 nA currents. Monepantel strongly enhanced the observed maximum current peak measured as well as the

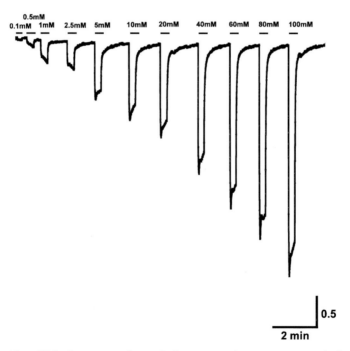

Figure 17.6 Current traces from a choline concentration–response curve obtained from a *X. laevis* oocyte expressing *Cel*-ACR-23 receptors. The bars indicate the time period of choline perfusion. Choline concentrations are indicated above the bars.

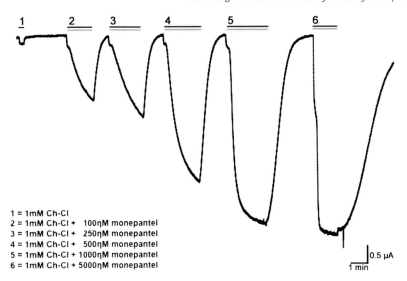

Figure 17.7 Monepantel can act as an ACR-23 channel modulator. Current amplitudes from a cumulative concentration-dependence of the potentiation by monepantel of currents elicited by 1 mM choline obtained from a X. laevis oocyte expressing Cel-ACR-23 receptors. The bars indicate the time period of choline (black) or monepantel (orange) perfusion. Choline and monepantel concentrations are indicated in the figure.

kinetic of the channel. The AAD-mediated potentiation of the current was measured at a concentration of 1 mM choline, which elicits only a small fraction of the maximal current amplitude. Coinjection of *Cel-acr-23* cRNA, with or without *Cel-ric-3*, did not significantly affect the modulation of *C. elegans* ACR-23 channels by monepantel (data not shown). The optical *R*-enantiomer of monepantel (AAD-2224), which has no antinematode effect, was inactive and failed to elicit or potentiate any current, either alone or in combination with choline chloride (data not shown).

Discovery of the *H. contortus* Monepantel-1 Gene

The first investigation to understand the mode of action of monepantel in *H. contortus* was performed using freshly harvested adult nematodes (maintained in Hank's balanced saline solution at 37 °C) exposed *in vitro* to various concentrations of monepantel. This experiment showed that the worms were almost completely paralyzed, but still able to move head and tail sections in a more or less normal fashion. This was an early hint that monepantel was targeting or interfering with the neuromuscular signal transmission.

In order to elucidate the molecular mechanism of monepantel, a forward genetic approach was followed. The primary step was to select a *H. contortus* population able to survive a full-dose treatment of monepantel in sheep. For this, a new "*in vitro* selection–*in vivo* propagation" protocol was developed [25], which allowed the successful selection of two independent AAD-mutant lines, *Hc*-CRA AAD^{M} and

Hc-Howick AAD^M, as reported [3, 26]. The discovery of ACR-23 in C. elegans allowed a search for homologous proteins in H. contortus via a tBLASTn search on the partially sequenced genome available online at: http://www.sanger.ac.uk/Projects/H_contortus. The two independent AAD mutant H. contortus lines were used to screen for mutations in the identified acetylcholine receptor genes of the DEG-3 subfamily. Two genes were affected: (i) H. contortus des-2 homolog, Hco-des-2, for which all AAD mutant H. contortus carried an insertion in the 5′-UTR introducing two additional, out-of-frame start codons, and (ii) monepantel-1 (Hco-mptl-1), for which a panel of different mutations was detected in AAD mutant (AAD^M) H. contortus. Apart from one nonsense mutation discovered in Hc-Howick AAD^M nematodes (Hco-MPTL-1-m5; Figure 17.8), the detected mutations all involved mis-splicing, resulting in loss of exon(s) from the mRNA as indicated by shortened reverse transcriptase-PCR products. Furthermore, the AAD mutants exhibited altered expression levels of the three DEG-3 subfamily genes, Hco-mptl-1, Hco-des-2, and Hco-deg-3, as quantified by real-time PCR. These results suggest that Hco-MPTL-1 and other DEG-3 subfamily subunit members are the most likely targets for AAD action against H. contortus. The loss-of-function mutations in the corresponding genes may be responsible for the loss of sensitivity to the AADs.

In a recent paper [27], it was demonstrated that monepantel sulfone (AAD-4670), the major metabolite of monepantel in sheep [28], potentiates the choline-activated currents mediated by H. contortus DEG-3/DES-2 receptors in a concentration-dependent way without opening the channels. Thus, it acts as a positive allosteric modulator with a threshold of approximately 0.3 μM and an EC$_{50}$ of approximately 4 μM.

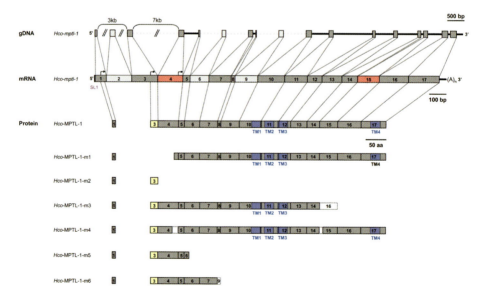

Figure 17.8 Hco-mptl-1 locus, mRNA, and protein (top), and mis-splicing mutations in the AAD mutants (bottom). (Adapted from [29].)

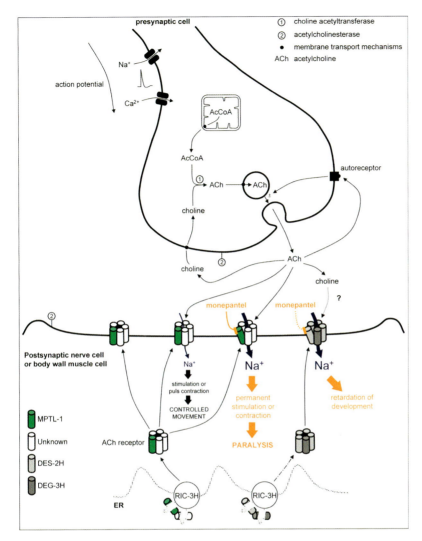

Figure 17.9 Hypothetical model of the interference of monepantel with acetylcholine receptors. An action potential arrives at the end of the presynaptic cell, opening the Na^+ and Ca^+ voltage-sensitive channels. This provokes the exocytosis of vesicles containing acetylcholine molecules in the synaptic region. Acetylcholine binds to the receptors present at the postsynaptic nerve cell or at the body wall muscle cell and opens the channel. An inflow of Na^+ ions enters the cell through the pore formed by the receptor and creates a depolarization of the cell membrane. This leads to the stimulation of the nerve cell or to the pulse contraction of the muscle cell. Hypothetically, if monepantel binds to the acetylcholine receptor containing a MPTL-1 subunit, it provokes a permanent stimulation or contraction that paralyzes the nematode. The last channel on the right is a DEG-3/DES-2 channel responding to choline [27] that is generated upon degradation of acetylcholine to choline and acetate by acetylcholinesterase. The DEG-3/DES-2 oligomer is not as sensitive as MPTL-1 (dotted line), but could still be involved in retarding the development observed at high monepantel concentrations. The ancillary protein RIC-3H, which is resident in the endoplasmic reticulum, is important for the correct assembly of the receptor containing MPTL-1 as well as the DEG-3H/DES-2H receptor. A downregulation of RIC-3H (dashed line) favors the incorporation of DES-2H subunits in the channel, thereby generating receptors with higher sensitivity to monepantel.

Developing a Model for the Mode of Action of Monepantel

With the discovery of *acr-23* in *C. elegans*, it was then possible to identify a potential homolog in the target parasite, *H. contortus*, named *mptl-1*. The apparent involvement of *acr-23* and *mptl-1* in AAD sensitivity has been demonstrated [25, 29] and it has also been shown that resistance to monepantel can be induced in nematodes [25]. With the knowledge gained from the use of *C. elegans* and *H. contortus*, the hypothetical AAD molecular mode of action could be as follows. An infected sheep is treated orally with monepantel, the drug is ingested, and may enter the nematode either by direct contact in the abomasum through passive diffusion or via the blood containing the drug. Monepantel reaches the acetylcholine receptors containing the MPTL-1 subunit at the neuromuscular junction and, upon binding, the AAD-sensitive receptors remain open, thus allowing an unrestricted inflow of cations that produces a constant depolarization of the cell membrane. This creates a spastic paralysis of the nematode and finally leads to the expulsion of the parasite from the host within the feces. The hypothetical interaction of monepantel with MPTL-1 and possibly DES-2 in the synaptic region is depicted in Figure 17.9. However, more work is needed to fully understand the molecular mode of action of AADs.

Conclusions

The discovery of monepantel and its development into the commercially available product Zolvix enables sheep farmers world-wide to regain control of nematode infections. Monepantel eliminates all major gastrointestinal nematodes including benzimidazole-, imidazothiazole-, macrocyclic lactone- and multiresistant isolates, due to the new mode of action. Therefore, monepantel is effective against nematode infections independent of the sensitivity status of worm populations to the classical anthelmintics.

Based on the description of the molecular target of monepantel, sensitive molecular tests should be developed to detect mutants in the field much earlier than using classical egg hatch tests. These tests would be of critical value in detecting resistance to AADs should it emerge in future. As ever, it is crucial to implement an integrated approach to worm control, including the judicious use of all available anthelmintics.

References

1 Ducray, P., Gauvry, N., Pautrat, F. *et al.* (2008) Discovery of amino-acetonitrile derivatives, a new class of synthetic anthelmintic compounds. *Bioorg. Med. Chem. Lett.*, **18**, 2935–2938.

2 van Wyk, J.A., Malan, F.S., and Randles, J.L., (1997) How long before resistance makes it impossible to control some field strains of *Haemonchus contortus* in South Africa with any of the modern anthelmintics? *Vet. Parasitol.*, **70**, 111–122.

3 Kaminsky, R., Gauvry, N., Schorderet, W.S. *et al.* (2008) Identification of the amino-acetonitrile derivative monepantel (AAD 1566) as a

new anthelmintic drug development candidate. *Parasitol. Res.*, **103**, 931–939.

4 Bustamante, M., Steffan, P.E., Morlan, J.B. *et al.* (2009) The efficacy of monepantel, an amino-acetonitrile derivative, against gastrointestinal nematodes of sheep in three countries of southern Latin America. *Parasitol. Res.*, **106**, 139–144.

5 Hosking, B.C., Kaminsky, R., Sager, H. *et al.* (2010) A pooled analysis of the efficacy of monepantel, an amino-acetonitrile derivative against gastrointestinal nematodes of sheep. *Parasitol. Res.*, **106**, 529–532.

6 Kaminsky, R., Mosimann, D., Sager, H. *et al.* (2009) Determination of the effective dose rate of monepantel (AAD 1566) against adult gastro-intestinal nematodes in sheep. *Int. J. Parasitol.*, **39**, 443–446.

7 Sager, H., Hosking, B.C., Bapst, B. *et al.* (2009) Efficacy of the amino-acetonitrile derivative, monepantel, against experimental and natural adult stage gastro-intestinal nematodes infections in sheep. *Vet. Parasitol.*, **159**, 49–54.

8 Kaminsky, R., Bapst, B., Stein, P.A. *et al.* (2011) Differences in efficacy of monepantel, derquantel and abamectin against multi-resistant nematodes of sheep. *Parasitol. Res.*, **109**, 19–23.

9 Malikides, N., Spencer, K., Mahoney, R. *et al.* (2009) Safety of an amino-acetonitrile derivative (AAD), monepantel, in ewes and their offspring following repeated oral administration. *NZ Vet. J.*, **57**, 193–202.

10 Malikides, N., Helbig, R., Roth, D.R. *et al.* (2009) Safety of an amino-acetonitrile derivative (AAD), monepantel, in weaned lambs following repeated oral administration. *NZ Vet. J.*, **57**, 10–15.

11 Malikides, N., Helbig, R., Mahoney, R. *et al.* (2009) Reproductive safety of an amino-acetonitrile derivative (AAD), monepantel, in rams following repeated oral administration. *NZ Vet. J.*, **57**, 16–21.

12 Lewis, J.A., Wu, C.H., Levine, J.H. *et al.* (1980) Levamisole-resistant mutants of the nematode *Caenorhabditis elegans* appear to lack pharmacological acetylcholine receptors. *Neuroscience*, **5**, 967–989.

13 Driscoll, M., Dean, E., Reilly, E. *et al.* (1989) Genetic and molecular analysis of a *Caenorhabditis elegans* beta-tubulin that conveys benzimidazole sensitivity. *J. Cell Biol.*, **109**, 2993–3003.

14 Nguyen, M., Alfonso, A., Johnson, C.D. *et al.* (1995) *Caenorhabditis elegans* mutants resistant to inhibitors of acetylcholinesterase. *Genetics*, **140**, 527–535.

15 Dent, J.A., Davis, M.W., and Avery, L. (1997) *avr-15* encodes a chloride channel subunit that mediates inhibitory glutamatergic neurotransmission and ivermectin sensitivity in *Caenorhabditis elegans*. *EMBO J.*, **16**, 5867–5879.

16 Dent, J.A., Smith, M.M., Vassilatis, D.K. *et al.* (2000) The genetics of ivermectin resistance in *Caenorhabditis elegans*. *Proc. Natl. Acad. Sci. USA*, **97**, 2674–2679.

17 Wicks, S.R., Yeh, R.T., Gish, W.R. *et al.* (2001) Rapid gene mapping in *Caenorhabditis elegans* using a high density polymorphism map. *Nat. Genet.*, **28**, 160–164.

18 Jones, A.K. and Sattelle, D.B. (2004) Functional genomics of the nicotinic acetylcholine receptor gene family of the nematode, *Caenorhabditis elegans*. *Bioessays*, **26**, 39–49.

19 Mongan, N.P., Baylis, H.A., Adcock, C. *et al.* (1998) An extensive and diverse gene family of nicotinic acetylcholine receptor alpha subunits in *Caenorhabditis elegans*. *Receptors Channels*, **6**, 213–228.

20 Rufener, L., Keiser, J., Kaminsky, R. *et al.* (2010) Phylogenomics of ligand-gated ion channels predicts monepantel effect. *PLoS Pathog.*, **6**, e1001091.

21 Mongan, N.P., Jones, A.K., Smith, G.R. *et al.* (2002) Novel alpha7-like nicotinic acetylcholine receptor subunits in the nematode *Caenorhabditis elegans*. *Protein Sci.*, **11**, 1162–1171.

22 Brown, L.A., Jones, A.K., Buckingham, S.D. *et al.* (2006) Contributions from *Caenorhabditis elegans* functional genetics to antiparasitic drug target identification and validation:

nicotinic acetylcholine receptors, a case study. *Int. J. Parasitol.*, **36**, 617–624.

23 Culetto, E., Baylis, H.A., Richmond, J.E. et al. (2004) The *Caenorhabditis elegans* unc-63 gene encodes a levamisole-sensitive nicotinic acetylcholine receptor alpha subunit. *J. Biol. Chem.*, **279**, 42476–42483.

24 Fleming, J.T., Squire, M.D., Barnes, T.M. et al. (1997) *Caenorhabditis elegans* levamisole resistance genes *lev-1, unc-29,* and *unc-38* encode functional nicotinic acetylcholine receptor subunits. *J. Neurosci.*, **17**, 5843–5857.

25 Kaminsky, R., Ducray, P., Jung, M. et al. (2008) A new class of anthelmintics effective against drug-resistant nematodes. *Nature*, **452**, 176–180.

26 Rufener, L., Kaminsky, R., and Maser, P. (2009) *In vitro* selection of *Haemonchus contortus* for benzimidazole resistance reveals a mutation at amino acid 198 of beta-tubulin. *Mol. Biochem. Parasitol.*, **168**, 120–122.

27 Rufener, L., Baur, R., Kaminsky, R. et al. (2010) Monepantel allosterically activates DEG-3/DES-2 channels of the gastrointestinal nematode *Haemonchus contortus. Mol. Pharmacol.*, **78**, 895–902.

28 Karadzovska, D., Seewald, W., Browning, A. et al. (2009) Pharmacokinetics of monepantel and its sulfone metabolite, monepantel sulfone, after intravenous and oral administration in sheep. *J. Vet. Pharmacol. Ther.*, **32**, 359–367.

29 Rufener, L., Maser, P., Roditi, I. et al. (2009) *Haemonchus contortus* acetylcholine receptors of the DEG-3 subfamily and their role in sensitivity to monepantel. *PLoS Pathog.*, **5**, e1000380.

18
Discovery, Mode of Action, and Commercialization of Derquantel

Debra J. Woods[*], *Steven J. Maeder, Alan P. Robertson, Richard J. Martin, Timothy G. Geary, David P. Thompson, Sandra S. Johnson, and George A. Conder*

Abstract

The frequent use of anthelmintics, particularly in geographic areas of intense parasite transmission, has led to the selection and spread of parasite strains that are resistant to them. Against that backdrop, Upjohn Animal Health (now Pfizer Animal Health) established a discovery program to identify compounds with novel modes of action and effective against several important nematode species, including strains resistant to the major classes of anthelmintics. This testing led to the discovery of 2-deoxy-paraherquamide (derquantel) – the first of the spiroindole class of anthelmintics with commercial utility. Derquantel was prepared semisynthetically by chemical reduction of paraherquamide, isolated from fermentation extracts of *Penicillium simplicissimum*. It was subsequently shown that derquantel is a nicotinic cholinergic antagonist. During clinical development, derquantel was combined with the macrocyclic lactone, abamectin. The combination of the new chemical with a second anthelmintic from a different chemical class in a single product (Startect®) provides a more complete spectrum of anthelmintic activity and efficacy against resistant strains. Additionally, the combination also offers a means of minimizing selection for resistance to derquantel through the use of abamectin with a second, distinct mode of action, thereby potentially enhancing the sustainability of worm control programs.

Introduction

The history of chemotherapy for all forms of infectious disease has been driven primarily by the remarkable capacity of infecting organisms to develop resistance to the drugs used against them. In general, resistance develops most rapidly and profoundly when the number of drugs is limited, frequency of dosing is high, and underdosing commonly practiced. Clearly, each of these conditions characterized chemotherapy for parasitic helminths in the second half of the twentieth century. The introduction of ivermectin [1] into veterinary usage in the early 1980s

---

[*] Corresponding Author.

Parasitic Helminths: Targets, Screens, Drugs and Vaccines, First Edition. Edited by Conor R. Caffrey.
© 2012 Wiley-VCH Verlag GmbH & Co. KGaA. Published 2012 by Wiley-VCH Verlag GmbH & Co. KGaA.

revolutionized the treatment of and market for anthelmintics, including both livestock and companion animals. At that time, drug resistance to the benzimidazoles and imidazolides, which were introduced at least 20 years earlier, was already widespread, especially in species that infect small ruminants [2]. The commercial accomplishment of ivermectin, coupled with emerging resistance in small ruminants, drove investment by animal health companies in the discovery of anthelmintics with novel mechanisms of action to compete with ivermectin and combat resistance. Following the success of the macrocyclic lactones, fungal metabolites were a proven rich source of anthelmintics, so it seemed a logical starting point in the search for new agents. Companies such as Merck, Meiji Seika (Bayer), and SmithKline Beecham followed this route, with the identification of cyclodepsipeptides [3] and paraherquamides [4–6]. A number of additional anthelmintic compounds emerged from these screens, particularly at Merck, but none was commercialized. Other animal health companies were also actively working on screening of natural product extracts and small molecules.

Discovery and Characterization of PNU-141962 (2-Deoxyparaherquamide)

Scientists at Upjohn Animal Health (now Pfizer Animal Health) initiated a discovery program based on screening of natural product extracts and small-molecule libraries against the free-living nematode *Caenorhabditis elegans*. They demonstrated that marcfortine A (first reported by Polonsky *et al.* [7] in 1980) had anthelmintic activity [8], although less potent than paraherquamide in their assays. Interestingly, this class of compounds is only weakly active in the screening format employed at Upjohn Animal Health at the time and was detected only because the fungal isolate serendipitously coproduced oligomycin A, which had weak anthelmintic activity. The anthelmintic activity of marcfortine A was identified following bioassay-guided fractionation.

As is clear from Figure 18.1a, the structures of marcfortine A and paraherquamide A (a metabolite of *Penicillium paraherquei*) are very similar, with the only differences occurring in the "G" ring. These observations led to a medicinal chemistry program, generating and screening over 300 analogs, to improve potency in a proprietary, patentable structure. As part of the analoging program, the marcfortine G ring was modified to incorporate some of the features found in the G ring of paraherquamide. This resulted in PNU-105775, which had similar activity to paraherquamide in the in-house jird anthelmintic model (an immunosuppressed jird, infected with ruminant gastrointestinal nematodes) [9].

The synthesis of PNU-105775 is a six-step process, with PNU-105774 being reduced to PNU-105775 in the final step (Figure 18.1b; more details can be found in Lee *et al.* [8]). Although potent and safe, this synthesis was too expensive to be cost-effective for a sheep anthelmintic. A small quantity of PNU-141400 was isolated from the final reduction, with loss of the oxygen at the 2 position (as shown in Figure 18.1b). This compound was as active as PNU-105775. This interesting reduction was then applied to paraherquamide (Figure 18.1c) to generate a novel,

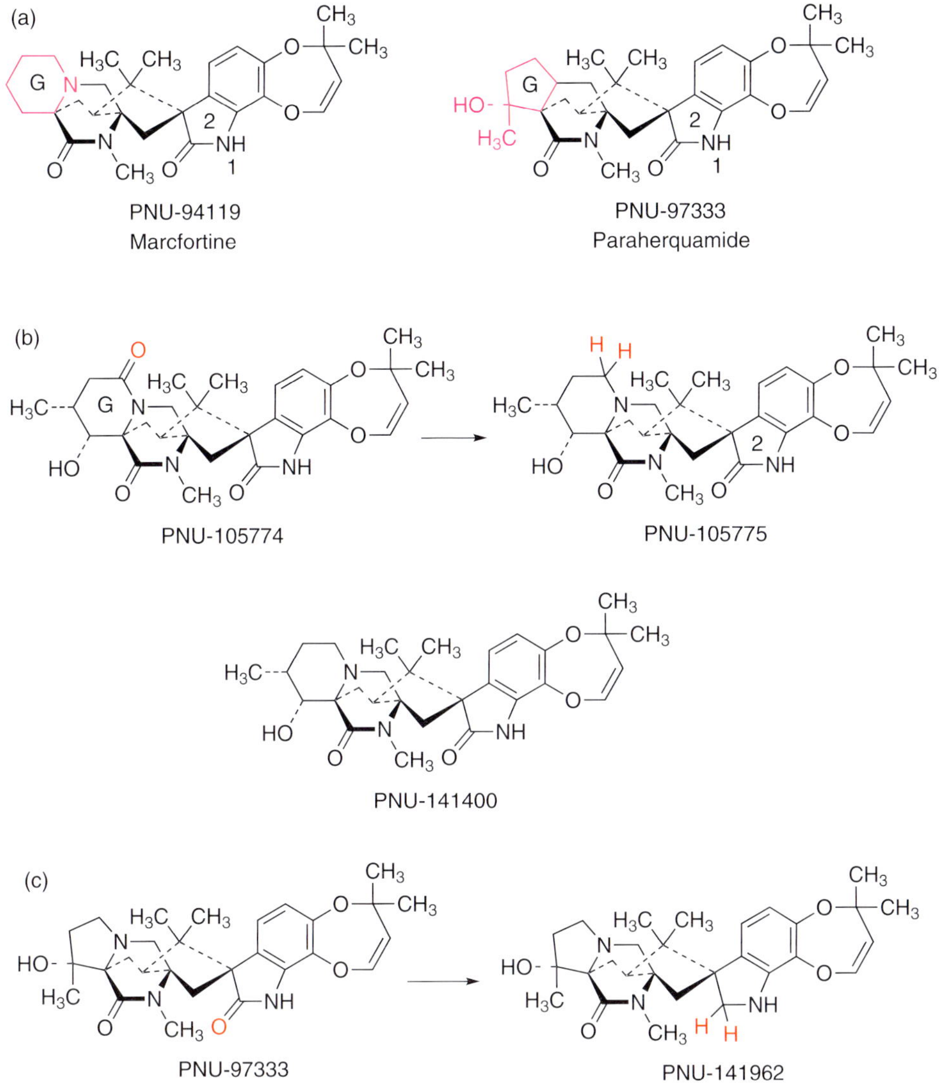

Figure 18.1 (a) Structures of marcfortine A and paraherquamide, illustrating the similarity in structure; only the G ring is different. (b) Final step in the synthesis of the potent marcfortine analog, PNU-105775. The over-reduced side-product, PNU-141400, is also shown. (c) Reduction of paraherquamide (PNU-97333) to 2-deoxy-paraherquamide (PNU-141962).

patentable molecule, PNU-141962 (2-deoxy-paraherquamide), now named derquantel. The compound was not tested in the *C. elegans* assay, due to the lack of activity of paraherquamide against *C. elegans* under standard screening conditions (as an interesting footnote, it has recently been demonstrated [10] that derquantel does have activity against *C. elegans*, but only in "cut worm" preparations). Derquantel was therefore tested directly in the jird anthelmintic model and shown to have equivalent activity to paraherquamide. Against *Haemonchus contortus*, *Trichostrongylus colubriformis*, and *Ostertagia ostertagi*, ED_{90} doses (single dosing) were 0.33, 0.11, and around 0.5 mg/jird (values in mg/kg are roughly 7.5, 2.5, and 12.5). These values were similar whether the drugs were given orally or via injection (intramuscular, intraperitoneal, and subcutaneous routes). Topical delivery provided slightly less potency. From accumulated data in this model, it was concluded that paraherquamide and derquantel are equipotent against these three major ruminant parasites. Furthermore, both were deliverable by all commercially useful routes.

Despite these exciting data, there were concerns about the toxicity of derquantel, since Merck had reported that paraherquamide is toxic to mice (estimated LD_{50} < 15 mg/kg) [11] and even more toxic in dogs, with death seen at doses as low as 0.5 mg/kg [12]. The toxicity is species-specific, as paraherquamide is quite safe for sheep, jirds, and rats. The toxicity of derquantel was therefore evaluated in mice and dogs. Doses up to 50 mg/kg had no untoward effects in mice. In dogs, 20 mg/kg produced only mild and reversible mydriasis.

Another key question at this early stage in the discovery process was whether derquantel was cross-resistant with existing commercial anthelmintics, a key factor to control of resistant nematodes in the field. As Table 18.1 shows, the molecule is essentially equipotent *in vitro* and *in vivo* against *H. contortus* strains multiply resistant to ivermectin and benzimidazoles or levamisole and benzimidazoles, compared to a susceptible strain. Similar studies in other species of nematodes consistently demonstrated equal efficacy in resistant and sensitive strains.

Studies were conducted in sheep (in-house, unpublished data), using both artificial (adult and fourth-stage (L4) larvae) and natural infections of intestinal nematodes, with oral drench doses of derquantel varying from 0.5 to 2.5 mg/kg. Excellent efficacy was achieved (greater than 5%) from doses of 1 mg/kg or above against adult and L4 larvae of *Trichostrongylus* spp. and *Cooperia curticei*; and

Table 18.1 *In vivo* (Jird) and *in vitro* effects of 2-deoxy-paraherquamide against macrocyclic lactone/benzimidazole- and levamisole/benzimidazole-resistant and -sensitive strains of *Haemonchus contortus*.

Strain	In vivo[a] ED_{95} (mg/jird)	In vitro[b] EC_{50} (µM)		
	Derquantel	Derquantel	Ivermectin	Levamisole
Sensitive	0.33	0.3	0.003	0.1
ML-R/BZ-R	0.33	0.3	0.03	0.1
Lev-R/BZ-R	0.33	0.3	0.003	2.0

a) Resistance factor *in vivo* for both resistant strains greater than 10-fold ($N = 4$ studies, 4 jirds per study).
b) EC_{50} values obtained following 24-h incubations; values averaged from three separate studies, eight culture tubes per concentration per study.

at 2 mg/kg against adult *H. contortus* and *Nematodirus spathiger*. Efficacy, however, was variable (70–95%) against *Teladorsagia circumcincta*, and poor (0–40%) against adult *Oesophagostomum columbianum* and *Trichuris ovis* at all doses tested.

Mode of Action of Derquantel: B-Subtype Nicotinic Acetylcholine Receptor Antagonist

Contraction assays using muscle strips from the parasitic nematode *Ascaris suum* show the presence of pharmacologically distinct types of nicotinic acetylcholine receptors (nAChRs), which are activated by different cholinergic anthelmintics [13–16]. Three subtypes of nAChR can be distinguished: an N-subtype that is preferentially activated by nicotine, an L-subtype that is preferentially activated by levamisole and antagonized in a competitive manner by paraherquamide, and a B-subtype that is preferentially activated by bephenium and antagonized by paraherquamide and derquantel (Figure 18.2; see also Chapters 1 and 14 for further perspectives on ligand-gated ion channels).

In addition to experiments conducted with muscle contraction assays, the effects of nicotine, levamisole, bephenium, paraherquamide, and derquantel have been examined under patch-clamp [17, 18] to test the hypothesis that the selectivity of the ligands is in fact different. With this approach, it was possible to describe the single-channel properties of the N-, L-, and B-subtypes of nAChRs and the different selective effects of the anthelmintics.

Initially, it was found that a high concentration of levamisole could activate three different types of nAChR ion channel that had conductances of around 24, 35, or 45 pS; however, levamisole preferentially activated the 35 pS channels [17]. Paraherquamide had no inhibitory effect on the 24 pS channels, but antagonized the 35- and 45-pS channels [18]. When bephenium was used as the agonist, it did not

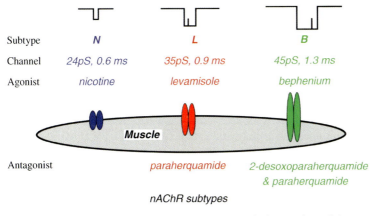

Figure 18.2 Summary diagram of channel properties and pharmacology of the N-, L-, and B-subtypes of nAChR receptor channel found on the muscle cell of *Ascaris* showing their mean conductance, mean open time, and selectivity of agonists and antagonists.

activate the 24- (N-subtype) or 35-pS (L-subtype) channels, but activated the 45-pS channels [18]. Derquantel was found to selectively inhibit the 45-pS channels [18]. These observations allowed the identification of the 45-pS channel as the B-subtype and that of the L-subtype as the 35-pS channel.

In addition to separation of the subtypes by pharmacology and conductance, it was found that there were significant differences in their mean open times [18]. The N-subtype (24 pS) had the briefest open time, 0.6 mS; the L-subtype (35 pS) had an intermediate open time, 0.9 ms; and the B-subtype (45 pS) had the longest open time, 1.3 ms, when levamisole was the agonist. These experiments allowed the identification and confirmation of at least three subtypes of muscle nAChR at the single-channel level and their pharmacology to be characterized.

The observations showed that derquantel was a more selective antagonist of the B-subtype of nAChR; this is clinically relevant because one type of levamisole resistance is associated with a loss of sensitivity of the L-subtype receptors with no loss in the sensitivity of the other subtypes [19]. This means that loss of the L-subtype with levamisole resistance might be overcome by using other cholinergic agonists (methyridine, oxantel; N-subtype) [16] or antagonists (derquantel; B-subtype) with selectivity for subtypes of nAChR other than the L-subtype.

Development of Startect®: A Novel Combination of Derquantel and Abamectin

At a dose rate of 2 mg/kg, derquantel was shown to display only mid-spectrum activity, with solid efficacy greater than 95% reduction in mean worm count against adults and L4 larvae of *Trichostrongylus* and *Nematodirus* spp., and the adult stage of *H. contortus*. At this dose it is, however, less effective against *T. circumcincta* (adults and L4 larvae), L4 larvae of *H. contortus*, and some large intestinal nematodes.

The urgent need for the development of a new anthelmintic family to overcome resistance to other anthelmintic families was clear, so experts were consulted to evaluate whether there was a way forward for development of derquantel as a new anthelmintic. The resistance in small ruminants in some geographic regions was so acute it was felt that there was indeed a need for development of a novel anthelmintic such as derquantel. It was, however, also concluded that development of a combination anthelmintic with a macrocyclic lactone would deliver activity against a broader spectrum of nematodes in addition to offering the potential to slow the development of resistance to both molecules [20–22]. The decision was made to combine derquantel with abamectin, resulting in the production of Startect (10 mg/ml derquantel and 1 mg/ml abamectin). The standard oral abamectin usage dose was chosen (0.2 mg/kg) and a dose of 2 mg/kg derquantel was selected.

To evaluate the efficacy of the combination product Startect, 11 dose confirmation studies were conducted in four countries (Australia, New Zealand, South Africa, and the United Kingdom [23, 24]) against natural or experimental infections of adult, L4 larvae and hypobiotic L4 larvae, with unknown or unconfirmed resistance. As recommended by VICH (International Cooperation on Harmonization of Technical Requirements for Registration of Veterinary Products), percent reduction in geometric worm count was compared to the negative control group. Group sizes of 10 animals were used, and animals blocked on fecal egg count and randomly allocated to group. Sheep were sacrificed 14 days after treatment and worms counted from samples of 5% aliquots (of total contents of abomasum and small intestine) or 10% aliquots (of total contents of large intestine). Consistently high efficacy (97% or above) was demonstrated against adult, L4, and hypobiotic L4 stages of a broad range of contemporary field strains of gastrointestinal (abomasum, small and large intestines) and respiratory nematodes of sheep in all four countries, with no negative interaction between the two active ingredients in the combination [24].

Seven studies were also conducted in the same four countries using anthelmintic resistant laboratory strains and one study was run in the United Kingdom with field isolates. The study design was similar to the dose confirmation studies, with the addition of reference groups to confirm the resistance profile of each parasite (reference group compounds were selected from the benzimidazole, imidazothiazole, macrocyclic lactone, salicylanilide, and organophosphate classes). Consistently high efficacy (greater than 99%) was demonstrated by Startect against these multidrug-resistant strains of economically important gastrointestinal nematodes of sheep with the single exception of 95.9% efficacy in one study against *Teladorsagia trifurcata* [24].

To evaluate field efficacy, 16 studies were run across a broad range of geographic regions, climate zones, sheep enterprises, breeds, ages, and nematode populations (in Australia, New Zealand, South Africa and the United Kingdom). The trials were run using a standard fecal egg count reduction test. Each study had two treatment groups: negative control and Startect with efficacy determined 14 days post-treatment by percent reduction in geometric mean of the test groups when compared to negative control. Group sizes were at least 20 animals and blocking was by fecal egg count with random allocation of animals to groups. These studies demonstrated consistently high efficacy of Startect (greater than 99%) against a broad range of naturally acquired gastrointestinal nematodes (Table 18.2).

Safety Studies

The safety of Startect in lambs and adult sheep was comprehensively evaluated in a series of target animal safety studies, including margin-of-safety, reproductive safety, and field safety studies. In addition, a study was conducted to evaluate the clinical safety of Startect when administered concurrently with other commonly used animal health products.

Pivotal Target Animal Safety Studies

Six pivotal safety studies were conducted in sheep, including three margin-of-safety studies (two in 6-month-old lambs dosed at 1.5, 4.5, or 7.5 times the recommended dose rate at weekly and monthly intervals, and the other in 6-week-old lambs dosed once at 1.5, 3, or 4.5 times the dose rate), two reproductive safety

Table 18.2 Summary of fecal egg count reduction test data for Startect following testing in 16 field studies run across a broad range of geographic regions, climate zones, sheep enterprises, breeds, ages, and nematode populations.

Country	Region	Nematode egg type			
		Strongyle		*Nematodirus* spp.	
		Control GM*	Reduction (%)	Control GM*	Reduction (%)
Australia	NSW – NE	1385	>99.9	11	100
	NSW – SE	595	99.9	—	—
	NSW – Central	674	100	20	100
	Victoria – SE	517	99.9	15	100
	Victoria – SW	977	100	88	100
	WA – Albany	303	100	—	—
	WA – Denmark	120	100	—	—
New Zealand	Manawatu (N)	707	99.9	32	100
	Pahiatua (N)	1536	>99.9	—	—
	Otago (S)	1179	100	79	100
	Southland (S)	733	100	—	—
	Canterbury (S)	358	99.2	3.4	100
South Africa	Limpopo	832	>99.9	—	—
	Mpumalanga	2934	99.9	—	—
United Kingdom	Scotland	125	100	3.2	100
	North Wales	345	>99.9	1.2	100

*GM: geometric mean.

studies with animals dosed at 3 times the recommended dose rate at weekly or monthly intervals for up to 217 days (one each in male and female sheep), and an overdose/repeat dose study in 9- to 13-week-old lambs dosed at 1.5 times (based on heaviest animal) the recommended dose rate twice 14 days apart. A study was also conducted in New Zealand to evaluate the clinical safety of Startect when given at registered dosage and administered concurrently with a multivalent clostridial vaccine (Glanvac® 6 Vaccine; Pfizer) and/or a mineralized combination lamb drench (First Drench Hi-Mineral™; Merial Ancare).

Startect was well tolerated in all age groups at doses up to 3 times the recommended label dose of 1 ml/5 kg; doses greater than 3 times were associated with toxicity in some animals. At doses up to 3 times the recommended label dose there were no adverse effects on the fertility of breeding rams or ewes and no effect on their offspring. The only treatment-related effect identified at the recommended usage dose was coughing immediately following administration; this was of a mild and transient nature, generally resolving within 30 s of dosing. The rate of coughing was 60–65% across all studies.

No adverse interactions were identified when Startect was administered concurrently with a multivalent clostridial vaccine and/or a mineralized combination lamb drench.

From these studies it was established that young lambs less than 15 kg should be accurately weighed and dosed. Where there is a large variation in size within the group, the dose rate should be based on label directions for each weight range. Care should be taken to avoid overdosing. The product should not be used in other species; Startect is extremely toxic to horses (Pfizer in-house data).

Commercialization

Derquantel Scale-Up

Key to the success of any drug is achieving an acceptable return on investment. For the animal health industry, cost of goods is often vital to the profitability of drug products, especially those aimed at the livestock sector.

Considerable investment by Pfizer scientists in a number of areas has made a significant impact on scale-up of derquantel to commercially viable quantities. Improvements in the efficiency of the fermentation, the producing microorganism, and recovery of paraherquamide has led to improved yields, including a 4- to 5-fold increase in the fermentation output, due to recent developments and an overall several hundred-fold increase from the original wild-type culture. Additionally, the conversion of paraherquamide to 2-deoxy-paraherquamide has been optimized. Further investments are being made in random and directed mutagenesis projects to make an even greater impact on the efficiency of the fermentation process.

Registration and Launch

Startect has been approved and launched in New Zealand and South Africa, and is currently under review by a number of other regulatory authorities

All animal studies were subject to animal welfare ethical review, and were conducted in compliance with local and national regulations.

Conclusions

This chapter highlights the challenges of bringing a new veterinary antiparasitic molecule to market and demonstrates that persistence, combined with timely and focused investment, can succeed in the end. Overcoming the major hurdle of controlling a broad spectrum of resistant parasites is only the first step. The drug has to be bioavailable in the target host species and to reach the predilection site of the parasite. The molecule must have an acceptable safety margin, from the perspective of target animal (sheep) safety, human food safety (residue levels), and user safety. Finally, the cost of producing the drug must be acceptable. In this case, combining a new chemical entity (derquantel) with a novel mechanism of action, not cross-resistant with existing drugs, with a second class (abamectin) utilizing a distinctly different mode of action proved to deliver excellent efficacy and safety, as well as providing the potential to minimize selection for resistance to both drugs in the combination.

References

1 Campbell, W.C., Fisher, M.H., Stanley, E.O., Albers-Schonberg, G., and Jacob, T.A. (1983) Ivermectin: a potent new antiparasitic agent. *Science*, **221**, 823–828.

2 Conder, G.A. and Campbell, W.C. (1995) Chemotherapy of nematode infections of veterinary importance, with special reference to drug resistance. *Adv. Parasitol.*, **35**, 1–84.

3 Sasaki, T., Takagi, M., Yaguchi, T., Miyadoh, S., Okada, T., and Koyama, M. (1992) A new anthelmintic cyclodepsipeptide, PF1022A. *J. Antibiot.*, **45**, 692–697.

4 Ostlind, D.A., Mickle, W.G., Ewaniw, D.V., Andriuli, F.J., Campbell, W.C., Hernandez, S., Mochales, S., and Munguira, E. (1990) Efficacy of paraherquamide against immature *Trichostrongylus colubriformis* in the gerbil (*Meriones unguiculatus*). *Res. Vet. Sci.*, **48**, 260–261.

5 Shoop, W.L., Egerton, J.R., Eary, C.H., and Suhayda, D. (1990) Anthelmintic activity of paraherquamide in sheep. *J. Parasitol.*, **76**, 349–351.

6 Blanchflower, S.E., Banks, R.M., Everett, J.R., Manger, B.R., and Reading, C. (1991) New paraherquamide antibiotics with anthelmintic activity. *J. Antibiot.*, **44**, 492–497.

7 Polonsky, J., Merrien, M.A., Prange, T., Pascard, C., and Moreau, S. (1980) Isolation and structure (X-ray analysis) of marcfortine A, a new alkaloid from *Penicillium roqueforti*. *J. Chem. Soc. Chem. Commun.*, **13**, 601–602.

8 Lee, B.H., Clothier, M.F., Dutton, F.E., Nelson, S.J., Johnson, S.S., Thompson, D.P., Geary, T.G. et al. (2002) Marcfortine and paraherquamide class of anthelmintics: discovery of PNU-141962. *Curr. Top. Med. Chem.*, **2**, 779–793.

9 Conder, G.A., Johnson, S.S., Guimond, P.M., Cox, D.L., and Lee, B.L. (1991) Concurrent infections with the ruminant nematodes *Haemonchus contortus* and *Trichostrongylus colubriformis* in jirds, *Meriones unguiculatus*, and use of this model for anthelmintic studies. *J. Parasitol.*, **77**, 621–623.

10 Ruiz-Lancheros, E., Viau, C., Walter, T.N., Francis, A., and Geary, T.G. (2011) Activity of novel nicotinic anthelmintics in cut preparations of *Caenorhabditis elegans*. *Int. J. Parasitol.*, **41**, 455–461.

11 Shoop, W.L., Haines, H.W., Eary, C.H., and Michael, B.F. (1992) Acute toxicity of paraherquamide and its potential as an anthelmintic. *Am. J. Vet. Res.*, **53**, 2032–2034.

12 Shoop, W.L., Eary, C.H., Michael, B.F., Haines, H.W., and Seward, R.L. (1991) Anthelmintic activity of paraherquamide in dogs. *Vet. Parasitol.*, **40**, 339–341.

13 Zinser, E.W., Wolf, M.L., Alexander-Bowman, S.J., Thomas, E.M., Davis, J.P., Groppi, V.E., Lee, B.H. et al. (2002) Anthelmintic paraherquamides are cholinergic antagonists in gastrointestinal nematodes and mammals. *J. Vet. Pharmacol. Ther.*, **25**, 241–250.

14 Robertson, A.P., Clark, C.L., Burns, T.A., Thompson, D.P., Geary, T.G., Trailovic and, S.M., and Martin, R.J. (2002) Paraherquamide and 2-deoxy-paraherquamide distinguish cholinergic receptor subtypes in *Ascaris* muscle. *J. Vet. Pharmacol. Ther.*, **302**, 853–860.

15 Martin, R.J., Bai, G., Clark, C.L., and Robertson, A.P. (2003) Methyridine (2-[2-methoxyethyl]-pyridine) and levamisole activate different ACh receptor subtypes in nematode parasites: a new lead for levamisole-resistance. *Br. J. Pharmacol.*, **140**, 1068–1107.

16 Martin, R.J., Clark, C.L., Trailovic, S.M., and Robertson, A.P. (2004) Oxantel is an N-type (methyridine and nicotine) agonist not an L-type (levamisole and pyrantel) agonist: classification of cholinergic anthelmintics in *Ascaris*. *Int. J. Parasitol.*, **34**, 1083–1090.

17 Levandoski, M.M., Robertson, A.P., Kuiper, S., Qian, H., and Martin, R.J. (2005) Single-channel properties of N- and L-subtypes of acetylcholine receptor in *Ascaris suum*. *J. Parasitol.*, **35**, 925–934.

18 Qian, H., Martin and, R.J., and Robertson, A.P. (2006) Pharmacology

of N-, L-, and B-subtypes of nematode nAChR resolved at the single-channel level in *Ascaris suum*. *FASEB J.*, **20**, 2606–2608.

19 Robertson, A.P., Bjorn, H.E., and Martin, R.J. (1999) Resistance to levamisole resolved at the single-channel level. *FASEB J.*, **13**, 749–760.

20 Anderson, N., Martin, P.J., and Jarrett, R.G. (1988) Mixtures of anthelmintics: a strategy against resistance. *Aust. Vet. J.*, **65**, 62–64.

21 Dobson, R.J., Besier, R.B., Barnes, E.H., Love, S.C.J., Vizard, A., Bell, K., and Le Jambre, L.F. (2001) Principles for the use of macrocyclic lactones to minimise selection for resistance. *Aust. Vet. J.*, **79**, 756–761.

22 Leathwick, D.M., Hosking, B.C., Bisset, S.A., and McKay, C.H. (2009) Managing anthelmintic resistance: Is it feasible in New Zealand to delay the emergence of resistance to a new anthelmintic class? *NZ Vet. J.*, **57**, 181–192.

23 Little, P.R., Hodge, A., Watson, T.G., Seed, J.A., and Maeder, S.J. (2010) Field efficacy and safety of an oral formulation of the novel combination anthelmintic, derquantel–abamectin, in sheep in New Zealand. *NZ Vet. J.*, **58**, 121–129.

24 Little, P.R., Hodge, A., Maeder, S.J., Wirtherle, N.C., Nicholas, D.R., Cox, G.G., and Conder, G.A. (2011) Efficacy of a combined oral formulation of derquantel-abamectin against the adult and larval stages of nematodes in sheep, including anthelmintic-resistant strains. *Vet. Parasitol.*, **181**, 180–193.

19
Praziquantel: Too Good to be Replaced?

Livia Pica-Mattoccia[*] *and Donato Cioli*

Abstract

Praziquantel (PZQ) was introduced in the 1970s for the chemotherapy of schistosomiasis and today it is practically the only drug used for the control of the disease. The undisputed strong points of PZQ are its effectiveness against all schistosome species, its safety, its affordable price, and its ease of administration as a single oral dose. Cure rates are of the order of 60–90% of those treated and the intensity of infection is usually reduced to levels that minimize the risks of serious morbidity. A weak point of PZQ is its lack of efficacy against immature stages of the parasite, which may result in low cure rates in high-transmission sites. In spite of about 30 years of intensive use and the current mass distribution of PZQ to many million people per year, no documented cases of PZQ resistance have been reported at the population level. Individual cases of PZQ failure have been repeatedly published, but no parasite isolates with a strong and stable drug resistance were obtained from such cases. A laboratory-derived schistosome strain with a decreased PZQ sensitivity has been described. The mechanism of PZQ action is still unresolved, current interpretations revolving around the toxic effects of calcium influx in the parasite and the corresponding involvement of schistosome calcium channels. These concepts have been recently challenged by the demonstration that high levels of calcium influx caused by PZQ are perfectly compatible with parasite survival in immature worms and in cytochalasin D-exposed schistosomes. However, an unexpected effect of PZQ on the regenerative polarity of a planarian worm was shown to depend on the activity of calcium channels. Research towards PZQ analogs and alternative antischistosomal compounds should be intensified because PZQ is not a perfect drug, and the possibility of resistance remains a serious threat, especially as PZQ is the only drug available for this global disease.

Praziquantel: A Success Story

The most valuable achievement in the field of schistosomiasis – possibly second only to the discovery of the parasite itself [1] – was the introduction of praziquantel (PZQ)

[*] Corresponding Author

Parasitic Helminths: Targets, Screens, Drugs and Vaccines, First Edition. Edited by Conor R. Caffrey
© 2012 Wiley-VCH Verlag GmbH & Co. KGaA. Published 2012 by Wiley-VCH Verlag GmbH & Co. KGaA.

for chemotherapy. The potency of the pyrazino isoquinoline ring system as an anthelmintic was discovered in 1972 at the laboratories of Bayer, Germany [2], but the chemical follow-up of this type of compounds was carried out at Merck, Germany, where over 400 analogs were synthesized [3]. The story started from an industrial motivation to discover antidepressants. Initial clinical trials against schistosomiasis were carried out in collaboration with the World Health Organization and these invariably gave very good results against all major schistosome species [4–6]. PZQ administered as a single oral dose of 40–60 mg/kg body weight proved to be well tolerated, with relatively few, mild, and transitory side-effects. Efficacy was also quite good, with cure rates in the range of 60–90%. The only initial problem was the high price, but market competition started even before the Bayer/Merck patent expired, when the Korean company Shin Poong obtained a process patent [7]. A rapid price decline ensued in the following years, reaching the present average cost of US$ 0.2 or 0.3 for the treatment of a child or an adult, respectively [8]. Efficacy against all schistosome species as well as against cestodes [9], safety, ease of administration, and low cost have made PZQ the drug of choice for the chemotherapy of schistosomiasis. In fact, alternative drugs like oxamniquine and metrifonate have practically disappeared from the market, thus leaving PZQ the only available antischistosomal drug [8, 10].

Limitations

From its discovery [2] it was clear that PZQ had very little efficacy against juvenile schistosomes, extending from 1 to 5 weeks after infection, with minimal efficacy around the fourth week. Activity is present in the first week and gradually returns to maximum levels after the fifth week postinfection. This biphasic curve of activity has been repeatedly observed *in vitro* [11], and in animal [11–13] and human studies [14, 15]. The biological basis of this phenomenon remains obscure, but a practical consequence is that in areas of intense disease transmission – where many individuals are likely to carry juvenile worms – the effectiveness of PZQ tends to be rather low and in some instances quite dramatically so [16]. As a countermeasure for this problem, it was proposed to administer two PZQ doses over an interval of a few weeks to permit the maturation of juvenile parasites [17]. The effectiveness of this approach in the field was confirmed [15, 18], but logistic and economic factors discourage its adoption in large-scale programs.

Even in the most successful campaigns of PZQ chemotherapy, complete cure is seldom, if ever, achieved. Apart from the problem of immature worms, it has been argued that the routinely employed PZQ dose is probably a subcurative one, even more so since the common Kato–Katz diagnostic technique used to assess cure is likely to miss uncured positive cases excreting a low number of eggs [19]. At the individual level, failure to achieve complete worm removal is mitigated by the fact that intensity of infection is generally reduced to levels that minimize the risks of serious late morbidity. At the population level, however, a subcurative dose may aggravate the risk of favoring drug resistant parasites [19].

Resistance

Mass distribution of PZQ is currently taking place in a number of endemic countries and results in the treatment of many millions of people every year, thanks to governmental and international programs [20]. Having learned the lesson from antibacterial and antimalarial chemotherapy, concern has been expressed that, under present circumstances, resistance to PZQ may develop, which could cause serious problems since we have essentially this single weapon for the control of schistosomiasis [21].

Alarming reports of possible PZQ resistance have indeed appeared in the literature, beginning with a focus in northern Senegal where the drug had poor cure rates in the range of 18–39% [16]. A reappraisal of this incident pointed to the high transmission rate of the infection in that focus, with the consequent high frequency of insensitive immature parasites in the population [14, 22]. This interpretation, however, was weakened by the fact that oxamniquine, which is also inactive against juvenile worms was normally effective in the same population [23] and by the fact that snails collected in the area carried a parasite isolate that proved partially insensitive to PZQ in the laboratory [24].

Additional evidence for the possible development of PZQ resistance has been found in Egypt where schistosome isolates derived from patients not cured after three rounds of chemotherapy showed a decreased PZQ sensitivity in laboratory animals [25] and *in vitro* [26] when compared to isolates derived from easily cured patients.

In 1994, a laboratory strain of *Schistosoma mansoni* repeatedly subjected to drug pressure over a number of mouse passages was reported to exhibit a decreased PZQ sensitivity when compared to the original unselected parasites [27]. Genetic crosses between selected and unselected parasites showed intermediate sensitivity in the hybrid progeny [28].

A number of schistosome isolates collected in different African countries were tested in a multicenter laboratory study and clear interisolate differences in PZQ sensitivity were recorded [29]. A general characteristic of the partially resistant isolates described in this study as well as in the previous studies is that the level of drug insensitivity was invariably modest, was mainly detectable at low doses, and was easily overcome with increased PZQ doses. The worrisome interpretation of such moderate levels of insensitivity is that this could represent the initial phase in the development of serious resistance (i.e., a phase where only a minority of parasites are resistant in the population, but will soon become the majority if kept under drug selection). However, in all reported occurrences of "PZQ resistance," repeated and prolonged drug pressure has never resulted in substantial increases of drug refractoriness beyond the initial level [30]. No schistosome isolate has been described so far that is unequivocally highly resistant. This failure to increase the mean level of insensitivity in a parasite population kept under drug pressure indicates that the majority of parasites is slightly insensitive, rather than the opposite scenario whereby only a few individuals are highly resistant and are the forerunners of a completely refractory population.

In a longitudinal study of 178 men occupationally exposed to schistosomes and repeatedly treated with PZQ, no pattern of failures consistent with development of clinical resistance to PZQ was found over a 12.5-year period [31]. A schistosome isolate obtained from a Kenyan car washer who was never fully cured after 18 rounds of treatment administered over several years proved partially insusceptible in *in vitro* and *in vivo* tests; in contrast, a subisolate that had not been kept under drug pressure was fully susceptible [32].

It has been speculated that the partial insensitivity to PZQ observed in some schistosome strains may not be due to a mutation in a drug target(s), but to a modulation of the influx–efflux mechanisms of the drug in the parasite, as suggested by the apparent conservation of a currently presumed target (a calcium channel β-subunit) in some "PZQ-resistant" isolates [33]. Another possibility is that the insensitivities measured in the laboratory [29, 30], usually after treatments given around the sixth to seventh week after infection, may be the result of slow parasite maturation in some geographical isolates, thus reflecting the previously described phenomenon of PZQ inefficacy against immature worms. This hypothesis, however, has not been confirmed in at least one case [34].

Over the years, several isolated instances of PZQ failure have been reported in the literature (reviewed in [35]). The number of failures is small when compared to the vast number of successfully treated people. In principle, some of these failures could be attributed to special metabolic characteristics of individual patients, to poor drug quality, to failed drug intake, to wrong diagnosis of persistent infection, and the like. Also, it is worth mentioning that the majority of reported failures concern returning travelers and are based on the finding of parasite eggs in locations other than the feces or urine, frequently dependent on indirect diagnostic methods, and these seem to occur more often with *Schistosoma haematobium* infections, for which egg clearance from the tissues after chemotherapy is known to be particularly slow [36].

The issue of drug quality deserves a brief statement. Of 34 PZQ samples tested at the user level, two were devoid of the active principle [37]. Also, a recent study detected significant differences in the bioavailability and antiparasitic effects among various PZQ brands [38].

In sum, we feel that no serious occurrence of PZQ resistance has been documented so far that might undermine the clinical value of the drug. This was confirmed by the normal PZQ efficacy in those Egyptian villages where schistosomes with decreased drug sensitivity had been isolated 10 years previously [39]. We think, however, based on theoretical considerations [40] and the previous experience with other drugs [41, 42], that the future development of PZQ resistance is a likely and alarming possibility, considering that this is the only available drug against an infection that affects large populations.

Mechanism of Action

It is certainly remarkable that, more than 30 years after the introduction of PZQ and so many millions of people successfully treated, the mechanism of action of PZQ is still essentially unknown [43, 44].

Any discussion on the mechanism of action of PZQ must begin with reference to the study by Pax et al. in 1978 [45]. The basic facts that characterize the mode of action of the drug are contained in that report, namely the spastic paralysis of the schistosome musculature and the influx of calcium into the parasite. The morphological alterations of the worm tegument that immediately follow exposure to PZQ (i.e., vacuolization and blebbing) were described soon afterwards [46]. It appeared obvious to attribute muscle contraction to the increased intraworm calcium concentration, but two crucial links remained obscure: how does PZQ cause calcium influx and how does this phenomenon eventually cause parasite death?

The discussion on the "upstream" link between PZQ and calcium initially stalled with the exclusion of a number of possible mechanisms, among which the opening of calcium channels by PZQ [43]. This possibility appeared in conflict with the fact that an inhibitor of calcium channel activity, methoxy-verapamil (also known as D600 or gallopamil) did not antagonize the schistosome muscle contraction or the Ca^{2+} accumulation induced by PZQ [47]. It was subsequently confirmed that methoxy-verapamil does not interfere with the effects of PZQ, but it was also shown that other calcium antagonists active on the same "L-type" channels of vertebrates (i.e., nicardipine and nifedipine) can antagonize PZQ's lethal activity in schistosomes [48].

Calcium channels were at the center of the discussion when Kohn et al. [49] showed that schistosomes possess, in addition to a canonical calcium channel β-subunit, a variant subtype of this protein lacking two highly conserved serine residues that potentially function as phosphorylation sites and that may be critical for the structural integrity of the subunit. When the variant schistosome β-subunit was expressed in Xenopus oocytes together with human or invertebrate α-chains, the resulting calcium channel proved unusually sensitive to PZQ (i.e., it produced an increased Ca^{2+} current in the presence of the drug). This uncommon PZQ sensitivity was not observed with the canonical schistosome β-subunit nor with the variant subunit mutated to restore the two conserved serines [50]. However, the hypersensitivity was again detected with a mammalian β-subunit mutagenized to eliminate the phosphorylation consensus sites represented by the two serines [51]. Based on these findings, the suggestion that Ca^{2+} channels may be the target of PZQ action [52] became clearly very attractive, especially since the variant β-subunit lacking the two serines is present in other PZQ-sensitive organisms like Taenia solium [53].

A recent study performed with the free-living flatworm, Dugesia japonica, provides indirect support for the calcium channel hypothesis [54], albeit conflicting with some of the data obtained with S. mansoni, as discussed below. In common with other planarians, D. japonica exhibits a remarkable regenerative capacity such that individual organisms simultaneously amputated of their heads and tails are able to reform both body ends. It was observed that the presence of PZQ during the regenerative process unexpectedly produced two-headed individuals in 100% of the worms. This phenomenon was accompanied by an increased calcium influx and was largely inhibited by the calcium channel blocker nicardipine. Most interestingly, the PZQ-evoked bipolarity was ablated to a large extent when the calcium channel β-subunit was targeted by RNA interference (RNAi). Surprisingly, however, suppression of bipolar regeneration was maximal when the canonical β-subunit – possessing the two serine residues that represent potential phosphorylation sites – was targeted for knockdown and less pronounced with the variant β-subunit that lacks the two serines, just the opposite of what had been observed in schistosomes. Also, PZQ proved lethal to *D. japonica*, although at much higher concentrations than observed *in vitro* with *S. mansoni*. RNAi of either, or both, calcium channel β-subunits did not abolish lethality, but prolonged flatworm survival [54]. Incidentally, the analogous experiment assessing PZQ activity upon RNAi silencing of β-subunits – although in principle experimentally feasible – has not been reported for *S. mansoni*.

Turning now to the other unresolved question – the link between intraworm calcium influx and schistosome death – the implicit assumption has been that lethality is simply due to high cytoplasmic concentrations of the free ion. This assumption was questioned by the recent observation that very high intraworm levels of calcium are perfectly compatible with schistosome survival [55], as outlined in the following experimental conditions. Schistosomes pre-exposed *in vitro* to cytochalasin D (CyD) – an agent known to disrupt the actin cytoskeleton and to block the activity of calcium channels in mammalian systems – proved to be strikingly insensitive to the otherwise lethal action of PZQ. Under the assumption that CyD had actually inhibited calcium entry into schistosomes, this result was interpreted as a confirmation of the calcium channel hypothesis [48]. However, subsequent experiments forced a complete revision of this conclusion, since it was found that CyD not only fails to inhibit the intraworm Ca^{2+} accumulation caused by PZQ, but actually contributes to increasing it, such that schistosomes pre-exposed to this agent are able to survive exposure to PZQ in spite of a massive calcium influx. The calcium blockers nicardipine and nifedipine also failed to prevent the calcium influx induced by PZQ, stressing the concept that invertebrate ion channels often appear to diverge from the rules that apply in vertebrates [56]. Similarly, a substantial calcium influx could be measured in 28-day-old worms exposed to PZQ, in accordance with their observable spastic paralysis and in spite of the fact that these immature worms are largely insensitive to the schistosomicidal effects of the drug [55]. Of possible relevance to the above results is that the use of radioactive calcium to measure this cation's concentration in whole worms, as currently performed [45, 55, 57], may be too crude an approach as it fails to take into account possible differences between tissues/compartments of the parasite (e.g., calcium stores) and does not consider the chemical status of the ion (free versus complexed).

A different hypothesis regarding PZQ's mechanism of action stems from the observation that the drug bears some structural similarity with adenosine, and that it inhibits the uptake of the nucleosides adenosine and uridine by schistosomes *in vitro*. This effect, which is absent in mammalian cells, is relevant since schistosomes cannot synthesize purine nucleosides *de novo* [58].

Other possible targets of PZQ action have been proposed, such as actin [59, 60] and the myosin light chain [61], but since these are among the most abundant proteins in the parasite, the danger of spurious results has been underlined [62].

A PZQ-binding site was identified in the crystal structure of glutathione S-transferase [63], but subsequent observations failed to substantiate this enzyme as the drug target [64].

PZQ was found to inhibit the turnover of inositol phosphates [65] and earlier reports pointed to alterations in the permeability or stability of schistosome surface bilayer membranes [66, 67]. There have been no follow-up studies regarding these hypotheses.

There is experimental evidence for a synergistic effect between PZQ and host antibodies *in vivo* [68–70] even though the drug is lethal *in vitro* in the absence of antibodies [11, 13]. Schistosomiasis patients with decreased $CD4^+$ T-cell counts as a consequence of HIV coinfection could be successfully treated with PZQ, as measured by egg excretion reduction [71], whereas, in a different study, somewhat reduced cure rates were observed in coinfected people when judging from circulating schistosome antigen levels [72].

Not Only Schistosomiasis

PZQ is effective in the treatment of human infections caused by a number of other trematodes, including *Opisthorchis (Clonorchis) sinensis*, *Opisthorchis viverrini*, *Paragonimus* spp., *Fasciolopsis buski*, *Heterophyes heterophyes*, and *Metagonimus yokogawai* [73]. These infections are usually treated with a 3-day course of PZQ at 25 mg/kg/day. A notable exception is *Fasciola* spp., against which the efficacy of PZQ *in vivo* is controversial. The location of this trematode in the bile ducts could be supposed to be the cause of poor effectiveness, but even *in vitro*, PZQ addition has little effect on *Fasciola* [46].

Animal and human infections with a number of cestodes are also sensitive to PZQ. In fact, veterinary cestode infections were treated with PZQ (under the tradename Droncit®) before the drug was introduced for use with humans as an antischistosomal [9]. As far as human cestode infections are concerned, *Hymenolepis* spp., *Taenia saginata*, and *Diphyllobothrium latum* are usually eradicated with a single low dose of PZQ [74]. The cysticercus stage of *T. solium*, especially in its localization in the brain (neurocysticercosis), can be treated with high doses of PZQ (50 mg/kg/day for 15 days), often in combination with corticosteroids [75] and cimetidine [76]. In hydatid disease caused by *Echinococcus* spp., PZQ is administered preoperatively (up to 75 mg/kg/day for 15–20 days), often in combination with albendazole [77].

Search for a Better PZQ

Beyond the original Bayer studies, some attempts have been made to modify the PZQ structure in order to improve its performance and to gain insights into structure–activity relationships [78–81]. As PZQ undergoes very rapid metabolic changes, with a plasma half-life in humans estimated between 1 and 3 h [82], efforts to increase metabolic stability of the original drug have met with marginal success [80]. Incidentally, it is possible that the rapid clearance of PZQ from the circulation, by avoiding any prolonged exposure of schistosomes to low drug concentrations, may actually be a crucial factor in delaying the appearance of drug resistance.

We are tempted to conclude that the results obtained so far suggest that no PZQ derivative has been found with an overall performance better than PZQ, even though occasional compounds showed some activity against immature forms [80].

A very promising variation on the original drug, however, is worth mentioning here – a project to produce stereochemically pure PZQ. In its present formulation, PZQ is a 50:50 mixture of two stereoisomers, only one of which (*levo*) has antischistosomal activity [78], whereas the other one is responsible for side-effects [83], for the unpleasant taste and smell of the drug [84], and adds to the bulk of the tablets that are difficult for small children to swallow [85]. Synthesis of the pure isomer has proved problematic so far, but an economically competitive method has been devised for the separation of the two components, with very favorable prospects [86].

Conclusions

A number of positive features clearly make PZQ hard to beat as a drug. It is effective after a single oral dose, it is very safe, it has a wide spectrum of activity, and it is reasonably priced. These considerations have probably discouraged the pharmaceutical industry, academic groups, and international agencies from a high-priority search for alternative drugs. Yet, there is a pressing need for new antischistosomal compounds (see also Chapter 20) because PZQ has its drawbacks (it is inactive against immature worms, occasionally produces low cure rates, has an unclear mechanism of action, and is only available as a racemate), and especially because drug resistance, after 30 years of massive usage, is a very realistic and disquieting threat.

References

1 Siebold, C.T. (1853) Ein Beitrag zur Helminthographia humana, aus brieflichen Mittheilungen des Dr. Bilharz in Kairo, nebst Bemerkungen von Prof. Th. v. Siebold. *Z. Wiss. Zool.*, **4**, 53–76.

2 Gönnert, R. and Andrews, P. (1977) Praziquantel, a new broad-spectrum antischistosomal agent. *Z. Parasitenkd.*, **52**, 129–150.

3 Seubert, J., Pohlke, R., and Loebich, F. (1977) Synthesis and properties of Praziquantel, a novel broad spectrum anthelmintic with excellent activity against Schistosomes and Cestodes. *Experientia*, **33**, 1036–1037.

4 Katz, N., Rocha, R., and Chaves, A. (1979) Preliminary trials with praziquantel in human infections due to *Schistosoma mansoni*. *Bull. World Health Organ.*, **57**, 781–785.

5 Davis, A., Biles, J.E., and Ulrich, A.M. (1979) Initial experiences with praziquantel in the treatment of human

infections due to *Schistosoma haematobium*. *Bull. World Health Organ.*, **57**, 773–779.

6 Ishizaki, T., Kamo, E., and Boehme, K. (1979) Double-blind studies of tolerance to praziquantel in Japanese patients with *Schistosoma japonicum* infections. *Bull. World Health Organ.*, **57**, 787–791.

7 Reich, M.R. and Govindaraj, R. (1998) Dilemmas in drug development for tropical diseases. Experiences with praziquantel. *Health Policy*, **44**, 1–18.

8 Fenwick, A., Savioli, L., Engels, D., Bergquist, N.R., and Todd, M.H. (2003) Drugs for the control of parasitic diseases: current status and development in schistosomiasis. *Trends Parasitol.*, **19**, 509–515.

9 Thomas, H. and Gönnert, R. (1977) The efficacy of praziquantel against cestodes in animals. *Z. Parasitenkd.*, **52**, 117–127.

10 Doenhoff, M.J. and Pica-Mattoccia, L. (2006) Praziquantel for the treatment of schistosomiasis: its use for control in areas with endemic disease and prospects for drug resistance. *Expert Rev. Anti Infect. Ther.*, **4**, 199–210.

11 Xiao, S.H., Catto, B.A., and Webster, L.T. (1985) Effects of praziquantel on different developmental stages of *Schistosoma mansoni in vitro* and *in vivo*. *J. Infect. Dis.*, **151**, 1130–1137.

12 Sabah, A.A., Fletcher, C., Webbe, G., and Doenhoff, M.J. (1986) *Schistosoma mansoni*: chemotherapy of infections of different ages. *Exp. Parasitol.*, **61**, 294–303.

13 Pica-Mattoccia, L. and Cioli, D. (2004) Sex- and stage-related sensitivity of *Schistosoma mansoni* to *in vivo* and *in vitro* praziquantel treatment. *Int. J. Parasitol.*, **34**, 527–533.

14 Gryseels, B., Mbaye, A., De Vlas, S.J., Stelma, F.F., Guissé, F., Van Lieshout, L., Faye, D. *et al.* (2001) Are poor responses to praziquantel for the treatment of *Schistosoma mansoni* infections in Senegal due to resistance? An overview of the evidence. *Trop. Med. Int. Health*, **6**, 864–873.

15 Barakat, R. and Morshedy, H.E. (2011) Efficacy of two praziquantel treatments among primary school children in an area of high *Schistosoma mansoni* endemicity, Nile Delta. *Egypt. Parasitol.*, **138**, 440–446.

16 Stelma, F.F., Talla, A., Sow, S., Kongs, A., Niang, M., Polman, K., Deelder, A.M., and Gryseels, B. (1995) Efficacy and side-effects of praziquantel in an epidemic focus of *Schistosoma mansoni*. *Am. J. Trop. Med. Hyg.*, **53**, 167–170.

17 Renganathan, E. and Cioli, D. (1998) An international initiative on praziquantel use. *Parasitol. Today*, **14**, 390–391.

18 N'Goran, E.K., Gnaka, H.N., Tanner, M., and Utzinger, J. (2003) Efficacy and side-effects of two praziquantel treatments against *Schistosoma haematobium* infection, among schoolchildren from Côte d'Ivoire. *Ann. Trop. Med. Parasitol.*, **97**, 37–51.

19 Doenhoff, M.J. (1998) Is schistosomicidal chemotherapy sub-curative? Implications for drug resistance. *Parasitol. Today*, **14**, 434–435.

20 Hotez, P.J. and Fenwick, A. (2009) Schistosomiasis in Africa: an emerging tragedy in our new global health decade. *PLoS Negl. Trop. Dis.*, **3**, e485.

21 Hudson, A. and Nwaka, S. (2007) The concept paper on the helminth drug initiative. Onchocerciasis/lymphatic filariasis and schistosomiasis: opportunities and challenges for the discovery of new drugs/diagnostics. *Expert Opin. Drug Discov.*, **2** (Suppl. 1), S3–S7.

22 Cioli, D. (2000) Praziquantel: is there real resistance and are there alternatives? *Curr. Opin. Infect. Dis.*, **13**, 659–663.

23 Stelma, F.F., Sall, S., Daff, B., Sow, S., Niang, M., and Gryseels, B. (1997) Oxamniquine cures *Schistosoma mansoni* infection in a focus in which cure rates with praziquantel are unusually low. *J. Infect. Dis.*, **176**, 304–307.

24 Fallon, P.G., Sturrock, R.F., Capron, A., Niang, M., and Doenhoff, M.J. (1995) Short report: diminished susceptibility to praziquantel in a Senegal isolate of *Schistosoma mansoni*. *Am. J. Trop. Med. Hyg.*, **53**, 61–62.

25 Ismail, M., Metwally, A., Farghaly, A., Bruce, J., Tao, L.F., and Bennett, J.L. (1996) Characterization of isolates of *Schistosoma mansoni* from Egyptian villagers that

tolerate high doses of praziquantel. *Am. J. Trop. Med. Hyg.*, **55**, 214–218.

26 Ismail, M., Botros, S., Metwally, A., William, S., Farghally, A., Tao, L.F., Day, T.A., and Bennett, J.L. (1999) Resistance to praziquantel: direct evidence from *Schistosoma mansoni* isolated from Egyptian villagers. *Am. J. Trop. Med. Hyg.*, **60**, 932–935.

27 Fallon, P.G. and Doenhoff, M.J. (1994) Drug-resistant schistosomiasis: resistance to praziquantel and oxamniquine induced in *Schistosoma mansoni* in mice is drug specific. *Am. J. Trop. Med. Hyg.*, **51**, 83–88.

28 Pica-Mattoccia, L., Doenhoff, M.J., Valle, C., Basso, A., Troiani, A.R., Liberti, P., Festucci, A. *et al.* (2009) Genetic analysis of decreased praziquantel sensitivity in a laboratory strain of *Schistosoma mansoni*. *Acta Trop.*, **111**, 82–85.

29 Cioli, D., Botros, S.S., Wheatcroft-Francklow, K., Mbaye, A., Southgate, V., Tchuem Tchuente, L.-A., Pica-Mattoccia, L. *et al.* (2004) Determination of ED_{50} values for praziquantel in praziquantel-resistant and -susceptible *Schistosoma mansoni* isolates. *Int. J. Parasitol.*, **34**, 979–987.

30 Sabra, A.N. and Botros, S.S. (2008) Response of *Schistosoma mansoni* isolates having different drug sensitivity to praziquantel over several life cycle passages with and without therapeutic pressure. *J. Parasitol.*, **94**, 537–541.

31 Black, C.L., Steinauer, M.L., Mwinzi, P.N., Secor, W.E., Karanja, D.M., and Colley, D.G. (2009) Impact of intense, longitudinal retreatment with praziquantel on cure rates of schistosomiasis mansoni in a cohort of occupationally exposed adults in western Kenya. *Trop. Med. Int. Health*, **14**, 450–457.

32 Melman, S.D., Steinauer, M.L., Cunningham, C., Kubatko, L.S., Mwangi, I.N., Wynn, N.B., Mutuku, M.W. *et al.* (2009) Reduced susceptibility to praziquantel among naturally occurring Kenyan isolates of *Schistosoma mansoni*. *PLoS Negl. Trop. Dis.*, **3**, e504.

33 Valle, C., Troiani, A.-R., Festucci, A., Pica-Mattoccia, L., Liberti, P., Wolstenholme, A., Francklow, K. *et al.* (2003) Sequence and level of endogenous expression of calcium channel β-subunits in *Schistosoma mansoni* displaying different susceptibilities to praziquantel. *Mol. Biochem. Parasitol.*, **130**, 111–115.

34 Fallon, P.G., Mubarak, J.S., Fookes, R.E., Niang, M., Butterworth, A.E., Sturrock, R.F., and Doenhoff, M.J. (1997) *Schistosoma mansoni*: maturation rate and drug susceptibility of different geographic isolates. *Exp. Parasitol.*, **86**, 29–36.

35 Guidi, A., Andolina, C., Makame Ame, S., Albonico, M., Cioli, D., and Juma Haji, H. (2010) Praziquantel efficacy and long-term appraisal of schistosomiasis control in Pemba Island. *Trop. Med. Int. Health*, **15**, 614–618.

36 Tchuem-Tchuenté, L.-A., Shaw, D.J., Polla, L., Cioli, D., and Vercruysse, J. (2004) Efficacy of praziquantel against *Schistosoma haematobium* infection in children. *Am. J. Trop. Med. Hyg.*, **71**, 778–782.

37 Sulaiman, S.M., Traoré, M., Engels, D., Hagan, P., and Cioli, D. (2001) Counterfeit praziquantel. *Lancet*, **358**, 666–667.

38 Botros, S., El-Lakkany, N., Seif el-Din, S.H., Sabra, A.N., and Ibrahim, M. (2011) Comparative efficacy and bioavailability of different praziquantel brands. *Exp. Parasitol.*, **127**, 515–521.

39 Botros, S., Sayed, H., Amer, N., El-Ghannam, M., Bennett, J.L., and Day, T.A. (2005) Current status of sensitivity to praziquantel in a focus of potential drug resistance in Egypt. *Int. J. Parasitol.*, **35**, 787–791.

40 Fong, I.W. and Drlica, K. (eds) (2010) *Antimicrobial Resistance and Implications for the 21st Century*, Springer, New York.

41 Gold, H.S. and Moellering, R.C. Jr (1996) Antimicrobial-drug resistance. *N. Engl. J. Med.*, **335**, 1445–1453.

42 Hayton, K. and Su, X.Z. (2004) Genetic and biochemical aspects of drug resistance in malaria parasites. *Curr. Drug Targets Infect. Disord.*, **4**, 1–10.

43 Day, T.A., Bennett, J.L., and Pax, R.A. (1992) Praziquantel: the enigmatic antiparasitic. *Parasitol. Today*, **8**, 342–344.

44 Caffrey, C.R. (2007) Chemotherapy of schistosomiasis: present and future. *Curr. Opin. Chem. Biol.*, **11**, 433–439.

45 Pax, R., Bennett, J.L., and Fetterer, R. (1978) A benzodiazepine derivative and praziquantel: effects on musculature of *Schistosoma mansoni* and *Schistosoma japonicum*. *Naunyn Schmiedebergs Arch. Pharmacol.*, **304**, 309–315.

46 Becker, B., Mehlhorn, H., Andrews, P., Thomas, H., and Eckert, J. (1980) Light and electron microscopic studies on the effect of praziquantel on *Schistosoma mansoni, Dicrocoelium dendriticum*, and *Fasciola hepatica* (Trematoda) *in vitro*. *Z. Parasitenkd.*, **63**, 113–128.

47 Fetterer, R.H., Pax, R.A., and Bennett, J.L. (1980) Praziquantel, potassium and 2,4-dinitrophenol: analysis of their action on the musculature of *Schistosoma mansoni*. *Eur. J. Pharmacol.*, **64**, 31–38.

48 Pica-Mattoccia, L., Valle, C., Basso, A., Troiani, A.-R., Vigorosi, F., Liberti, P., Festucci, A., and Cioli, D. (2007) Cytochalasin D abolishes the schistosomicidal activity of praziquantel. *Exp. Parasitol.*, **115**, 344–351.

49 Kohn, A.B., Anderson, P.A., Roberts-Misterly, J.M., and Greenberg, R.M. (2001) Schistosome calcium channel beta subunits. Unusual modulatory effects and potential role in the action of the antischistosomal drug praziquantel. *J. Biol. Chem.*, **276**, 36873–36876.

50 Kohn, A.B., Roberts-Misterly, J.M., Anderson, P.A., Khan, N., and Greenberg, R.M. (2003) Specific sites in the beta interaction domain of a schistosome Ca^{2+} channel beta subunit are key to its role in sensitivity to the anti-schistosomal drug praziquantel. *Parasitology*, **127**, 349–356.

51 Kohn, A.B., Roberts-Misterly, J.M., Anderson, P.A., and Greenberg, R.M. (2003) Creation by mutagenesis of a mammalian Ca^{2+} channel beta subunit that confers praziquantel sensitivity to a mammalian Ca^{2+} channel. *Int. J. Parasitol.*, **33**, 1303–1308.

52 Greenberg, R.M. (2005) Are Ca^{2+} channels targets of praziquantel action? *Int. J. Parasitol.*, **35**, 1–9.

53 Jeziorski, M.C. and Greenberg, R.M. (2006) Voltage-gated calcium channel subunits from platyhelminths: potential role in praziquantel action. *Int. J. Parasitol.*, **36**, 625–632.

54 Nogi, T., Zhang, D., Chan, J.D., and Marchant, J.S. (2009) A novel biological activity of praziquantel requiring voltage-operated Ca^{2+} channel beta subunits: subversion of flatworm regenerative polarity. *PLoS Negl. Trop. Dis.*, **3**, e464.

55 Pica-Mattoccia, L., Orsini, T., Basso, A., Festucci, A., Liberti, P., Guidi, A., Marcatto-Maggi, A.-L. *et al.* (2008) *Schistosoma mansoni*: lack of correlation between praziquantel-induced intra-worm calcium influx and parasite death. *Exp. Parasitol.*, **119**, 332–335.

56 Mendonça-Silva, D.L., Novozhilova, E., Cobbett, P.J., Silva, C.L., Noel, F., Totten, M.I., Maule, A.G., and Day, T.A. (2006) Role of calcium influx through voltage-operated calcium channels and of calcium mobilization in the physiology of *Schistosoma mansoni* muscle contractions. *Parasitology*, **133**, 67–74.

57 William, S. and Botros, S. (2004) Validation of sensitivity to praziquantel using *Schistosoma mansoni* worm muscle tension and Ca^{2+} uptake as possible *in vitro* correlates to *in vivo* ED_{50} determination. *Int. J. Parasitol.*, **34**, 971–977.

58 Angelucci, F., Basso, A., Bellelli, A., Brunori, M., Pica-Mattoccia, L., and Valle, C. (2007) The anti-schistosomal drug praziquantel is an adenosine antagonist. *Parasitology*, **134**, 1215–1221.

59 Tallima, H. and El Ridi, R. (2007) Praziquantel binds *Schistosoma mansoni* adult worm actin. *Int. J. Antimicrob. Agents*, **29**, 570–575.

60 Tallima, H. and El Ridi, R. (2007) Re: Is actin the praziquantel receptor? *Int. J. Antimicrob. Agents*, **30**, 566–567.

61 Gnanasekar, M., Salunkhe, A.M., Mallia, A.K., He, Y.K., and Ramaswamy, K. (2009) Praziquantel affects the regulatory myosin light chain of *Schistosoma mansoni*. *Antimicrob. Agents Chemother.*, **53**, 1054–1060.

62 Troiani, A.R., Pica-Mattoccia, L., Valle, C., Cioli, D., Mignogna, G., Ronketti, F., and

Todd, M. (2007) Is actin the praziquantel receptor? *Int. J. Antimicrob. Agents*, **30**, 280–281.

63 McTigue, M.A., Williams, D.R., and Taine, J.A. (1995) Crystal structures of a schistosomal drug and vaccine target: glutathione S-transferase from *Schistosoma japonica* and its complex with the leading antischistosomal drug praziquantel. *J. Mol. Biol.*, **246**, 21–27.

64 Milhon, J.L., Thiboldeaux, R.L., Glowac, K., and Tracy, J.W. (1997) *Schistosoma japonicum* GSH S-transferase Sj26 is not the molecular target of praziquantel action. *Exp. Parasitol.*, **87**, 268–274.

65 Wiest, P.M., Li, Y., Olds, R., and Bowen, W.D. (1992) Inhibition of phosphoinositide turnover by praziquantel in *Schistosoma mansoni*. *J. Parasitol.*, **78**, 753–755.

66 Harder, A., Goossens, J., and Andrews, P. (1988) Influence of praziquantel and Ca^{2+} on the bilayer-isotropic-hexagonal transition of model membranes. *Mol. Biochem. Parasitol.*, **29**, 55–60.

67 Schepers, H., Brasseur, R., Goormaghtigh, E., Duquenoy, P., and Ruysschaert, J.M. (1988) Mode of insertion of praziquantel and derivatives into lipid membranes. *Biochem. Pharmacol.*, **37**, 1615–1623.

68 Sabah, A.A., Fletcher, C., Webbe, G., and Doenhoff, M.J. (1985) *Schistosoma mansoni*-reduced efficacy of chemotherapy in infected T-cell deprived mice. *Exp. Parasitol.*, **60**, 348–354.

69 Brindley, P.J. and Sher, A. (1987) The chemotherapeutic effect of praziquantel against *Schistosoma mansoni* is dependent on host antibody response. *J. Immunol.*, **139**, 215–220.

70 Doenhoff, M.J., Sabah, A.A., Fletcher, C., Webbe, G., and Bain, J. (1987) Evidence of an immune-dependent action of praziquantel on *Schistosoma mansoni* in mice. *Trans. R. Soc. Trop. Med. Hyg.*, **81**, 947–951.

71 Karanja, D.H.S., Boyer, A.E., Strand, M., Colley, D.G., Nahlen, B.L., Ouma, J.H., and Secor, W.E. (1998) Studies on schistosomiasis in western Kenya: II. Efficacy of praziquantel for treatment of schistosomiasis in persons coinfected with human immunodeficiency virus-1. *Am. J. Trop. Med. Hyg.*, **59**, 307–311.

72 Kallestrup, P., Zinyama, R., Gomo, E., Butterworth, A.E., van Dam, G.J., Gerstoft, J., Erikstrup, C., and Ullum, H. (2006) Schistosomiasis and HIV in rural Zimbabwe: efficacy of treatment of schistosomiasis in individuals with HIV coinfection. *Clin. Infect. Dis.*, **42**, 1781–1789.

73 Wegner, D.H. (1984) The profile of the trematodicidal compound praziquantel. *Arzneimittelforschung*, **34**, 1132–1136.

74 Craig, P. and Ito, A. (2007) Intestinal cestodes. *Curr. Opin. Infect. Dis.*, **20**, 524–532.

75 Bale, J.F. Jr (2000) Cysticercosis. *Curr. Treat. Options Neurol.*, **2**, 355–360.

76 Overbosch, D. (1992) Neurocysticercosis. An introduction with special emphasis on new developments in pharmacotherapy. *Schweiz. Med. Wochenschr.*, **122**, 893–898.

77 Cobo, F., Yarnoz, C., Sesma, B., Fraile, P., Aizcorbe, M., Trujillo, R., Diaz-de-Liano, A., and Ciga, M.A. (1998) Albendazole plus praziquantel versus albendazole alone as a pre-operative treatment in intra-abdominal hydatisosis caused by *Echinococcus granulosus*. *Trop. Med. Int. Health*, **3**, 462–466.

78 Andrews, P., Thomas, H., Pohlke, R., and Seubert, J. (1983) Praziquantel. *Med. Res. Rev.*, **3**, 147–200.

79 Ronketti, F., Ramana, A.V., Chao-Ming, X., Pica-Mattoccia, L., Cioli, D., and Todd, M.H. (2007) Praziquantel derivatives I: modification of the aromatic ring. *Bioorg. Med. Chem. Lett.*, **17**, 4154–4157.

80 Dong, Y., Chollet, J., Vargas, M., Mansour, N.R., Bickle, Q., Alnouti, Y., Huang, J. *et al.* (2010) Praziquantel analogs with activity against juvenile *Schistosoma mansoni*. *Bioorg. Med. Chem. Lett.*, **20**, 2481–2484.

81 Laurent, S.A.-L., Boissier, J., Coslédan, F., Gornitzka, H., Robert, A., and Meunier, B. (2008) Synthesis of "Trioxaquantel" derivatives as potential new antischistosomal drugs. *Eur. J. Org. Chem.*, **2008**, 895–913.

82 Mandour, M.E., el Turabi, H., Homeida, M.M., el Sadig, T., Ali, H.M., Bennett, J.L., Leahey, W.J., and Harron, D.W. (1990) Pharmacokinetics of praziquantel in healthy volunteers and patients with schistosomiasis. *Trans. R. Soc. Trop. Med. Hyg.*, **84**, 389–393.

83 Wu, M.H., Wei, C.C., Xu, Z., Yuan, H.C., Lian, W.N., Yang, Q.J., Chen, M. *et al.* (1991) Comparison of the therapeutic efficacy and side effects of a single dose of levopraziquantel with mixed isomer praziquantel in 278 cases of schistosomiasis japonica. *Am. J. Trop. Med. Hyg.*, **45**, 345–349.

84 Meyer, T., Sekljic, H., Fuchs, S., Bothe, H., Schollmeyer, D., and Miculka, C. (2009) Taste, a new incentive to switch to (*R*)-praziquantel in schistosomiasis treatment. *PLoS Negl. Trop. Dis.*, **3**, e357.

85 Fleming, F.M., Fenwick, A., Tukahebwa, E.M., Lubanga, R.G., Namwangye, H., Zaramba, S., and Kabatereine, N.B. (2009) Process evaluation of schistosomiasis control in Uganda, 2003 to 2006: perceptions, attitudes and constraints of a national programme. *Parasitology*, **136**, 1759–1769.

86 Woelfle, M., Seerden, J.-P., de Gooijer, J., Pouwer, K., Olliaro, P., and Todd, M.H. (2011) Resolution of Praziquantel. *PLoS Negl. Trop. Dis.*, **5**, e1260. (DOI:10.1371/journal.pntd.0001260).

20
Drug Discovery for Trematodiases: Challenges and Progress

Conor R. Caffrey[*], *Jürg Utzinger, and Jennifer Keiser*

Abstract

Treatment of the millions of people parasitized by pathogenic nematodes has always benefited from drugs originally developed in the animal health sector. The relentless emergence of resistance by nematodes of veterinary importance and the considerable profit margins provide the necessary stimuli to develop new nematicides that often cross-over to human medicine. The same is not true for flatworms, including trematodes. The smaller veterinary market for trematocidal drugs, and the considerable investment to discover, develop, and market drugs, provide little incentive to develop new entities, even in the face of mounting drug resistance to the current trematocide, triclabendazole. Thus, for the hundreds of millions of people afflicted with schistosomiasis and other flatworm infections, and who depend entirely on just two drugs (praziquantel and triclabendazole) for treatment, the animal health industry alone cannot be relied upon to supply the next generation of drugs. Encouragingly, over the last decade, governmental, not-for-profit organizations, and academic drug discovery centers have begun to address this shortfall as part of an overall effort to discover new drugs for neglected tropical diseases, including those caused by trematodes. We review the latest infrastructural, technological, and chemical developments that are influencing and accelerating the discovery of new trematocides. This chapter is intended to provide an overview of the current drug discovery landscape and the important changes taking place.

Trematodiases

This chapter focuses on those important trematodes that parasitize humans, namely blood flukes that cause schistosomiasis, and liver, lung, and intestinal flukes that are the causative agents of various food-borne trematodiases (phylum Platyhelminthes). Schistosomiasis is the most widespread trematode infection. An estimated 800 million people are at risk and more than 200 million people are infected, with about half of them showing clinical manifestations of disease. Although difficult to quantify, the global burden due to schistosomiasis has been

---

[*] Corresponding Author

Parasitic Helminths: Targets, Screens, Drugs and Vaccines, First Edition. Edited by Conor R. Caffrey.
© 2012 Wiley-VCH Verlag GmbH & Co. KGaA. Published 2012 by Wiley-VCH Verlag GmbH & Co. KGaA.

estimated at 1.7–4.5 million disability-adjusted life years (DALYs). Recent assessments are even more alarming: as many as 550–650 million may live with some form of the disease, and the global burden might be as high as 70 million DALYs when factoring in inadequate field testing, misdiagnosis of infection, and the long-term sequelae due to previously active disease [1, 2]. Severe morbidity incapacitates an estimated 20 million individuals and the annual death toll might be as high as 280 000 [3, 4]. More than 95% of schistosomiasis cases are concentrated in Africa, but the disease also occurs in parts of South America, the Middle East, and Asia [5].

With regard to food-borne trematodiasis, liver fluke infections (i.e., clonorchiasis, fascioliasis, and opisthorchiasis) and lung fluke infections (paragonimiasis) are the most widespread. Indeed, between 80 million people (opisthorchiasis) and up to 600 million people (clonorchiasis) are at risk, with some 70 million individuals actively infected [6]. Intestinal fluke infections are the least understood; perhaps 40–50 million people are infected. The highest infection prevalences of food-borne trematodes have been reported from Southeast Asia and the Americas. A recent systematic review and meta-analysis suggests that 7.9 million people suffer from severe sequelae due to food-borne trematodiasis causing an annual mortality rate of 7200 and a global burden of 665 000 DALYs [7].

Current Therapy

Treatment of human trematode infection still relies entirely on two drugs – praziquantel (PZQ) and triclabendazole (TCBZ). Both drugs are also widely used in veterinary medicine. PZQ was discovered in the early 1970s through the collaborative efforts of Merck and Bayer in Germany, and marketed as a broad-spectrum flukicide for companion animals and livestock [8] (see also Chapter 19). In the late 1970s, PZQ was moved by the World Health Organization (WHO) into a series of clinical trials against the major human schistosome species [9–12], followed by open-label clinical trials launched in Asia to assess its efficacy against *Clonorchis sinensis* and *Opisthorchis viverrini* [13, 14] before full-scale use in the early 1980s [15]. As ivermectin was to become for human nematodiases [16, 17], PZQ was the "wonder drug" for treatment of the three major schistosome species infecting humans [18, 19] and other trematodiases, with the exception of fascioliasis [6]. The excellent safety and good efficacy profiles of PZQ, its operational ease of administration (single oral dose), and its plummeting price are key factors explaining PZQ's success as an antischistosomal [20, 21]. For human schistosomiasis, a single oral dose of 40 mg/kg usually decreases parasite burdens (as measured by egg outputs in stool or urine) by 60–90% [22].

For clonorchiasis, opisthorchiasis, paragonimiasis, and intestinal fluke infection, PZQ is the drug of choice. The recommended therapy of clonorchiasis and opisthorchiasis is 3×25 mg/kg PZQ on 2 consecutive days. Therapy of paragonimiasis consists of 3×25 mg/kg PZQ on at least 2 consecutive days. An alternative regimen for clonorchiasis and paragonimiasis is a single 40 mg/kg dose of PZQ [23]. For food-borne trematodiases, current treatment regiments of PZQ result in cure rates (CRs) of 76–97% [24].

TCBZ is the drug of choice for fascioliasis and also is active against paragonimiasis. Discovered by Ciba Geigy in 1978, TCBZ has been on the market since 1983 (Novartis Animal Health). The WHO recommends the following regimens: 10 mg/kg TCBZ (in case of treatment failures: 2×10 mg/kg) for fascioliasis and 2×10 mg/kg TCBZ for paragonimiasis [23]. TCBZ is well tolerated. For the treatment of fascioliasis in sheep and cattle, alternative therapy employs clorsulon, rafoxanide, closantel, and diamphenethide [25, 26].

Despite the prolonged and widespread use of PZQ and TCBZ in man, particularly PZQ within the framework of preventive chemotherapy targeting schistosomiasis, clinically relevant resistance has not been recorded [27–29]. However, an isolated report of a small trial with Vietnamese patients infected with *C. sinensis* documented a low CR of only 29% following PZQ treatment (25 mg/kg daily for 3 consecutive days) [30]. Despite the absence of TCBZ resistance in humans, resistance is now widespread in sheep and cattle, posing a considerable veterinary public health problem in Europe, Australia, and, more recently, in South America [24, 31]. Changes in drug influx/efflux mechanisms and in the metabolism of TCBZ might be involved [25], although the exact resistance mechanism(s) is unclear.

Overall, given the deteriorating value of TCBZ as an animal health drug and the tenuous situation of PZQ as the only drug to treat the tens of millions of school-aged children at risk of schistosomiasis, particularly in Africa, new drugs are very much needed.

Challenges Confronting Drug Discovery for Trematodiases

Simply put, and in spite of the enormous prevalence and public health impact, helminth diseases, including trematodiases, are just not as prominent in the public mind as other infectious (tropical) diseases and certainly not on a par with the "big three" (i.e., HIV/AIDS, tuberculosis, and malaria) [32–34]. Neither are helminthiases a major focus of donor-supported public–private partnerships of the type that have arisen since 2000, such as the Medicines for Malaria Venture (MMV; http://www.mmv.org) and the Drugs for Neglected Diseases *initiative* (http://www.dndi.org). This is understandable given the frightening mortality associated with viral, bacterial, and protozoal diseases, and the real need for safe, effective, oral, and short-course therapies. By contrast, safe and reasonable effective therapies are in place for helminthiases, which are, in any case, more commonly responsible for chronic and morbid conditions rather than acute, fatal disease. We have the animal health industry to thank for the development and provision of the bulk of the current armamentarium of anthelmintics [35–37] (see also Chapters 8 and 14). However, drug development efforts focus on nematodes rather than flatworms (trematodes and cestodes); thus, the present and near-future therapeutic options for flatworm diseases, including trematodiases, are extremely limited.

A second challenge to trematode drug development, specifically for schistosomiasis, is the therapeutic success of PZQ, which, when coupled with its operational simplicity and affordability as a generic drug (also donated by Merck; see their corporate web site: http://www.merck.com), has essentially cornered the market and stifled interest in investing in other chemical entities [19, 22]. The operational simplicity provided by PZQ as a safe, single-dose, oral drug underpins the drug delivery campaigns such as those now being implemented in sub-Saharan Africa (e.g., by the Carter Center (http://www.cartercenter.org/index.html) and the Schistosomiasis Control Initiative (http://www3.imperial.ac.uk/schisto)). Efforts are underway to expand preventive chemotherapy for food-borne trematodiases [33] and there is movement to integrate the treatment of multiple tropical diseases [33, 38, 39]. The establishment of a PZQ monotherapy was further cemented by the contraction of the pharmaceutical industry in general from antiparasitic/infective drug development, going hand-in-hand with the loss of the necessary financial clout, expertise, and infrastructure to continue to identify other (and better) drugs. The result today is that much of the basic identification and validation of drug targets and chemical agents is performed in the academic setting, which, traditionally, has not been best suited to taking compounds forward preclinically. Yet, this situation is changing [40–42], as discussed below.

Other factors detracting from the development of new trematocidal drugs (and anthelmintics in general) are technological; not least (i) the expense and expertise required to maintain complex cycles and the absence of fully defined *in vitro* culture systems, organism clones, or cell lines (as a note, continuous *in vitro* culture has been established for the cestode, *Echinococcus multilocularis* (see research by Brehm *et al.*, e.g., [43])), (ii) the relative lack of validated molecular targets with which target-based drug discovery programs can be engaged, and (iii) the lack of robust reverse genetics tools (e.g., targeted gene disruption and transgenic parasites (although RNA interference (RNAi) is useful (see below)) with which targets can be genetically validated. Such limitations have made schistosomes and flatworms in general unattractive for basic and applied drug discovery research for which the hypothesis-driven and protein target-centric paradigm of "rational drug design" (RDD) has been the central strategy for drug discovery over the last 20 years, including for parasitic protozoa [44]. In contrast, anthelmintic drug discovery has and still relies on the "intellectually unattractive" [36] activity of "phenotypic" (e.g., bioactivity, whole-organism, or physiological) screening to fish out compounds that demonstrate activity *in vitro* and/or *in vivo*. That stated, phenotypic screening is of proven merit as virtually all of the anthelmintics (or their prototypes, including PZQ) that are on the market today [36, 45] have been identified in animal models of infection or in culture. As for RDD, academic centers have moved to fill the gap left by the withdrawal of the pharmaceutical industry from anti-infectives/antiparasitics and the consolidation of the animal health industry around the still lucrative market [46] for therapies to treat a prescribed set of endo- and ectoparasitic diseases.

New Infrastructures to Reinvigorate Trematode Drug Discovery

Drug discovery to combat trematodiases is carried out in various academic institutions world-wide. Examples include the Sandler Center for Drug Discovery at the University of California San Francisco (UCSF Sandler Center), the Swiss Tropical and Public Health Institute (Swiss TPH; http://www.swisstph.ch), and the London School of Hygiene and Tropical Medicine (LSHTM; http://www.lshtm.ac.uk).

At the Swiss TPH, the life cycles of *S. mansoni* and *Echinostoma caproni* are maintained, and efforts are underway to establish the life cycles of *Schistosoma haematobium* and *Fasciola hepatica*. Currently, infected *Bulinus* snails are obtained from the US National Institutes of Health's National Institute of Allergy and Infectious Diseases, (NIH–NIAID) Schistosomiasis Resource Center (http://www.schisto-resource.org/schistohome.html) for subsequent infections of hamsters with *S. haematobium*. For *F. hepatica*, metacercariae are purchased from Baldwin Aquatics (Monmouth, OR). *Opisthorchis viverrini* and *C. sinensis* metacercariae are provided by collaborators in endemic countries. Screens first employ larval stages (newly excysted worms or schistosomula as described below) followed by adult stages. Whereas adult schistosomes, echinostomes, *O. viverrini*, and *C. sinensis* are collected from rodent models of infection, adult *F. hepatica* are obtained from local slaughterhouses. Chemical hits obtained from *in vitro* studies are progressed into *in vivo* investigations. Screening activities involve collaborations with a number of academic partners. The trematocidal activities of various antimalarial drugs such as the artemisinins, synthetic peroxides (1,2,4-trioxolanes), and mefloquine have been studied at the Swiss TPH (see below). Compounds demonstrating efficacy *in vivo* are then studied in more detail preclinically and might progress into exploratory open-label phase II clinical testing. The Swiss TPH maintains long-term partnerships with health research and development centers in sub-Saharan Africa and Asia with which clinical trials can be jointly conducted. For example, exploratory phase II trials have been carried out with mefloquine and the artemisinins in *S. mansoni-*, *S. haematobium-*, *F. hepatica-*, and *O. viverrini*-infected individuals [47, 48].

The UCSF Sandler Center houses the infrastructure and expertise to preclinically prosecute lead compounds for a number of tropical infectious diseases through to filing for investigational new drug (IND) status at the US Food and Drug Administration (http://www.fda.gov) [41]. The center maintains its own *S. mansoni* life cycle, and has been active in the discovery of antischistosomal lead chemistries [49] and the development of screening automation and assay tools [50, 51]. The center pioneered the use of microtiter plate-formatted schistosomula as part of its screening platform to triage large collections of many thousands of compounds prior to tests with adults *in vitro* or in a murine model of infection. Compound collections are available in-house (http://smdc.ucsf.edu/documents/index.htm) or through an extensive network of industry and academic collaborators, and include drugs approved for human use, natural products and various target (e.g., protease, kinase)-specific and diverse small molecules. Thus far, the platform has discovered a variety of schistosomicidal compounds with *in vitro* and/or *in vivo* bioactivity, including nematicides, antiprotozoals, and natural products [50]. Whenever possible, results of screening campaigns are made available on a free registration basis (for academia) through Collaborative Drug Discovery Inc.'s web site (https://www.collaborativedrug.com).

Finally, and in our view a critical step forward that will ultimately facilitate new treatments for schistosomiasis, food-borne trematodiasis, and other tropical diseases, is the establishment, in 2009, of the Therapeutics for Rare and Neglected Diseases (TRND) program by the NIH (http://nctt.nih.gov/trnd/). TRND coordinates the necessary expertise and infrastructure to support the preclinical development of drugs through to IND status. Proposals for support are reviewed by TRND staff, and those successful enter the TRND development pipeline that involves both NIH intramural and extramural expertise. One of the first pilot projects to be adopted by TRND was the development of the oxadiazole-2-oxide compound series of antischistosomals [52, 53] (see below).

Repurposing Drugs and New Drug Leads

Repurposing or repositioning approved drugs for new medical indications provides a potentially quicker and cost-effective route to bringing therapeutics to market. The strategy has been investigated for a number of years in the neglected and rare diseases arena (for reviews, see [54, 55]), including for trematodiases (see below and as referenced in [40]). Evidence from randomized controlled trials with the artemisinins and artemisinin-based combination therapies against schistosomiasis and the prevention of patent *Schistosoma* infection has been summarized [33]. More recently, for *F. hepatica*, a study in Egypt found low-to-moderate CRs and egg reduction rates (ERRs) after administration of artemether using two different malaria dosing regimens (6×80 mg over 3 consecutive days and 3×200 mg within 24 h) [56]. In Vietnam, patients suffering from acute fascioliasis were more likely to be free of abdominal pain compared to TCBZ-treated patients following a 10-day treatment with artesunate [57]. In Lao People's Democratic Republic, tribendimidine, mefloquine–artesunate, and mefloquine were tested in an exploratory open-label trial targeting *O. viverrini* [48]. Artesunate (10 mg/kg as three split doses within 12 h) resulted in low-to-moderate CR (33%) and ERR (32%). Tribendimidine performed slightly better than PZQ in terms of CR (70 versus 56%), whereas high ERRs were found with both drugs (98–99%). No effect was observed with the mefloquine–artesunate combination (100 mg artesunate plus 250 mg mefloquine once daily for 3 consecutive days) or mefloquine (25 mg/kg) in *O. viverrini*-infected patients [48]. The finding with mefloquine–artesunate contrasts the results obtained in *S. haematobium*-infected children treated in Côte d'Ivoire where ERRs above 95% and a CR of 61% were recorded [47]. Considerably lower CRs and ERRs (21 and 74%, respectively) were observed in children who had received mefloquine alone.

Further studies on the effect of tribendimidine on Asian liver flukes (e.g., phase I dose-finding, including determination of pharmacokinetic parameters and assessment of the effect against *C. sinensis*) have been designed and will be launched as soon as ethical approval from the respective authorities is obtained. This project is currently funded by a UK Department for International Development/Medical Research Council/Wellcome Trust grant. For *S. haematobium*, as synergistic effects were observed with a mefloquine–PZQ combination in *S. mansoni*-infected mice and *in vitro* [58], a proof-of-concept study has been launched to assess the therapeutic benefit of mefloquine–PZQ and mefloquine–artesunate–PZQ in *S. haematobium*-infected children. Note that drugs will be administered on subsequent days, as potential interactions between these drugs have yet to be determined.

In terms of new drug leads, and as noted above, the NIH-funded TRND program is now helping guide the antischistosomal oxadiazole-2-oxide lead series of compounds through preclinical development. The original compound, furoxan, was discovered in a high-throughput chemical screen of the molecular target, thioredoxin glutathione reductase (TGR), using the NIH Molecular Libraries Small Molecule Repository [59]. In a mouse model of *S. mansoni* infection, furoxan offered a better pharmacological profile over that of PZQ by killing all relevant stages of *S. mansoni* (skin and lung stages, juveniles and adults) [52]. Parasite death by furoxan is associated with the donation of the nitric oxide radical (NO•) in the presence of TGR and NADPH [52]. More recent research has identified the basic molecular pharmacophore as 3-cyano-1,2,5-oxadiazole-2-oxide and that *S*-nitrosylation of TGR occurs upon donation of nitric oxide until the enzyme is inactivated; TGR must be active for this to occur [53]. Metabolic tests *in vitro* with a number of oxadiazole-2-oxide analogs have shown that they are reasonably stable in the presence of liver microsomes with acceptable CYP (cytochrome P450 superfamily enzymes) and hERG (human ether-a-go-go related gene; the $K_v 11.1$ potassium ion channel involved in coordinating the heartbeat) profiles. The long-term goal is to identify orally active compounds [53].

Two further groups of compounds should be discussed. First, the aryl hydantoins, as represented by Ro 13-3978 and nilutamide (the latter marketed as an androgen receptor antagonist), might offer a starting point to identify lead antischistosomals. Administration of a singe 400 mg/kg oral dose of nilutamide to experimentally infected mice decreased worm burdens by 85% [60]. Second, potential drug candidates might stem from a group of synthetic peroxides, the 1,2,4-trioxolanes, and related derivatives. One such compound, termed MT04, cured *F. hepatica* juvenile and adult infections in rats at single doses of 50–100 mg/kg. In the *S. mansoni*-mouse model, selected 1,2,4-trioxolanes achieved worm burden reductions of 60% and up to 100% at single doses of 200–400 mg/kg against juvenile and adult infections, respectively [61].

Phenotypic Screens: Assay Development and Automation

Phenotypic screening has really come into its own over the last decade with the revolution in automated high-throughput robotics and high-content imaging technologies. These technologies have together facilitated the measurement of responses of cells, tissues, and whole organisms to genetic and/or chemical perturbation (e.g., [62–64]). For helminths, specifically, *Caenorhabditis elegans*, a number of high-throughput roboticized systems have been developed [65, 66] and high-content imaging techniques have also rapidly evolved to measure multiparametric biological responses to chemical stimuli or as a result of genetic modulation (e.g., [67, 68]). Indeed, the (re-)emergence of whole-organism screening and its contribution to identifying antiparasitic compounds of interest is evident, for example, in the drug development portfolio of the MMV. All of this activity is filtering into the realm of drug discovery for helmintic and trematodal diseases.

For schistosomes, the last few years have seen the exploration of a number of quantitative (in most cases microtiter plate formatted) assays. Although not strictly high-content in approach, they have at least been designed to measure end-points for parasite vitality rather than rely on visual scoring approaches. The assays tested include use of "live/death" fluorometry with propidium iodide and fluorescein diacetate [69], fluorescently labeled albumin ingested by the parasite as a readout for development [70], the vital dye, Alamar Blue [71], the xCELLigence system (Roche) that measures electrical impedance across interdigitated microelectrodes integrated on the bottom of tissue culture "E-Plates" [72], and isothermal microcalorimetry to measure (in real-time) changes in heat flow in organisms [73]. Microcalorimetry was also employed to detect drug effects on adult *F. hepatica* [74]. A significant step forward has been the *de novo* development of an image (video)-based high-content system to identify and track *S. mansoni* schistosomula, and then sort phenotypes based on appearance, shape, and motion [51] (see also Chapter 10). The goal here is to merge this and similar high-content systems into the high-throughput automation under development for phenotypic screening first reported in [50].

All of the above assay approaches have advantages and limitations, but collectively represent encouraging progress towards quantifying trematode responses to environmental perturbation and, in some cases, in an automated screening environment. Which, if any, fits the bill for ease of use, robustness, throughput adaptability, and cost is not yet clear, and will depend on the preferences of the individual research teams. Apart from the assay, the considerable logistical challenges associated with the supply of flatworm parasites and chemistries remain, but can be overcome if the necessary resources and expertise are to hand.

Improving Genomics and Functional Genomics Tools

With the arrival and ongoing refinement of annotated schistosome genome sequences [75–77], target-focused RDD can now be entertained for schistosomes. Significant genomic (e.g., synteny, gene copy number, molecular pathway analyses, and metabolic reconstruction to identify chokepoints) and transcriptomic (e.g., life-stage expression and splice variation; see [78] for references) context is now at hand with which the importance of gene products can be assessed as potential targets for chemical (or immunological) intervention. This is as much true for schistosome protein groups already validated as drug targets (e.g., redox enzymes [53] (and references therein) and cysteine proteases [49, 79]), as it is for those more putative targets such as kinases [80] and G-protein-coupled receptors [81] that are "druggable" [82] in other biomedical contexts, including against nematodes [83].

The reader is encouraged to review the above-cited genome and transcriptome reports and their extensive supplementary information that display annotated lists of druggable targets that include G-protein-coupled receptors, ligand- and voltage-gated ion channels, proteases, kinases, and neuropeptides. Subsequent analyses of the *S. mansoni* genome information have also described the complement of proteases ("degradome") [84] and kinases ("kinome") [85].

In addition to particular proteins or protein classes of interest, *in silico*, global, and comparative genomics have identified ("prevalidated") potential drug targets for *S. mansoni* [86, 87]. Both studies focused on orthology between schistosome genes and those from the model organisms *Saccharomyces cerevisiae* (http://www.yeastgenome.org), *C. elegans* (http://www.wormbase.org), and/or *Drosophila melanogaster* (http://www.flybase.org) to generate partially overlapping lists of potentially essential and druggable genes. In the first case, in-house software and expertise was used [86]; in the second report, a publicly available relational database (http://www.tdrtargets.org) maintained by the Special Programme for Research and Training in Tropical Diseases (TDR) and which is based at the WHO, was employed [88]. This database incorporates a number of filters with adjustable weightings that the user can modulate to produce lists of "priority" targets (see also Chapter 3). Over the next year, the Schistodb database (http://www.schistodb.net) will be upgraded to offer improved query functionality and graphical user interfaces similar to those incorporated into the EuPathDB family of genome databases [89]. Soon, it should be possible to perform comparative genomics with other platyhelminth genomes, including *Taenia solium* [90], *Schmidtea mediterranea* [91], *F. hepatica*, *Echinoccocus* spp., and *Hymenolepis microstoma* (research ongoing for the last three parasites at the Wellcome Trust Sanger Institute). These advances are in addition to the next-generation sequencing technologies being put to work to elucidate the transcriptomes of a number of platyhelminths of medical and agricultural importance (see Chapter 5).

In the above *in silico* studies [86, 87], orthologous genes were actively sought rather than unique or genus-specific genes. Recent analyses have shown that organism-specific genes tend to suffer a decreased probability of being essential [92], whereas conserved and essential genes are more likely to yield the most severe phenotypes upon disruption [92, 93]. Additionally, sufficient physiological, parasitological, and/or structural circumstances usually exist to negate initial fears that targeting genes conserved between parasite and host would generate toxicity (outlined in [86]). Finally, knowing that very short-course therapies are required for the success of any new anthelmintic drug, "off-target" toxicity would be, in any case, limited.

The biggest hurdle is not so much the comparative genomics or the identification of potential drug targets, but rather the limited options available to experimentally test the hypotheses that the genes of interest are indeed essential. In the absence of target-specific chemistries, a first recourse might be the use of RNAi, which, as described in Chapter 7, has been useful to validate potential drug targets. A second issue of concern is how relevant outputs derived for *S. mansoni* are for *S. haematobium*, as the latter is the more prevalent of the two species in sub-Saharan Africa [94]. In this regard, the very recent release of a draft of the

S. haematobium genome sequence [95] should facilitate the search for drug targets common to both species. However, for any new antischistosomal drug to be successful, it must offer at least the same spectrum of activity and operational simplicity as PZQ. It is not clear how even subtle sequence differences between *S. mansoni* and *S. haematobium* targets identified *in silico* or otherwise (especially in the ligand binding site) would impact the eventual development of a single chemical entity.

Target Validation Through Reverse Genetics: RNAi

Transient RNAi has been valuable in defining gene function in parasitic flatworms, including *Schistosoma*, and, more recently, *F. hepatica*, *O. viverrini*, and some cestodes (see also Chapter 7). Consideration is being given to attempting large-scale screens of *S. mansoni* using RNAi (e.g., [78]), but it is clear that not all genes are (robustly) suppressed by the current approaches using transient RNAi with either plasmid-derived double-stranded RNA or synthetic small interfering RNA ([78] and references therein). Also, a standard protocol for RNAi in schistosomes is not yet in place, including but not limited to the choice of culture medium and method of delivery. Rather, smaller-scale gene-, pathway-, or tissue-specific RNAi may be preferable, given the parasite resources demanded and the associated running costs (e.g., purchase of two to three small interfering RNA molecules per gene target). Often phenotypes are not recorded in schistosomes even after robust gene suppression [96], including of more than one gene at the same time [78], and this might be in part due to a lack of "environmental challenge" of parasites in rich culture media. However, there are examples where RNAi has generated lethal phenotypes, such as with peroxiredoxin [97] and TGR [98]. In the latter case, the cognate protein was subsequently chemically validated as a drug target [52], as reviewed above. Apart from transient RNAi, there are no routine reverse genetics strategies for flatworm parasites, although transgenesis via particle bombardment [99] and viruses [100] is under study. Vector-based delivery of small hairpin RNAs has also shown promise in schistosomes [101, 102].

Recent Advances with Metabolic Profiling

Metabolic profiling employs a combination of analytical tools (e.g., capillary electrophoresis, mass spectrometry, and nuclear magnetic resonance spectroscopy) and multivariate statistical analyses (e.g., principal component analysis and projection to latent structure-discriminant analysis) to investigate the dynamics of biochemical responses of living systems to pathophysiological stimuli [103]. Metabolic profiling offers exciting opportunities to assess drug safety, gene function, disease diagnosis, and physiological monitoring, and perform metabolome-wide association studies [104, 105]. Progress has been made with metabolic profiling for discovery and identification of biomarkers in rodents experimentally infected with trematodes [106], including *S. mansoni* in the mouse [107], *S. japonicum* in the hamster [108], *E. caproni* in the mouse [109], and *F. hepatica* in the rat [110]. Most recently, the temporal dynamics of metabolic alterations in mouse urine, blood, and feces due to *S. mansoni* infection have been studied at the systems level. In total, 13 plasma metabolites, 12 urinary biomarkers, and five metabolites in fecal extracts were found that distinguished between *S. mansoni*-infected and uninfected control mice. The most consistent plasma metabolites separating the two groups were lipid components, particularly D-3-hydroxybutyrate and glycerophosphorylcholine. With regard to urinary metabolites, hippurate, phenylacetylglycine (PAG), and 2-oxoadipate were particularly robust in terms of indicating disease progression. In terms of chemical composition, fecal extracts showed the greatest variability with 5-aminovalerate being the most stable metabolite that showed a positive correlation with urinary PAG [111]. Interestingly, alterations in a range of gut bacteria-related metabolites were noted both in urine and in fecal extracts of *S. mansoni*-infected mice (e.g., trimethylamine, PAG, acetate, butyrate, propionate, and hippurate), whereas in the plasma, *S. mansoni* infection was characterized by changes in metabolites related to energy homeostasis (e.g., elevated levels of lipids and decreased levels of glucose) [106, 107, 111]. Recently, Balog *et al.* presented corroborating evidence that findings obtained from a *S. mansoni*–mouse model are indeed transferable to humans. In a well-characterized cohort of 447 *S. mansoni*-infected individuals from Uganda who were given PZQ, infection-related metabolites were primarily linked to changes in gut microflora, energy metabolism, and liver function [112].

Conclusions

In spite of the economic and structural challenges described above, encouraging changes are afoot in providing the necessary resources to discover and deliver new trematocidal compounds. Academia, together with governmental and not-for-profit institutions, are actively engaged, not just in the identification and validation of drug targets, but also in the preclinical and clinical prosecution of small molecules, both novel and those arising from drug repurposing investigations. New tools and technologies are and will be key to facilitating the lengthy process of drug discovery. Bearing in mind the current reliance on just two drugs to treat the many millions afflicted with trematodiases, these changes are both welcome and necessary, and may, ultimately, prove crucial.

Acknowledgments

C.R.C. is currently supported by the Sandler Foundation and NIH-NIAID grant 1R01A1089896. J.U. (project no. IZ70Z0_123900) and J.K. (project nos. PPOOA-114941 and PP00P3_135170) acknowledge financial support by the Swiss National Science Foundation.

References

1 King, C.H. (2010) Parasites and poverty: the case of schistosomiasis. *Acta Trop.*, **113**, 95–104.
2 Hotez, P.J. and Fenwick, A. (2009) Schistosomiasis in Africa: an emerging tragedy in our new global health decade. *PLoS Negl. Trop. Dis.*, **3**, e485.
3 Hotez, P.J., Molyneux, D.H., Fenwick, A., Ottesen, E., Ehrlich Sachs, S., and Sachs, J.D. (2006) Incorporating a rapid-impact package for neglected tropical diseases with programs for HIV/AIDS, tuberculosis, and malaria. *PLoS Med.*, **3**, e102.
4 Steinmann, P., Keiser, J., Bos, R., Tanner, M., and Utzinger, J. (2006) Schistosomiasis and water resources development: systematic review, meta-analysis, and estimates of people at risk. *Lancet. Infect. Dis.*, **6**, 411–425.
5 World Health Organization (2011) Schistosomiasis. *Wkly Epidemiol. Rec.*, **86**, 73–80.
6 Keiser, J. and Utzinger, J. (2009) Food-borne trematodiases. *Clin. Microbiol. Rev.*, **22**, 466–483.
7 Fürst, T., Keiser, J. and Utzinger, J. (2012) Global burden of human food-borne trematodiasis: a systematic review and meta-analysis. *Lancet Infect Dis.*, **12**, 210–221.
8 Gönnert, R. and Andrews, P. (1977) Praziquantel, a new board-spectrum antischistosomal agent. *Z. Parasitenkd.*, **52**, 129–150.
9 Davis, A., Biles, J.E., and Ulrich, A.M. (1979) Initial experiences with praziquantel in the treatment of human infections due to *Schistosoma haematobium*. *Bull. World Health Organ.*, **57**, 773–779.
10 Davis, A. and Wegner, D.H. (1979) Multicentre trials of praziquantel in human schistosomiasis: design and techniques. *Bull. World Health Organ.*, **57**, 767–771.
11 Katz, N., Rocha, R.S., and Chaves, A. (1979) Preliminary trials with praziquantel in human infections due to *Schistosoma mansoni*. *Bull. World Health Organ.*, **57**, 781–785.
12 Santos, A.T., Blas, B.L., Nosenas, J.S., Portillo, G.P., Ortega, O.M., Hayashi, M., and Boehme, K. (1979) Preliminary clinical trials with praziquantel in *Schistosoma japonicum* infections in the Philippines. *Bull. World Health Organ.*, **57**, 793–799.
13 Rim, H.J., Lyu, K.S., Lee, J.S., and Joo, K.H. (1981) Clinical evaluation of the therapeutic efficacy of praziquantel (Embay 8440) against *Clonorchis sinensis* infection in man. *Ann. Trop. Med. Parasitol.*, **75**, 27–33.
14 Bunnag, D. and Harinasuta, T. (1981) Studies on the chemotherapy of human opisthorchiasis: III. Minimum effective dose of praziquantel. *Southeast Asian J. Trop. Med. Public Health*, **12**, 413–417.
15 Andrews, P., Thomas, H., Pohlke, R., and Seubert, J. (1983) Praziquantel. *Med. Res. Rev.*, **3**, 147–200.
16 Campbell, W.C. (1993) Ivermectin, an antiparasitic agent. *Med. Res. Rev.*, **13**, 61–79.
17 Omura, S. (2008) Ivermectin: 25 years and still going strong. *Int. J. Antimicrob. Agents*, **31**, 91–98.
18 Cioli, D. and Pica-Mattoccia, L. (2003) Praziquantel. *Parasitol. Res.* **90** (Suppl. 1), S3–S9.
19 Caffrey, C.R. (2007) Chemotherapy of schistosomiasis: present and future. *Curr. Opin. Chem. Biol.*, **11**, 433–439.
20 Doenhoff, M.J., Hagan, P., Cioli, D., Southgate, V., Pica-Mattoccia, L., Botros, S., Coles, G. et al. (2009) Praziquantel: its use in control of schistosomiasis in sub-Saharan Africa and current research needs. *Parasitology*, **136**, 1825–1835.
21 Fenwick, A. and Webster, J.P. (2006) Schistosomiasis: challenges for control, treatment and drug resistance. *Curr. Opin. Infect. Dis.*, **19**, 577–582.
22 Doenhoff, M.J. and Pica-Mattoccia, L. (2006) Praziquantel for the treatment of schistosomiasis: its use for control in areas with endemic disease and prospects for drug resistance. *Expert Rev. Anti Infect. Ther.*, **4**, 199–210.
23 World Health Organization (2011) *Report of the WHO Expert Consultation on*

Foodborne Trematode Infections and Taeniasis/Cysticercosis, WHO, Geneva.

24 Keiser, J. and Utzinger, J. (2010) The drugs we have and the drugs we need against major helminth infections. *Adv. Parasitol.*, **73**, 197–230.

25 Fairweather, I. (2009) Triclabendazole progress report, 2005–2009: an advancement of learning? *J. Helminthol.*, **83**, 139–150.

26 Fairweather, I. and Boray, J.C. (1999) Fasciolicides: efficacy, actions, resistance and its management. *Vet. J.*, **158**, 81–112.

27 Black, C.L., Steinauer, M.L., Mwinzi, P.N., Secor, E.W., Karanja, D.M., and Colley, D.G. (2009) Impact of intense, longitudinal retreatment with praziquantel on cure rates of schistosomiasis mansoni in a cohort of occupationally exposed adults in western Kenya. *Trop. Med. Int. Health*, **14**, 450–457.

28 Botros, S., Sayed, H., Amer, N., El-Ghannam, M., Bennett, J.L., and Day, T.A. (2005) Current status of sensitivity to praziquantel in a focus of potential drug resistance in Egypt. *Int. J. Parasitol.*, **35**, 787–791.

29 Guidi, A., Andolina, C., Makame Ame, S., Albonico, M., Cioli, D., and Juma Haji, H. (2010) Praziquantel efficacy and long-term appraisal of schistosomiasis control in Pemba Island. *Trop. Med. Int. Health*, **15**, 614–618.

30 Tinga, N., De, N., Vien, H.V., Chau, L., Toan, N.D., Kager, P.A., and Vries, P.J. (1999) Little effect of praziquantel or artemisinin on clonorchiasis in Northern Vietnam. A pilot study. *Trop. Med. Int. Health*, **4**, 814–818.

31 Olaechea, F., Lovera, V., Larroza, M., Raffo, F., and Cabrera, R. (2011) Resistance of *Fasciola hepatica* against triclabendazole in cattle in Patagonia (Argentina). *Vet. Parasitol.*, **178**, 364–366.

32 Molyneux, D.H. (2008) Combating the "other diseases" of MDG 6: changing the paradigm to achieve equity and poverty reduction? *Trans. R. Soc. Trop. Med. Hyg.*, **102**, 509–519.

33 Utzinger, J., N'Goran, E.K., Caffrey, C.R., and Keiser, J. (2011) From innovation to application: social–ecological context, diagnostics, drugs and integrated control of schistosomiasis. *Acta Trop.*, **120** (Suppl. 1), S121–S137.

34 Hotez, P.J., Fenwick, A., Savioli, L., and Molyneux, D.H. (2009) Rescuing the bottom billion through control of neglected tropical diseases. *Lancet*, **373**, 1570–1575.

35 Geary, T.G., Woo, K., McCarthy, J.S., Mackenzie, C.D., Horton, J., Prichard, R.K., de Silva, N.R. *et al.* (2010) Unresolved issues in anthelmintic pharmacology for helminthiases of humans. *Int. J. Parasitol.*, **40**, 1–13.

36 Geary, T.G., Woods, D.J., Williams, T., and Nwaka, S. (2009) Target identification and mechanism-based screening for anthelmintics: application of veterinary antiparasitic research programs to search for new antiparasitic drugs for human indications. In: *Antiparasitic and Antibacterial Drug Discovery: From Molecular Targets to Drug Candidates Drug Discovery in Infectious Diseases* (ed. P.M. Selzer), Wiley-VCH Verlag GmbH, Weinheim, pp. 3–15.

37 Woods, D.J., Lauret, C., and Geary, T.G. (2007) Anthelmintic discovery and development in the animal health industry. *Expert Opin. Drug Discov.*, **2**, 1–8.

38 Mohammed, K.A., Haji, H.J., Gabrielli, A.F., Mubila, L., Biswas, G., Chitsulo, L., Bradley, M.H. *et al.* (2008) Triple co-administration of ivermectin, albendazole and praziquantel in Zanzibar: a safety study. *PLoS Negl. Trop. Dis.*, **2**, e171.

39 Molyneux, D.H., Hotez, P.J., and Fenwick, A. (2005) "Rapid-impact interventions": how a policy of integrated control for Africa's neglected tropical diseases could benefit the poor. *PLoS Med.*, **2**, e336.

40 Caffrey, C.R. and Secor, W.E. (2011) Schistosomiasis: from drug deployment to drug development. *Curr. Opin. Infect. Dis.*, **24**, 410–417.

41 Caffrey, C.R. and Steverding, D. (2008) Recent initiatives and strategies to developing new drugs for tropical

parasitic diseases. *Expert Opin. Drug Discov.*, **3**, 173–186.

42 Frearson, J.A. and Collie, I.T. (2009) HTS and hit finding in academia-from chemical genomics to drug discovery. *Drug Discov. Today*, **14**, 1150–1158.

43 Spiliotis, M., Mizukami, C., Oku, Y., Kiss, F., Brehm, K., and Gottstein, B. (2010) *Echinococcus multilocularis* primary cells: improved isolation, small-scale cultivation and RNA interference. *Mol. Biochem. Parasitol.*, **174**, 83–87.

44 Frearson, J.A., Wyatt, P.G., Gilbert, I.H., and Fairlamb, A.H. (2007) Target assessment for antiparasitic drug discovery. *Trends Parasitol.*, **23**, 589–595.

45 Harder, A. (2002) Milestones of helmintic research at Bayer. *Parasitol. Res.*, **88**, 477–480.

46 Selzer, P.M. (ed.) (2009) *Antiparasitic and Antibacterial Drug Discovery: From Molecular Targets to Drug Candidates Drug Discovery in Infectious Diseases*, Wiley-VCH Verlag GmbH, Weinheim.

47 Keiser, J., N'Guessan, N.A., Adoubryn, K.D., Silue, K.D., Vounatsou, P., Hatz, C., Utzinger, J., and N'Goran, E.K. (2010) Efficacy and safety of mefloquine, artesunate, mefloquine–artesunate, and praziquantel against *Schistosoma haematobium*: randomized, exploratory open-label trial. *Clin. Infect. Dis.*, **50**, 1205–1213.

48 Soukhathammavong, P., Odermatt, P., Sayasone, S., Vonghachack, Y., Vounatsou, P., Hatz, C., Akkhavong, K., and Keiser, J. (2010) Efficacy and safety of mefloquine, artesunate, mefloquine–artesunate, tribendimidine, and praziquantel in patients with *Opisthorchis viverrini*: a randomised, exploratory, open-label, phase 2 trial. *Lancet Infect. Dis.*, **11**, 110–118.

49 Abdulla, M.H., Lim, K.C., Sajid, M., McKerrow, J.H., and Caffrey, C.R. (2007) Schistosomiasis mansoni: novel chemotherapy using a cysteine protease inhibitor. *PLoS Med.*, **4**, e14.

50 Abdulla, M.H., Ruelas, D.S., Wolff, B., Snedecor, J., Lim, K.C., Xu, F., Renslo, A.R. et al. (2009) Drug discovery for schistosomiasis: hit and lead compounds identified in a library of known drugs by medium-throughput phenotypic screening. *PLoS Negl. Trop. Dis.*, **3**, e478.

51 Lee, H., Moody-Davis, A., Saha, U., Suzuki, B.M., Asarnow, D., Chen, S., Arkin, M., Caffrey, C.R., and Singh, R. (2012) Quantification and clustering of phenotypic screening data using time-series analysis for chemotherapy of schistosomiasis. *BMC Genomics*, **13**, (Suppl 1): S4.

52 Sayed, A.A., Simeonov, A., Thomas, C.J., Inglese, J., Austin, C.P., and Williams, D.L. (2008) Identification of oxadiazoles as new drug leads for the control of schistosomiasis. *Nat. Med.*, **14**, 407–412.

53 Rai, G., Sayed, A.A., Lea, W.A., Luecke, H.F., Chakrapani, H., Prast-Nielsen, S., Jadhav, A. et al. (2009) Structure mechanism insights and the role of nitric oxide donation guide the development of oxadiazole-2-oxides as therapeutic agents against schistosomiasis. *J. Med. Chem.*, **52**, 6474–6483.

54 Ekins, S. and Williams, A.J. (2011) Finding promiscuous old drugs for new uses. *Pharm. Res.*, **28**, 1785–1791.

55 Ekins, S., Williams, A.J., Krasowski, M.D., and Freundlich, J.S. (2011) In silico repositioning of approved drugs for rare and neglected diseases. *Drug Discov. Today*, **16**, 298–310.

56 Keiser, J., Sayed, H., El-Ghanam, M., Sabry, H., Anani, S., El-Wakeel, A., Hatz, C. et al. (2011) Efficacy and safety of artemether in the treatment of chronic fascioliasis in Egypt: exploratory phase-2 trials. *PLoS Negl. Trop. Dis.*, **5**, e1285.

57 Hien, T.T., Truong, N.T., Minh, N.H., Dat, H.D., Dung, N.T., Hue, N.T., Dung, T.K. et al. (2008) A randomized controlled pilot study of artesunate versus triclabendazole for human fascioliasis in central Vietnam. *Am. J. Trop. Med. Hyg.*, **78**, 388–392.

58 Keiser, J., Manneck, T., and Vargas, M. (2011) Interactions of mefloquine with praziquantel in the *Schistosoma mansoni* mouse model and *in vitro*. *J. Antimicrob. Chemother.*, **66**, 1791–1797.

59 Simeonov, A., Jadhav, A., Sayed, A.A., Wang, Y., Nelson, M.E., Thomas, C.J., Inglese, J. et al. (2008) Quantitative high-throughput screen identifies inhibitors of the *Schistosoma mansoni* redox cascade. *PLoS Negl. Trop. Dis.*, **2**, e127.

60 Keiser, J., Vargas, M., and Vennerstrom, J.L. (2010) Activity of antiandrogens against juvenile and adult *Schistosoma mansoni* in mice. *J. Antimicrob. Chemother.*, **65**, 1991–1995.

61 Keiser, J., Ingram, K., Vargas, M., Chollet, J., Wang, X., Dong, Y., and Vennerstrom, J.L. (2012) *In vivo* activity of aryl ozonides against *Schistosoma* species. *Antimicrob. Agents Chemother.*, **56**, 1090–1092.

62 Niederlein, A., Meyenhofer, F., White, D., and Bickle, M. (2009) Image analysis in high-content screening. *Comb. Chem. High Throughput Screen.*, **12**, 899–907.

63 Peravali, R., Gehrig, J., Giselbrecht, S., Lütjohann, D.S., Hadzhiev, Y., Müller, F., and Liebel, U. (2011) Automated feature detection and imaging for high-resolution screening of zebrafish embryos. *Biotechniques*, **50**, 319–324.

64 Wlodkowic, D., Khoshmanesh, K., Akagi, J., Williams, D.E., and Cooper, J.M. (2011) Wormometry-on-a-chip: innovative technologies for *in situ* analysis of small multicellular organisms. *Cytometry A*, **79**, 799–813.

65 Chung, K., Crane, M.M., and Lu, H. (2008) Automated on-chip rapid microscopy, phenotyping and sorting of *C. elegans*. *Nat. Methods*, **5**, 637–643.

66 Stirman, J.N., Brauner, M., Gottschalk, A., and Lu, H. (2010) High-throughput study of synaptic transmission at the neuromuscular junction enabled by optogenetics and microfluidics. *J. Neurosci. Methods*, **191**, 90–93.

67 Green, R.A., Kao, H.L., Audhya, A., Arur, S., Mayers, J.R., Fridolfsson, H.N., Schulman, M. et al. (2011) A high-resolution *C. elegans* essential gene network based on phenotypic profiling of a complex tissue. *Cell*, **145**, 470–482.

68 Albrecht, D.R. and Bargmann, C.I. (2011) High-content behavioral analysis of *Caenorhabditis elegans* in precise spatiotemporal chemical environments. *Nat. Methods*, **8**, 599–605.

69 Peak, E., Chalmers, I.W., and Hoffmann, K.F. (2010) Development and validation of a quantitative, high-throughput, fluorescent-based bioassay to detect *Schistosoma* viability. *PLoS Negl. Trop. Dis.*, **4**, e759.

70 Holtfreter, M.C., Loebermann, M., Frei, E., Riebold, D., Wolff, D., Hartung, G., Kinzelbach, R., and Reisinger, E.C. (2010) Schistosomula, pre-adults and adults of *Schistosoma mansoni* ingest fluorescence-labelled albumin *in vitro* and *in vivo*: implication for a drug-targeting model. *Parasitology*, **137**, 1645–1652.

71 Mansour, N.R. and Bickle, Q.D. (2010) Comparison of microscopy and Alamar blue reduction in a larval based assay for schistosome drug screening. *PLoS Negl. Trop. Dis.*, **4**, e795.

72 Smout, M.J., Kotze, A.C., McCarthy, J.S., and Loukas, A. (2010) A novel high throughput assay for anthelmintic drug screening and resistance diagnosis by real-time monitoring of parasite motility. *PLoS Negl. Trop. Dis.*, **4**, e885.

73 Manneck, T., Braissant, O., Haggenmüller, Y., and Keiser, J. (2011) Isothermal microcalorimetry to study drugs against *Schistosoma mansoni*. *J. Clin. Microbiol.*, **49**, 1217–1225.

74 Kirchhofer, C., Vargas, M., Braissant, O., Dong, Y., Wang, X., Vennerstrom, J.L., and Keiser, J. (2011) Activity of OZ78 analogues against *Fasciola hepatica* and *Echinostoma caproni*. *Acta Trop.*, **118**, 56–62.

75 The *Schistosoma japonicum* Genome Sequencing and Functional Analysis Consortium (2009) The *Schistosoma japonicum* genome reveals features of host–parasite interplay. *Nature*, **460**, 345–351.

76 Berriman, M., Haas, B.J., LoVerde, P.T., Wilson, R.A., Dillon, G.P., Cerqueira, G.C., Mashiyama, S.T. et al. (2009) The genome of the blood fluke *Schistosoma mansoni*. *Nature*, **460**, 352–358.

77 Tsai, I., Otto, T.D., and Berriman, M. (2010) Improving draft assemblies by

78 Stefanić, S., Dvořák, J., Horn, M., Braschi, S., Sojka, D., Ruelas, D.S., Suzuki, B. *et al.* (2010) RNA interference in *Schistosoma mansoni* schistosomula: selectivity, sensitivity and operation for larger-scale screening. *PLoS Negl. Trop. Dis.*, **4**, e850.

79 Jílková, A., Rezácová, P., Lepsik, M., Horn, M., Váchová, J., Fanfrlík, J., Brynda, J. *et al.* (2011) Structural basis for inhibition of the cathepsin B drug target from the human blood fluke, *Schistosoma mansoni*. *J. Biol. Chem.*, **286**, 35770–35781.

80 Dissous, C. and Grevelding, C.G. (2010) Piggy-backing the concept of cancer drugs for schistosomiasis treatment: a tangible perspective? *Trends Parasitol.*, **27**, 59–66.

81 Fitzpatrick, J.M., Peak, E., Perally, S., Chalmers, I.W., Barrett, J., Yoshino, T.P., Ivens, A.C., and Hoffmann, K.F. (2009) Anti-schistosomal intervention targets identified by lifecycle transcriptomic analyses. *PLoS Negl. Trop. Dis.*, **3**, e543.

82 Hopkins, A.L. and Groom, C.R. (2002) The druggable genome. *Nat. Rev. Drug Discov.*, **1**, 727–730.

83 Saeger, B., Schmitt-Wrede, H.P., Dehnhardt, M., Benten, W.P., Krucken, J., Harder, A., Von Samson-Himmelstjerna, G. *et al.* (2001) Latrophilin-like receptor from the parasitic nematode *Haemonchus contortus* as target for the anthelmintic depsipeptide PF1022A. *FASEB J.*, **15**, 1332–1334.

84 Bos, D.H., Mayfield, C., and Minchella, D.J. (2009) Analysis of regulatory protease sequences identified through bioinformatic data mining of the *Schistosoma mansoni* genome. *BMC Genomics*, **10**, 488.

85 Andrade, L.F., Nahum, L.A., Avelar, L.G.A., Lopes, L., Zerlotini, A., Ruiz, J.C., and Oliveira, G.E. (2011) Eukaryotic protein kinases (ePKs) of the helminth parasite *Schistosoma mansoni*. *BMC Genomics*, **12**, 215.

86 Caffrey, C.R., Rohwer, A., Oellien, F., Marhofer, R.J., Braschi, S., Oliveira, G., McKerrow, J.H., and Selzer, P.M. (2009) A comparative chemogenomics strategy to predict potential drug targets in the metazoan pathogen, *Schistosoma mansoni*. *PLoS One*, **4**, e4413.

87 Crowther, G.J., Shanmugam, D., Carmona, S.J., Doyle, M.A., Hertz-Fowler, C., Berriman, M., Nwaka, S. *et al.* (2010) Identification of attractive drug targets in neglected-disease pathogens using an *in silico* approach. *PLoS Negl. Trop. Dis.*, **4**, e804.

88 Agüero, F., Al-Lazikani, B., Aslett, M., Berriman, M., Buckner, F.S., Campbell, R.K., Carmona, S. *et al.* (2008) Genomic-scale prioritization of drug targets: the TDR targets database. *Nat. Rev. Drug Discov.*, **7**, 900–907.

89 Aurrecoechea, C., Brestelli, J., Brunk, B.P., Fischer, S., Gajria, B., Gao, X., Gingle, A. *et al.* (2010) EuPathDB: a portal to eukaryotic pathogen databases. *Nucleic Acids Res.*, **38**, D415–D419.

90 Aguilar-Diaz, H., Bobes, R.J., Carrero, J.C., Camacho-Carranza, R., Cervantes, C., Cevallos, M.A., Davila, G. *et al.* (2006) The genome project of *Taenia solium*. *Parasitol. Int.*, **55** (Suppl.), S127–S130.

91 Robb, S.M., Ross, E., and Sanchez Alvarado, A. (2008) SmedGD: the *Schmidtea mediterranea* genome database. *Nucleic Acids Res.*, **36**, D599–D606.

92 Doyle, M.A., Gasser, R.B., Woodcroft, B.J., Hall, R.S., and Ralph, S.A. (2010) Drug target prediction and prioritization: using orthology to predict essentiality in parasite genomes. *BMC Genomics*, **11**, 222.

93 McCarter, J.P. (2004) Genomic filtering: an approach to discovering novel antiparasitics. *Trends Parasitol.*, **20**, 462–468.

94 Rollinson, D. (2009) A wake up call for urinary schistosomiasis: reconciling research effort with public health importance. *Parasitology*, **136**, 1593–1610.

95 Young, N.D., Jex, A.R., Li, B., Liu, S., Yang, L., Xiong, Z., and Li, Y. *et al.* (2012) Whole-genome sequence of *Schistosoma haematobium*. *Nat. Genet.*, **44**, 221–225.

96 Krautz-Peterson, G., Radwanska, M., Ndegwa, D., Shoemaker, C.B., and Skelly, P.J. (2007) Optimizing gene suppression in schistosomes using RNA interference. *Mol. Biochem. Parasitol.*, **153**, 194–202.

97 Sayed, A.A., Cook, S.K., and Williams, D.L. (2006) Redox balance mechanisms in *Schistosoma mansoni* rely on peroxiredoxins and albumin and implicate peroxiredoxins as novel drug targets. *J. Biol. Chem.*, **281**, 17001–17010.

98 Kuntz, A.N., Davioud-Charvet, E., Sayed, A.A., Califf, L.L., Dessolin, J., Arner, E.S., and Williams, D.L. (2007) Thioredoxin glutathione reductase from *Schistosoma mansoni*: an essential parasite enzyme and a key drug target. *PLoS Med.*, **4**, e206.

99 Dvořák, J., Beckmann, S., Lim, K.C., Engel, J.C., Grevelding, C.G., McKerrow, J.H., and Caffrey, C.R. (2010) Biolistic transformation of *Schistosoma mansoni*: studies with modified reporter-gene constructs containing regulatory regions of protease genes. *Mol. Biochem. Parasitol.*, **170**, 37–40.

100 Tchoubrieva, E.B., Ong, P.C., Pike, R.N., Brindley, P.J., and Kalinna, B.H. (2010) Vector-based RNA interference of cathepsin B1 in *Schistosoma mansoni*. *Cell Mol. Life Sci.*, **67**, 3739–3748.

101 Ayuk, M.A., Suttiprapa, S., Rinaldi, G., Mann, V.H., Lee, C.M., and Brindley, P.J. (2011) *Schistosoma mansoni* U6 gene promoter-driven short hairpin RNA induces RNA interference in human fibrosarcoma cells and schistosomules. *Int. J. Parasitol.*, **41**, 783–789.

102 Zhao, Z.R., Lei, L., Liu, M., Zhu, S.C., Ren, C.P., Wang, X.N., and Shen, J.J. (2008) *Schistosoma japonicum*: inhibition of Mago nashi gene expression by shRNA-mediated RNA interference. *Exp. Parasitol.*, **119**, 379–384.

103 Nicholson, J.K., Connelly, J., Lindon, J.C., and Holmes, E. (2002) Metabonomics: a platform for studying drug toxicity and gene function. *Nat. Rev. Drug Discov.*, **1**, 153–161.

104 Lindon, J.C., Holmes, E., Bollard, M.E., Stanley, E.G., and Nicholson, J.K. (2004) Metabonomics technologies and their applications in physiological monitoring, drug safety assessment and disease diagnosis. *Biomarkers*, **9**, 1–31.

105 Bictash, M., Ebbels, T.M., Chan, Q., Loo, R.L., Yap, I.K., Brown, I.J., de Iorio, M. et al. (2010) Opening up the "Black Box": metabolic phenotyping and metabolome-wide association studies in epidemiology. *J. Clin. Epidemiol.*, **63**, 970–979.

106 Wang, Y., Li, J.V., Saric, J., Keiser, J., Wu, J., Utzinger, J., and Holmes, E. (2010) Advances in metabolic profiling of experimental nematode and trematode infections. *Adv. Parasitol.*, **73**, 373–404.

107 Wang, Y.L., Holmes, E., Nicholson, J.K., Cloarec, O., Chollet, J., Tanner, M., Singer, B.H., and Utzinger, J. (2004) Metabonomic investigations in mice infected with *Schistosoma mansoni*: an approach for biomarker identification. *Proc. Natl. Acad. Sci. USA*, **101**, 12676–12681.

108 Wang, Y., Utzinger, J., Xiao, S.H., Xue, J., Nicholson, J.K., Tanner, M., Singer, B.H., and Holmes, E. (2006) System level metabolic effects of a *Schistosoma japonicum* infection in the Syrian hamster. *Mol. Biochem. Parasitol.*, **146**, 1–9.

109 Saric, J., Li, J.V., Wang, Y., Keiser, J., Bundy, J.G., Holmes, E., and Utzinger, J. (2008) Metabolic profiling of an *Echinostoma caproni* infection in the mouse for biomarker discovery. *PLoS Negl. Trop. Dis.*, **2**, e254.

110 Saric, J., Li, J.V., Swann, J.R., Utzinger, J., Calvert, G., Nicholson, J.K., Dirnhofer, S. et al. (2010) Integrated cytokine and metabolic analysis of pathological responses to parasite exposure in rodents. *J. Proteome Res.*, **9**, 2255–2264.

111 Li, J.V., Saric, J., Wang, Y., Keiser, J., Utzinger, J., and Holmes, E. (2011) Chemometric analysis of biofluids from mice experimentally infected with *Schistosoma mansoni*. *Parasit. Vectors*, **4**, 179.

112 Balog, C.I., Meissner, A., Goraler, S., Bladergroen, M.R., Vennervald, B.J., Mayboroda, O.A., and Deelder, A.M. (2011) Metabonomic investigation of human *Schistosoma mansoni* infection. *Mol. Biosyst.*, **7**, 1473–1480.

Part Four
Vaccines

21
Barefoot thru' the Valley of Darkness: Preclinical Development of a Human Hookworm Vaccine

Jeffrey M. Bethony[*], *Maria Victoria Periago, and Amar R. Jariwala*

Abstract

Hookworm is considered a neglected tropical disease, which is a group of parasitic and related infectious diseases that are common infections in low-income countries, where they produce a disease burden equivalent to HIV/AIDS or malaria. Despite their importance, progress on developing vaccines for neglected tropical diseases such as hookworm has lagged because of critical technical hurdles. These include the lack of relevant animal models for efficacy testing, an absence of correlates of protection in humans, and minimal experience in the development technologies to bring these vaccines to the clinic. Herein, we review the current status of a vaccine against an important NTD the human hookworm, *Necator americanus*, as a cautionary tale of hurdles for the preclinical development of vaccines for this important group of diseases.

Introduction

This chapter focuses on a little discussed but critical phase in the development of neglected tropical disease (NTD) vaccines: the preclinical development stage. In current Good Manufacturing Practice (cGMP), the term "preclinical development" refers to the studies that test a vaccine on animals or in other nonhuman test systems to gain data about the vaccine's efficacy and safety before tests on humans can begin (a good example of a preclinical study is a "toxicology study"). However, in the current chapter, the term preclinical development specifically refers to the diverse set of tasks prior to the clinical testing of a biologic in humans. This definition enables us to show that many of the obstacles encountered in the discovery of candidate antigens for NTD vaccines carry-over into the more prosaic world of NTD vaccine development. In fact, many of the problems that have hindered the discovery of vaccines antigens against this wide array of pathogens pose the same problems for NTD vaccine

[*] Corresponding Author

development. The best examples of this and the focus of the current chapter are the preclinical tests used to determine the "biological effect" of the vaccine formulation or its "potency." Although numerous reports describe the economic, social, and scientific barriers to developing NTDs, few discuss the routine "nut-and-bolts" problems encountered by groups attempting to develop NTD vaccine candidates into NTD vaccines. Herein, we discuss one of the critical tests for any vaccine and a near insurmountable challenge for NTD vaccines – the heretofore little-known potency testing program.

Potency Testing Program

Potency assays usually come close to the end of preclinical development when a process for the manufacturing of the vaccine has (possibly) been developed and the large-scale production of the vaccine contemplated under the guidance of cGMP. For a new biological (the "vaccine"), potency is one of a battery of biophysical, biochemical, and immunological tests required to determine whether the drug product (the finished dosage form of the biologic) can be "released" for phase I first-in-humans testing. For a biological already in use (e.g., a marketed vaccine), the potency test is one of a battery of tests used to evaluate the stability of the biologic over time or to compare the lot-to-lot manufacture of the vaccine, which is crucial due to the "batch-like" product of biologics produced in "living systems" systems such *Escherichia coli* or *Pichia pastoris*.

Potency Assay: Yesterday and Today

Yesterday
Most new vaccines are derived from a living organism (e.g., fermentation in *P. pastoris*) in a batch-wise procedure. Due to this manufacturing process, a key aspect of the quality of a biologic is the assurance of its "consistent" production – that each batch (or lot) of the vaccine manufactured is as pure, safe, and effective (potent) as the previous one. This "consistency principle" [1, 2] is implicit in the licensing and regulatory process for biological products, and forms the basis of contemporary quality systems for vaccine manufacturing, such as cGMP. Henriksen [1, 2] traces the origins of modern vaccine potency testing to Erlhich's "indirect protection test" for standardizing lots of antiserum against diphtheria or tetanus toxin, whereby serial dilutions of the antiserum were mixed with fixed amounts of toxin and then injected into an animal model [1, 3]. The parameter evaluated was the lowest serum dilution to still show toxin neutralization by survival of the immunized animal. Erlhich subsequently standardized the indirect test by comparing the toxin neutralization levels of a newly derived antiserum with the neutralization levels of an antiserum known to be protective in humans – the first use of a standard reference serum. An important modification to the indirect test came with Prigge (1937; quoted in [1, 3]),

who is credited with designing the immunization challenge protocol for potency testing:

... several groups of guinea pigs [are] injected with increasing amounts of antigen, ranging from a dose that is ineffective in all animals to a dose that is effective in all. Next the percentage of animals which is protected when injected with the toxin in determined.

The "immunization challenge model" remains the method of choice for potency testing, and is still used for pertussis, tetanus, diphtheria, rabies, leptospira, and clostridial vaccines. Prigge is also credited with being the first to use contemporary potency test parameters such as "linearity," "parallelism," and the vaccine dose that induces protection in 50% of immunized animals (the median effective dose or ED_{50}) [1, 3].

Today
Although the US Code of Federal Regulations (CFRs) mandates potency testing of each newly manufactured lot of vaccine, it defines "potency" in the broadest sense:

... the specific ability or capacity of the product, as indicated by appropriate laboratory tests or by adequately controlled clinical data obtained through the administration of the product in the manner intended, to effect a given result. (21 CFR §600.3 [s])

The International Conference on Harmonization (ICH) also provides a broad but more precise definition for potency testing, even though it is not intended strictly for vaccines (biologics):

... [a] measure of the biological activity using a suitably quantitative biological assay [also called a potency assay or bioassay], based on the attribute of the product which is linked to the relevant biological properties. (ICH Q6B)

Hence, potency testing measures attributes essential for the clinical efficacy of a vaccine; in other words, the qualities needed to "effect a given result," which in most cases is protection against lethal challenge. As discussed above, in traditional potency testing a parameter often estimated was the protective dose 50 (PD_{50}) or the dose of manufactured vaccine that results in protection of 50% of the test animals against the targeted pathogenic entity. However, the immunization challenge model requires the following [3]:

i) A dose of the pathogen that is uniformly lethal.
ii) An animal model that replicates human infections (including lethality) with the target pathogen.
iii) A correlate of protection (CoP) using the vaccine in humans.

The immunization challenge model is not feasible for a hookworm and many other NTD vaccines for the same reasons:

i) The target pathogen does not result in a lethal infection.
ii) There is no animal model that replicates the pathology seen in the human infection.
iii) There is no known CoP in humans as this vaccine has never undergone clinical testing and natural infection does not result in protection against subsequent challenge.

The traditional "potency assay" measures the ability of the vaccine in an animal assay (formally known as a "bioassay") to predict the behavior of the vaccine in the target population (humans resident in endemic areas). It is used to determine the level of an immune response that is "associated with" or "directly correlates" with the protection offered by the vaccine – a level that must be achieved in order to demonstrate that each manufacture of the vaccine produces an effective formulation of the vaccine. However, NTD pathogens have a number of important characteristics that make the development of a traditional potency assay extremely difficult, including but not limited to:

i) A lack of reliable animal models to test an efficacious response that may parallel the human immune response.
ii) Few (if any) known immune CoPs in humans infected with the pathogen.

As with many things involved in the development of NTD vaccines, we will need to redefine the term "potency" and its use in vaccine development.

Box 1 The Preclinical Challenges for NTD Vaccines

The preclinical of NTD vaccines may prove to be an even greater hurdle than antigen discovery.

A Cautionary Tale for NTD Vaccines: Hookworm Disease

Helminths are common infections of humans in developing regions of the world. An estimated 1 billion people are infected with one or more helminths and the epidemiology of hookworm infection as it relates to a rationale for a hookworm vaccine can be found in a number of reports [4–6]. The most common helminth infections are caused by intestinal worms, including ascariasis (*Ascaris lumbricoides*), trichuriasis (*Trichus trichuria*), and the hookworms (*Necator americanus* and *Anclyostoma doudenale*). Current control efforts utilize anthelmintic drugs of the benzimidazole class, usually albendazole or mebendazole [4–6]. Although anthelmintics are effective at eliminating an existing helminth infection, they fail to confer lasting protection, resulting in rapid reinfection of individuals in areas of active transmission. For this reason, the extensive use of the benzimidazole drugs has failed to limit parasite transmission as individuals become reinfected to their previous levels of infection within 12 months [4–6]. The application of mass drug administration has also raised concerns about drug failure (mebendazole) and drug resistance as has been witnessed in the veterinary field.

Natural History of Hookworm Infection

The life cycle of N. americanus and A. duodenale as they relate to vaccine development has been reviewed extensively elsewhere [4–6] and we briefly synthesize these reports here. Individuals become infected with hookworms when third-stage infective larvae (L3) penetrate through the skin, migrate into subcutaneous venules and lymphatics and then enter the pulmonary capillary bed. From there, the L3 enter the respiratory tree through the alveolae and ascend the bronchioles, before passing into the intestinal tract. In the lumen, the L3 can live for 5 years or more. The adult worms, approximately 1 cm in length, attach to the mucosa and submucosa, and feed on host blood and mucosal tissues. The hookworms mate and produce thousands of eggs that exit the body in the feces. The eggs hatch in soil with adequate moisture and high temperatures.

Intestinal blood loss is the major clinical manifestation of human hookworm infection [4–6]. Heavily and even moderately infected patients with underlying nutritional deficiencies can develop hookworm disease – the iron deficiency and microcytic, hypochromic anemia (iron deficiency anemia (IDA)) caused by hookworms feeding on blood [4–6]. In resource-poor regions in which school-aged children and adults possess lower iron stores than those in developed countries, there is a well-established relationship between the intensity of hookworm infection, intestinal blood loss, and host anemia [4–6].

Human Immune Response
As with other human helminths, a robust immune response is induced by hookworm infection, but it fails to protect against established or incoming infections. This relationship has been extensively reviewed elsewhere [7] and has important consequences for the development of a helminth vaccine as well for the development of the potency assay referred to above. The major hurdle is that we have never seen what protection against these helminths may look like in a human – a crucial impediment to the making of a prophylactic vaccine.

Box 2 The Major Hurdle

The major hurdle is that we have never seen what protection against many NTDs may look like in a human – a crucial impediment to the making of a prophylactic vaccine (for a classic review of these challenges, see [8]).

An important reason for the "lack of knowledge" is the epidemiology of hookworm infections, which are chronic (often lifelong) and highly prevalent in endemic areas. Accordingly, it is difficult to find individuals who have not been infected for months, years, or even decades. As such, it is difficult to monitor individuals resident in endemic areas for incident or "new" infection and then monitor them longitudinally to determine how the human immune response evolves over time to the infection. The limitations of cross-sectional studies are obvious:

- Only a snapshot of a failed immunological situation can be taken, in which the parasite has successfully colonized its human host for months, years, or decades.
- A difficulty in classifying humans into the different phases of the infection: exposure, prepatency, patency, and postpatency.
- Moreover, it is ethically not possible to follow hookworm patients over a long period of time without drug intervention.
- The most common study design for hookworm immune responses comes from the rather unnatural situation of the treatment and reinfection study in high-transmission areas (i.e., patients are treated for their established infections and the immune response monitored as they become reinfected).

In short, as with most NTDs, our knowledge of the human immune responses against hookworms comes from chronically infected individuals (i.e., individuals who have failed to mount a protective immune response against the pathogen). This leaves us with no immune response to predict protection induced by a vaccine in humans – what vaccinologists refer to as a correlate of protection or a "CoP," which has very specific consequences for preclinical development [9, 10]. The lack of a CoP profoundly affects the ability to determine the potency of a human hookworm vaccine a problem that we predict will occur with many of the NTD vaccines.

However, from the little that we know about the host immune response to hookworm infection, the response is robust and comprehensive. Naturally infected humans mount antibody responses involving all isotypes and IgG subclasses, with IgE exhibiting the greatest increases. These responses are mounted to all of the stages of the pathogen as it migrates through the host (L3, L4, and L5) [11, 12]. As seen with other helminth infections, hookworm is associated with a systemic down-modulation of immune responsive, with measurable attenuation of responses to bystander antigens. This "spill-over" suppression can extend to responses to unrelated antigens, including vaccines. It is well accepted that helper T cell T_h2 responses are elicited during helminth infections, including by schistosomes and filarids [8, 13–16]. As part of this T_h2 response, individuals develop elevated levels of total and parasite-specific IgE, as well as increased levels of interleukin (IL)-4, IL-5, and IL-13, with concomitant increases in eosinophils and mast cells. There has been a long-standing hypothesis that parasite-specific IgE can have a partially protective effect against helminth infection, especially by *Schistosoma* spp. [17, 18]. Elevated levels of IgE to recombinant *Ac*-ASP-2, the *Ancylostoma caninum* homolog of *Na*-ASP-2 (ASP = *Ancylostoma* Secreted Protein), were associated with a decreased risk of heavy hookworm infection [19].

The T_h2 response during helminth infection is induced against a background of potent, parasite-induced immunoregulation, referred to as a "modified" T_h2 response [8, 13–16]. This modified T_h2 response can consist of alternatively activated macrophages, Foxp3$^+$ CD4 regulatory T cells (T_{reg}), and CD4$^+$ T_{reg}1 IL-10-producing T cells [8, 13–16]. This response generates an immune environment that is so extensively downregulated that it should protect the host, not only from the strong inflammatory effects of helminth infections, but also from the effects of other IgE-mediated disorders such as atopy, asthma, and anaphylaxis [16]. Reduced allergic responses have been shown in mice infected with various helminth infections (see [20] for a review). Moreover, epidemiological evidence suggests that hookworm infection is associated with reduced skin reactivity to common allergens and a lowered risk of extrinsic asthma [21].

Preclinical Testing of an NTD Vaccine
The only possible laboratory animal models to study hookworm infection are canines and hamsters. Canines can be experimentally infected with *A. caninum*, which closely resembles human *Necator* hookworm infection [22]. The hamster *Mesocricetus auratus* can be infected with *Ancylostoma ceylanicum* and *N. americanus*. Although these animal models are extremely valuable for antigen discovery, they are of limited use in a bioassay for potency of a recombinant hookworm vaccine for the following reasons:

i) Neither animal model has been shown to be entirely permissive for hookworm.
ii) Although initially permissive to infection with third stage infective larvae (L3), both models become "refractory" to the infection over time [23–25]. For example, canines develop natural resistance to hookworm infection after 20 weeks of infection [24, 25]. This makes the immunization-and-challenge model difficult to mount and a long-term pathological end-point such as anemia difficult to induce by hookworm infection in such a short time span of infection.
iii) Neither canines nor hamsters easily reproduce the clinical end-points of human hookworm disease; specifically, the reduction in IDA. The relationship between worm burden and blood loss is not straightforward in either model, probably due to the method of infection (a single bolus challenge of infective larvae), which has to be given over a short timeframe to permissively infect a large group of animals.
iv) Finally, the hamster model has the further limitation that less than 20% of the infective larvae become adults in the gastrointestinal tract.

No CoP (as defined by Qin *et al.* [26] or Plotkin [9, 10]) has been found for human hookworm infection. The fact that the immune system reacts vigorously to hookworm infection but fails to harm the parasite not only hampers identification of target vaccine molecules for antigen discovery (about which much has been written [4–6, 8, 27]), but also provides challenges for vaccine product and clinical development.

Potency Testing for NTD Vaccines

The development of potency assays is divided into three areas:
i) Design of the potency assay.
ii) Development of the components of the potency assay, including a unique set of reagents.
iii) Determination of the performance of the potency assay.

Potency testing relies heavily on statistical analyses, especially those used to determine the reproducibility of the assay, and standard and dose–response curves, including the problems of linearity (for lines that are essentially nonlinear) and parallelism (for lines that are essentially not parallel). Finally, the potency test holds a unique position in vaccine development. It stands at the nexus of product and clinical development; as such, it is one of the few areas of vaccine development that requires an interdisciplinary knowledge of the vaccine and the pathogen as well as knowledge of process development, cGMP manufacture, and even clinical trials.

As mentioned above, the essential attribute determined by potency testing is the induction of a protective immune response in an animal model (bioassay) against the target pathogen [1–3].

> **Box 3 Summary of Technical Challenges for Potency Testing of NTD Vaccines**
>
> - Difficulty in maintaining developmental stages of NTD pathogens *in vitro*.
> - Paucity of laboratory animal models permissive to the NTD pathogens or that can accurately reproduce human disease or protective immunity.
> - Paucity of *in vitro* functional tests to test different lots of the manufactured vaccine.
> - Few if any correlates of protection in naturally-infected humans.
> - No examples of vaccine-induced immunity in humans.

Thru' the Valley of Darkness

We developed a potency test that would be appropriate for preclinical development of a candidate NTD vaccine formulation [28]. Most NTD vaccines will probably require neutralizing antibodies to be protective and these antibodies will have to have the correct conformation in order to elicit this protective response. However, the correlation of these responses with clinical protection will often not be established and, therefore, could not be used to claim that the potency test was measuring an "attribute essential for effect" as required by most regulatory bodies (e.g., US Food and Drug Administration (FDA), European Medicines Agency, etc.). Hence, following a paradigm outlined by Giersing *et al.* for recombinant malaria vaccines [29], we decided that the potency assay for many NTD vaccines would not measure a correlate of vaccine efficacy, but instead would measure antibody response in mice immunized with a predetermined dose of the NTD vaccine as an indicator of manufacturing consistency (for release) and drug product stability over time. The NTD potency assay is, therefore, one among many analytical procedures and cGMP quality assurance measures, and is not designed to predict or reflect clinical efficacy *per se*. Essentially, this potency assay would measure an animal immune response as an indicator of vaccine manufacturing consistency. Although the antibodies measured in the animal assay would not be those directly involved in protection, the rationale here is that if the molecule is presented to the immune system in a consistent form and quantity, the immune system will respond reproducibly. In this sense, vaccine potency for many NTD vaccines could not be used to conclude that the vaccine is "biologically effective". Rather, it refers to only one of the parameters (i.e., immunogenicity) that is employed to demonstrate that the manufacturing process yields a material of consistent quality and quantity.

> **Box 4 Thru' the Valley of Darkness**
>
> Following a paradigm outlined by Giersing *et al.* for recombinant malaria vaccines [29], the potency assay for many NTD vaccines would not measure a correlate of vaccine efficacy, but instead would measure an IgG response in mice immunized with a predetermined dose as an indicator of manufacturing consistency and product stability over time. The NTD potency assay is, therefore, one assay among many analytical procedures and cGMP quality assurance measures and is not designed to predict or reflect clinical efficacy *per se*. Hence, it would measure an animal immune response as an indicator of vaccine manufacturing consistency [28].

The NTD potency assay should be able to measure the capacity of the vaccine to trigger an immune response that is determined to be of sufficient strength so as to be different from baseline and in a range that is likely to be clinically meaningful. This would provide confirmation that a sufficient amount of one or more selected antigens is present. In addition, the recombinant NTD antigens that are not considered to be sufficiently immunogenic for use alone must be formulated to enhance their immunogenicity. Hence, the NTD potency assay would test the antigen in a formulated "drug product" (i.e., the molecule would be assessed in the presence of other components to demonstrate that the antigen is still potent by nonbiological means). For this reason, *in vivo* biological assays that measure the antigen's immunogenicity are often the only method to assess the conformation and behavior of the vaccine formulation.

Potency Assays for NTDs: Setting Specifications with Few Assumptions

We based our NTD potency assay on the median effective dose (ED_{50}) method because it is a standardized method to measure potency, and has been applied for vaccines to polio, malaria, hepatitis B, hepatitis A, and human papilloma virus (Gardasil®) [29]. Potency is reported as an ED_{50} of antigen in micrograms (Figure 21.1). As a vaccine loses potency, a larger dose will be required to seroconvert 50% of the animals. The specifications for potency are designed to detect a loss or gain in vaccine potency over time. There are many ways to set specification limits for potency. One of the methods used to measure potency is to set the specification around the "relative potency" of the vaccine, which is obtained by dividing the ED_{50} of the test vaccine lot by that of the reference lot [29]. However, relative potency mandates the use of a reference vaccine. In the initial

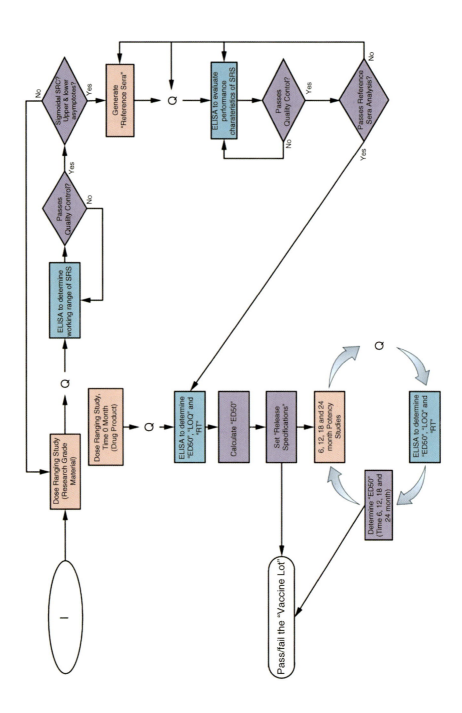

phase of clinical development, it is often difficult to obtain a clinically proven lot of "known vaccine potency " (i.e., if a vaccine has never been tested in humans, it is difficult to assume the level of antibody that the vaccine must generate to induce protection). In lieu of relative potency, there are other ways to set specifications. Many guidelines explain the methods of setting limits. Some use standard deviation while others use dynamic tolerance intervals with confidence limits. Also, there are no strict rules on choosing the right time to set limits on potency assays. Once doses for potency assays are finalized, specification could be potentially defined as a one-sided potency limit (i.e., the maximum dose required to seroconvert half of the immunized animals in the test group). In other words,

Figure 21.1 Development of a potency testing program for a hypothetical NTD vaccine. Each color represents one event. The pink boxes represent bioassays (or animal studies), the blue boxes represent immunoassay studies (enzyme-linked immunosorbent assays (ELISAs)), and the violet boxes represent statistical analyses. The term "I" refers to initiation of the potency testing program and "Q" represents the qualification of immunoassays. As discussed, the potency assay is based on a quantal response or the minimal concentration of the NTD vaccine formulation that induces an antigen-specific antibody response in 50% of the animals in a dose group (the median effective dose (ED_{50})). A critical step in the quantal assays method is the determination of a threshold of IgG against NTD vaccine formulation above which one could assign an individual murine serum as being "positive" (seroconversion). Hence, a critical first step in the development of a potency testing program is the establishment of a detection limit or a "reactivity threshold." There are a number of different "detection limits" that can be used and include the limit of quantification (LOQ) as shown here. In order to determine the LOQ, one first has to generate an "in-house" reagent referred to as a standard reference serum (SRS) that would be assayed on each ELISA plate, with its statistical representation (four-parameter logistic log modeling) termed a standard calibration curve (SCC). The SRS and the SCC have two functions. The first is to establish the LOQ and the second is that the optical densities of test sera at a chosen dilution (e.g., 1/100) are interpolated onto this curve to derived the arbitrary units of antibody against the NTD vaccine formulation. This calibration method utilizes "homologous interpolation," such that the SRS that is used to derive the SCC is developed using the exact same reagents as the test sera (e.g., same plates, same animal model, same antigen lot, same secondary antibody). The term "qualification" refers to the protocol used and the performance characteristics: precision (reproducibility), linearity, and ruggedness. By analyzing performance characteristics, we will set forth criteria with which to accept or reject an ELISA performed under these conditions. The term "release" refers to specifications that must be met to use a vaccine in clinical development. This usually consists of "release criteria," which are a combination of physical, chemical, biological, and immunological tests that determine whether a final drug product is suitable for use in clinical testing. These are predefined, and include chemical, physical, biological, and environmental characteristics for testing a product or system, and can include, but are not limited to, starting materials, packaging materials, intermediate, bulk, drug substance, or drug product. The term "stability" is used for the ability of a drug product or drug substance to stay within chemical, physical, microbiological, and biopharmaceutical specified limits during its whole shelf-life. A stability program, of which potency is a part, refers to the planned and documented program assessing the stability profile of materials and products to establish their retest periods or shelf-life and storage directions. (Adapted from reference [28]) the ED_{50} must be less than or equal to a defined maximum dose used in the study; in our case, it would be 50 μg. Others use a one-sided upper fiducial limit of ED_{50} as an internal one-sided specification limit. In the initial stages of clinical development this is perhaps the best and easiest way to set empirical acceptability criteria. For our example, on day 28, the upper one-sided 95% fiducial limit would be 12.07 μg (i.e., if the ED_{50} exceeds 12.07 μg in subsequent testing then that lot fails the potency test and will warrant further investigation). As the vaccine undergoes clinical development, more stringent specifications would be applied as potency values for lots with known clinical efficacies become available.

Conclusions

Over the next decade, a new generation of vaccines to combat parasitic infections will be forthcoming. For many of these vaccines, the CoPs are poorly defined or difficult to evaluate in animal models for the same reasons that they are difficult for hookworm, principally because few NTD induce sterilizing immunity. The crucial goal of most NTD vaccines is to reduce morbidity and decrease the chronic debilitation caused by these infections – outcomes that are hard to measure in traditional potency testing models. Moreover, traditional potency testing, which focuses on measuring the reproducibility of a CoP in laboratory animals, usually with an immunization-and-challenge model, cannot be used for most NTD vaccines for reasons stated above. Nevertheless, potency testing will remain an essential component of the product development of anti-NTD vaccines, not only because the FDA and other regulatory agencies mandate potency testing for the purposes of product release and monitoring of vaccines, but also because potency testing represents one of the few product release assays that truly assesses the essential biological activity of the drug product (i.e., the ability of a vaccine to perform its principal function of eliciting an immune response).

A new paradigm for potency testing is needed such as the one outlined here. We believe that the process and methods stated here will prove useful for those involved in vaccine efforts for other NTDs, many of which are based on the same paradigm (i.e., using a recombinant protein to produce nonsterilizing protection by inducing high levels of antibody to prevent chronic debilitation).

References

1 Hendriksen, C., Arciniega, J.L., Bruckner, L., Chevalier, M., Coppens, E., Descamps, J., Duchene, M. et al. (2008) The consistency approach for the quality control of vaccines. *Biologicals*, **36**, 73–77.

2 Hendriksen, C.F. (2002) Refinement, reduction, and replacement of animal use for regulatory testing: current best scientific practices for the evaluation of safety and potency of biologicals. *ILAR J.*, **43** (Suppl.), S43–S48.

3 Hendriksen, C.F. (2009) Replacement, reduction and refinement alternatives to animal use in vaccine potency measurement. *Expert Rev. Vaccines*, **8**, 313–322.

4 Bethony, J.M., Cole, R.N., Guo, X., Kamhawi, S., Lightowlers, M.W., Loukas, A., Petri, W. et al. (2011)

Vaccines to combat the neglected tropical diseases. *Immunol. Rev.*, **239**, 237–270.

5 Hotez, P.J., Bethony, J.M., Diemert, D.J., Pearson, M., and Loukas, A. (2010) Developing vaccines to combat hookworm infection and intestinal schistosomiasis. *Nat. Rev. Microbiol.*, **8**, 814–826.

6 Hotez, P.J., Bethony, J.M., Oliveira, S.C., Brindley, P.J., and Loukas, A. (2008) Multivalent anthelminthic vaccine to prevent hookworm and schistosomiasis. *Expert Rev. Vaccines*, **7**, 745–752.

7 Loukas, A., Constant, S.L., and Bethony, J.M. (2005) Immunobiology of hookworm infection. *FEMS Immunol. Med. Microbiol.*, **43**, 115–124.

8 Maizels, R.M., Holland, M.J., Falcone, F.H., Zang, X.X., and Yazdanbakhsh, M. (1999) Vaccination against helminth parasites – the ultimate challenge for vaccinologists? *Immunol. Rev.*, **171**, 125–147.

9 Plotkin, S.A. (2001) Immunologic correlates of protection induced by vaccination. *Pediatr. Infect. Dis. J.*, **20**, 63–75.

10 Plotkin, S.A. (2010) Correlates of protection induced by vaccination. *Clin. Vaccine Immunol.*, **17**, 1055–1065.

11 Geiger, S.M., Caldas, I.R., Mc Glone, B.E., Campi-Azevedo, A.C., De Oliveira, L.M., Brooker, S., Diemert, D. *et al.* (2007) Stage-specific immune responses in human *Necator americanus* infection. *Parasite Immunol.*, **29**, 347–358.

12 Geiger, S.M., Fujiwara, R.T., Santiago, H., Correa-Oliveira, R., and Bethony, J.M. (2008) Early stage-specific immune responses in primary experimental human hookworm infection. *Microbes Infect.*, **10**, 1524–1535.

13 Maizels, R.M., Pearce, E.J., Artis, D., Yazdanbakhsh, M., and Wynn, T.A. (2009) Regulation of pathogenesis and immunity in helminth infections. *J. Exp. Med.*, **206**, 2059–2066.

14 Maizels, R.M. and Yazdanbakhsh, M. (2008) T-cell regulation in helminth parasite infections: implications for inflammatory diseases. *Chem. Immunol. Allergy*, **94**, 112–123.

15 Maizels, R.M. and Yazdanbakhsh, M. (2003) Immune regulation by helminth parasites: cellular and molecular mechanisms. *Nat. Rev. Immunol.*, **3**, 733–744.

16 Yazdanbakhsh, M., van den Biggelaar, A., and Maizels, R.M. (2001) T_h2 responses without atopy: immunoregulation in chronic helminth infections and reduced allergic disease. *Trends Immunol.*, **22**, 372–377.

17 Hagan, P. (1993) IgE and protective immunity to helminth infections. *Parasite Immunol.*, **15**, 1–4.

18 Hagan, P., Blumenthal, U.J., Dunn, D., Simpson, A.J., and Wilkins, H.A. (1991) Human IgE, IgG4 and resistance to reinfection with *Schistosoma haematobium*. *Nature*, **349**, 243–245.

19 Bethony, J., Loukas, A., Smout, M., Brooker, S., Mendez, S., Plieskatt, J., Goud, G. *et al.* (2005) Antibodies against a secreted protein from hookworm larvae reduce the intensity of hookworm infection in humans and vaccinated laboratory animals. *FASEB J.*, **19**, 1743–1745.

20 Erb, K.J. (2007) Helminths allergic disorders and IgE-mediated immune responses: where do we stand? *Eur. J. Immunol.*, **37**, 1170–1173.

21 Leonardi-Bee, J., Pritchard, D., and Britton, J. (2006) Asthma and current intestinal parasite infection: systematic review and meta-analysis. *Am. J. Respir. Crit. Care Med.*, **174**, 514–523.

22 Fujiwara, R.T., Geiger, S.M., Bethony, J., and Mendez, S. (2006) Comparative immunology of human and animal models of hookworm infection. *Parasite Immunol.*, **28**, 285–293.

23 Diemert, D.J., Bethony, J.M., and Hotez, P.J. (2008) Hookworm vaccines. *Clin. Infect. Dis.*, **46**, 282–288.

24 Miller, T.A. (1971) Vaccination against the canine hookworm diseases. *Adv. Parasitol.*, **9**, 153–183.

25 Miller, T.A. (1978) Industrial development and field use of the canine hookworm vaccine. *Adv. Parasitol.*, **16**, 333–342.

26 Qin, L., Gilbert, P.B., Corey, L., McElrath, M.J., and Self, S.G. (2007) A

framework for assessing immunological correlates of protection in vaccine trials. *J. Infect. Dis.*, **196**, 1304–1312.

27 Loukas, A., Bethony, J., Brooker, S., and Hotez, P. (2006) Hookworm vaccines: past, present, and future. *Lancet Infect. Dis.*, **6**, 733–741.

28 Jariwala, A.R., Oliveira, L.M., Diemert, D.J., Keegan, B., Plieskatt, J.L., Periago, M.V., Bottazzi, M.E. et al. (2010) Potency testing for the experimental *Na*-GST-1 hookworm vaccine. *Expert Rev. Vaccines*, **9**, 1219–1230.

29 Giersing, B.K., Dubovsky, F., Saul, A., Denamur, F., Minor, P., and Meade, B. (2006) Potency assay design for adjuvanted recombinant proteins as malaria vaccines. *Vaccine*, **24**, 4264–4270.

22
Vaccines Linked to Chemotherapy: A New Approach to Control Helminth Infections

Sara Lustigman[*], *James H. McKerrow, and Maria Elena Bottazzi*

Abstract

Currently, chemotherapy is the dominant application among the tools available for the control or elimination of human helminth infections. Single-drug agents are available for mass drug administration (MDA), but recent evidence suggests that some drugs previously thought to be effective now appear less so. Recent progress in vaccine development for human parasitic infections holds promise for the control of several diseases. While the goal of chemotherapy is to temporarily cure or reduce infection intensities, morbidity, and transmission, vaccines would also reduce worm burdens and, ideally, induce long-lasting protective host immune responses. In so doing, these vaccines might obviate the need for repeated MDA, and reduce the risk of both drug failure and reinfection. Some vaccines might also influence transmission through targeting the intermediate or reservoir host when the infection is zoonotic. Since biological targets are, in many cases, different from those of anthelmintic drugs, vaccination would also be synergistic with drug therapy. This would justify the use of effective vaccines as a long-term solution presently lacking in most of the control strategies. The repositioning of vaccines, to complement chemotherapy, would be a novel revitalizing concept to control activities that have remained focused on morbidity and/or transmission reduction. Antihelminth vaccines would thus aid in achieving the UN Millennium Development Goals regarding poverty reduction, education, and child and maternal health. The benefits of a new vaccine strategy would require long-term support and advocacy to maintain preclinical and clinical development.

Introduction

Drug-dependent control measures have made considerable progress in reducing the prevalence and intensity of tropical diseases in many low- and middle-income countries. However, without the long-term protection a vaccine could offer, this approach runs the risk of having to be continued indefinitely. For most of the prevalent human helminth infections (i.e., soil transmitted helminthiases (STHs),

[*] Corresponding Author

schistosomiasis, and onchocerciasis) there is only a single anthelmintic drug available. To provide impact, these drugs must be deployed via mass drug administration (MDA) and target millions of people living in low- and middle-income countries. In most cases, the approach is designed to decrease morbidity rather than eliminate disease *per se*. However, high rates of post-treatment reinfection, the declining efficacy with repeated treatment, rebound morbidity, and the potential for the emergence of anthelmintic drug resistance undermine the sustainability of MDA as the only form of control [4–6]. The one exception is for lymphatic filariasis, for which several rounds of MDA using albendazole in combination with diethylcarbamazine or ivermectin, have been effective in eliminating the development of disease and transmission [7–10].

An alternative or complementary approach – vaccinating following anthelmintic therapy – has long been advocated for schistosomiasis, spearheaded by Robert Bergquist *et al.* [11, 12]. As was stated in the reports, an entirely vaccine-based approach to schistosomiasis control is unrealistic, but acceptable protection could be achieved by chemotherapy followed by vaccination aimed at reducing, or markedly delaying, the development of pathology. In their opinion, the issue is not vaccines versus chemotherapy, but how to graft a vaccine approach onto current schistosomiasis control programs. As many other helminths have been targeted for control or elimination, to meet this challenge, the repositioning of vaccines through the combined use of chemotherapy and vaccination is highly recommended as the basis for a novel, more versatile approach to control [13].

The goal of vaccine development against human helminth infections includes the identification of a vaccine capable of inducing effective and long-lasting immunity to significantly reduce worm burden. Vaccination as an adjunct to chemotherapy would also reduce the likelihood that vaccinated individuals would develop severe infections, thus reducing the burden of disease throughout the world. Several vaccine candidates are currently under development. Even though the induction of a consistent, high-level protection in humans has not been recorded yet, the 40–50% commonly reported protection levels of these candidates in experimental animals in our opinion still justify the application of a combined chemotherapy/vaccine approach. Vaccines are still the most economical, efficient, and effective tools for controlling infectious diseases. They remain the only way to guarantee control and elimination of helminth infections as envisioned by the World Health Organization (WHO) [14]. There is also evidence that vaccination-induced immune responses are increased following anthelmintic chemotherapy, possibly due to the reversal of immune suppression induced by the adult worms [3, 6, 9, 10, 15, 16], or because of the release and immunological presentation of helminth antigens following the treatment [17].

The research foundations supporting the feasibility of developing antihelminth vaccines for clinical use have been already established. These are listed in Box 1. Moreover, the tools for the development and testing of vaccines linked to chemotherapy are already available and could be put to the test in clinical trials in a reasonable time frame. Thus, an integrated approach, which includes the follow-up of initial drug treatment with vaccination to achieve long-term protection, has much to offer [12]. Antihelminth vaccines are considered a key technology for poverty reduction. When linked to chemotherapy, these vaccines are now considered a critical path toward achieving the UN Millennium Development Goals (MDGs) [14]. To realize these, it is crucial that support and funding be secured for process development and clinical trials of the repository of specific vaccines that may prove most effective against these infectious agents.

> **Box 1 Conceptual Underpinnings to Support the Feasibility of Developing Antihelminth Vaccines for Clinical Use**
>
> - Humans living in endemic areas develop against several of these diseases a degree of natural protection with some becoming immune or resistant to disease [1, 2].
> - Irradiated vaccines containing infective stages of the parasites confer up to 80% protection in experimental animal models [3].
> - Promising vaccine candidates that produce partial but significant protection in animal models already exist (see the other chapters relevant to vaccine development in this volume).
> - Recombinant protein vaccines have been shown to elicit antienzyme neutralizing antibodies, which reduce parasite metabolism and pathogenicity [19–22].
> - Effective recombinant veterinary vaccines against taeniid cestodes have been developed [24, 25], and support the development and testing of vaccine antigens for other human helminth infections.

Current Progress in Helminth Vaccine Development

Onchocerca volvulus

Approximately 120 million people are at risk for onchocerciasis; 37 million people are infected in 36 tropical countries of Africa and Latin America. Of these, 270 000 individuals have been blinded and an additional 500 000 are visually impaired, making onchocerciasis the second leading cause of infectious blindness world-wide. Onchocerciasis causes 46 000 new cases of blindness annually [18] (htp://www.apoc.bf/en). Although major onchocerciasis control programs (Onchocerciasis Control Programme, the African Programme for Onchocerciasis Control, and the Onchocerciasis Elimination Program in the Americas) have been successful in controlling infections and onchocerciasis as a public health problem in some endemic areas, there is a consensus among the global public health community that onchocerciasis in Africa will not be eliminated by MDA with ivermectin. This is due primarily to logistic considerations, and the ominous discovery of possible ivermectin resistance after many years of treatments in some communities in Ghana and Cameroon [23].

Therefore, if ivermectin resistance is confirmed and spreads, the potential for success by MDA with ivermectin as a stand-alone strategy decreases substantially. To support the onchocerciasis control measures, a new control tool, such as a vaccine, is warranted.

Feasibility and preclinical studies for developing an *Onchocerca* vaccine are ongoing. They are based on a number of elements, including:

i) Clear demonstration of protective immunity against *O. volvulus* larvae in humans, cattle, and mice.

ii) Identification and characterization of a defined set of *O. volvulus* recombinant vaccine molecules and their homologs that induce protection in more than one model of filarial nematode infection.

iii) Development of an innovative strategy of *O. volvulus* vaccine antigen selection based on screening for efficacy in two complementary small animal models. Based on this rational scoring system, the top-ranking eight *O. volvulus* protective antigens (*Ov*-CPI-2, *Ov*-ALT-1, *Ov*-RAL-2, *Ov*-ASP-1, *Ov*-103, *Ov*-RBP-1, *Ov*-CHI-1, and *Ov*-B20; CPI = cysteine proteinase inhibitor; ALT = abundant larval transcript; ASP = activation-associated secreted protein; RBP = retinol-binding protein; CHI = chitinase) have been selected for a preclinical evaluation and further prioritization (S. Lustigman, unpublished).

iv) Reports in the last decade of additional antigens with protective properties (e.g., *Ov*-FBA-1 [26], *Ov*-GAPDH [27], *Ov*-AST-1 [28], and paramyosin [29]; FBA = aldolase; GAPDH = glyceraldehyde-3-phosphate dehydrogenase; AST = astacin-like metalloproteinase) have been reported;

v) Recent reports using the cow model and *Onchocerca ochengi* demonstrate the possibility of developing vaccines against *O. volvulus* [30].

A vaccine aimed at preventing infection with L3 would be an essential addition to the effort to control onchocerciasis, as it will support additional reduction in microfilariae burdens and thus reduce transmission potential. Vaccine development against infection with *O. volvulus* has been the subject of much thought and work in the past through the funding of the Edna McConnell Clark Foundation (1985–1999) [31]. The need for *O. volvulus* vaccine development has also been endorsed by the "Conference on the Eradicability of Onchocerciasis" [32] and a conference on the global program to eliminate lymphatic filariasis [33]. In essence, an anti-L3 vaccine does not depend on MDA with ivermectin, but it will be administered in communities that have most likely already gone through rounds of MDA with ivermectin. Therefore, such a vaccine would complement this control measure and support the same goal – elimination of onchocerciasis as a public health problem in sub-Sahara Africa.

Lymphatic Filariasis

There are approximately 120 million cases of lymphatic filariasis in more than 90 countries throughout the world. The Global Alliance for the Elimination of Lymphatic Filariasis aims to eliminate the disease within the next 20 years. Like control strategies for onchocerciasis, this plan is based on the utilization of MDA using albendazole in combination with diethylcarbamazine or ivermectin. These drugs targeting the microfilariae can block transmission. However, there are also drawbacks, such as inadequate drug coverage, reappearance of infection through migration of infected people into controlled areas, and partial success leading to reduced compliance. The potential for the development of drug resistance has been raised and the benzimidazole resistance allele has been identified at an increased frequency in microfilariae loads of *Wuchereria bancrofti* from patients in MDA areas [34]. Subsequent modeling studies have raised serious concern for the future acquisition and spread of resistance against albendazole and ivermectin [35]. This has led to a call for complementary approaches that include both improved chemotherapy models and vaccine development, and the continued consideration of a vaccine against lymphatic filariasis is still strongly advocated [33].

Importantly, protective mechanisms against infection by the early filarial L3 stages and the target molecules involved have been evolutionarily preserved, even though the disease processes caused by adult worms and microfilariae of the various filarial parasites are quite different [36–39]. The protective immune responses to human lymphatic filariae and the epidemiologic outcomes of exposure to these parasites are, therefore, similar to those described for *O. volvulus*. These include (i) the description of individuals without signs of patent, microfilariae-positive, infection (the so-called endemic normals or putatively immune) in areas endemic for *W. bancrofti* or *Brugia malayi* infections [1], (ii) the age-acquired resistance to superinfection with adult worms [40], and (iii) the anti-L3 concomitant protective humoral [41] and cellular [42] immunity in infected individuals. Moreover, several *B. malayi* and other proteins have been cloned and tested for protective immunity. As detailed in Chapter 23, it appears that many of the lymphatic filariasis vaccine candidates are highly similar to the *O. volvulus* protective antigens (*Bm*-ALT-1, r*Bm*-ASP-1, *Ls*-cystatin, *Bm*-SXP-1, and *Bm*-chitinase) [43–46]. In addition, it was shown that the *O. volvulus* recombinant proteins *Ov*-RBP-1 and *Ov*-B20 also induced protection against a challenge with *Acanthocheilonema viteae* in jirds [47]. Other vaccine candidates that were experimentally shown to protect through antibody-dependent cellular cytotoxicity are glutathione *S*-transferase (GST) [48], myosin [49], a microfilarial soluble 38-kDa protease [50], and a 175-kDa collagenase [51].

Large-scale, proteomic analyses to identify the excretory/secretory products of the L3, L3 to L4 molting, adult male, adult female, and microfilarial stages of *B. malayi* have recently been published [52]. These provide extended insight into the host–parasite interaction and the reported abundance of a number of previously characterized immunomodulatory proteins in the excretory/secretory products of microfilariae increases the chances of identifying novel vaccine candidates.

Currently, and with the support of the National Institutes of Health, collaborative preclinical studies of *O. volvulus* and *B. malayi* vaccine antigens are underway in four institutions: New York Blood Center, Thomas Jefferson University, Louisiana State University, and Baylor College of Medicine. It is projected that out of the eight top-ranking antigens described above, the two most effective vaccine candidates of *O. volvulus* and *B. malayi* will be selected and fully evaluated. This will include identification of their immune protection correlates which will be followed by process development and manufacturing under Good Manufacturing Practice (GMP), and then phase I clinical testing using the Global Access Strategy developed by the Sabin Vaccine Institute [53].

Schistosomiasis

There are 800 million people in 74 countries at risk and more than 200 million infected [54, 55]. However, additional studies suggest that more than 400 million people may suffer from schistosomiasis at any one time, resulting in a disease burden that is comparable to HIV/AIDS, tuberculosis, or malaria [56]. Initial progress in the control of schistosomiasis led some to suggest that it may be "consigned to history" by 2015 – the target stated in the MDGs [57]. Since the 1990s, the major approach to schistosomiasis control has been periodic treatment with praziquantel. Recent versions of control suggest the integration of praziquantel treatment into the other NTD control programs [58–60]. However, the sustainability of praziquantel treatment for the long-term control of schistosomiasis is a cause for concern because of the variable efficacy of praziquantel, high rates of post-treatment reinfection, and the ongoing concern regarding eventual drug resistance. The last possibility alone reinforces the need for alternatives to single drug treatment (for more on praziquantel and drug development for schistosomiasis, see Chapters 19 and 20).

The case for schistosomiasis vaccine development is based on the understanding that vaccination, even if not 100% effective, would contribute to long-term reduction of egg excretion from the host. An effective vaccine might also ameliorate the aggressive inflammatory response that has been observed following interrupted chemotherapy in children living in high-transmission areas. The underlying reason for this "rebound morbidity" is unclear. It may be due to partial interruption in the naturally developed immune modulation during chronic infection [61, 62].

The arguments supporting the utility of a vaccine against schistosomiasis, based on more than 50 years of laboratory and field research, are strong. For example, it is well known that humans living in schistosome-endemic areas develop some degree of protection naturally [63]. Also, injection of mice with irradiated schistosome cercariae consistently induces 60–85% protection [6]. Despite the fact that the *Schistosoma haematobium* GST (*Sh*28-GST) is the current lead candidate, the great majority of *Schistosoma* candidate vaccine antigens under evaluation are derived from *Schistosoma mansoni*. The most well researched are *Sm*28-GST and *Sh*28-GST [64], paramyosin [65], *Sm*28-TPI [66], *Sm*37-GADPH [67], *Sm*14-FABP [68, 69], and *Sm*p80-calpain [70, 71] (TPI = triose phosphate isomerase; GADPH = glyceralde-hyde-3-phosphate dehydrogenase; FABP = fatty acid-binding protein). There are also multiple antigenic peptide constructs made from various integrated membrane antigens, such as *Sm*10, *Sm*23, *Sm*28-TPI, and *Sm*28-GST [72, 73]. All of the above antigens show an average protection of 50% (in some cases higher) and have been tested either as native full-length antigens, recombinant antigens, multiple antigenic peptide constructs, or as DNA vaccines in various animal models. Notably, national funds have been invested in Brazil and France supporting clinical trials for two of these antigens, *Sm*14-FABP and *Sh*28-GST, respectively [13]. Industrial scale-up was first achieved for *Sh*28-GST, which is now in clinical trials under the name of Bilhvax [64]. This vaccine candidate has successfully passed phase I/II clinical trials. It has been shown to be entirely safe producing helper T cell T_h2 cytokines (interleukin-5 and -13) followed by high titers of neutralizing antibodies after three injections. Treatment followed by immunization was felt to be the most appropriate modality and the best time to give the vaccine seems to be about 3 months after treatment when patients have switched to the T_h2-type of response, which takes time to occur and is generally not seen until after drug treatment (http://www.rnas.org.cn/upload/inFile/2008-9-25161018-Strategy.pdf). The phase II trials of Bilhvax were based on this model, including both primary clinical and secondary parasitological end-points in measuring efficacy [13].

Industrial scale-up has also been achieved for the *Schistosoma* FABP, *Sm*14-FABP [69] (see Chapter 26). Interestingly, thanks to it being a shared antigen between *Fasciola* and *Schistosoma*, both natural infection and experimental animal research show cross-protection [68]. The former parasite causes great losses in sheep and cattle breeding, and can also infect humans. Commercial interest in a vaccine for veterinary applications has helped move this vaccine candidate into advanced veterinary field trials, which in turn made it possible to explore the use of the same molecule in the development of a human vaccine against schistosomiasis [69]. A collaborative initiative in Brazil for the GMP scale-up of stable and properly folded *Sm*14-FABP was established between the Oswaldo Cruz Foundation (FIOCRUZ), a government-funded research center, and Instituto Butantan, a producer of vaccines for the Brazilian Ministry of Health. Plans are underway for phase I safety trials [74].

More recently, the *S. mansoni* tegumental surface tetraspanin known as *Sm*-TSP-2 has shown promise as a vaccine for intestinal schistosomiasis (see Chapter 25). The following studies provided the basis for selecting the extracellular domain of *Sm*-TSP-2 as a candidate vaccine: sera from putatively resistant individuals residing in an endemic area of Brazil contain high levels of anti-*Sm*-TSP-2 IgG1 and IgG3 [75]; also, schistosomes exposed to RNA interference of the *Sm-tsp-2* transcript fail to generate a proper surface tegument and do not become adult worms [76]. When the extracellular domain of *Sm*-TSP-2 is expressed as a recombinant protein in bacteria (and more recently yeast), the resulting 9-kDa polypeptide is an effective immunogen resulting in 40–60% reductions in *S. mansoni* worm burdens in mice [75]. It has undergone process development, scale-up, and formulation by the product development partnerships (PDP) of the Sabin Vaccine Institute. There are current plans to produce pilot amounts of the recombinant protein formulated in alum at Instituto Butantan prior to anticipated phase I trials in Brazil [22]. Efforts are also in progress to identify and develop *S. haematobium* orthologs as vaccines.

Vaccine development was originally focused on *S. mansoni* and *S. haematobium*, but a panel of well-characterized *Schistosoma japonicum* antigens (e.g., *Sj*97, *Sj*TPI, *Sj*ASP (aspartic protease), *Sj*23, *Sj*28GST, *Sj*14-3-3, *Sj*14, *Sj*Serpin, *Sj*Fer (ferritin), *Sj*SVLBP (*S. japonicum* very-low-density lipoprotein-binding protein)) have also shown protective efficacy in animals justifying support for further consideration (reviewed in [17]). As *S. japonicum* is a zoonosis, it presents an added challenge for control programs [77]. However, the diverse host spectrum permits a step-wise path that might start with a "transmission-blocking" veterinary product [78] before moving on to a human vaccine, thus offering a shortcut in the development of vaccines for China and the Philippines. The possibility that this approach could pay off is supported by studies in China showing that the animal–snail–human transmission cycle is more prominent than the human–snail–human cycle in sustaining the infection in endemic areas [79]. An additional advantage of the *S. japonicum* vaccine development is the access to full-size animal models, which overcomes the limitations of the mouse model [80].

Based on the notion that reduced schistosome infection in water buffaloes would also reduce disease transmission to humans, randomized double-blind trials in water buffaloes using DNA vaccines encoding well-researched S. *japonicum* antigens (*Sj*28-TPI, *Sj*23) have taken place in China and showed close to 50% protection, which exceeds the hypothetical level predicted by mathematical modeling that is needed to achieve a significant reduction in schistosome transmission [81]. Such transmission-blocking *S. japonicum* vaccines are currently in field trials [81, 82]. The recent publication of the *S. japonicum* genome [83] as well as recent transcriptome and proteome studies [84, 85] will definitely contribute to increased activities focused on vaccine development against this species.

Hookworm Infections and Other STHs

The STHs are among the most common and persistent parasitic infections worldwide. According to the latest estimates, 800 million people are infected with roundworm (*Ascaris lumbricoides*), 600 million with whipworm (*Trichuris trichiura*), and 600 million with hookworm (*Necator americanus, Ancylostoma duodenale*) [4, 86, 87], with most of the infections caused by *A. duodenale*. *N. americanus* is the major hookworm found in sub-Saharan Africa, Southeast Asia, and Latin America and the Caribbean [88]. Hookworm is also a leading cause of maternal and child morbidity in the developing countries of the tropics and subtropics [88, 89].

Interventions for the control of STHs involve MDA and/or chemotherapy of individuals, as well as improved sanitation and education. MDA programs for STHs (and schistosomes) are most often directed at school-aged children as they are the population group most at risk of acquiring heavy infection and developing associated morbidity, and the most accessible group for intervention through school-based programs. However, some mass chemotherapy programs are directed at whole communities in highly endemic areas. The focus of MDA for STHs is on achieving long-term reductions in infection prevalence and intensity, and hence in the associated morbidity, rather than attempting to eliminate the reservoir of infection [90]. There has also been increased recent awareness that, apart from *A. lumbricoides*, the current anthelmintics for control of STHs (albendazole, mebendazole, ivermectin, pyrantel, and levamisole) are not particularly effective against hookworms and, especially, whipworms [91]. Recently, the genetic polymorphisms in β-tubulin, which cause benzimidazole resistance in livestock parasites, have been found in *T. trichiura* and *N. americanus* [92].

Vaccine research targets have been evaluated from both the larval and adult stages of the hookworms. Initially, a promising larval vaccine candidate was the *Na*-ASP-2 antigen, first shown in secretions from *Anyclostoma*, but later isolated from *N. americanus* [93]. Well-controlled studies initially showed this candidate to be safe in animals, and capable of inducing protective responses consisting both of specific IgG antibodies and cellular immune responses [93, 94]. Furthermore, a phase I safety trial completed in the United States showed evidence of safety and immunogenicity [94]. However, subsequent phase I trials in a hookworm-endemic area of Brazil had to be stopped for safety concerns due to evidence of an allergic response in association with prevaccination IgE [22] (Bethony and Diemert, personal communication; also see Chapter 21).

Vaccine development is now focused on targeting adult hookworm antigens as a means to reduce host worm burdens and blood loss. During an intensive investigation of their preclinical efficacy (which includes safety experiments to ensure absence of prevaccination IgE in endemic populations), two adult *N. americanus* vaccine antigens (i.e., *Na*-GST-1 and *Na*-APR-1) have emerged as the non-IgE naturally inducing candidates for the antihookworm vaccines. The putative adult worm vaccine antigens were identified based on the knowledge of the mechanisms of worm feeding, and the ability to interfere with those enzymes involved in the degradation and detoxification of hemoglobin [22]. Among these were a cysteine protease [95], an aspartic protease (APR) [19], and a GST [96]. Vaccination with *Na*-APR-1 and *Na*-GST-1 recombinant vaccines significantly reduces adult hookworm burdens, parasite blood loss, and fecal egg counts in dogs and/or hamsters challenged with either *Ancylostoma caninum* and/or *N. americanus* [21, 96]. The *Na*-GST-1 hookworm vaccine is already in phase I trial [22] and *Na*-APR-1 is currently being manufactured. A combination of these two antigens has been proposed as an eventual human hookworm vaccine in order to prevent moderate and heavy hookworm infections caused by *N. americanus*. Such a vaccine could be incorporated into existing deworming programs that target preschool and school-aged children living in areas of high transmission to reduce the morbidity – primarily anemia and protein malnutrition – attributed to this parasite. Antihookworm vaccine development is being conducted in partnership with vaccine manufacturers in middle-income endemic countries, such as Brazil, and in partnership with the corresponding health ministries, in order to ensure that the populations who most need the vaccine will have timely access to it once efficacy is shown in phase III testing.

Finally, there is a strong rationale to combine hookworm and schistosome antigens in the development of a multivalent antihelminth vaccine against parasites that are coendemic and induce similar pathologies, including anemia [97]. Such a vaccine would target two of the most prevalent and insidious helminth diseases.

Product Development Strategies that Involve Manufacturing Partners in Disease-Endemic Countries

The adverse consequences of the NTDs and other conditions on child development, pregnancy outcome, worker productivity, and malaria and HIV/AIDS coinfections offer a powerful basis for developing new antihelminth vaccines. However, this requires long-term commitment and sustainable development. Until a few years ago, antigen discovery and preclinical development of these vaccines had not progressed much beyond early development. There are two major reasons for this situation. (i) For eukaryotic pathogens, such as protozoa and worms, it had not been generally possible to exploit high-throughput reverse vaccinology approaches because of the requirements for complex eukaryotic expression vectors and animal models for vaccine testing. (ii) Clinical development had not progressed for many of the antipoverty vaccines because of the absence of commercial markets and, therefore, industry interest. However, over the last 10 years several nonprofit organizations (see below) have created product development partnerships, and focused their activities on the development and testing of recombinant vaccines for helminth infections, including hookworm, schistosomiasis, and onchocerciasis [22, 53]. In addition, the Institut Pasteur and the French Institut National de la Santé et de la Recherche Médicale, are developing a vaccine for urogenital schistosomiasis caused by *S. haematobium*. Table 22.1 summarizes the current stages of vaccine development of the various antihelminth vaccines.

Progress has been particularly strong in the field of schistosomiasis vaccines. This does not mean it is an easier parasite to work with, but it is rather a reflection of the financial support that has been available for research on this parasite in the 1980s and 1990s [98]. This support includes nationally available funds invested in Brazil and France, and the interest in China that has facilitated trials in water buffaloes with *S. japonicum* antigens. Similarly, advances in *O. volvulus* and *B. malayi* vaccine studies (basic research of protective immunity, vaccine antigen discovery, animal model development, etc.) were supported by the Edna McConnell Clark Foundation [31] and by the National Institutes of Health in the 1980s and early 1990s [10]. The hookworm vaccine candidates are being developed by the PDP of the Sabin Vaccine Institute and funded by the Bill & Melinda Gates Foundation, together with the Dutch Ministry of Foreign Affairs. A similar group of partners is also advancing the *Sm*-TSP-2 recombinant vaccine for intestinal schistosomiasis in Brazil. The successful TSOL18 porcine vaccine for cysticercosis [99] shows that it is indeed possible to create a highly effective vaccine against a multicellular parasite (see Chapter 29). Proof-of-concept of the feasibility of eliminating *Taenia solium* transmission in a wide endemic area of Peru and in Cameroon has been also provided [24, 25]. Regrettably, it seems that, despite the availability of excellent vaccines, they will not be widely applied without a commercial incentive. This can only be remedied by convincing governments, international donor agencies, and private foundations to support large-scale vaccination projects and/or by the provision of vaccines as a public health measure through local production in the endemic countries themselves.

In the case of the hookworm and intestinal schistosomiasis vaccines, an important strategy is to pursue vaccine manufacture through partnerships with innovative

Table 22.1 Overview of candidates under development as antihelminth vaccines.

Parasite	Antigen discovery[a]	Scale-up and manufacturing	Phase I trial	Phase II trial	Phase III trial	Registration
Hookworm	>25	3	1 in 2007; 1 started in 2011 and 1 anticipated in 2012			
W. bancrofti	>10					
B. malayi	>10					
O. volvulus	>10					
S. mansoni	>100[b]	3	1 anticipated in 2012			
S. haematobium	>10[b]			1		
S. japonicum	<100[b]					

a) Although the number of antigens discovered cannot be more than approximate, the table highlights where the lead products are.
b) Corresponding antigens exist in the various species; only a few are species-specific. However, not all antigens in each species have been developed into vaccine candidates.

developing countries (IDCs). IDCs are middle-income countries, such as Brazil, Cuba, China, and India, with modest to strong economies and sustained levels of innovation in biotechnology based on their per capita numbers of peer-reviewed papers, international patents, and production of drugs, vaccines, and diagnostics [100]. Many of the IDCs are highly endemic for the major NTDs, including helminth infections, and this provides an opportunity to partner with IDCs, both to develop and clinically test vaccine candidates.

Therefore, PDP–IDC liaisons hold promise for the development and testing of the antipoverty vaccines. For example, a partnership involving the Sabin Vaccine Institute, FIOCRUZ, the vaccine manufacturers Instituto Butantan and FIO-CRUZ-Biomanguinhos, and the Brazilian Ministry of Health has been critical for the transition from proof-of-concept to product development and clinical trials of the hookworm and schistosomiasis vaccines. The further development of global strategies to ensure that the world's poorest people have access to these innovations is essential. Therefore, the Sabin Vaccine Institute has developed a unique Global Access Strategy to ensure that vulnerable populations receive the human hookworm vaccine at an extremely low cost [53].

In order to further ensure timely vaccine introduction, efforts should also be in place to establish international consensus on the use of these helminth vaccines. This process should be done under the auspices of the WHO and its Department of Neglected Tropical Diseases. Other organizations such as the Global Network for Neglected Tropical Disease Control, an alliance of the major NTD public-private partnerships, should be engaged. In 2005, the WHO called for the development of new control tools for hookworms, especially a vaccine [101]. As part of an international consensus on hookworm controls, the idea of distributing human hookworm vaccine in conjunction with the school-based deworming programs that have already been mandated by a 2001 World Health Assembly resolution should be strongly promoted. For this reason, the global access and development strategy of the "Human Hookworm Vaccine" PDP strategy is to link vaccination with deworming ("chemotherapy-linked vaccination") and to recommend that vaccination occur after deworming school-aged children with an anthelmintic medication, typically a benzimidazole anthelmintic. Since 2001, however, preschool children aged 1–5 have emerged as an important target population for deworming [102] and global efforts at reaching this population through Child Health Days have so far been more successful than efforts to reach school-aged children [102]. Therefore, the Sabin Vaccine Institute is now exploring promotion of the human hookworm vaccine for both preschool children and school-aged children. The process will maximize the likelihood of vaccine integration into an existing healthcare system currently devoted to worm control; this would also complement the use of benzimidazoles for disease control and, possibly, forestall the emergence of drug resistance. Ultimately, the vaccine will be used in a strategy targeting low-income populations. It will be combined with other low-cost interventions including MDA for schistosomiasis, lymphatic filariasis, onchocerciasis, and trachoma, as well as micronutrients, vitamin A, bed net distribution, and health education [90].

As a component of their national immunization programs, most industrialized and middle-income countries have policies for vaccinating both preschool children and schoolchildren. Through Child Health Days, millions of preschool children currently receive measles vaccine along with vitamin A, deworming tablets, and antimalaria bed nets. With respect to school-aged children, several hookworm-endemic nations, including Brazil, Colombia, Nicaragua, Panama, Peru, Namibia, India, Malaysia, and Papua New Guinea, currently deliver vaccines in schools. Building a school-based program for delivery of hookworm and other future anti-helminth vaccines may employ similar efforts recently proposed for human papilloma virus (HPV) vaccines in some countries. In time, a program of school-based vaccine delivery could offer low-income countries the opportunity not only to deliver a package of the WHO's Expanded Programme on Immunization vaccines, but also allow for the introduction of new vaccines to prevent HIV/AIDS, hookworm, HPV, tuberculosis, and other infections, including the major human helminth infections. In many countries, Child Health Days and school-based programs are not mutually exclusive, as it is common to use schools as the host venue for delivery of vaccines in Child Health Days [103, 104].

Conclusions

The economic benefits of combining vaccines and drug interventions are many and represent a potentially powerful tool for improving public health problems. The expansion of parasite sequence resources (see also Chapters 3–5) is providing a fresh start by permitting a more rational approach to vaccine discovery. A range of new vaccines can be expected during the next few years so long as international donor organizations and private foundations can agree on a joint, major NTD vaccine initiative. The task ahead is to assure product delivery by convincing potential donors that vaccine production in the developing world is a realistic goal worth supporting.

The development of vaccines will require careful analyses of cost-effectiveness, which in turn is based on a number of parameters, including transmission dynamics, disease burden, and healthcare delivery systems. The cost and effort to introduce and sustain a vaccine for decades requires the development of credible models of cost-effectiveness. For example, to better estimate the global burden of hookworm disease, the PDP of the Sabin Vaccine Institute has embarked on a global health impact analysis involving several activities. It is refining models of hookworm transmission dynamics, rederiving new disability-adjusted life years estimates based on local studies conducted in Brazil, performing a meta-analysis of the attributable burden of anemia ascribable to hookworm in different developing countries, and conducting a detailed analysis of the projected use of the human hookworm vaccine in different settings. An initial cost analysis of the human hookworm vaccine conducted in Uganda indicates that the most important determinants of overall costs are vaccine price and the number of doses of vaccine. The costs of distribution and delivery of the human hookworm vaccine are comparable to the outlays for deworming, particularly in the setting of Child Health Days. National and international funding mechanisms will be required to purchase vaccines for countries unable to finance their own procurement. For the Americas, the Sabin Vaccine Institute is exploring the Pan American Health Organization Revolving Fund for Vaccine Procurement mechanism. Elsewhere, especially in low-income sub-Saharan Africa, identifying the procurement funds and mechanisms for the large-scale purchase and distribution of a human hookworm vaccine in high transmission areas will be a major impediment to global access. Currently, the United Nations Children's Fund purchases traditional childhood vaccines for developing countries, which covers about 65% of the world's children.

Similar to the MDA programs, which employ drugs that are donated or available at low cost, we believe that once antihelminth vaccines are ready for distribution, they will be incorporated into the existing control measures [53]. The ultimate goal will be to provide sustainable reductions in and eventually eliminate the global burden of human helminth infections, not least in the poorest countries of Africa, Asia, and the Americas.

Acknowledgment

The authors wish to thank Dr. Peter Hotez for critical reading of the chapter.

References

1 Kazura, J.W. (2000) Resistance to infection with lymphatic-dwelling filarial parasites, in *Lymphatic Filariasis* (ed. T.B. Nutman), Imperial College Press, London, pp. 83–102.

2 Bethony, J., Loukas, A., Smout, M., Brooker, S., Mendez, S., Plieskatt, J., Goud, G. *et al.* (2005) Antibodies against a secreted protein from hookworm larvae reduce the intensity of hookworm

infection in humans and vaccinated laboratory animals. *FASEB J.*, **19**, 1743–1745.

3 Oothuman, P., Denham, D.A., McGreevy, P.B., Nelson, G.S., and Rogers, R. (1979) Successful vaccination of cats against *Brugia pahangi* with larvae attenuated by irradiation with 10 krad cobalt 60. *Parasite Immunol.*, **1**, 209–216.

4 Hotez, P.J., Bethony, J.M., Oliveira, S.C., Brindley, P.J., and Loukas, A. (2008) Multivalent anthelminthic vaccine to prevent hookworm and schistosomiasis. *Expert Rev. Vaccines*, **7**, 745–752.

5 Prichard, R.K. (2007) Ivermectin resistance and overview of the Consortium for Anthelmintic Resistance SNPs. *Expert Opin. Drug Discov.*, **2**, S41–S52.

6 Dean, D.A. (1983) *Schistosoma* and related genera: acquired resistance in mice. *Exp. Parasitol.*, **55**, 1–104.

7 Molyneux, D.H. (2009) 10 years of success in addressing lymphatic filariasis. *Lancet*, **373**, 529–530.

8 Bockarie, M.J. and Molyneux, D.H. (2009) The end of lymphatic filariasis? *Br. Med. J.*, **338**, b1686.

9 Boag, P.R., Parsons, J.C., Presidente, P.J., Spithill, T.W., and Sexton, J.L. (2003) Characterisation of humoral immune responses in dogs vaccinated with irradiated *Ancylostoma caninum*. *Vet. Immunol. Immunopathol.*, **92**, 87–94.

10 Lustigman, S. and Abraham, D. (2009) Onchocerciasis, in *Vaccines for Biodefense and Emerging and Neglected Diseases* (eds A.D.T. Barrett and L.R. Stanberry), Academic Press, New York, pp. 1379–1400.

11 Bergquist, N.R., Leonardo, L.R., and Mitchell, G.F. (2005) Vaccine-linked chemotherapy: can schistosomiasis control benefit from an integrated approach? *Trends Parasitol.*, **21**, 112–117.

12 Bergquist, R., Utzinger, J., and McManus, D.P. (2008) Trick or treat: the role of vaccines in integrated schistosomiasis control. *PLoS Negl. Trop. Dis.*, **2**, e244.

13 Bergquist, R. and Lustigman, S. (2010) Control of important helminthic infections: vaccine development as part of the solution. *Adv. Parasitol.*, **73**, 297–326.

14 Hotez, P.J. and Ferris, M.T. (2006) The antipoverty vaccines. *Vaccine*, **24**, 5787–5799.

15 Ghosh, K., Wu, W., Antoine, A.D., Bottazzi, M.E., Valenzuela, J.G., Hotez, P.J., and Mendez, S. (2006) The impact of concurrent and treated *Ancylostoma ceylanicum* hookworm infections on the immunogenicity of a recombinant hookworm vaccine in hamsters. *J. Infect. Dis.*, **193**, 155–162.

16 Allen, J.E., Adjei, O., Bain, O., Hoerauf, A., Hoffmann, W.H., Makepeace, B.L., Schulz-Key, H. et al. (2008) Of mice, cattle, and humans: the immunology and treatment of river blindness. *PLoS Negl. Trop. Dis.*, **2**, e217.

17 McManus, D.P. and Loukas, A. (2008) Current status of vaccines for schistosomiasis. *Clin. Microbiol. Rev.*, **21**, 225–242.

18 Noma, M., Nwoke, B.E., Nutall, I., Tambala, P.A., Enyong, P., Namsenmo, A., Remme, J. et al. (2002) Rapid epidemiological mapping of onchocerciasis (REMO): its application by the African Programme for Onchocerciasis Control (APOC). *Ann. Trop. Med. Parasitol.*, **96** (Suppl. 1), S29–S39.

19 Loukas, A., Bethony, J.M., Mendez, S., Fujiwara, R.T., Goud, G.N., Ranjit, N., Zhan, B. et al. (2005) Vaccination with recombinant aspartic hemoglobinase reduces parasite load and blood loss after hookworm infection in dogs. *PLoS Med.*, **2**, e295.

20 Loukas, A., Bethony, J., Brooker, S., and Hotez, P. (2006) Hookworm vaccines: past, present, and future. *Lancet Infect. Dis.*, **6**, 733–741.

21 Pearson, M.S., Bethony, J.M., Pickering, D.A., de Oliveira, L.M., Jariwala, A., Santiago, H., Miles, A.P. et al. (2009) An enzymatically inactivated hemoglobinase from *Necator americanus* induces neutralizing antibodies against multiple hookworm species and protects dogs against heterologous hookworm infection. *FASEB J.*, **23**, 3007–3019.

22 Hotez, P.J., Bethony, J.M., Diemert, D.J., Pearson, M., and Loukas, A. (2010) Developing vaccines to combat hookworm infection and intestinal schistosomiasis. *Nat. Rev. Microbiol.*, **8**, 814–826.

23 Osei-Atweneboana, M.Y., Awadzi, K., Attah, S.K., Boakye, D.A., Gyapong, J.O., and Prichard, R.K. (2011) Phenotypic evidence of emerging ivermectin resistance in *Onchocerca volvulus*. *PLoS Negl. Trop. Dis.*, **5**, e998.

24 Lightowlers, M.W. (2010) Eradication of *Taenia solium* cysticercosis: a role for vaccination of pigs. *Int. J. Parasitol.*, **40**, 1183–1192.

25 Assana, E., Kyngdon, C.T., Gauci, C.G., Geerts, S., Dorny, P., De Deken, R., Anderson, G.A. *et al.* (2010) Elimination of *Taenia solium* transmission to pigs in a field trial of the TSOL18 vaccine in Cameroon. *Int. J. Parasitol.*, **40**, 515–519.

26 McCarthy, J.S., Wieseman, M., Tropea, J., Kaslow, D., Abraham, D., Lustigman, S., Tuan, R. *et al.* (2002) *Onchocerca volvulus* glycolytic enzyme fructose-1,6-bisphosphate aldolase as a target for a protective immune response in humans. *Infect. Immun.*, **70**, 851–858.

27 Erttmann, K.D., Kleensang, A., Schneider, E., Hammerschmidt, S., Buttner, D.W., and Gallin, M. (2005) Cloning, characterization and DNA immunization of an *Onchocerca volvulus* glyceraldehyde-3-phosphate dehydrogenase (*Ov*-GAPDH). *Biochim. Biophys. Acta*, **1741**, 85–94.

28 Borchert, N., Becker-Pauly, C., Wagner, A., Fischer, P., Stocker, W., and Brattig, N.W. (2007) Identification and characterization of onchoastacin, an astacin-like metalloproteinase from the filaria *Onchocerca volvulus*. *Microbes Infect.*, **9**, 498–506.

29 Erttmann, K.D. and Buttner, D.W. (2009) Immunohistological studies on *Onchocerca volvulus* paramyosin. *Parasitol. Res.*, **105**, 1371–1374.

30 Makepeace, B.L., Jensen, S.A., Laney, S.J., Nfon, C.K., Njongmeta, L.M., Tanya, V.N., Williams, S.A. *et al.* (2009) Immunisation with a multivalent, subunit vaccine reduces patent infection in a natural bovine model of onchocerciasis during intense field exposure. *PLoS Negl. Trop. Dis.*, **3**, e544.

31 Cook, J.A., Steel, C., and Ottesen, E.A. (2001) Towards a vaccine for onchocerciasis. *Trends Parasitol.*, **17**, 555–558.

32 Dadzie, Y., Neira, M., and Hopkins, D. (2003) Final report of the Conference on the Eradicability of Onchocerciasis. *Filaria J.*, **2**, 2.

33 Hoerauf, A. and Steel, C. (2004) Towards a strategic plan for research to support the global program to eliminate lymphatic filariasis. 3.2 Protective immunity – vaccines. *Am. J. Trop. Med. Hyg.*, **71** (Suppl.), 34–36.

34 Schwab, A.E., Boakye, D.A., Kyelem, D., and Prichard, R.K. (2005) Detection of benzimidazole resistance-associated mutations in the filarial nematode *Wuchereria bancrofti* and evidence for selection by albendazole and ivermectin combination treatment. *Am. J. Trop. Med. Hyg.*, **73**, 234–238.

35 Schwab, A.E., Churcher, T.S., Schwab, A.J., Basáñez, M.G., and Prichard, R.K. (2007) An analysis of the population genetics of potential multi-drug resistance in *Wuchereria bancrofti* due to combination chemotherapy. *Parasitology*, **134**, 1025–1040.

36 Lawrence, R.A. and Devaney, E. (2001) Lymphatic filariasis: parallels between the immunology of infection in humans and mice. *Parasite Immunol.*, **23**, 353–361.

37 Devaney, E. and Osborne, J. (2000) The third-stage larva (L3) of *Brugia*: its role in immune modulation and protective immunity. *Microbes Infect.*, **2**, 1363–1371.

38 Maizels, R.M., Blaxter, M.L., and Scott, A.L. (2001) Immunological genomics of *Brugia malayi*: filarial genes implicated in immune evasion and protective immunity. *Parasite Immunol.*, **23**, 327–344.

39 Blaxter, M., Daub, J., Guiliano, D., Parkinson, J., and Whitton, C. (2002) The *Brugia malayi* genome project: expressed sequence tags and gene discovery. *Trans. R. Soc. Trop. Med. Hyg.*, **96**, 7–17.

40 Day, K.P., Gregory, W.F., and Maizels, R.M. (1991) Age-specific acquisition of immunity to infective larvae in a bancroftian filariasis endemic area of Papua New Guinea. *Parasite Immunol.*, **13**, 277–290.

41 Kurniawan-Atmadja, A., Sartono, E., Partono, F., Yazdanbakhsh, M., and Maizels, R.M. (1998) Antibody responses to filarial infective larvae are not dominated by the IgG4 isotype. *Parasite Immunol.*, **20**, 9–17.

42 Sartono, E., Kruize, Y.C., Kurniawan, A., Maizels, R.M., and Yazdanbakhsh, M. (1997) Depression of antigen-specific interleukin-5 and interferon-gamma responses in human lymphatic filariasis as a function of clinical status and age. *J. Infect. Dis.*, **175**, 1276–1280.

43 Gregory, W.F., Atmadja, A.K., Allen, J.E., and Maizels, R.M. (2000) The abundant larval transcript-1 and -2 genes of *Brugia malayi* encode stage-specific candidate vaccine antigens for filariasis. *Infect. Immun.*, **68**, 4174–4179.

44 Pfaff, A.W., Schulz-Key, H., Soboslay, P.T., Taylor, D.W., MacLennan, K., and Hoffmann, W.H. (2002) *Litomosoides sigmodontis* cystatin acts as an immunomodulator during experimental filariasis. *Int. J. Parasitol.*, **32**, 171–178.

45 Wang, S.H., Zheng, H.J., Dissanayake, S., Cheng, W.F., Tao, Z.H., Lin, S.Z., and Piessens, W.F. (1997) Evaluation of recombinant chitinase and SXP1 antigens as antimicrofilarial vaccines. *Am. J. Trop. Med. Hyg.*, **56**, 474–481.

46 Adam, R., Kaltmann, B., Rudin, W., Friedrich, T., Marti, T., and Lucius, R. (1996) Identification of chitinase as the immunodominant filarial antigen recognized by sera of vaccinated rodents. *J. Biol. Chem.*, **271**, 1441–1447.

47 Taylor, M.J., Abdel-Wahab, N., Wu, Y., Jenkins, R.E., and Bianco, A.E. (1995) *Onchocerca volvulus* larval antigen, OvB20, induces partial protection in a rodent model of onchocerciasis. *Infect. Immun.*, **63**, 4417–4422.

48 Veerapathran, A., Dakshinamoorthy, G., Gnanasekar, M., Reddy, M.V., and Kalyanasundaram, R. (2009) Evaluation of *Wuchereria bancrofti* GST as a vaccine candidate for lymphatic filariasis. *PLoS Negl. Trop. Dis.*, **3**, e457.

49 Vedi, S., Dangi, A., Hajela, K., and Misra-Bhattacharya, S. (2008) Vaccination with 73kDa recombinant heavy chain myosin generates high level of protection against *Brugia malayi* challenge in jird and mastomys models. *Vaccine*, **26**, 5997–6005.

50 Krithika, K.N., Dabir, P., Kulkarni, S., Anandharaman, V., and Reddy, M.V. (2005) Identification of 38kDa *Brugia malayi* microfilarial protease as a vaccine candidate for lymphatic filariasis. *Indian J. Exp. Biol.*, **43**, 759–768.

51 Pokharel, D.R., Rai, R., Nandakumar Kodumudi, K., Reddy, M.V., and Rathaur, S. (2006) Vaccination with *Setaria cervi* 175kDa collagenase induces high level of protection against *Brugia malayi* infection in jirds. *Vaccine*, **24**, 6208–6215.

52 Bennuru, S., Meng, Z., Ribeiro, J.M., Semnani, R.T., Ghedin, E., Chan, K., Lucas, D.A. et al. (2011) Stage-specific proteomic expression patterns of the human filarial parasite *Brugia malayi* and its endosymbiont *Wolbachia*. *Proc. Natl. Acad. Sci. USA*, **108**, 9649–9654.

53 Bottazzi, M.E. and Brown, A.S. (2008) Model for product development of vaccines against neglected tropical diseases: a vaccine against human hookworm. *Expert Rev. Vaccines*, **7**, 1481–1492.

54 Steinmann, P., Keiser, J., Bos, R., Tanner, M., and Utzinger, J. (2006) Schistosomiasis and water resources development: systematic review, meta-analysis, and estimates of people at risk. *Lancet Infect. Dis.*, **6**, 411–425.

55 World Health Organization (2008) *Elimination of Schistosomiasis from Low-Transmission Areas: Report of a WHO Informal Consultation*. WHO, Geneva.

56 King, C.H. (2010) Parasites and poverty: the case of schistosomiasis. *Acta Trop.*, **113**, 95–104.

57 Fenwick, A. (2006) Waterborne infectious diseases – could they be consigned to history? *Science*, **313**, 1077–1081.

58 Hotez, P.J., Molyneux, D.H., Fenwick, A., Ottesen, E., Ehrlich Sachs, S., and Sachs, J.D. (2006) Incorporating a rapid-impact package for neglected tropical diseases with programs for HIV/AIDS, tuberculosis, and malaria. *PLoS Med.*, **3**, e102.

59 Hotez, P., Ottesen, E., Fenwick, A., and Molyneux, D. (2006) The neglected tropical diseases: the ancient afflictions of stigma and poverty and the prospects for their control and elimination. *Adv. Exp. Med. Biol.*, **582**, 23–33.

60 Lammie, P.J., Fenwick, A., and Utzinger, J. (2006) A blueprint for success: integration of neglected tropical disease control programmes. *Trends Parasitol.*, **22**, 313–321.

61 Olveda, R.M., Daniel, B.L., Ramirez, B.D., Aligui, G.D., Acosta, L.P., Fevidal, P., Tiu, E. *et al.* (1996) Schistosomiasis japonica in the Philippines: the long-term impact of population-based chemotherapy on infection, transmission, and morbidity. *J. Infect. Dis.*, **174**, 163–172.

62 Reimert, C.M., Tukahebwa, E.M., Kabatereine, N.B., Dunne, D.W., and Vennervald, B.J. (2008) Assessment of *Schistosoma mansoni* induced intestinal inflammation by means of eosinophil cationic protein, eosinophil protein X and myeloperoxidase before and after treatment with praziquantel. *Acta Trop.*, **105**, 253–259.

63 Butterworth, A.E., Capron, M., Cordingley, J.S., Dalton, P.R., Dunne, D.W., Kariuki, H.C., Kimani, G. *et al.* (1985) Immunity after treatment of human schistosomiasis mansoni. II. Identification of resistant individuals, and analysis of their immune responses. *Trans. R. Soc. Trop. Med. Hyg.*, **79**, 393–408.

64 Capron, A., Riveau, G., Capron, M., and Trottein, F. (2005) Schistosomes: the road from host–parasite interactions to vaccines in clinical trials. *Trends Parasitol.*, **21**, 143–149.

65 Pearce, E.J., James, S.L., Hieny, S., Lanar, D.E., and Sher, A. (1988) Induction of protective immunity against *Schistosoma mansoni* by vaccination with schistosome paramyosin (Sm97), a nonsurface parasite antigen. *Proc. Natl. Acad. Sci. USA*, **85**, 5678–5682.

66 Harn, D.A., Gu, W., Oligino, L.D., Mitsuyama, M., Gebremichael, A., and Richter, D. (1992) A protective monoclonal antibody specifically recognizes and alters the catalytic activity of schistosome triose-phosphate isomerase. *J. Immunol.*, **148**, 562–567.

67 Goudot-Crozel, V., Caillol, D., Djabali, M., and Dessein, A.J. (1989) The major parasite surface antigen associated with human resistance to schistosomiasis is a 37-kD glyceraldehyde-3P-dehydrogenase. *J. Exp. Med.*, **170**, 2065–2080.

68 Vilar, M.M., Barrientos, F., Almeida, M., Thaumaturgo, N., Simpson, A., Garratt, R., and Tendler, M. (2003) An experimental bivalent peptide vaccine against schistosomiasis and fascioliasis. *Vaccine*, **22**, 137–144.

69 Tendler, M. and Simpson, A.J. (2008) The biotechnology-value chain: development of Sm14 as a schistosomiasis vaccine. *Acta Trop.*, **108**, 263–266.

70 Siddiqui, A.A., Pinkston, J.R., Quinlin, M.L., Kavikondala, V., Rewers-Felkins, K.A., Phillips, T., and Pompa, J. (2005) Characterization of protective immunity induced against *Schistosoma mansoni* via DNA priming with the large subunit of calpain (Sm-p80) in the presence of genetic adjuvants. *Parasite*, **12**, 3–8.

71 Ahmad, G., Zhang, W., Torben, W., Haskins, C., Diggs, S., Noor, Z., Le, L., and Siddiqui, A.A. (2009) Prime-boost and recombinant protein vaccination strategies using Sm-p80 protects against *Schistosoma mansoni* infection in the mouse model to levels previously attainable only by the irradiated cercarial vaccine. *Parasitol. Res.*, **105**, 1767–1777.

72 Argiro, L., Henri, S., Dessein, H., Kouriba, B., Dessein, A.J., and Bourgois, A. (2000) Induction of a protection against *S. mansoni* with a MAP containing epitopes of Sm37-GAPDH and Sm10-DLC. Effect of coadsorption with GM-CSF on alum. *Vaccine*, **18**, 2033–2038.

73 Ribeiro de Jesus, A., Araujo, I., Bacellar, O., Magalhaes, A., Pearce, E., Harn, D., Strand, M., and Carvalho, E.M. (2000) Human immune responses to *Schistosoma mansoni* vaccine candidate antigens. *Infect. Immun.*, **68**, 2797–2803.

74 Ramos, C.R., Spisni, A., Oyama, S. Jr., Sforca, M.L., Ramos, H.R., Vilar, M.M., Alves, A.C. et al. (2009) Stability improvement of the fatty acid binding protein Sm14 from *S. mansoni* by Cys replacement: structural and functional characterization of a vaccine candidate. *Biochim. Biophys. Acta*, **1794**, 655–662.

75 Tran, M.H., Pearson, M.S., Bethony, J.M., Smyth, D.J., Jones, M.K., Duke, M., Don, T.A. et al. (2006) Tetraspanins on the surface of *Schistosoma mansoni* are protective antigens against schistosomiasis. *Nat. Med.*, **12**, 835–840.

76 Tran, M.H., Freitas, T.C., Cooper, L., Gaze, S., Gatton, M.L., Jones, M.K., Lovas, E. et al. (2010) Suppression of mRNAs encoding tegument tetraspanins from *Schistosoma mansoni* results in impaired tegument turnover. *PLoS Pathog.*, **6**, e1000840.

77 Utzinger, J., Zhou, X.N., Chen, M.G., and Bergquist, R. (2005) Conquering schistosomiasis in China: the long march. *Acta Trop.*, **96**, 69–96.

78 McManus, D.P. (2005) Prospects for development of a transmission blocking vaccine against *Schistosoma japonicum*. *Parasite Immunol.*, **27**, 297–308.

79 Gray, D.J., Williams, G.M., Li, Y., Chen, H., Forsyth, S.J., Li, R.S., Barnett, A.G. et al. (2009) A cluster-randomised intervention trial against *Schistosoma japonicum* in the Peoples' Republic of China: bovine and human transmission. *PLoS One*, **4**, e5900.

80 Zhu, Y., Si, J., Harn, D.A., Xu, M., Ren, J., Yu, C., Liang, Y. et al. (2006) *Schistosoma japonicum* triose-phosphate isomerase plasmid DNA vaccine protects pigs against challenge infection. *Parasitology*, **132**, 67–71.

81 Da'dara, A.A., Li, Y.S., Xiong, T., Zhou, J., Williams, G.M., McManus, D.P., Feng, Z. et al. (2008) DNA-based vaccines protect against zoonotic schistosomiasis in water buffalo. *Vaccine*, **26**, 3617–3625.

82 McManus, D.P., Li, Y., Gray, D.J., and Ross, A.G. (2009) Conquering 'snail fever': schistosomiasis and its control in China. *Expert Rev. Anti. Infect. Ther.*, **7**, 473–485.

83 Zhou, Y., Zheng, H., Chen, Y., Zhang, L., Wang, K., Guo, J., Huang, Z. et al. (2009) The *Schistosoma japonicum* genome reveals features of host-parasite interplay. *Nature*, **460**, 345–351.

84 Hong, Y., Peng, J., Jiang, W., Fu, Z., Liu, J., Shi, Y., Li, X., and Lin, J. (2011) Proteomic Analysis of *Schistosoma japonicum* schistosomulum proteins that are differentially expressed among hosts differing in their susceptibility to the infection. *Mol. Cell Proteomics*, **10**, M110.006098.

85 Liu, F., Chen, P., Cui, S.J., Wang, Z.Q., and Han, Z.G. (2008) SjTPdb: integrated transcriptome and proteome database and analysis platform for *Schistosoma japonicum*. *BMC Genomics*, **9**, 304.

86 Hotez, P.J., Brindley, P.J., Bethony, J.M., King, C.H., Pearce, E.J., and Jacobson, J. (2008) Helminth infections: the great neglected tropical diseases. *J. Clin. Invest.*, **118**, 1311–1321.

87 Hotez, P.J. and Kamath, A. (2009) Neglected tropical diseases in sub-saharan Africa: review of their prevalence, distribution, and disease burden. *PLoS Negl. Trop. Dis.*, **3**, e412.

88 Hotez, P.J., Brooker, S., Bethony, J.M., Bottazzi, M.E., Loukas, A., and Xiao, S. (2004) Hookworm infection. *N. Engl. J. Med.*, **351**, 799–807.

89 Brooker, S., Hotez, P.J., and Bundy, D.A. (2008) Hookworm-related anaemia among pregnant women: a systematic review. *PLoS Negl. Trop. Dis.*, **2**, e291.

90 Hotez, P.J. (2009) Mass drug administration and integrated control for the world's high-prevalence neglected tropical diseases. *Clin. Pharmacol. Ther.*, **85**, 659–664.

91 Keiser, J. and Utzinger, J. (2008) Efficacy of current drugs against soil-transmitted helminth infections: systematic review and meta-analysis. *J. Am. Med. Assoc.*, **299**, 1937–1948.

92 Diawara, A. (2008) *Development of DNA Assays for the Detection of Single Nucleotide*

Polymorphism Associated with Benzimidazole Resistance, in Human Soil-Transmitted Helminths, McGill University, Montreal.

93 Diemert, D.J., Bethony, J.M., and Hotez, P.J. (2008) Hookworm vaccines. *Clin. Infect. Dis.*, **46**, 282–288.

94 Bethony, J.M., Simon, G., Diemert, D.J., Parenti, D., Desrosiers, A., Schuck, S., Fujiwara, R. *et al.* (2008) Randomized, placebo-controlled, double-blind trial of the *Na*-ASP-2 hookworm vaccine in unexposed adults. *Vaccine*, **26**, 2408–2417.

95 Loukas, A., Bethony, J.M., Williamson, A.L., Goud, G.N., Mendez, S., Zhan, B., Hawdon, J.M. *et al.* (2004) Vaccination of dogs with a recombinant cysteine protease from the intestine of canine hookworms diminishes the fecundity and growth of worms. *J. Infect. Dis.*, **189**, 1952–1961.

96 Zhan, B., Perally, S., Brophy, P.M., Xue, J., Goud, G., Liu, S., Deumic, V. *et al.* (2010) Molecular cloning, biochemical characterization, and partial protective immunity of the heme-binding glutathione S-transferases from the human hookworm *Necator americanus*. *Infect. Immun.*, **78**, 1552–1563.

97 Hotez, P.J., Bottazzi, M.E., Franco-Paredes, C., Ault, S.K., and Periago, M.R. (2008) The neglected tropical diseases of Latin America and the Caribbean: a review of disease burden and distribution and a roadmap for control and elimination. *PLoS Negl. Trop. Dis.*, **2**, e300.

98 Bergquist, N.R. and Colley, D.G. (1998) Schistosomiasis vaccine: research to development. *Parasitol. Today*, **14**, 99–104.

99 Garcia, H.H., González, A.E., Del Brutto, O.H., Tsang, V.C., Llanos-Zavalaga, F., Gonzalvez, G., Romero, J., and Gilman, R.H. (2007) Strategies for the elimination of taeniasis/cysticercosis. *J. Neurol. Sci.*, **262**, 153–157.

100 Morel, C.M., Acharya, T., Broun, D., Dangi, A., Elias, C., Ganguly, N.K., Gardner, C.A. *et al.* (2005) Health innovation networks to help developing countries address neglected diseases. *Science*, **309**, 401–404.

101 World Health Organization (2004) *Deworming for Health and Development: Report of the Third Global Meeting of the Partners for Parasite Control*, WHO, Geneva.

102 World Health Organization (2008) Soil-transmitted, helminthiasis. Progress report on number of children treated with anthelminthic drugs: an update towards the 2010 global target. *Wkly Epidemiol. Rec.*, **82**, 237–252.

103 Mackroth, M.S., Irwin, K., Vandelaer, J., Hombach, J., and Eckert, L.O. (2010) Immunizing school-age children and adolescents: experience from low- and middle-income countries. *Vaccine*, **28**, 1138–1147.

104 Kane, M.A., Sherris, J., Coursaget, P., Aguado, T., and Cutts, F. (2006) Chapter 15: HPV vaccine use in the developing world. *Vaccine*, **24** (Suppl. 3), 132–139.

23
Antifilarial Vaccine Development: Present and Future Approaches

Sara Lustigman[*], *David Abraham, and Thomas R. Klei*

Abstract

Human onchocerciasis and lymphatic filariasis are serious neglected tropical diseases causing blindness and chronic disability in the developing world. *Onchocerca volvulus*, which causes onchocerciasis, and *Wuchereria bancrofti* and *Brugia malayi*, which cause lymphatic filariasis, are the center of the long-term objective of elimination through mass drug administration (MDA) programs directed at reducing parasite transmission and morbidity. However, formidable technical and logistical obstacles, including the possible emergence of drug resistance, must be overcome before the goal of elimination can be attained. This has led to a call for complementary approaches that include vaccine development that targets the infective-stage larvae. Importantly, protective immunity against *Onchocerca* and lymphatic filariae larvae has now been definitively demonstrated in humans, cattle, and animal models, thereby providing the conceptual underpinnings that vaccines can be produced against these infections. Moreover, several recombinant vaccine antigens have been identified that are capable of inducing a significant yet partial reduction in the survival of challenge larvae using experimental animal models. The recent advances and future prospective for the development of vaccines against both onchocerciasis and lymphatic filariasis are reviewed.

General Aspects of Human Filarial Infection and Disease

A large number of filarial nematodes infect animals and humans throughout the world. The major parasites of humans are those causing river blindness, *Onchocerca volvulus*, and those which cause lymphatic filariasis, *Wuchereria bancrofti* and *Brugia malayi*. Infection with the heartworm of dogs, *Dirofilaria immitis*, may result in fatal disease and is a significant veterinary health problem. Study of *D. immitis* has provided important information on the diagnosis, treatment, and control of human filarial parasites. The focus of this chapter is on *O. volvulus* and the lymphatic filarial parasites, primarily *B. malayi*.

[*] Corresponding author.

It is important to note that most filarial nematodes, including those to be discussed here, serve as a host for an endosymbiotic *Rickettsia*-like bacteria in the genus *Wolbachia*. *Wolbachia* is essential for worm survival and a target of chemotherapeutic control [1, 2] (see Chapter 15). The endosymbiont has also been important in the pathogenesis of the inflammatory conditions associated with onchocerciasis eye pathology [3] and likely lymphatic disease [4].

Geographic Distribution, Incidence, and Disease Presentation

Approximately 120 million people are at risk for onchocerciasis. Adult worms can live for over a decade in nodules under the skin and release millions of microfilariae. Circulating microfilariae of *O. volvulus* cause persistent, debilitating itching, severe dermatitis, and ocular lesions resulting in blindness [5]. Disease manifestations are caused to some degree by the immune response to the parasite [6, 7]. According to the World Health Organization, an estimated 37 million people are infected in 36 tropical countries of Africa and Latin America [8] (http://ww.apoc.bf/en). Of these, 270 000 individuals have been blinded and an additional 500 000 are visually impaired, making onchocerciasis the second leading cause of infectious blindness world-wide. Onchocerciasis causes 46 000 new cases of blindness annually (http://ww.apoc.bf/en).

Approximately 1.3 billion people are at risk for infection with lymphatic filarial nematodes in 83 endemic countries. There are an estimated 120 million cases of lymphatic filariasis throughout the world. Roughly 40 million individuals infected with *W. bancrofti* and *B. malayi* exhibit clinical disease, which may include elephantiasis of the limbs or genitals, acute filarial fever, and potentially extensive subclinical disease involving the kidney, lung, and other organs [9].

Immunity

The long-standing observation that individuals living in endemic areas and exposed to bites of filarial-infected vectors remain free of infection has led to the supposition that naturally acquired immunity occurs in a significant portion of the population. These individuals have been classified as putatively immune or endemic normal. Using cells and sera from these individuals, and comparing their responses to specific molecules with those of infected individuals, is a standard approach to identifying antigens important in naturally acquired protective resistance (reviewed in [10]). In addition, it appears that the infected individuals are possibly protected from further new infections by concomitant immunity (i.e., newly introduced infective third-stage larvae (L3) are eliminated while adult worms and microfilariae are left unaffected) [11]. The concept of concomitant immunity was recently verified experimentally using the *Acanthocheilonema viteae* jird model [12]. Although immune responses are directed at all stages of the parasite in specific ways (reviewed in [7]) the important target of protective immune responses is likely to be L3 and/or the molting L3.

The most striking and direct results demonstrating protective mechanisms *in vitro* have come from using sera from putatively immune and infected individuals.

There have been consistent demonstrations that antibody-dependent cell-mediated cytotoxicity (ADCC) is an important aspect of protective resistance to *O. volvulus* and lymphatic filariasis. These studies showed *in vitro* a granulocyte-dependent killing of *O. volvulus* L3 using sera from both putatively immune and infected individuals [13, 14]. Studies in animal models have supported the significance of anti-L3 ADCC responses (reviewed in [15] and [16]). Other support for the importance of antibody in protection is the increase in anti-L3 IgG3 and IgE in aging patients, and the presence of L3 surface-specific antibodies in putatively immune sera [17].

Understanding the significance of specific cellular responses and cytokine release has been challenging. Early studies in human and animal models demonstrated that filarial nematodes induce a dominant helper T cell T_h2 cellular response promoting interleukin (IL)-4, -5, and -10, and their associate effects such as eosinophilia, and IgE production [7, 18]. However, in comparing the cellular responses of putatively immune and infected individuals to *O. volvulus* L3 and molting L3 antigens, significantly higher IL-5 and interferon-γ responses were seen in the putatively immune group (reviewed in [10]), indicating that a mixed T_h1/T_h2 response occurred in these individuals. Mixed T_h1/T_h2 responses have also been reported in some animal model systems (reviewed in [7]).

An important aspect of the cellular immune response to *O. volvulus* and lymphatic filariasis is the induction of a complex system for immune regulation. A focus of this regulation is the cytokines IL-10 and transforming growth factor-β. Cells involved include T regulatory cells and alternately activated macrophages, among others [19]. This nematode-induced immune regulatory system has been studied in detail and shown to also downregulate a number of inflammatory diseases, such as colitis, reactive airway disease, encephalitis, and diabetes [20]. Experimental filarial infections have also been shown to downregulate the proinflammatory induced gastric lesions associated with *Helicobacter pylori* [21]. It is possible that existing filarial infections and the associated immune regulatory networks they induce may have untoward impacts on homologous vaccinations. However, this has not been yet considered experimentally in the context of vaccination against filarial parasite.

Pathology

Filarial infections induce a spectrum of clinical presentations in patient populations ranging from exposed, apparently uninfected individuals with no easily demonstrable disease, to individuals with overt clinical disease [7, 18]. This range of disease manifestations is determined by host genetics and a complex series of immune regulatory mechanisms controlled by the presence of specific cytokines [7, 18]. The lesions and clinical signs associated with infections are often parasite stage-specific such as onchocercal blindness or pulmonary tropical eosinophilia, which are associated with microfilariae. Adult worms of lymphatic filariasis living in the lymphatics and lymph nodes induce obstructive granulomatous responses, which produce the lymphadenitis and lymphangiectasia seen in lymphatic filariasis. The immunologically mediated inflammatory responses that induce the lesions are diverse and parasite stage-specific in different infections. Some of these inflammatory responses are mediated by proinflammatory cytokines and others by IgE [7, 18]. These pathological responses might present a challenge for the development of successful protective immunization protocols if they induce concomitant immune-mediated pathology.

Treatment and Control

Mass drug administration (MDA) programs using donated drugs and directed at reducing parasite transmission and morbidity have had a major positive impact on controlling both *O. volvulus* and lymphatic filariasis, and are the center of the long-term objective of elimination [22]. The MDA programs aim to achieve a high level of coverage (65–90%) of the eligible population. For onchocerciasis, the only drug available for safe mass treatment remains ivermectin. For lymphatic filariasis, mass chemotherapy uses diethylcarbamazine plus albendazole or diethylcarbamazine alone outside of sub-Saharan Africa, whereas ivermectin plus albendazole is used in sub-Saharan Africa because of contraindications for diethylcarbamazine in patients heavily infected with *O. volvulus*. Currently, tens of millions of people in hyper- and mesoendemic areas are under annual or semiannual treatment for onchocerciasis, while hundreds of millions of people are under annual treatment for lymphatic filariasis.

There are emerging questions regarding the continued feasibility and effectiveness of these control programs. MDA has some deficiencies, which include the absence of an effective drug against the adult parasites that can be administered easily in endemic areas, difficulties inherent with the necessity of regular long-term treatments of large portions of the infected and at-risk populations, and the possibility that susceptibility to reinfection may return post-treatment [23, 24]. The most recent concern is the potential development of resistance to ivermectin [25]. In addition to the drugs currently available for MDA, the use of antibacterial agents such as doxycycline targeting *Wolbachia* have shown some promise as a macrofilaricidal agent in human trials against *O. volvulus* and lymphatic filariasis [26]. Current efforts to identify new antibacterial agents and combining these with MDA approaches may prove beneficial [27] (see also Chapter 15).

Natural Host–Parasite Systems for Onchocerciasis and Lymphatic Filariasis

Bovine Onchocerciasis: *Onchocerca ochengi* in Cattle

Studies of natural and experimental bovine infections with *O. ochengi* have demonstrated the existence of naturally occurring immunity against the L3, which is analogous to humans characterized as putatively immune. When this subset of cattle was exposed to natural challenge they were significantly less susceptible to infection than naïve control cows (reviewed in [23]). Experimental infections with *O. ochengi* have also revealed the kinetics of the immune response in relation to parasite development, and demonstrated analogous responses to those reported in

O. volvulus infection in humans and chimpanzees (reviewed in [23]), including antibody responses to some of the *O. volvulus* vaccine candidates, *Ov*-CPI-2 (Ov7), *Ov*-103 and *Ov*-B20 [28]. Moreover, vaccination with *O. ochengi* irradiation attenuated L3 (xL3) conferred resistance to severe and prolonged field challenge of cattle with *O. ochengi* L3 (53% reduction in mean adult load and a significant reduction in microfilarial prevalence and density). Cattle immunized with xL3 also had significant levels of protective immunity against experimental challenge with L3 (84% reduction in mean adult load) [29]. These results provided the first direct evidence of protective immunity in onchocerciasis and showed that immunoprophylaxis is feasible. Eight recombinant proteins, which were homologs of the *O. volvulus* vaccine candidates, were tested for efficacy in cows against a natural challenge in Cameroon [30]. The recombinant proteins were highly immunogenic and reduced patent infections in vaccinated animals by 58% on average; however, the frequency of nodules or recovery of adult worms was not significantly reduced by the vaccination. Nonetheless, the feasibility of testing vaccine candidates was demonstrated. However, logistical and economic limitations prevent the use of cows as a primary screening model for preclinical development of a recombinant *O. volvulus* vaccine.

Feline filariasis: *Brugia* spp. in Cats

The most extensive experimental studies of a natural host parasite model of lymphatic filariasis is *Brugia pahangi* in cats [31, 32]. Patterns of infections in cats with *B. pahangi* closely mimic the population patterns described for human infections with *W. bancrofti* and *B. malayi*. Infections are long-lived and repeated infections develop concomitant immunity [32]. Development of lymph edema is associated with repeated infections and immunity. Vaccination studies are limited, but xL3 have been shown to induce an 80% reduction in worm recovery in immunized cats [33]. As immunologic reagents are now more readily available for cats [34, 35], experimental studies in this system, while difficult, may be useful in the future.

Vaccinology

The fact that protective immunity develops in humans to infection with *O. volvulus* and lymphatic filariasis, and the presence of protective immunity in animals to filarial worms, suggests that vaccines against these infections are feasible. Filarial worms cannot be grown in culture, which makes live-attenuated vaccines impractical and recombinant vaccines the only viable approach to large-scale immunization. Vaccines developed against *O. volvulus* and lymphatic filariasis infections of humans may have significantly different goals, such as preventing infection or disease, respectively, and therefore specific vaccines will be required to achieve these objectives through the use of stage-specific immunity. An anti-L3 vaccine may be administered in communities that have gone through several rounds of MDA, thereby complementing the existing control measures that have the same goal of preventing *O. volvulus* and lymphatic filariasis infections. Moreover, these vaccines, when linked to chemotherapy, might avoid the need for repeated MDA and reduce the risk of drug failure or reinfection.

Prophylactic Vaccines

The objective of these vaccines will be to prevent the development of all stages of the infection in immunized hosts, including L3, fourth-stage larvae (L4), adults, and microfilariae. Clearly, the optimal method to achieve this goal would be a multivalent vaccine with components directed at eliminating both the L3 and the L4. This will prevent the development of all subsequent stages and it represents an achievable goal based on the relative size of the L3/L4 compared to the effector cells of the immune response. L3 and L4 are antigenically and physiologically distinct [36], so a vaccine directed at controlling both of these stages may be possible, and would result in a two-hit process that would potentially enhance its efficacy and reduce vaccine failure. This vaccine could be used in uninfected endemic children and travelers as a prophylaxis against acquiring primary infections. In addition, these vaccines may be used in adults living in endemic regions that have received treatment with ivermectin. Use of ivermectin in yearly MDA has little effect on adult worms of *O. volvulus* [37] and lymphatic filariasis [38]. Therefore, vaccination of treated individuals with the anti-L3/L4 vaccine would induce concomitant immunity, in that protective immunity develops to reinfection while leaving the adults from the current infection intact. This would prevent an increase in adult worm infection levels and diminish the chronicity of the infection. It is acknowledged that filarial infections induce a spectrum of disease manifestations related to the level and type of immune responses induced [39]. Within the spectrum of disease presentations, there may be some forms for which this vaccine would not be appropriate, such as patients with hypo- or hyper-reactivity to some of the filarial vaccine antigens.

Antipathology Vaccine

The objective of this vaccine would be to eliminate the stage of the parasite that causes pathology in the host. An advantage of this approach is that sterile immunity is not required for the vaccine to be effective. For lymphatic filariasis, the primary source of pathology is the presence of adult worms in the lymphatic vessels [40]. A prophylactic vaccine that eliminated L3/L4 would also eliminate adult worms. Although there has been some success with this approach, targeting antigens found in the worm's intestine [41], the relative size and location of the adult worms make this approach formidable. Pathology associated with infection with *O. volvulus* is caused by the presence of microfilariae in the skin or eyes [42]. The target of an antipathology vaccine designed for *O. volvulus* would be the elimination of the microfilariae, with the goal of killing these worms in a manner that does not cause or exacerbate pathology. This vaccine would be appropriate for use in uninfected individuals to prevent infection and thus the development of disease, and would likely be counterproductive in infected individuals because of the danger of aggravating the immune response to the microfilariae. As an alternative approach, the antipathology vaccine could be directed at the *Wolbachia* found in the adult and microfilariae. Treatment of infected individuals with doxycycline to eliminate *Wolbachia* in adult worms results in reduced fecundity of the female worms and thereby reduced numbers of microfilariae reaching the eyes [26]. In addition, reducing the immune response to *Wolbachia* released by microfilariae in the eye or altering the type of immune response to the bacteria would also eliminate or reduce pathology. Vaccine-induced immune responses against *Wolbachia* resulted in enhanced survival of *Litomosoides sigmodontis* in mice [43], thus exacerbating rather than preventing disease – obviously, an unappealing vaccine approach.

Antitransmission Vaccine

Infections with *O. volvulus* and lymphatic filariasis caused by *W. bancrofti* are restricted to human hosts. The fact that these are not zoonoses means that reducing infection in the human population will have a direct and dramatic effect on transmission. The altruistic antitransmission vaccine would target the microfilariae or *Wolbachia*, as described above. This vaccine would have limited use in *O. volvulus* populations because of the possibility of exacerbated disease, but may be of use in the control of lymphatic filariasis.

Panhelmintic Vaccine

One of the interesting observations noted in analyzing the antigens that have been used in vaccines against filarial worms is that the antigens that have efficacy against *O. volvulus* usually have homologs that are efficacious against lymphatic filariasis and vice versa (see below). In addition, many of the antigens functional in filarial vaccines have homologs that have proven useful in vaccines against other helminths. It is therefore possible to conjecture that there are shared antigens between filarial worms and other helminths that could be used in panhelminthic vaccines. Specific critical epitopes that are shared between the worms would be used as the vaccine targets. Advantages using this approach would be to vaccinate against several filarial worms and other nematodes with a single injection. Also, the memory response would be maintained by environmental boosting by a variety of parasites. This approach also highlights a potential risk with filarial vaccines if the vaccine antigens are shared with other parasites. There is the danger that an immune response that is protective against the filarial worm may induce immunopathological responses to other parasites with shared antigens.

Current Status of Filarial Vaccine Development

Animal Models

The selection of animal models for the development of human vaccines is complicated and controversial. In the ideal situation, one would be able to use the parasite species that is the target of the vaccine in a fully permissive host that develops lesions and clinical symptoms similar to those in humans. Furthermore, such systems would allow detailed immunologic measurements and manipulations. However, for the most part, filarial nematodes possess a marked degree of host specificity, thus limiting the numbers of animal models that can be used to study immunity and/or vaccines (reviewed in [23, 44]). Consequently, compromises must be made that either involve using (i) nonhuman parasites in mice, (ii) human parasites that will develop in mice for at least part of their life cycle, or (iii) human parasites in nonmurine hosts that lack the advantage of access to inbred strains and the depth of immunologic analyses available for mice.

Animal Models Used for Lymphatic Filariae Vaccine Studies
Aside from humans, *W. bancrofti* only infects the silvered leaf monkey [45, 46], which has allowed for some studies on pathogenesis, although it is not a suitable model for vaccine development because of the scarcity of parasite material and host. Both the human parasite, *B. malayi*, and the natural parasite of dogs and cats, *B. pahangi*, infect a wide range of hosts, including rhesus macaques [47], dogs [48, 49], cats [32], short-term infections in some strains of mice [50, 51], rats [52], ferrets [53], hamsters [54], and the multimammate mouse, *Mastomys* spp. [55]. The permissive Mongolian gerbil or jird, *Meriones unguicualtus*, has been used extensively in vaccine studies using *B. malayi* and *B. pahangi*. A significant protective immune response was mounted in jirds following immunization with *Brugia* xL3 [56, 57], and antibody to surface antigens and ADCC reactions were associated with protective immunity in these studies [57, 58]. The *Brugia*–jird model has also been effectively used to test protection induced by single recombinant molecules (Table 23.1). Marked reduction of worm burden (76%) was seen using *Bm*-ALT-1 in Freund's Complete adjuvant (FCA) [59]. *Bm*-ALT-2 decreased L3 survival by 72% when placed in peritoneal diffusion chambers [60]. More than a 90% reduction in microfilariae production was seen after immunization with *Bm*-SXP-1 or *Bm*-chitinase [61, 62]. *Bm*-ASP-1 decreased L3 survival in diffusion chambers by 62% [60]. A 76% protection against *B. malayi* challenge was also seen following immunization with a native collagenase purified from *Setaria cervi* – a filarial nematode of bovines [63]. Jird antibodies to this protein inhibited enzymatic activity and promoted an ADCC reaction using jird peritoneal exudate cells *in vitro*. In diffusion chambers implanted inside immunized jirds, host cells migrated and adhered to the microfilariae and L3, killing a significant number within 48 h [64]. Protection against *B. malayi* L3 and microfilariae was 67–69% after immunization of jirds with *Bm*-37 – a recombinant protein recognized by putatively immune/endemic normal sera [65]. The importance of glutathione S-transferase (GST) to parasite survival in jirds was also tested; vaccination decreased a *B. malayi* challenge infection by 61%. Moreover, human and mouse anti-GST antibodies had a cytotoxic effect in an ADCC assay against L3 [66]. Immunization with *B. malayi* recombinant myosin resulted in a 76% reduction in microfilarial burden and a 54–58% lower adult worm burden, conferred through the induction of both humoral and cellular immunity [67]. In addition, a microfilarial derived 38-kDa protease isolated from

Table 23.1 Analogous O. volvulus and lymphatic filariae vaccine candidates.

O. volvulus (accession/gene name)	Percent protection [model, adjuvant] (reviewed in [15, 72])	Lymphatic filariae (accession/gene name)	Percent protection lymphatic filariae models [animal model, adjuvant]	Protection in other helminth models [model, adjuvant]
Ov-CPI-2 (M37105)	43–49 [mice, alum/BC]	Bm-CPI-1 (AAC47623)	Ls-cystatin 50% reduction in patent infection [Ls mouse model, alum and Pam3Cys] [117]	Ac-cystatin; 22% reduction in worm burden [Ac dog model, AS03] (P.J. Hotez, unpublished)
Ov-ASP-1 (AF020586)	44 [mice, alum/FCA]	Bm-ASP-1	62% reduction in survival of L3 in chamber [jird, alum] [60]	Ac-ASP-2; 26% reduction in worm burden; 69% reduction in egg output; 60% reduction in L3 migration in vitro using serum from the vaccinated dogs [Ac dog model, AS03] [118]
Ov-RAL-2 (U00693)	51–60 [mice, BC/FCA]	(Bm-VAL-1/WbVAH) (Bm1_14040) Bm-SXP-1 (Bm1_42870)	Bm-ASP-1 + Bm-ALT-2: 79% reduction in worm burden [jird, alum] [60] rWb-SXP/Bm14; 30% reduction of L3 survival within chambers [mice, FCA] [119] rBm-SXP-1; >90% reduction in microfilaremia and 35% in adult worm burden [jird, FCA, alum] [61]	rAs16; 64% reduction in A. suum L3 [mice, cholera toxin] rAs16; 58% reduction in A. suum lung–stage L3s [pigs, cholera toxin] rAc-16; 25% reduction in worm burden, 64% reduction in egg count [Ac dog model; AS03] (P.J. Hotez, unpublished)
Ov-ALT-1 (U96176)	39–62 [mice, alum]	Bm-ALT-1 (AF183572)	Bm-ALT-1; 76% reduction in worm burden [jird, FCA] [59]	ALT-1 and ALT-2 are filariae-specific proteins

(Continued)

Table 23.1 (Continued)

O. volvulus (accession/gene name)	Percent protection [model, adjuvant] (reviewed in [15, 72])	Lymphatic filariae (accession/gene name)	Percent protection lymphatic filariae models [animal model, adjuvant]	Protection in other helminth models [model, adjuvant]
		Bm-ALT-2 (U84723)	Bm-ALT-2; 72% reduction in survival of L3 in chamber [jird, alum] [60, 119] Bm-ALT-2 + Bm-ASP-1; 79% reduction in worm burden [jird, alum] [60, 119]	
Ov-103 (M55155)	69 [mice, alum]	Bm1_01550	ND	Ac-SAA-1; antibodies inhibited (46%) migration of L3 [Ac, FCA] [90]
Ov-B20 (L41928)	39 [mice, alum];	AAL91105/AAL91104	49–60% [Av jird, FCA] [81, 120]	ND
Ov-RBP-1 (L27686)	42 [mice, BC]	Bm1_41425	36–55% [Av jird, FCA] [81, 120]	ND
Ov-CHI-1 (U14639)	53 [mice, DNA]	Bm-chitinase (Bm1_28620/ Bm1_17035)	48% reduction in worm burden and >90% in microfilariae [Av jird, FCA, alum] [61, 62]	ND
Ov-GST (L28771)	was not protective	Wb-GST (HM590636)	61% reduction in worm burden [Bm jird, alum] [66]	Na-GST-1: 32–39% reductions in adult hookworm burdens [Na, hamster, alum] [91] Ac-GST-1 39% worm burden reduction [Ac, dog, alum]; Ac-GST-1 51–54% worm burden reduction [Na, hamster, alum] [91, 92]

ND, not done; ALT, abundant larval transcript; ASP, activation-associated secreted protein; CHI, chitinase; CPI, cysteine proteinase inhibitor; GST, glutathione S-transferase; RAL, rabbit antilarvae; RBP, retinol-binding protein; SAA, surface-associated antigen; VAH, venom allergen antigen homolog; VAL, VAH/ASP-like.

B. malayi [68] and a zinc-containing 175-kDa collagenase [63] also induced significant protection against *B. malayi* in jirds.

Animal Models Used for O. volvulus Vaccine Studies
Chimpanzees are susceptible to *O. volvulus* infection, but these nonhuman primates are not suitable for large-scale investigations [69]. Comprehensive studies on immunity to *O. volvulus* L3 were done in mice using xL3s (reviewed in [23]). Although *O. volvulus* L3 do not develop into adult worms in mice, it is possible to study antilarval immunity by placing *O. volvulus* L3 in diffusion chambers. Protective immunity induced by xL3s in the *O. volvulus*–mouse model (around 50%) was dependent on T_h2 cytokines, IgE, eosinophils, and a direct contact between host cells and the parasites (reviewed in [10] and [70]).

Although mice are not permissive hosts for *O. volvulus*, the *O. volvulus*–mouse model employing *O. volvulus* L3 in diffusion chambers has nonetheless demonstrated the antilarval protective efficacy and immunological correlates using recombinant *O. volvulus* antigens (r*Ov*Ags). Fifteen out of 44 proteins tested in the *O. volvulus*–mouse model induced partial, but statistically significant, protection (30–69%) against L3 challenge in the presence of the adjuvants block copolymer (BC), alum, or FCA (reviewed in [71, 72]). Of these, 12 were identified by immunoscreening and the other three proteins were cloned using polymerase chain reaction (PCR) approaches (reviewed in [10, 72]). Only one additional antigen with protective properties, *Ov*-GAPDH, which was cloned using immunoscreening, has been recently reported [73].

Notably, the putative mechanisms of protective immunity elicited by vaccination with the r*Ov*Ags were more similar to those described in protected humans than in the xL3-vaccine model. Both T_h2 and/or T_h1 protective immunity was induced in mice by the r*Ov*Ags, and the protective T_h2 response did not appear to require IgE or eosinophils. This conclusion was based on the type of adjuvant used to induce protective immunity (alum as a T_h2 adjuvant and FCA as a T_h1 adjuvant) and the induced antibody isotype response (reviewed in [71, 72]). The recombinant antigens *Ov*-CPI-2, *Ov*-ALT-1, *Ov*-103, *Ov*-B20, *Ov*-B8, *Ov*-TMY-1, and *Av*-ABC were protective only in the presence of alum. The antibody responses were dominated by IgG1 with minimal IgE levels, which suggested a T_h2 response that does not appear to require IgE [71]. No increase in either eosinophil numbers or levels of eotaxin in the diffusion chambers was observed after immunization with *Ov*-CPI-2, *Ov*-ALT-1, *Ov*-B8, or *Ov*-103. In contrast, *Ov*-RAL-2, *Ov*-FBA-1, and *Av*-UBI were protective only in the presence of FCA, with an apparent T_h1 response based on an elevated IgG2a antibody response [72, 74]. *Ov*-ASP-1 was protective in the presence of alum or FCA [75]. The mechanisms of protective immunity induced by the two adjuvants with *Ov*-ASP-1 differed in that IgG1 dominated the response induced by alum and IgG2a dominated that induced by FCA. The ability of *Ov*-RBP-1, *Ov*-CAL-1, and OI5/OI3 to induce significant protection was only tested using BC as the adjuvant. *Ov*-CHI-1 effectively induced protection using DNA immunization [62]. Therefore, individual r*Ov*Ags can induce immunity through T_h1, T_h2, or mixed T_h1/T_h2 responses that do not appear to require IgE or eosinophils.

Although the discrepancies between responses to xL3 and rOvAgs may be due to differences in the immunization protocols, it was hypothesized that they may actually reflect intrinsic immunological properties of these vaccine antigens. This was supported by the observation that four of the native L3 proteins recognized by rOvAg-specific antibodies were not recognized by anti-xL3 antibodies; however, all of them are recognized by IgG1 and/or IgG3 cytophilic antibodies from putatively immune or individuals who developed concomitant immunity [10]. Therefore, the rOvAg-induced protective responses in mice are apparently quite similar to those observed in humans – a finding that confirms the O. volvulus–mouse model as a reliable system to evaluate O. volvulus vaccine antigens for antilarval protective immunity.

Models Using Nonhuman Parasites in Rodents
Two host–parasite systems have been employed as models for O. volvulus and lymphatic filariasis to study immunity and vaccination. While neither infection produces lesions similar to the human parasites, both host–parasite systems have provided considerable data on antifilarial immunity. A. viteae infects a number of laboratory rodent hosts including gerbils, multimammate rats, and hamsters [76]. In hamsters a strong protective antibody-dependent response develops against microfilariae [77], while jirds and multimammate rats support prolonged microfilaremia. Vaccination with xL3 induced protective immunity against infection in hamsters and jirds [78]. Eosinophil-mediated killing of L3 [23] occurred in the subcutaneous tissues of the vaccinated hosts, and recombinant A. viteae tropomyosin [79], O. volvulus tropomyosin [80], and Ov-B20 [81] antigens offered some protection in the jirds. L. sigmodontis, a natural parasite of cotton rats, completes its life cycle in mice with varying degrees of development depending on strain. This system has been used in studies of protective immunity and immune regulation (reviewed in [44]). Protective immunity can be induced by xL3 vaccination and appears to target incoming L3 (reviewed in [44]). Studies with gene-deficient mice showed that vaccination success depends on IL-5 and antibody [82, 83], which is consistent with the observations made for O. volvulus in mice [70]. Immune protection generated by L. sigmodontis xL3 leads to rapid destruction of the challenge larvae in the subcutaneous tissue [84, 85] and long-lived protection [86]. Gene expression data from L. sigmodontis have shown clearly that the most abundantly expressed genes from the L3 stage of B. malayi and O. volvulus are also highly abundant in L. sigmodontis [87]. Powerful genomic and proteomic tools are now available ([87] and http://www.nematodes.org/nembase4/libSpec.php), which will help to identify both targets of immunity and potential immune regulators.

Comparative Vaccine Studies
Interestingly, seven of the 15 O. volvulus protecting antigens are also protective for B. malayi in jirds, L. sigmodontis in mice, and/or A. viteae in jirds (Table 23.1). Moreover, three of seven of the O. volvulus and lymphatic filariasis vaccine candidates were also tested for protection in other nematode host–parasite systems and found to decrease worm burdens or provide other evidence of protective immunity, such as

reduction of blood loss or the induction of antibodies that reduce larva migration through the skin. These include (i) *Ov*-ASP-1 and *Bm*-ASP-1 homologs to the hookworms vaccine, *Na*-ASP-2 [88]; (ii) *Ac*-cystatin, the hookworm homolog of *Ov*-CPI-2 and Ls-cystatin; and (iii) r*Ac*-16 and r*As*-16, the hookworm and *A. suum* homologs, respectively, of *Ov*-RAL-2 and *Bm*-SXP-1 [89] (Table 23.1). In addition, the hookworm homolog of *Ov*-103, *Ac*-SAA-1, induced a partial protection against hookworm infection (25%), a 64% decrease in egg count, and a significant decrease in blood loss [90]. Finally, the hookworm homologs of *Wb*-GST, *Ac*-GST-1 and *Na*-GST-1, decreased worm burdens after challenge with canine and human hookworms [91, 92]. These comparative vaccine studies suggest that functionally conserved nematode L3 proteins are essential for the establishment of infection by filarial worms and, therefore, are ideal components of vaccines against these infections.

Multivalent Vaccines

Multivalent vaccines have been produced for various pathogens with the objective of overcoming antigenic variability in the organism [93] or host variability in epitope recognition [94]. Among the approaches taken has been inclusion of both B- and T-cell epitopes in the vaccine [95]. The complex life cycle of *O. volvulus* and *B. malayi*, with multiple stages having unique characteristics and the multicellular nature of the parasite, makes the multivalent vaccine approach reasonable. It has also been proposed that multivalent recombinant vaccines can target two pathogens such as hookworms and *Schistosoma* when a majority of the endemic area's individuals are coinfected [96]. Initial attempts to combine *O. volvulus* vaccine proteins based on the T_h1 (FCA) or T_h2 (alum) adjuvant used for inducing protection demonstrated that the individual antigens when combined within the immunization protocol had immunodominant or immunosuppressive properties [71]. Support for the multivalent vaccine approach is found in vaccine studies using *B. malayi* vaccine antigens. The combination of *Bm*-ALT-2 and *Bm*-VAH (also known as *Bm*-ASP-1) induced enhanced immune responses and protection in jirds when compared with single-antigen vaccination of the jirds [60, 97]. More recent studies have shown that a combination of three proteins, *Wb*-HSP, *Wb*-ALT-2, and *Wb*-TSP, shown to be protective individually or as a combination of two [98–100], were highly effective when used as a multivalent protein or DNA vaccine and can induce almost 100% protection (Ramaswamy K., unpublished results).

Discovery of New Vaccine Candidates

Protective immunity in humans against lymphatic filariasis and *O. volvulus* L3 is associated with T_h1 and T_h2 responses and ADCC [10]. Importantly, the function of antibodies in protective immunity provided the rationale for the most used strategy to clone putative lymphatic filariasis and *O. volvulus* antigens for use in vaccine studies, namely immunoscreening of cDNA libraries using immune sera from human or animal hosts (reviewed in [15, 44, 72]). Although this approach was used with success, it does not take into account carbohydrate and other nonprotein determinants, important in other helminth systems [101–104] and which could be crucial for the generation of protective immunity.

A second strategy for cloning vaccine candidates is to isolate molecules thought to be vital in the infection process. These would include proteins with vital metabolic functions or defense properties, which permit the parasite to survive in immunocompetent hosts. Targeting such molecules would block the establishment of the parasite in the host. In addition, antigens that are not normally seen by the host but that are, nevertheless, accessible to host immune effector molecules and cells, the "hidden antigens," would also be potentially useful as vaccine targets [105]. Isolation of the gene encoding the protein of interest was achieved by (i) screening a cDNA library using a heterologous probe [106], (ii) PCR cloning using degenerate primers [106], (iii) purifying the protein followed by partial amino acid sequencing and molecular cloning [107], or (iv) identifying the gene of interest by searching the *O. volvulus* and *B. malayi* expressed sequence tag databases as well as the available filarial genomic databases [108, 109].

Infections with filarial worms are successful because of their ability to control regulatory pathways. Bypassing this regulation may be the key to development of a vaccine and future disease control. This will require a thorough understanding of how the parasite induces regulation and identification of the targets and processes that mediate a protective but nonpathological response. A large-scale, proteomic analysis of the excretory/secretory (ES) products of the L3, L3 to L4 molting, adult male, adult female, and microfilariae stages of the filarial parasite *B. malayi* provides extended insight into the host–parasite interaction [110, 111]. The reported abundance of a number of previously characterized immunomodulatory proteins in the ES products of microfilariae increases the chances of identifying novel vaccine candidates that will either alter the immune response from tolerant to effector or change an immunopathological response into one that is protective [110].

The recent availability of comprehensive genomic, proteomic, and transcriptomic datasets from human and nonhuman filarial parasites provides new opportunities for vaccine discovery [109–112]. These databases can be mined to identify promising vaccine candidate antigens by proteome-wide screening of antibody and T-cell reactivity using specimens from individuals exposed to filariae, but protected from chronic infections and disease. The existence of the *B. malayi* genome [109] and partial genomes for *O. volvulus, O. ochengi, W. bancrofti* and *Loa loa* (http://www.sanger.ac.uk/sequencing/Onchocerca/volvulus; http://xyala.cap.ed.ac.uk/downloads/959nematodegenomes/blast/blast.php; http://www.broadinstitute.org/annotation/genome/filarial_worms/GenomesIndex.html), when combined with technology platforms such as protein arrays, high-throughput protein production, and epitope prediction algorithms, should provide opportunities to identify antigens that, either alone or in combination, function as targets for a naturally acquired immunity against filariae. These approaches permit large-scale seroepidemiological, longitudinal, and sero-surveillance analyses, and measure immunoreactive responses at various stages of the infectious process in a manner not previously possible [113]. Immunomic approaches that enable the selection of the best possible targets by prioritizing antigens according to clinically relevant criteria may overcome the problem of poorly immunogenic, poorly protective vaccines that has plagued antiparasitic vaccine development [114].

Conclusions

It is clear that the development of vaccines against infection by filarial worms remains an achievable goal. Despite the progress outlined herein, there is no vaccine currently in human trials. However, significant progress has been made in the development of vaccines against *Taenia solium* for use in pigs [115, 116] (see also Chapter 29), hookworm for use in humans (see also Chapter 21), and *Schistosoma* spp. for use in humans [96] (see also Chapter 25). These advances encourage the development of filarial vaccines for use in humans. Moreover, new filarial antigens are being identified using the *O. ochengi*–cattle model and *L. sigmodontis* in mice (http://filaria.eu/projects/projects/epiaf.html), which might provide new and more effective vaccine components. Importantly, new adjuvants are being developed and tested for safety and potency in humans, and these will be valuable.

Multivalent vaccines are an attractive, alternative approach to single-antigen vaccines based on the broad range of targets that may potentiate vaccine efficacy and result in high levels of protective immunity. Decreased adult worm burdens will reduce the number of microfilariae produced by the adult female worms, and, thus, both pathology and the rates of transmission. As the majority of the populations at risk might already be participants in MDA programs, it is anticipated that these vaccines will be deployed in conjunction with the relevant chemotherapy and, thus, support global elimination while helping sustain the limited anthelminthic pharmacopeia currently available (see also Chapter 22).

References

1. Slatko, B.E., Taylor, M.J., and Foster, J.M. (2010) The *Wolbachia* endosymbiont as an anti-filarial nematode target. *Symbiosis*, **51**, 55–65.
2. Taylor, M.J., Hoerauf, A., and Bockarie, M. (2010) Lymphatic filariasis and onchocerciasis. *Lancet*, **376**, 1175–1185.
3. Pearlman, E. and Gillette-Ferguson, I. (2007) *Onchocerca volvulus*, *Wolbachia* and river blindness. *Chem. Immunol. Allergy*, **92**, 254–265.
4. Taylor, M.J., Bandi, C., and Hoerauf, A. (2005) *Wolbachia* bacterial endosymbionts of filarial nematodes. *Adv. Parasitol.*, **60**, 245–284.
5. Richards, F.O. Jr, Boatin, B., Sauerbrey, M., and Seketeli, A. (2001) Control of onchocerciasis today: status and challenges. *Trends Parasitol.*, **17**, 558–563.
6. Ottesen, E.A. (1995) Immune responsiveness and the pathogenesis of human onchocerciasis. *J. Infect Dis.*, **171**, 659–671.
7. Hoerauf, A. and Brattig, N. (2002) Resistance and susceptibility in human onchocerciasis – beyond T_h1 vs. T_h2. *Trends Parasitol.*, **18**, 25–31.

8. Noma, M., Nwoke, B.E., Nutall, I., Tambala, P.A., Enyong, P., Namsenmo, A., Remme, J. et al. (2002) Rapid epidemiological mapping of onchocerciasis (REMO): its application by the African Programme for Onchocerciasis Control (APOC). *Ann. Trop. Med. Parasitol.*, **96** (Suppl. 1), S29–S39.

9. World Health Organization (2002) *TDR Strategic Direction for Research: Lymphatic Filariasis*, WHO, Geneva.

10. Lustigman, S., MacDonald, A.J., and Abraham, D. (2003) $CD4^+$ dependent immunity to *Onchocerca volvulus* third-stage larvae in humans and the mouse vaccination model: common ground and distinctions. *Int. J. Parasitol.*, **33**, 1161–1171.

11. Trees, A.J., Graham, S.P., Renz, A., Bianco, A.E., and Tanya, V. (2000) *Onchocerca ochengi* infections in cattle as a model for human onchocerciasis: recent developments. *Parasitology*, **120** (Suppl.), S133–S142.

12. Rajakumar, S., Bleiss, W., Hartmann, S., Schierack, P., Marko, A., and Lucius, R. (2006) Concomitant immunity in a rodent model of filariasis: the infection of *Meriones unguiculatus* with *Acanthocheilonema viteae*. *J. Parasitol.*, **92**, 41–45.

13. Day, K.P., Gregory, W.F., and Maizels, R.M. (1991) Age-specific acquisition of immunity to infective larvae in a bancroftian filariasis endemic area of Papua New Guinea. *Parasite Immunol.*, **13**, 277–290.

14. Johnson, E.H., Irvine, M., Kass, P.H., Browne, J., Abdullai, M., Prince, A.M., and Lustigman, S. (1994) *Onchocerca volvulus*: *in vitro* cytotoxic effects of human neutrophils and serum on third-stage larvae. *Trop. Med. Parasitol.*, **45**, 331–335.

15. Lustigman, S. and Abraham, D. (2009) Onchocerciasis, in *Vaccines for Biodefense and Emerging and Neglected Diseases* (eds A.D.T. Barrett and L.R. Stanberry), Academic Press, New York, pp. 1379–1400.

16. Cho-Ngwa, F., Liu, J., and Lustigman, S. (2010) The *Onchocerca volvulus* cysteine proteinase inhibitor, *Ov*-CPI-2, is a target of protective antibody response that increases with age. *PLoS Negl. Trop. Dis.*, **4**, e800.

17. MacDonald, A.J., Turaga, P.S., Harmon-Brown, C., Tierney, T.J., Bennett, K.E., McCarthy, M.C., Simonek, S.C. et al. (2002) Differential cytokine and antibody responses to adult and larval stages of *Onchocerca volvulus* consistent with the development of concomitant immunity. *Infect. Immun.*, **70**, 2796–2804.

18. Ottesen, E.A. (1992) The Wellcome Trust Lecture. Infection and disease in lymphatic filariasis: an immunological perspective. *Parasitology*, **104** (Suppl.), S71–S79.

19. Hoerauf, A., Satoguina, J., Saeftel, M., and Specht, S. (2005) Immunomodulation by filarial nematodes. *Parasite Immunol.*, **27**, 417–429.

20. Elliott, D.E., Summers, R.W., and Weinstock, J.V. (2007) Helminths as governors of immune-mediated inflammation. *Int. J. Parasitol.*, **37**, 457–464.

21. Martin, H.R., Shakya, K.P., Muthupalani, S., Ge, Z., Klei, T.R., Whary, M.T., and Fox, J.G. (2010) *Brugia filariasis* differentially modulates persistent *Helicobacter pylori* gastritis in the gerbil model. *Microbes Infect.*, **12**, 748–758.

22. Hoerauf, A., Pfarr, K., Mand, S., Debrah, A.Y., and Specht, S. (2011) Filariasis in Africa – treatment challenges and prospects. *Clin. Microbiol. Infect.*, **17**, 977–985.

23. Abraham, D., Lucius, R., and Trees, A.J. (2002) Immunity to *Onchocerca* spp. in animal hosts. *Trends Parasitol.*, **18**, 164–171.

24. Njongmeta, L.M., Nfon, C.K., Gilbert, J., Makepeace, B.L., Tanya, V.N., and Trees, A.J. (2004) Cattle protected from onchocerciasis by ivermectin are highly susceptible to infection after drug withdrawal. *Int. J. Parasitol.*, **34**, 1069–1074.

25. Osei-Atweneboana, M.Y., Awadzi, K., Attah, S.K., Boakye, D.A., Gyapong, J.O.,

and Prichard, R.K. (2011) Phenotypic evidence of emerging ivermectin resistance in *Onchocerca volvulus*. *PLoS Negl. Trop. Dis.*, **5**, e998.

26 Hoerauf, A. (2008) Filariasis: new drugs and new opportunities for lymphatic filariasis and onchocerciasis. *Curr. Opin. Infect. Dis.*, **21**, 673–681.

27 Kazura, J.W. (2010) Higher-dose, more frequent treatment of *Wuchereria bancrofti*. *Clin. Infect. Dis.*, **51**, 1236–1237.

28 Graham, S.P., Lustigman, S., Trees, A.J., and Bianco, A.E. (2000) *Onchocerca volvulus*: comparative analysis of antibody responses to recombinant antigens in two animal models of onchocerciasis. *Exp. Parasitol.*, **94**, 158–162.

29 Tchakoute, V.L., Graham, S.P., Jensen, S.A., Makepeace, B.L., Nfon, C.K., Njongmeta, L.M., Lustigman, S. *et al.* (2006) In a bovine model of onchocerciasis, protective immunity exists naturally, is absent in drug-cured hosts, and is induced by vaccination. *Proc. Natl. Acad. Sci. USA*, **103**, 5971–5976.

30 Makepeace, B.L., Jensen, S.A., Laney, S.J., Nfon, C.K., Njongmeta, L.M., Tanya, V.N., Williams, S.A. *et al.* (2009) Immunisation with a multivalent, subunit vaccine reduces patent infection in a natural bovine model of onchocerciasis during intense field exposure. *PLoS Negl. Trop. Dis.*, **3**, e544.

31 Denham, D.A. and Fletcher, C. (1987) The cat infected with *Brugia pahangi* as a model of human filariasis. *Ciba Found Symp.*, **127**, 225–235.

32 Grenfell, B.T., Michael, E., and Denham, D.A. (1991) A model for the dynamics of human lymphatic filariasis. *Parasitol. Today*, **7**, 318–323.

33 Oothuman, P., Denham, D.A., McGreevy, P.B., Nelson, G.S., and Rogers, R. (1979) Successful vaccination of cats against *Brugia pahangi* with larvae attenuated by irradiation with 10 krad cobalt 60. *Parasite Immunol.*, **1**, 209–216.

34 Harley, R., Helps, C.R., Harbour, D.A., Gruffydd-Jones, T.J., and Day, M.J. (1999) Cytokine mRNA expression in lesions in cats with chronic gingivostomatitis. *Clin. Diagn. Lab. Immunol.*, **6**, 471–478.

35 Reinero, C.R. (2009) Feline immunoglobulin E: historical perspective, diagnostics and clinical relevance. *Vet. Immunol. Immunopathol.*, **132**, 13–20.

36 Irvine, M., Johnson, E.H., and Lustigman, S. (1997) Identification of larval-stage-specific antigens of *Onchocerca volvulus* uniquely recognized by putative immune sera from humans and vaccination sera from animal models. *Ann. Trop. Med. Parasitol.*, **91**, 67–77.

37 Awadzi, K., Attah, S.K., Addy, E.T., Opoku, N.O., and Quartey, B.T. (1999) The effects of high-dose ivermectin regimens on *Onchocerca volvulus* in onchocerciasis patients. *Trans. R. Soc. Trop. Med. Hyg.*, **93**, 189–194.

38 Dreyer, G., Addiss, D., Santos, A., Figueredo-Silva, J., and Noroes, J. (1998) Direct assessment *in vivo* of the efficacy of combined single-dose ivermectin and diethylcarbamazine against adult *Wuchereria bancrofti*. *Trans. R. Soc. Trop. Med. Hyg.*, **92**, 219–222.

39 Ottesen, E.A. (1980) Immunopathology of lymphatic filariasis. *Springer Semin. Immunopathol.*, **2**, 373–385.

40 Dreyer, G., Noroes, J., Figueredo-Silva, J., and Piessens, W.F. (2000) Pathogenesis of lymphatic disease in bancroftian filariasis: a clinical perspective. *Parasitol. Today*, **16**, 544–548.

41 McGonigle, S., Yoho, E.R., and James, E.R. (2001) Immunisation of mice with fractions derived from the intestines of *Dirofilaria immitis*. *Int. J. Parasitol.*, **31**, 1459–1466.

42 Connor, D.H., George, G.H., and Gibson, D.W. (1985) Pathologic changes of human onchocerciasis: implications for future research. *Rev. Infect. Dis.*, **7**, 809–819.

43 Lamb, T.J., Harris, A., Le Goff, L., Read, A.F., and Allen, J.E. (2008) *Litomosoides sigmodontis*: vaccine-induced immune responses against *Wolbachia* surface protein can enhance the survival of filarial nematodes during primary infection. *Exp. Parasitol.*, **118**, 285–289.

44 Allen, J.E., Adjei, O., Bain, O., Hoerauf, A., Hoffmann, W.H.,

Makepeace, B.L., Schulz-Key, H. et al. (2008) Of mice, cattle, and humans: the immunology and treatment of river blindness. *PLoS Negl. Trop. Dis.*, **2**, e217.

45 Palmieri, J.R., Connor, D.H., and Purnomo and Marwoto, H.A. (1983) Bancroftian filariasis. *Wuchereria bancrofti* infection in the silvered leaf monkey (*Presbytis cristatus*). *Am. J. Pathol.*, **112**, 383–386.

46 Dube, A., Murthy, P.K., Puri, S.K., and Misra-Bhattacharya, S. (2004) *Presbytis entellus*: a primate model for parasitic disease research. *Trends Parasitol.*, **20**, 358–360.

47 Dennis, V.A., Lasater, B.L., Blanchard, J.L., Lowrie, R.C. Jr, and Campeau, R.J. (1998) Histopathological, lymphoscintigraphical, and immunological changes in the inguinal lymph nodes of rhesus monkeys during the early course of infection with *Brugia malayi*. *Exp. Parasitol.*, **89**, 143–152.

48 Schacher, J.F., Edeson, J.F., Sulahian, A., and Rizk, G. (1973) An 18-month longitudinal lymphographic study of filarial diseases in dogs infected with *Brugia pahangi* (Buckley and Edeson, 1956). *Ann. Trop. Med. Parasitol.*, **67**, 81–94.

49 Miller, S., Snowden, K., Schreuer, D., and Hammerberg, B. (1990) Selective breeding of dogs for segregation of limb edema from microfilaremia as clinical manifestations of *Brugia* infections. *Am. J. Trop. Med. Hyg.*, **43**, 489–497.

50 Lawrence, R.A. and Devaney, E. (2001) Lymphatic filariasis: parallels between the immunology of infection in humans and mice. *Parasite Immunol.*, **23**, 353–361.

51 Rajan, T.V., Ganley, L., Paciorkowski, N., Spencer, L., Klei, T.R., and Shultz, L.D. (2002) Brugian infections in the peritoneal cavities of laboratory mice: kinetics of infection and cellular responses. *Exp. Parasitol.*, **100**, 235–247.

52 Bell, R.G., Adams, L., Coleman, S., Negrao-Correa, D., and Klei, T.R. (1999) *Brugia pahangi*: quantitative analysis of infection in several inbred rat strains. *Exp. Parasitol.*, **92**, 120–130.

53 Hines, S.A., Crandall, R.B., Crandall, C.A., and Thompson, J.P. (1989) Lymphatic filariasis. *Brugia malayi* infection in the ferret (*Mustela putorius furo*). *Am. J. Pathol.*, **134**, 1373–1376.

54 Carraway, J.H. and Malone, J.B. (1985) *Brugia pahangi*: comparative susceptibility of the Mongolian jird, *Meriones unguiculatus*, and the PD4 inbred hamster, *Mesocricetus auratus*. *Exp. Parasitol.*, **59**, 68–73.

55 Shakya, S., Singh, P.K., Kushwaha, S., and Misra-Bhattacharya, S. (2009) Adult *Brugia malayi* approximately 34kDa (BMT-5) antigen offers T_h1 mediated significant protection against infective larval challenge in *Mastomys coucha*. *Parasitol. Int.*, **58**, 346–353.

56 Yates, J.A. and Higashi, G.I. (1985) *Brugia malayi*: vaccination of jirds with ^{60}cobalt-attenuated infective stage larvae protects against homologous challenge. *Am. J. Trop. Med. Hyg.*, **34**, 1132–1137.

57 Weil, G.J., Li, B.W., Liftis, F., and Chandrashekar, R. (1992) *Brugia malayi*: antibody responses to larval antigens in infected and immunized jirds. *Exp. Parasitol.*, **74**, 315–323.

58 Yates, J.A. and Higashi, G.I. (1986) Ultrastructural observations on the fate of *Brugia malayi* in jirds previously vaccinated with irradiated infective stage larvae. *Am. J. Trop. Med. Hyg.*, **35**, 982–987.

59 Gregory, W.F., Atmadja, A.K., Allen, J.E., and Maizels, R.M. (2000) The abundant larval transcript-1 and -2 genes of *Brugia malayi* encode stage-specific candidate vaccine antigens for filariasis. *Infect. Immun.*, **68**, 4174–4179.

60 Anand, S.B., Krithika, K.N., Murugan, V., Reddy, M.V., and Kaliraj, P. (2006) Comparison of immuno prophylactic efficacy of Bm rALT2 or Bm rVAH or rALT+rVAH by single and multiple antigen vaccination mode. *Am. Soc. Trop. Med. Hyg.*, **75**, 295.

61 Wang, S.H., Zheng, H.J., Dissanayake, S., Cheng, W.F., Tao, Z.H., Lin, S.Z., and Piessens, W.F. (1997) Evaluation of recombinant chitinase and

SXP1 antigens as antimicrofilarial vaccines. *Am. J. Trop. Med. Hyg.*, **56**, 474–481.

62 Adam, R., Kaltmann, B., Rudin, W., Friedrich, T., Marti, T., and Lucius, R. (1996) Identification of chitinase as the immunodominant filarial antigen recognized by sera of vaccinated rodents. *J. Biol. Chem.*, **271**, 1441–1447.

63 Pokharel, D.R., Rai, R., Nandakumar Kodumudi, K., Reddy, M.V., and Rathaur, S. (2006) Vaccination with *Setaria cervi* 175 kDa collagenase induces high level of protection against *Brugia malayi* infection in jirds. *Vaccine*, **24**, 6208–6215.

64 Srivastava, Y., Rathaur, S., Bhandari, Y.P., Reddy, M.V., and Harinath, B.C. (2004) Adult 175 kDa collagenase antigen of *Setaria cervi* in immunoprophylaxis against *Brugia malayi* in jirds. *J. Helminthol.*, **78**, 347–352.

65 Dabir, P., Dabir, S., Krithika, K.N., Goswami, K., and Reddy, M.V. (2006) Immunoprophylactic evaluation of a 37-kDa *Brugia malayi* recombinant antigen in lymphatic filariasis. *Clin. Microbiol. Infect.*, **12**, 361–368.

66 Veerapathran, A., Dakshinamoorthy, G., Gnanasekar, M., Reddy, M.V., and Kalyanasundaram, R. (2009) Evaluation of *Wuchereria bancrofti* GST as a vaccine candidate for lymphatic filariasis. *PLoS Negl. Trop. Dis.*, **3**, e457.

67 Vedi, S., Dangi, A., Hajela, K., and Misra-Bhattacharya, S. (2008) Vaccination with 73kDa recombinant heavy chain myosin generates high level of protection against *Brugia malayi* challenge in jird and mastomys models. *Vaccine*, **26**, 5997–6005.

68 Krithika, K.N., Dabir, P., Kulkarni, S., Anandharaman, V., and Reddy, M.V. (2005) Identification of 38kDa *Brugia malayi* microfilarial protease as a vaccine candidate for lymphatic filariasis. *Indian J. Exp. Biol.*, **43**, 759–768.

69 Prince, A.M., Brotman, B., Johnson, E.H. Jr, Smith, A., Pascual, D., and Lustigman, S. (1992) *Onchocerca volvulus*: immunization of chimpanzees with X-irradiated third-stage (L3) larvae. *Exp. Parasitol.*, **74**, 239–250.

70 Abraham, D., Leon, O., Schnyder-Candrian, S., Wang, C.C., Galioto, A.M., Kerepesi, L.A., Lee, J.J., and Lustigman, S. (2004) Immunoglobulin E and eosinophil-dependent protective immunity to larval *Onchocerca volvulus* in mice immunized with irradiated larvae. *Infect. Immun.*, **72**, 810–817.

71 Abraham, D., Leon, O., Leon, S., and Lustigman, S. (2001) Development of a recombinant antigen vaccine against infection with the filarial worm *Onchocerca volvulus*. *Infect. Immun.*, **69**, 262–270.

72 Lustigman, S., James, E.R., Tawe, W., and Abraham, D. (2002) Towards a recombinant antigen vaccine against *Onchocerca volvulus*. *Trends Parasitol.*, **18**, 135–141.

73 Erttmann, K.D., Kleensang, A., Schneider, E., Hammerschmidt, S., Buttner, D.W., and Gallin, M. (2005) Cloning, characterization and DNA immunization of an *Onchocerca volvulus* glyceraldehyde-3-phosphate dehydrogenase (Ov-GAPDH). *Biochim. Biophys. Acta*, **1741**, 85–94.

74 McCarthy, J.S., Wieseman, M., Tropea, J., Kaslow, D., Abraham, D., Lustigman, S., Tuan, R. *et al.* (2002) *Onchocerca volvulus* glycolytic enzyme fructose-1,6-bisphosphate aldolase as a target for a protective immune response in humans. *Infect. Immun.*, **70**, 851–858.

75 MacDonald, A.J., Tawe, W., Leon, O., Cao, L., Liu, J., Oksov, Y., Abraham, D., and Lustigman, S. (2004) Ov-ASP-1, the *Onchocerca volvulus* homologue of the activation associated secreted protein family is immunostimulatory and can induce protective anti-larval immunity. *Parasite Immunol.*, **26**, 53–62.

76 Lucius, R., Kapaun, A., and Diesfeld, H.J. (1987) *Dipetalonema viteae* infection in three species of rodents: species specific patterns of the antibody response. *Parasite Immunol.*, **9**, 67–80.

77 Neilson, J.T., Crandall, C.A., and Crandall, R.B. (1981) Serum immunoglobulin and antibody levels and the passive transfer of resistance in

hamsters infected with *Dipetalonema viteae*. *Acta Trop.*, **38**, 309–318.

78 Lucius, R., Textor, G., Kern, A., and Kirsten, C. (1991) *Acanthocheilonema viteae*: vaccination of jirds with irradiation-attenuated stage-3 larvae and with exported larval antigens. *Exp. Parasitol.*, **73**, 184–196.

79 Hartmann, S., Sereda, M.J., Sollwedel, A., Kalinna, B., and Lucius, R. (2006) A nematode allergen elicits protection against challenge infection under specific conditions. *Vaccine*, **24**, 3581–3590.

80 Taylor, M.J., Jenkins, R.E., and Bianco, A.E. (1996) Protective immunity induced by vaccination with *Onchocerca volvulus* tropomyosin in rodents. *Parasite Immunol.*, **18**, 219–225.

81 Taylor, M.J., Abdel-Wahab, N., Wu, Y., Jenkins, R.E., and Bianco, A.E. (1995) *Onchocerca volvulus* larval antigen, OvB20, induces partial protection in a rodent model of onchocerciasis. *Infect. Immun.*, **63**, 4417–4422.

82 Martin, C., Saeftel, M., Vuong, P.N., Babayan, S., Fischer, K., Bain, O., and Hoerauf, A. (2001) B-cell deficiency suppresses vaccine-induced protection against murine filariasis but does not increase the recovery rate for primary infection. *Infect. Immun.*, **69**, 7067–7073.

83 Martin, C., Al-Qaoud, K.M., Ungeheuer, M.N., Paehle, K., Vuong, P.N., Bain, O., Fleischer, B., and Hoerauf, A. (2000) IL-5 is essential for vaccine-induced protection and for resolution of primary infection in murine filariasis. *Med. Microbiol. Immunol.*, **189**, 67–74.

84 Le Goff, L., Martin, C., Oswald, I.P., Vuong, P.N., Petit, G., Ungeheuer, M.N., and Bain, O. (2000) Parasitology and immunology of mice vaccinated with irradiated *Litomosoides sigmodontis* larvae. *Parasitology*, **120**, 271–280.

85 Le Goff, L., Marechal, P., Petit, G., Taylor, D.W., Hoffmann, W., and Bain, O. (1997) Early reduction of the challenge recovery rate following immunization with irradiated infective larvae in a filaria mouse system. *Trop. Med. Int. Health*, **2**, 1170–1174.

86 Babayan, S.A., Attout, T., Harris, A., Taylor, M.D., Le Goff, L., Vuong, P.N., Renia, L. *et al.* (2006) Vaccination against filarial nematodes with irradiated larvae provides long-term protection against the third larval stage but not against subsequent life cycle stages. *Int. J. Parasitol.*, **36**, 903–914.

87 Allen, J.E., Daub, J., Guiliano, D., McDonnell, A., Lizotte-Waniewski, M., Taylor, D.W., and Blaxter, M. (2000) Analysis of genes expressed at the infective larval stage validates utility of *Litomosoides sigmodontis* as a murine model for filarial vaccine development. *Infect. Immun.*, **68**, 5454–5458.

88 Bethony, J.M., Simon, G., Diemert, D.J., Parenti, D., Desrosiers, A., Schuck, S., Fujiwara, R. *et al.* (2008) Randomized, placebo-controlled, double-blind trial of the Na-ASP-2 hookworm vaccine in unexposed adults. *Vaccine*, **26**, 2408–2417.

89 Tsuji, N., Miyoshi, T., Islam, M.K., Isobe, T., Yoshihara, S., Arakawa, T., Matsumoto, Y., and Yokomizo, Y. (2004) Recombinant *Ascaris* 16-kilodalton protein-induced protection against *Ascaris suum* larval migration after intranasal vaccination in pigs. *J. Infect. Dis.*, **190**, 1812–1820.

90 Zhan, B., Wang, Y., Liu, Y., Williamson, A., Loukas, A., Hawdon, J.M., Xue, H.C. *et al.* (2004) Ac-SAA-1, an immunodominant 16kDa surface-associated antigen of infective larvae and adults of *Ancylostoma caninum*. *Int. J. Parasitol.*, **34**, 1037–1045.

91 Zhan, B., Liu, S., Perally, S., Xue, J., Fujiwara, R., Brophy, P., Xiao, S. *et al.* (2005) Biochemical characterization and vaccine potential of a heme-binding glutathione transferase from the adult hookworm *Ancylostoma caninum*. *Infect. Immun.*, **73**, 6903–6911.

92 Xiao, S., Zhan, B., Xue, J., Goud, G.N., Loukas, A., Liu, Y., Williamson, A. *et al.* (2008) The evaluation of recombinant hookworm antigens as vaccines in hamsters (*Mesocricetus auratus*) challenged with human hookworm, *Necator americanus*. *Exp. Parasitol.*, **118**, 32–40.

93 Carlos, M.P., Yamamura, Y., Diaz-Mitoma, F., and Torres, J.V. (1999) Antibodies from HIV-positive and AIDS patients bind to an HIV envelope multivalent vaccine. *J. Acquir. Immune. Defic. Syndr.*, **22**, 317–324.

94 Zevering, Y., Khamboonruang, C., and Good, M.F. (1998) Human and murine T-cell responses to allelic forms of a malaria circumsporozoite protein epitope support a polyvalent vaccine strategy. *Immunology*, **94**, 445–454.

95 Londono, J.A., Gras-Masse, H., Dubeaux, C., Tartar, A., and Druilhe, P. (1990) Secondary structure and immunogenicity of hybrid synthetic peptides derived from two *Plasmodium falciparum* pre-erythrocytic antigens. *J. Immunol.*, **145**, 1557–1563.

96 Hotez, P.J., Bethony, J.M., Diemert, D.J., Pearson, M., and Loukas, A. (2010) Developing vaccines to combat hookworm infection and intestinal schistosomiasis. *Nat. Rev. Microbiol.*, **8**, 814–826.

97 Anand, S.B., Kodumudi, K.N., Reddy, M.V., and Kaliraj, P. (2011) A combination of two *Brugia malayi* filarial vaccine candidate antigens (BmALT-2 and BmVAH) enhances immune responses and protection in jirds. *J. Helminthol.*, **85**, 442–452.

98 Gnanasekar, M., Anand, S.B., and Ramaswamy, K. (2008) Identification and cloning of a novel tetraspanin (TSP) homologue from *Brugia malayi*. *DNA Seq.*, **19**, 151–156.

99 Samykutty, A., Gajalakshmi, D., and Ramaswamy, K. (2010) Multivalent vaccine for lymphatic filariasis. *Proc. Vaccinol.*, **3**, 12–18.

100 Ramaswamy, K. and Padmavathi, B. (2011) Multivalent vaccine formulation with BmVAL-1 and BmALT-2 confer significant protection against challenge infections with *Brugia malayi* in mice and jirds. *Res. Rep. Trop. Med.*, **2**, 45–56.

101 van Der Kleij, D., Tielens, A.G., and Yazdanbakhsh, M. (1999) Recognition of schistosome glycolipids by immunoglobulin E: possible role in immunity. *Infect. Immun.*, **67**, 5946–5950.

102 Ellis, L.A., Reason, A.J., Morris, H.R., Dell, A., Iglesias, R., Ubeira, F.M., and Appleton, J.A. (1994) Glycans as targets for monoclonal antibodies that protect rats against *Trichinella spiralis*. *Glycobiology*, **4**, 585–592.

103 McVay, C.S., Tsung, A., and Appleton, J. (1998) Participation of parasite surface glycoproteins in antibody-mediated protection of epithelial cells against *Trichinella spiralis*. *Infect. Immun.*, **66**, 1941–1945.

104 McVay, C.S., Bracken, P., Gagliardo, L.F., and Appleton, J. (2000) Antibodies to tyvelose exhibit multiple modes of interference with the epithelial niche of *Trichinella spiralis*. *Infect. Immun.*, **68**, 1912–1918.

105 Sher, A. (1988) Vaccination against parasites: special problems imposed by the adaptation of parasitic organisms to the host immune response, in *The Biology of Parasitism* (eds P.T. Englund and A. Sher), Alan R. Liss, New York, pp. 169–182.

106 Henkle-Duhrsen, K. and Kampkotter, A. (2001) Antioxidant enzyme families in parasitic nematodes. *Mol. Biochem. Parasitol.*, **114**, 129–142.

107 Wu, Y., Adam, R., Williams, S.A., and Bianco, A.E. (1996) Chitinase genes expressed by infective larvae of the filarial nematodes, *Acanthocheilonema viteae* and *Onchocerca volvulus*. *Mol. Biochem. Parasitol.*, **75**, 207–219.

108 Lizotte-Waniewski, M., Tawe, W., Guiliano, D.B., Lu, W., Liu, J., Williams, S.A., and Lustigman, S. (2000) Identification of potential vaccine and drug target candidates by expressed sequence tag analysis and immunoscreening of *Onchocerca volvulus* larval cDNA libraries. *Infect. Immun.*, **68**, 3491–3501.

109 Ghedin, E., Wang, S., Spiro, D., Caler, E., Zhao, Q., Crabtree, J., Allen, J.E. *et al.* (2007) Draft genome of the filarial nematode parasite *Brugia malayi*. *Science*, **317**, 1756–1760.

110 Bennuru, S., Semnani, R., Meng, Z., Ribeiro, J.M., Veenstra, T.D., and Nutman, T.B. (2009) *Brugia malayi* excreted/secreted proteins at the host/

parasite interface: stage- and gender-specific proteomic profiling. *PLoS Negl. Trop. Dis.*, **3**, e410.

111 Bennuru, S., Meng, Z., Ribeiro, J.M., Semnani, R.T., Ghedin, E., Chan, K., Lucas, D.A. *et al.* (2011) Stage-specific proteomic expression patterns of the human filarial parasite *Brugia malayi* and its endosymbiont *Wolbachia*. *Proc. Natl. Acad. Sci. USA*, **108**, 9649–9654.

112 Brindley, P.J., Mitreva, M., Ghedin, E., and Lustigman, S. (2009) Helminth genomics: The implications for human health. *PLoS Negl. Trop. Dis.*, **3**, e538.

113 Bacarese-Hamilton, T., Bistoni, F., and Crisanti, A. (2002) Protein microarrays: from serodiagnosis to whole proteome scale analysis of the immune response against pathogenic microorganisms. *Biotechniques*, Suppl., 24–29.

114 Doolan, D.L. (2010) Plasmodium immunomics. *Int. J. Parasitol.*, **41**, 3–20.

115 Lightowlers, M.W. (2010) Eradication of *Taenia solium* cysticercosis: a role for vaccination of pigs. *Int. J. Parasitol.*, **40**, 1183–1192.

116 Assana, E., Kyngdon, C.T., Gauci, C.G., Geerts, S., Dorny, P., De Deken, R., Anderson, G.A. *et al.* (2010) Elimination of *Taenia solium* transmission to pigs in a field trial of the TSOL18 vaccine in Cameroon. *Int. J. Parasitol.*, **40**, 515–519.

117 Pfaff, A.W., Schulz-Key, H., Soboslay, P.T., Taylor, D.W., MacLennan, K., and Hoffmann, W.H. (2002) *Litomosoides sigmodontis* cystatin acts as an immunomodulator during experimental filariasis. *Int. J. Parasitol.*, **32**, 171–178.

118 Goud, G.N., Zhan, B., Ghosh, K., Loukas, A., Hawdon, J., Dobardzic, A., Deumic, V. *et al.* (2004) Cloning, yeast expression, isolation, and vaccine testing of recombinant *Ancylostoma*-secreted protein (ASP)-1 and ASP-2 from *Ancylostoma ceylanicum*. *J. Infect. Dis.*, **189**, 919–929.

119 Ramachandran, S., Kumar, M.P., Rami, R.M., Chinnaiah, H.B., Nutman, T., Kaliraj, P., and McCarthy, J. (2004) The larval specific lymphatic filarial ALT-2: induction of protection using protein or DNA vaccination. *Microbiol. Immunol.*, **48**, 945–955.

120 Jenkins, R.E., Taylor, M.J., Gilvary, N., and Bianco, A.E. (1996) Characterization of a secreted antigen of *Onchocerca volvulus* with host-protective potential. *Parasite Immunol.*, **18**, 29–42.

24
Proteases as Vaccines Against Gastrointestinal Nematode Parasites of Sheep and Cattle

David Knox

Abstract

Parasitic nematodes contain and secrete various proteases (proteolytic enzymes) that are known or proposed to facilitate the penetration of host tissue barriers, the digestion of host protein for nutrients, and the evasion of the host antiparasite immune responses, in addition to their functions in internal processes such as tissue catabolism and apoptosis. These key functions underscore the reasons why proteases have been targeted as vaccine components. Several excreted/secreted (ES) proteases are known to be targeted by host-protective humoral immune responses and have been evaluated as vaccine candidates against nematode parasites of livestock. In particular, ES cysteine proteases are associated with vaccination-induced protective immunity in cattle and sheep against the abomasal parasites *Ostertagia ostertagi* and *Haemonchus contortus*, respectively. Moreover, proteases found on the intestinal surface of the latter are among the most effective vaccine antigens identified to date for any helminth parasite. These proteases include a variety of endo- and exopeptidases required to digest hemoglobin in the blood meal – a process that involves a partly conserved cascade or network of proteases also found in hookworms, schistosomes, and *Plasmodium* spp. In addition to cysteine proteases, other intestinal proteases include aspartic and metalloproteases, aminopetidases, and dipeptidyl peptidases. In general, protection by protease vaccines is mediated by antibody inhibition of enzyme activity that blocks either parasite invasion of the host or digestion, leading to parasite expulsion and/or death. A major barrier to vaccine production is that recombinant protease vaccines lack the efficacy of their native counterparts for a variety of reasons, including incorrect protein folding and/or the lack of, or inappropriate, post-translational modifications such as glycosylation. These issues have been addressed by the use of eukaryotic expression systems such as insect cells and recent work indicates that the free-living nematode, *Caenorhabditis elegans*, can be also engineered to produce functional heterologous nematode parasite proteases.

Introduction

The ubiquity of proteases (proteolytic enzymes) and their function in parasites of man and livestock is underlined in several review articles (e.g., [1, 2]). Antibody

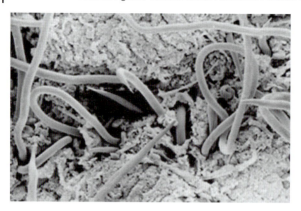

Figure 24.1 Scanning electron micrograph of adult *T. circumcincta* in the abomasal (gastric) glands of an infected lamb.

inhibition of protease activity or function is likely to have direct effects on parasite establishment and survival within the host, suggesting that these enzymes are appropriate vaccine targets.

Infection with any the major gastrointestinal nematodes of livestock commences when the infective third larval stage (L3) is ingested during grazing. These larvae are small (less than 1 mm in length) yet grow rapidly within the host to become adult parasites ranging in size from around 0.5 to 3.5 cm depending on species and sex (Figure 24.1). Even subclinical infection levels can have profound effects on livestock, including impaired growth (Figure 24.2), meat quality, and milk production.

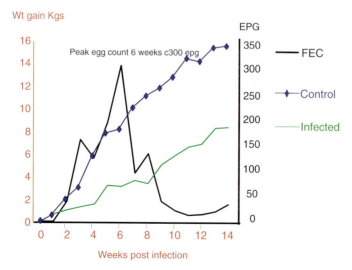

Figure 24.2 Impact of a moderate *T. circumcincta* infection on growth rate in postweaning lambs. Infection virtually halves the growth rate and this is evident within 14 days.

Together, these reduce production efficiency, which is an increasing cause for concern at a time when global food security is more challenging.

Irrespective of the species, the increase in size from L3 to adult is dramatic in a short period of time and insinuates the need for very efficient nutrient acquisition to fuel this growth. In turn, this would imply that the developing parasite is dependent on a range of proteases to facilitate the breakdown of ingested proteins into sufficiently small units (e.g., amino acids or dipeptides) to allow rapid nutrient turnover [2, 3]. Proteases are central to key nematode processes such as collagen processing and cuticle turnover [4]. Larval and adult stages may need to breakdown host tissue barriers and to evade host antiparasite immune responses [5], and numerous nematodes excrete/secrete proteases (e.g., [6–8]). The accumulating body of evidence linking proteases to key parasite processes and survival has led to proteases being viewed as vaccine targets. For me, this view was stimulated by work on the rodent intestinal nematode, *Nippostrongylus muris* [9, 10], and studies with the dog hookworm, *Ancylostoma caninum* [11, 12]. Protease activity in extracts of the esophagus from the adult *A. caninum* was inhibited by immune serum [11] and, of greater importance, dogs could be partially protected against *A. caninum* infection by injection of parasite esophageal extracts prior to challenge with the same parasite [12].

Proteases of Gastrointestinal Nematodes of Livestock – Overview

Dependency on proteases occurs at the earliest stages of infection, and is associated with egg hatching and larval ecdysis. Leucine aminopeptidase and aspartyl proteases [13–15] have been implicated in egg hatching, while metalloproteases mediate ecdysis in sheathed *Haemonchus contortus* L3 [16, 17]. The cuticle is crucial to the development and survival of all nematodes. Made up of collagen, its correct formation requires the coordinated action of numerous enzymes. In *Caenorhabditis elegans*, an astacin-like metalloprotease is particularly important in cuticular synthesis [4]. This protease is expressed in the gut and secretory system of *C. elegans*, and mutation of the gene results in severe cuticle defects. Once in contact with the host, the parasite must reach its predilection site and, again, the gastrointestinal nematodes seem to utilize proteases to breakdown host tissues (e.g., [18–23]). Proteases are found in the excreted/secreted (ES) products of all the common nematode species infecting ruminants studied to date [6, 7], and, in all cases, there is a degree of species- and stage-specificity.

In addition to facilitating penetration of host tissues, proteases are also central to nutrient acquisition. For example, in common with other blood-feeding parasites, *H. contortus* utilizes a cascade of differing proteases to digest blood proteins and to prevent blood coagulation [24–29]. These are usually expressed on the luminal surface of the intestinal cells.

When specifically sought, host antibody inhibition of parasite proteases is evident (e.g., [18, 23, 24, 35]) and has been correlated to the induction of protective immunity [24, 35]. However, this is not always the case. Parasite proteases can cleave host immunoglobulin [25] and it is possible that the proteases have to be saturated by host antibody to induce, presumably, starvation of the worm. Is the cleavage of IgG simply because a protease has been mixed with a protein substrate in an artificial laboratory situation or is it true evidence of a specific function? Immature *Fasciola hepatica*, an important trematode parasite of ruminants and a zoonosis, release a cathepsin B-like cysteine protease that can cleave immunoglobulin of mouse, rat, rabbit, and sheep origin *in vitro* [30]. Further analyses [31] showed that, contrary to the extensive degradation produced by cathepsins on digested proteins, the action on IgG subclasses was specific and restricted, and the authors suggested that the peptide fragments produced could be involved in the mechanisms used by the parasite to evade the host immune response.

The importance of proteases in nematode invasion of the host is underlined by the many gene sequencing initiatives that now employ new technologies to allow whole transcriptomes to be readily sampled (see also Chapter 4). These projects have identified numerous proteases, many of which are likely secreted as they possess signal peptides. However, the majority are unlikely to be useful vaccine components because they are expressed internally within the parasite and, thus, are not accessible to the host immune response. The biologist/parasitologist must make informed choices from these datasets that includes the incorporation of knowledge derived from all aspects of the parasite biology.

In adult female *H. contortus*, cathepsin B-like cysteine protease genes (*cbl*) comprised 17% of all protein-coding expressed sequence tags (ESTs) analyzed [32]. Jasmer et al. [33] used the available *H. contortus* ESTs to assess both the size and diversity of the *H. contortus cbl* gene family. Contig analysis of 686 *cbl* ESTs from a isolate identified in the United States resolved 123 clusters. The *cbl* genes were extremely diverse compared to other genes investigated. Of note, when considering cathepsins B as vaccine targets, is that 60% of the *cbl* clusters from a UK isolate were shared with those identified in the US isolate, suggesting a conservation of *cbl* gene repertoires across regions, although minor to moderate geographic variation could not be excluded. Of more concern was the observation that the *cbl* genes showed great potential for antigenic diversity [33].

Desirable Vaccine Efficacy

This has been considered using a computer model that simulates most genetic and management conditions for any environment in sheep flocks [34]. The model was used to estimate the required efficacy of vaccines based on (i) conventional antigens that are recognized by the host immune system during infection and (ii) concealed or hidden antigen vaccines that are not recognized by the humoral immune response in the course of natural infection. Conventional antigens include ES components and substantial worm control can be achieved using a vaccine with 60% efficacy in 80% of the flock. The required efficacy with a concealed antigen vaccine is predicted to be higher (80% in 80% of the flock). It is highly desirable to have an idea of what efficacy is required before undertaking vaccine trials so that a baseline is available against which success can be judged.

Gut-Expressed Proteases as Vaccine Antigens

Many of the most effective protective antigens identified to date have been isolated from the intestine of the blood-feeding nematode parasite of sheep and goats, *H. contortus*. Almost without exception, these prototype vaccines comprise mixtures of proteins as judged by sodium dodecyl sulfate–polyacrylamide gel electrophoresis (SDS–PAGE) analysis. The nature and presumed function of these proteins was undefined when they were first evaluated in protection trials. Subsequent gene and functional analyses have shown that the inherent proteases are required to digest the blood meal are, therefore, potentially effective vaccines.

Microsomal Aminopeptidase from the Intestine of *H. contortus*: H11

The most effective antigen described to date from any parasitic nematodes is the H11 protein, which is found on the microvillar surface of the intestinal cells of fourth-stage larvae (L4) and adults [35]. Reductions of worm burdens by greater than 90% have been recorded in a range of sheep breeds, in very young lambs and pregnant ewes, and in animals infected with anthelmintic-resistant strains of *H. contortus* (reviewed in [36]). It was termed H11 because the major protein component of the vaccine migrated as a doublet at 110 kDa in SDS–PAGE gels. Sequence analysis (of cDNA) indicated that this protein is an aminopeptidase – a suggestion confirmed by enzymatic characterization of purified native protein that showed H11 had both aminopeptidase A and M activity. To date, five distinct isoforms have been identified from the extensive EST and genome sequence data available for *H. contortus* (Britton, personal communication). H11 is predicted to have a structure typical of a type II integral membrane protein with a short N-terminal cytoplasmic tail, a transmembrane region, and an extracellular region organized into four domains [37]. It is glycosylated and the glycan component contains core fucose elements [38] that are highly immunogenic. H11 has an HEXXHXW sequence motif followed by a glutamic acid, which is characteristic of the zinc-binding sequence of microsomal aminopeptidases. Enzyme activity is localized exclusively to the microvilli, and is inhibited by the specific aminopeptidase inhibitors, bestatin and amastatin, and also by the chelating agent, phenanthroline [37]. Antisera to H11 inhibit aminopeptidase activity *in vitro* [35] and the inhibition measured closely correlates with protection. Vaccine efficacy of H11 was decreased by dissociation and/or denaturation [35], indicative of the involvement of conformational epitopes in the induction of immunity.

The extracellular domains of H11-1, -2, and -3 isoforms were expressed as active recombinant enzymes in insect cells, but were not protective in trials despite inducing antibodies that inhibited enzyme activity of both the recombinant and native H11 proteins [36]. Worms recovered from sheep immunized with native H11 had a coating of sheep antibody bound to the microvillar surface of the intestine, whereas those recovered from sheep immunized with insect cell-expressed H11 did not [36] – an observation that could be ascribed to the differing glycan components in the two vaccine candidates. A potentially important finding from recent proteomic analyses is that the native H11 preparation also contained traces of other known protective antigens, particularly metalloprotease components of the *Haemonchus* galactose-containing glycoprotein complex (H-gal-GP; see below; Sherlock and Smith, unpublished). Hence, a combination recombinant vaccine may be required. However, RNA interference (RNAi) of the *h11-1* gene isoform in infective larvae prior to infection resulted in a 57% reduction in fecal egg count, a 40% reduction in worm burden, and a 64% decrease in aminopeptidase activity compared to larvae presoaked in control double-stranded RNA [39]. In addition, H11 has been expressed in insect cells as an active protein that showed aminopeptidase A activity alone, unlike the native H11 protein extracts that possessed both A- and M-type activity [37, 40]. Nonetheless, the latter [40] recombinant protein did stimulate protective immunity against *H. contortus* challenge in Merino sheep given a single bolus challenge of 15 000 L3s. Final worm burdens in vaccinates were reduced by 30% compared to controls [40]. Moreover, DNA vaccines expressing H11 antigen have shown greater than 50% efficacy, as judged by worm burdens, in goats [41].

H-gal-GP

This antigen complex was identified by specific labeling of glycoproteins on the luminal surface of the gut of adult *H. contortus* with a panel of lectins [42]. Using peanut lectin–agarose affinity chromatography H-gal-GP was purified from detergent-solubilized extracts of the membrane protein fraction from adult parasites [42]. It is an effective vaccine in both housed (e.g., [42, 43]) and field trials (e.g., [44] and Smith, unpublished) with typical reductions in worm burden and fecal egg count of 70 and 90%, respectively (Figure 24.3). Like the H11 vaccinates, the microvillar surface of the intestinal cells of worms retrieved from lambs vaccinated with H-gal-GP is coated with sheep immunoglobulin and the systemic antibody titer correlates with protection [42].

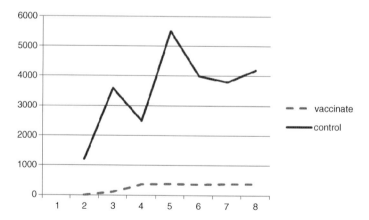

Figure 24.3 Typical impact on *H. contortus* egg output by vaccinating lambs with TSBP purified from adult parasites prior to a bolus challenge of 5000 L3. Egg output is usually reduced by around 50% with a corresponding reduction in worm numbers. However, these levels of reduction are not sufficient to control infection in the field based on efficacy predictions derived from computer modeling [67].

H-gal-GP migrates with an apparent molecular weight of above 1000 kDa in native PAGE gels and, using nonreducing SDS–PAGE, separates into groups of peptides at 35, 45, 170, and 230 kDa under reducing conditions [42]. The complex contains aspartic proteases (pepsin-like, PEP1 [45, 46]) and metalloproteases (MEP1, 2, and 3 [47, 48]), a galectin [49], a cystatin [50], and a thrombospondin [51]. The H-gal-GP complex has proven resistant to fractionation using a variety of chromatographic techniques, under native conditions. In recent work (Trinnick and Smith, unpublished), the complex has been visualized using electron microscopy, being the size of a small virus particle, and is similar in size to bacterial proteosomes.

H-gal-GP readily digests ovine hemoglobin and albumin – the two most abundant proteins in the parasite's blood meal [24]. Antibodies from H-gal-GP-immunized sheep reduced the rate of hemoglobin digestion by H-gal-GP by 70–90% compared to only 30% when nonprotective IgG from sheep immunized with denatured H-gal-GP was added. IgG from worm-free sheep had no effect. These results support the theory that the mechanism of protection in sheep vaccinated with H-gal-GP is by specific antibodies impairing the parasites ability to digest its blood meal.

So what is the protective component(s) of H-gal-GP? This question has been addressed in several ways. When separated from the rest of the complex by gel filtration in 8 M urea, the fraction containing the pepsin-like components significantly reduced *H. contortus* egg counts by 48% and worm numbers by 36% in vaccinated and challenged lambs compared to controls [52]. Similarly, the metalloproteases, either MEP3 alone or MEP1, 2, and 4 in combination, reduced egg counts by about 33% [53]. These studies implicated both the aspartic proteases and metalloproteases in the induction of protective immunity, but protection fell well short of the 70–90% protection obtained with the native complex. An antigen cocktail containing MEP1, 3, and 4 expressed as soluble recombinant proteins in insect cells, and recombinant PEP1 expressed in *Escherichia coli*, and then refolded, was evaluated as a vaccine [54]. Groups of sheep were immunized with either native H-gal-GP, this cocktail, or adjuvant alone (Quil A in phosphate-buffered saline) and challenged with 5000 infective larvae 1 week after the final vaccination. High levels of serum antibodies that recognized H-gal-GP were detected in both the native antigen and recombinant cocktail-immunized groups by the time of challenge, but protective immunity was only observed in the group immunized with native H-gal-GP.

Field Efficacy of H11 and H-gal-P

This is the "acid test" for any vaccine. In housed trials of vaccines against gastrointestinal nematodes, the parasite challenge is delivered orally either as a single challenge bolus or at regular dosing intervals designed to mimic field exposure. Parasite challenge on pasture can vary dramatically with larval contamination being dependent on climatic conditions and host immunological status. A native protein vaccine comprising H11, H-gal-GP, cysteine proteases, and other proteins from the *Haemonchus* intestine was tested in a trial lasting 11 months in South Africa where sheep were allowed to graze on pasture contaminated with *H. contortus* [55]. On average, during one 4-month period of the trial, the vaccine reduced egg output by greater than 82%, and decreased anemia and mortality compared to unvaccinated controls. Vaccine immunity did not persist throughout the trial period, but a booster vaccination cleared newly acquired infections and restored protection.

In another field trial in New South Wales, Australia, grazing Merino sheep were vaccinated with 100 μg each of H11 and H-gal-GP, and the ability to control the parasite challenge resulting from grazing was assessed using fecal egg counts and blood packed cell volumes [56]. The level of larval contamination on pasture was estimated from the worm counts of tracer sheep introduced monthly to the paddocks. Fecal egg counts and anemia were significantly reduced in vaccinated animals compared to controls, and all the latter required salvage treatment with anthelmintic. Moreover, enzyme-linked immunosorbent assay analyses indicated that protection by H11/H-gal-GP was probably mediated by antibodies, particularly IgG1.

The data from these field trials [55, 56] indicate that if similar protective effects could be obtained with recombinant versions of the proteins present in either H11 or H-gal-GP, then the prospects for a commercial *Haemonchus* vaccine are real.

However, as noted above, producing recombinant proteins that have the same vaccine efficacy has proven elusive. In very recent work, vaccine dose–response assessments have shown that the levels of protective immunity described above can be stimulated with very low protein doses (5 μg/dose), indeed to the extent that it is feasible to produce the native vaccine, on a regional basis, from adult parasites harvested from a relatively limited number of donor lambs (Smith, unpublished). This approach to control is being tested in further field trials in Australia, South Africa, and South America – regions where *Haemonchus* is a the major threat to sheep, goat, and cattle production.

H. contortus Cysteine Proteases

Cysteine proteases assist in the digestion of blood proteins by blood-feeding nematodes, including *Haemonchus* (e.g., [25]), and, as with other hematophagous endo- and ectoparasites (e.g., hookworms, schistosomes, *Plasmodium*, and ticks), they are central to hemoglobinolysis [57–60]. An analysis of ESTs to assess both the size and diversity of the *H. contortus* cathepsin B gene family was undertaken [61]. Contig analysis of 686 ESTs from a American isolate resolved into 123 clusters indicative of extreme diversity, although 60% of the clusters were shared with those from a UK isolate, suggesting conservation across different geographic regions. These sequence comparisons also provided evidence for antigenic diversity among cathepsin B-like proteins and this has potential negative implications for developing a defined cathepsin B vaccine candidate. The authors noted that, compared to other parasitic nematodes of mammals, this level of transcript abundance and diversity appears to be a relative specialization for *H. contortus* [61]. Despite these potential confounding factors, cysteine protease vaccines against *Haemonchus* have shown some promise.

A 35-kDa cysteine protease purified from water-soluble extracts of adult *H. contortus* induced substantial, but variable, levels of protective immunity against challenge infection in immunized lambs [62]. The protease was not detectable by immunoblot in the three larval parasitic developmental stages of *H. contortus*, but Northern blots showed that the mRNA transcript was present at low levels in a mixed population of L3 and L4 larvae, and in high abundance in adult worms [63]. This expression pattern correlates with blood-feeding. The protease is one of a gene family (designated AC-1 to -5; 64–77% identity) that is expressed in the adult parasite [64]. The primary sequence differences noted between the proteases suggest that they may differ in their substrate specificities and precise physiological functions [65]. All contained potential signal sequences for secretion. However, no localization data was reported. A similar small gene family has been demonstrated in *Ostertagia ostertagi* (CP-1 to -3), and, again, two of these are tandemly linked and have closer homology to the *Haemonchus* AC sequences than to mammalian cathepsin B [66].

Membrane extracts from adult *H. contortus* can be enriched for cysteine protease activity by passage over a thiol-Sepharose affinity column yielding a protein fraction designated thiol-Sepharose-binding proteins (TSBPs [67]). This fraction also contains serine and metalloprotease activities. A limited number of the peptide components are glycosylated. Vaccinated lambs that had been challenged with a single bolus of 5000 *Haemonchus* L3 had reduced fecal egg counts and worm burdens (overall means of 77 and 47%, respectively, from three trials; Figure 24.4) compared to challenge controls. Antibody in sera from vaccinated lambs almost exclusively bound to the surface of the parasite gut, suggesting that protection may have been mediated by the inhibition of parasite digestion. Unlike H11 and H-gal-GP, protection has never consistently correlated with antibody inhibition of enzyme activity (Redmond and Knox, unpublished). In the study [67], it was surprising that a TSBP fraction from a saline extract of adult worms was not an effective immunogen. Cysteine proteases enriched from water-soluble, adult *Haemonchus* extracts were effective against a

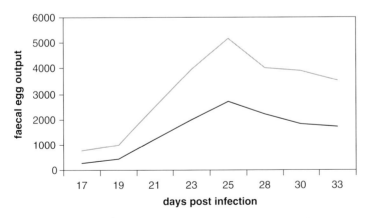

Figure 24.4 Impact of a native protein vaccine against *H. contortus* in young, growing lambs. The dramatic (around 90%) reduction in egg output is paralleled by a 70% reduction in worm burdens. These reductions *are* sufficient to control infection in the field ([34] © 1995 Elsevier).

challenge infection in goats with fecal egg counts and worm burdens reduced by 89 and 68%, respectively, compared to challenge controls [68].

The major protein components of TSBP were identified by cDNA expression library immunoscreening with anti-TSBP serum. Three novel cysteine protease-encoding cDNAs, designated hmcp1, 4, and 6, were identified [69]. Their expression coincided with the onset of blood feeding and all were expressed at the luminal surface of the intestinal cells [69]. The cysteine proteases of adult *H. contortus* TSBP were specifically purified by affinity chromatography using recombinant *H. contortus* cystatin – a potent cysteine protease inhibitor [70]. All the cysteine protease activity bound to cystatin-Sepharose, representing 1.5% of the total TSBP protein content. Sheep immunized with less than 3 μg protein per dose with Quil A as adjuvant had reduced fecal egg counts of 48 and 28% and worm burdens of 44 and 46% compared to adjuvant alone controls over two trials [70]. The predicted mature forms of the three cysteine proteases identified in TSBP [70] were expressed in bacteria as insoluble, glutathione S-transferase (GST)-fusion proteins [70]. The resultant recombinant proteins were solubilized in urea/dithiothreitol (DTT) and the protective capacity of this cocktail of recombinant proteins evaluated in sheep. Worm burdens in vaccinated sheep were significantly reduced (38%) compared to controls, although fecal egg count was unaffected [70]. In a repeat trial [71], similar results were reported and the protection obtained was compared to that induced by vaccination with the predicted mature forms of hmcp1, 4, and 6 expressed in bacteria as nonfusion proteins. Sheep immunized with a cocktail of these nonfusion proteins had reduced fecal egg counts of 27% and worm burdens of 29% compared to controls. High levels of host serum IgG were detected in GST–hmcp and nonfusion hmcp-immunized animals, although no correlation with protection could be determined. Sera from these groups bound to the microvillar surface of the gut of *H. contortus*.

The ES components from adult *H. contortus* have notable vaccine potential inducing 65–90% protection against haemonchosis in sheep [72, 73]. Cysteine proteases are the most prominent protease class evident in the ES components of *H. contortus* [74] and are likely to be involved in the induction of protective immunity. The cysteine protease component of adult parasite ES product was isolated using thiol-Sepharose chromatography and the bound proteins eluted with 25 mM cysteine followed by 25 mM DTT [75]. Sheep vaccinated with the DTT-eluted fraction showed the highest level of protection with fecal egg counts and worm burdens being reduced by 52 and 50%, respectively, compared to the adjuvant control group [75]. Subsequently, cysteine proteases were purified from adult ES product [76] using a recombinant *H. contortus* cystatin-affinity column [70]. A single 43-kDa peptide band was identified as AC-5 after SDS–PAGE and mass spectrometry. AC-5 is a cathepsin B-like cysteine protease not previously identified in the ES products of *H. contortus* [76]. Lambs vaccinated with the cystatin-binding fraction 3 times prior to a single bolus challenge of 10 000 L3 *H. contortus* had 36 and 32% lower worm burdens and fecal egg counts, respectively, compared to controls; vaccination also induced local and systemic ES-specific IgA and IgG responses [76].

O. ostertagi Cysteine Proteases

O. ostertagi infects the bovine abomasum (true stomach) and, unlike *H. contortus*, is not an obligate blood-feeder. Geldhof *et al.* [7] partially characterized and showed that cysteine proteases predominate in ES product. Thiol-Sepharose chromatography was then used to obtain cysteine protease-enriched fractions from membrane-bound protein extracts (S3-thiol) and ES product (ES-thiol) of adults [77]. These fractions were tested in a vaccination experiment [77] in which calves were vaccinated with antigen in Quil A 3 times prior to challenge with a trickle infection of 25 000 infective larvae given over 25 days at 1000 L3/day, 5 days/week. Fecal egg count from the ES-thiol group was reduced by 60% compared to the controls. No reduction in egg output was observed in the S3-thiol group. At necropsy, calves immunized with ES-thiol had a significantly higher percentage of inhibited L4 larvae (9.8%) and had 18% less worms than the control calves. Adult worm size was reduced and there were less eggs per female worm in the ES-thiol group. *Ostertagia*-specific antibody levels in the abomasal mucosa were increased following vaccination, and had a significant negative correlation with the size of the adult worms, the number of eggs per female worm, and the cumulative fecal egg counts. However, these correlations were quite weak and did not appear to be isotype-specific. The major protein component of ES-thiol was an activation-associated secreted protein (ASP), whereas cysteine proteases only represented a small fraction of the total protein content [78].

In an extension of the work described in [79], *O. ostertagi* ES-thiol was subfractionated by anion-exchange chromatography to determine whether the ASP and/or the cysteine proteases were responsible for the induced protection. Groups of calves injected with the ASP-enriched, the cysteine protease-enriched, and the rest of the fraction demonstrated a reduction in cumulative fecal egg count of 74, 80, and 70%, respectively [79]. There were no significant reductions in worm burdens, but worm size was significantly reduced compared to controls. These data underlined the protective potential of the cysteine protease components of ES-thiol [78].

Confirmation of the Efficacy of Vaccine Targets and Approaches to Antigen Production and Delivery

DNA Vaccines

To date, there is only one report of successful DNA vaccination against a nematode in livestock [41]. This report targeted *Haemonchus* in goats with pcDNA 4 vaccine constructs expressing H11-1 with or without interleukin (IL)-2. Transcription of H11 and IL-2 was confirmed in muscle biopsies using the reverse transcription-polymerase chain reaction 10 days after primary immunization and translation of H11 was detected by Western blot analysis 7 days after the second immunization. Animals given the combined H11 and IL-2 DNA vaccine responded with high serum IgG, nonspecific serum IgA, and mucosal IgA. In addition, CD4$^+$ T-lymphocytes, CD8$^+$ T-lymphocytes, and B-lymphocytes were produced. Both egg output and final worm burdens were reduced by more than 40% in goats given H11-1 alone or in combination with IL-2 [41].

Production of Recombinant Nematode Proteases

The production of recombinant proteases that show the same level of vaccine efficacy as the native form has proven problematic. A key indicator of correct expression is enzymatic activity in the recombinant protein. Bacterial expression is generally useful for producing recombinant protein in quantity, but folding is often incorrect such that the protein is enzymatically inactive [80]. However, there are successes as exemplified by the recent description of a membrane-associated metalloprotease from the cestode *Taenia solium* metacestode [81]. The protease was expressed in *E. coli*, was proteolytically active with a pH optimum at 7.5 with activity being enhanced by low concentrations of Zn^{2+}. The most consistent expression system used to date for the expression of functionally active helminth proteases has been the yeast, *Pichia pastoris*, with over 30 examples described in the literature, including cysteine (e.g., [82–84]) and aspartic proteases [85]. Insect cell expression using baculovirus transfection has also proven useful for helminths proteases [86–90]. When tested in vaccine trials, these recombinant proteases have often stimulated a modest level of protective immunity, mostly reflected in a reduction in parasite egg output [90–92].

It is worthy of note that, with the exception of the work described for *H. contortus* and *O. ostertagi*, it has not been possible usually to obtain parasite biomass in sufficient quantity to allow purification of the target protease in native form for vaccine trials. Therefore, it is a distinct possibility that protection noted with the recombinant proteases outlined above could be enhanced by the use of a different expression system. For example, protection obtained with enzymically active forms of H11 expressed in bacteria, yeast, or insect cells has never approached the efficacy of the native protein. This interpretation should be viewed with caution because the native proteases used in vaccine trials to date have usually contained other proteins. Even though these represented a small percentage of the total protein, we know that small amounts of a protective protein can be, nevertheless, effective [70, 71]. The development of *in vivo* RNAi (see below) will be of immense value here because, theoretically at least, it will provide a measure of what level could be achieved targeting a single antigen or even a combination.

Expression of Vaccine Antigens in *Caenorhabditis elegans*

The frequent failure of recombinant proteins to stimulate the same degree of protective immunity as their native antigen counterparts has been generally ascribed to incorrect post-translational processing, be it folding or glycosylation. One possible solution being pursued is the use of *C. elegans* to express the target antigen given that it is a clade V nematode (like *H. contortus*) and that post-translational processing is likely to be similar. This approach was stimulated by a report that used *C. elegans* as a model to study the mechanism of resistance against benzimidazole drugs in *H. contortus* [93]. The gonad of *C. elegans* was transfected with plasmid constructs carrying *H. contortus* benzimidazole-sensitive and benzimidazole-resistant alleles, and mutagenized β-tubulin gene constructs. Importantly, the benzimidazole sensitivity of the progeny correlated with the nature of the construct delivered [93].

Using *C. elegans* to express heterologous nematode proteins was also explored in [94] in which the authors isolated a 4-kb genomic sequence encoding an aspartic protease component of H-gal-GP. This contained eight introns ranging in size from 54 to 1475 base pairs and, together with the 3′ noncoding DNA region containing a polyadenylation signal sequence, was cloned into the Bluescript SK$^+$ vector immediately downstream of the *C. elegans* intestinal cysteine protease (*cpr-5*) gene promoter. The plasmid was injected into *C. elegans* and two transgenic lines were established. Immunohistochemistry showed expression of the *Haemonchus* protein in the gut of transgenic *C. elegans*, with reactivity evident in the larval and adult stages. This work was extended when a *C. elegans* cathepsin L-like gene (*Ce-cpl-1*), known to be essential for embryonic development could be replaced by transgenic expression of the *H. contortus* (*Hc*) *cpl-1* gene that rescued the embryonic lethality arising from the *Ce-cpl-1* null mutant [95]. In a further extension of this work, *C. elegans* was evaluated as an expression system for the *Hc-cpl-1* with the aim of producing sufficient functionally active recombinant protein to conduct downstream biochemical analyses and vaccine trials [96]. *Hc-cpl-1*, containing a polyhistidine tag at the C-terminus, was expressed in *C. elegans* with optimal expression being evident under the control of the promoter of the endogenous *Ce-cpl-1*. The recombinant protein (Figure 24.5) was purified from liquid cultures by nickel chelation chromatography, and was functionally active and glycosylated. The product was tested as a vaccine, but no protective immunity was observed. Nevertheless, this work [96] showed that active, post-translationally modified parasitic nematode proteases can be expressed in *C. elegans* and that this approach could be extended to other known

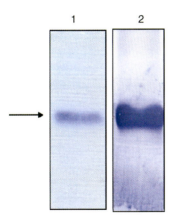

Figure 24.5 Expression of *H. contortus* cathepsin L in *C. elegans*. The protein (lane 1) is antigenically similar to its native counterpart (lane 2, an immunoblot probed with anticathepsin L antibody), and is functionally active and glycosylated. Heterologous nematode proteases can be produced in this system in sufficient quantity for vaccination studies ([96] © 1997 Elsevier).

protective antigens. Indeed, this has now been accomplished for two *Haemonchus* H11 isoforms (Roberts *et al.*, unpublished). The recombinant proteins exhibited aminopeptidase activity, possessed glycan modifications similar to those of the native protein, and were produced in sufficient quantities for vaccine trials, the outcome of which is awaited.

RNAi

Gene silencing by RNAi has been successful in *C. elegans* to study gene function and identify genes that are essential for survival. However, the technique has proven less effective in parasitic nematodes (see also Chapter 6). In *H. contortus*, previous studies showed reproducible silencing of β-tubulin [97], but not of other genes targeted [98]. RNAi in *Haemonchus* [99] and *O. ostertagi* [100] only works on a limited number of genes, and in some cases the effect is small and difficult to reproduce. The reasons for this have been discussed, and include factors such as the mode of delivery of double-stranded RNA to the parasite, the developmental stage targeted, and, perhaps of most importance, whether the RNAi pathway (as defined by studies in *C. elegans*) is fully functional in some parasitic nematodes [98]. A recent study examined whether the level of target transcript or site of gene expression influence susceptibility to RNAi by soaking [101]. Genes expressed in sites accessible to the environment appeared to be more likely to be susceptible to RNAi by soaking and these genes included that encoding the highly protective gut aminopeptidase H11. The study assessed whether RNAi of H11 could mimic H11 vaccination in reducing worm and egg counts *in vivo*. RNAi targeting the H11-1 isoform gene in L3s prior to infection resulted in 57 and 40% reductions in fecal egg count and worm burdens, respectively, with a 64% decrease in aminopeptidase activity in recovered adult worms compared to worms soaked in control double-stranded RNA (Figure 24.6) [101]. Future work will measure

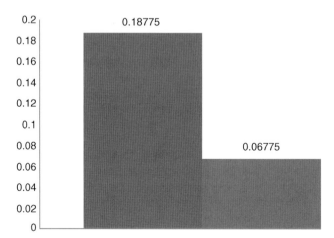

Figure 24.6 RNAi of the H11-1 isoform decreases aminopeptidase activity in whole-worm extracts of adult *H. contortus* [39]. Enzyme activity in H11-1 RNAi-treated worms (red) was reduced compared to controls (blue) – data which suggest that H11-1 is a good vaccine target.

the effects of RNAi on a variety of genes expressed in the intestine of livestock nematode parasites, including proteases. RNAi offers the possibility of precise target definition when protection is stimulated using a mixture of proteases such as the *Haemonchus* H-gal-GP or TSBP discussed above. In addition, it provides a pathway to exploit the genome and transcriptome sequencing projects being undertaken for several livestock nematode parasites (see Chapter 4).

Conclusions

At the start of this chapter, I stated that antibody inhibition of protease function is likely to affect parasite establishment and survival within the host. This has made these enzymes lead vaccine targets for nematode infections. I hope the preceding discussion has supported this view convincingly. The challenge that remains is to reproduce the protective effects of native proteins with recombinant versions. This is being addressed in innovative ways, such the engineering of *C. elegans* [98] and *P. pastoris* to produce appropriate expression levels of proteins with the correct type of glycans [102, 103]. RNAi will hopefully become a more reliable tool to defining gene products that are essential for nematode survival. This will allow precise definition of the target's essentiality and the level of protection that can be produced by vaccination. With this information, it will then be possible to accurately assess the performance of a recombinant protein-based vaccine. Of course, the latter is dependent on the accessibility of the target protein to the host immune response and the timing of expression. Therefore, in this genomics-centric era, we must not lose sight of the need for basic underpinning research on gene function, site of expression, and the nature of the target protein.

Acknowledgments

The author would like to acknowledge the support received for his work over a number of years from the Scottish Government, European Union, and a number of commercial companies. The preparation of this chapter was supported by funding from the European Commission Framework VII programme (project **265862**).

References

1 McKerrow, J.H., Caffrey, C., Kelly, B., Loke, P., and Sajid, M. (2006) Proteases in parasitic diseases. *Annu. Rev. Pathol.*, **1**, 497–536.

2 Tort., J., Brindley, P.J., Knox., D., Wolfe, K.H., and Dalton, J.P. (1999) Proteinases and associated genes of parasitic helminths. *Adv. Parasitol.*, **43**, 161–266.

3 Williamson, A.L., Brindley, P.J., Knox, D.P., Hotez, P.J., and Loukas, A. (2003) Digestive proteases of blood-feeding nematodes. *Trends Parasitol.*, **19**, 417–423.

4 Stepek, G., McCormack, G., and Page, A.P. (2010) Collagen processing and cuticle formation is catalysed by the astacin metalloprotease DPY-31 in free-living and parasitic nematodes. *Int. J. Parasitol.*, **40**, 533–542.

5 Knox, D.P. (1994) Parasite enzymes and the control of roundworm and fluke infestation in domestic animals. *Br. Vet. J.*, **150**, 319–337.

6 Knox, D.P. and Jones, D.G. (1990) Studies on the presence and release of proteolytic enzymes (proteinases) in gastro-intestinal nematodes of ruminants. *Int. J. Parasitol.*, **20**, 243–249.

7 Geldhof, P., Claerebout, E., Knox, D.P., Jagneessens, J., and Vercruysse, J. (2000) Proteinases released *in vitro* by the parasitic stages of the bovine abomasal nematode *Ostertagia ostertagi*. *Parasitology*, **121**, 639–647.

8 Redmond, D.L., Smith, S.K., Halliday, A., Smith, W.D., Jackson, F., Knox, D.P., and Matthews, J.B. (2006) An immunogenic cathepsin F secreted by the parasitic stages of *Teladorsagia circumcincta*. *Int. J. Parasitol.*, **36**, 277–286.

9 Thorson, R.E. (1953) Studies on the mechanism of immunity in the rat to the nematode, *Nippostrongylus muris*. *Am. J. Hygiene*, **58**, 1–15.

10 Thorson, R.E. (1954) Effect of immune serum from rats on infective larvae of *Nippostrongylus muris*. *Exp. Parasitol.*, **3**, 9–15.

11 Thorson, R.E. (1956) Proteolytic activity in extracts of the oesophagus of adults of *Ancylostoma caninum* and the effect of immune serum on this activity. *J. Parasitol.*, **42**, 21–25.

12 Thorson, R.E. (1956) The stimulation of acquired immunity in dogs by injections of extracts of the oesophagus of adult hookworms. *J. Parasitol.*, **42**, 501–504.

13 Rogers, W.P. and Brooks, F. (1977) The mechanism of hatching of eggs of *Haemonchus contortus*. *Int. J. Parasitol.*, **7**, 61–65.

14 Rinaldi, G., Morales, M.E., Alrefaei, Y.N., Cancela, M., Castillo, E., Dalton, J.P., Tort, J.F., and Brindley, P.J. (2009) RNA interference targeting leucine aminopeptidase blocks hatching of *Schistosoma mansoni* eggs. *Mol. Biochem. Parasitol.*, **167**, 118–126.

15 González-Páez, G.E., Argüello-García, R., and Alba-Hurtado, F. (2007) *Toxocara canis*: proteinases in perivitelline fluid from hatching eggs. *Vet. Parasitol.*, **147**, 332–335.

16 Gamble, H.R., Purcell, J.P., and Fetterer, R.H. (1989) Purification of a 44 kilodalton protease which mediates the ecdysis of infective *Haemonchus contortus* larvae. *Mol. Biochem. Parasitol.*, **33**, 49–58.

17 Gamble, H.R., Fetterer, R.H., and Mansfield, L.S. (1996) Developmentally regulated zinc metalloproteinases from third- and fourth-stage larvae of the ovine nematode *Haemonchus contortus*. *J. Parasitol.*, **82**, 197–202.

18 Knox, D.P. and Kennedy, M.W. (1988) Proteinases released by the parasitic larval stages of *Ascaris suum*, and their inhibition by antibody. *Mol. Biochem. Parasitol.*, **28**, 207–216.

19 Rhoads, M.L. and Fetterer, R.H. (1996) Extracellular matrix degradation by *Haemonchus contortus*. *J. Parasitol.*, **82**, 379–383.

20 De Cock, H., Knox, D.P., Claerebout, E., and De Graaf, D.C. (1993) Partial characterization of proteolytic enzymes in different developmental stages of *Ostertagia ostertagi*. *J. Helminthol.*, **67**, 271–278.

21 Young, C.J., McKeand, J.B., and Knox, D.P. (1995) Proteinases released *in vitro* by the parasitic stages of *Teladorsagia circumcincta*, an ovine abomasal nematode. *Parasitology*, **110**, 465–471.

22 MacLennan, K., Gallagher, M.P., and Knox, D.P. (1997) Stage-specific serine and metallo-proteinase release by adult and larval *Trichostrongylus vitrinus*. *Int. J. Parasitol.*, **27**, 1031–1036.

23 Todorova, V.K., Knox, D.P., and Kennedy, M.W. (1995) Proteinases in the excretory/secretory products (ES) of adult *Trichinella spiralis*. *Parasitology*, **111**, 201–208.

24 Ekoja, S.E. and Smith, W.D. (2010) Antibodies from sheep immunized against *Haemonchus contortus* with H-gal-GP inhibit the haemoglobinase

activity of this protease complex. *Parasite Immunol.*, **32**, 731–738.
25. Knox, D.P., Redmond, D.L., and Jones, D.G. (1993) Characterization of proteinases in extracts of adult *Haemonchus contortus*, the ovine abomasal nematode. *Parasitology*, **106**, 395–404.
26. Cox, G.N., Pratt, D., Hageman, R., and Boisvenue, R.J. (1990) Molecular cloning and primary sequence of a cysteine protease expressed by *Haemonchus contortus* adult worms. *Mol. Biochem. Parasitol.*, **41**, 25–34.
27. Geldhof, P. and Knox, D. (2008) The intestinal contortin structure in *Haemonchus contortus*: An immobilised anticoagulant? *Int. J. Parasitol.*, **38**, 1579–1588.
28. Fetterer, R.H. and Rhoads, M.L. (1997) The *in vitro* uptake and incorporation of haemoglobin by adult *Haemonchus contortus*. *Vet. Parasitol.*, **69**, 77–87.
29. Fetterer, R.H. and Rhoads, M.L. (1997) The *in vitro* uptake of albumin by adult *Haemonchus contortus* is altered by extracorporeal digestion. *Vet. Parasitol.*, **73**, 249–256.
30. Chapman, C.B. and Mitchell, G.F. (1982) Proteolytic cleavage of immunoglobulin by enzymes released by *Fasciola hepatica*. *Vet. Parasitol.*, **11**, 165–178.
31. Berasain, P., Carmona, C., Frangione, B., Dalton, J.P., and Goñi, F. (2000) *Fasciola hepatica*: parasite-secreted proteinases degrade all human IgG subclasses: determination of the specific cleavage sites and identification of the immunoglobulin fragments produced [erratum in *Exp. Parasitol.* (2002), 100(3), 208]. *Exp. Parasitol.*, **94**, 99–110..
32. Jasmer, D.P., Roth, J., and Myler, P.J. (2001) Cathepsin B-like cysteine proteases and *Caenorhabditis elegans* homologues dominate gene products expressed in adult *Haemonchus contortus* intestine. *Mol. Biochem. Parasitol.*, **116**, 159–169.
33. Jasmer, D.P., Mitreva, M.D., and McCarter, J.P. (2004) mRNA sequences for *Haemonchus contortus* intestinal cathepsin B-like cysteine proteases display an extreme in abundance and diversity compared with other adult mammalian parasitic nematodes. *Mol. Biochem. Parasitol.*, **137**, 297–305.
34. Barnes, E.H., Dobson, R.J., and Barger, I.A. (1995) Worm control and anthelmintic resistance: adventures with a model. *Parasitol. Today*, **11**, 56–63.
35. Munn, E.A., Smith, T.S., Smith, H., James, F.M., Smith, F.C., and Andrews, S.J. (1997) Vaccination against *Haemonchus contortus* with denatured forms of the protective antigen H11. *Parasite Immunol.*, **19**, 243–248.
36. Newton, S.E. and Munn, E.A. (1999) The development of vaccines against gastrointestinal nematode parasites, particularly *Haemonchus contortus*. *Parasitol. Today*, **15**, 116–122.
37. Smith, T.S., Graham, M., Munn, E.A., Newton, S.E., Knox, D.P., Coadwell, W.J., McMichael-Phillips, D., Smith, H. Smith, W.D., and Oliver, J.J. (1997) Cloning and characterization of a microsomal aminopeptidase from the intestine of the nematode *Haemonchus contortus*. *Biochim. Biophys. Acta*, **1338**, 295–306.
38. Haslam, S.M., Coles, G.C., Munn, E.A., Smith, T.S., Smith, H.F., Morris, H.R., and Dell, A. (1996) *Haemonchus contortus* glycoproteins contain *N*-linked oligosaccharides with novel highly fucosylated core structures. *J. Biol. Chem.*, **271**, 30561–30570.
39. Samarasinghe, B., Knox, D.P., and Britton, C. (2011) Factors affecting susceptibility to RNA interference in *Haemonchus contortus* and *in vivo* silencing of an H11 aminopeptidase gene. *Int. J. Parasitol.*, **41**, 51–59.
40. Reszka, N., Rijsewijk, F.A., Zelnik, V., Moskwa, B., and Bieńkowska-Szewczyk, K. (2007) *Haemonchus contortus*: characterization of the baculovirus expressed form of aminopeptidase H11. *Exp. Parasitol.*, **117**, 208–213.
41. Zhao, G., Yan, R., Muleke, C.I., Sun, Y., Xu, L., and Li, X. (2012) Vaccination of goats with DNA vaccines encoding H11 and IL-2 induces partial protection against *Haemonchus contortus* infection. *Vet. J.*, **191**, 94–100.

42 Smith, W.D., Smith, S.K., and Murray, J.M. (1994) Protection studies with integral membrane fractions of *Haemonchus contortus*. *Parasite Immunol.*, **16**, 231–241.

43 Smith, S.K., Pettit, D., Newlands, G.F., Redmond, D.L., Skuce, P.J., Knox, D.P., and Smith, W.D. (1999) Further immunization and biochemical studies with a protective antigen complex from the microvillar membrane of the intestine of *Haemonchus contortus*. *Parasite Immunol.*, **21**, 187–199.

44 LeJambre, L.F., Windon, R.G., and Smith, W.D. (2008) Vaccination against *Haemonchus contortus*: performance of native parasite gut membrane glycoproteins in Merino lambs grazing contaminated pasture. *Vet. Parasitol.*, **153**, 302–312.

45 Smith, W.D., Skuce, P.J., Newlands, G.F., Smith, S.K., and Pettit, D. (2003) Aspartyl proteases from the intestinal brush border of *Haemonchus contortus* as protective antigens for sheep. *Parasite Immunol.*, **25**, 521–530.

46 Longbottom, D., Redmond, D.L., Russell, M., Liddell, S., Smith, W.D., and Knox, D.P. (1997) Molecular cloning and characterisation of a putative aspartate proteinase associated with a gut membrane protein complex from adult *Haemonchus contortus*. *Mol. Biochem. Parasitol.*, **88**, 63–72.

47 Redmond, D.L., Knox, D.P., Newlands, G., and Smith, W.D. (1997) Molecular cloning and characterisation of a developmentally regulated putative metallopeptidase present in a host protective extract of *Haemonchus contortus*. *Mol. Biochem. Parasitol.*, **85**, 77–87.

48 Newlands, G.F., Skuce, P.J., Nisbet, A.J., Redmond, D.L., Smith, S.K., Pettit, D., and Smith, W.D. (2006) Molecular characterization of a family of metalloendopeptidases from the intestinal brush border of *Haemonchus contortus*. *Parasitology*, **133**, 357–368.

49 Newlands, G.F., Skuce, P.J., Knox, D.P., Smith, S.K., and Smith, W.D. (1999) Cloning and characterization of a beta-galactoside-binding protein (galectin) from the gut of the gastrointestinal nematode parasite *Haemonchus contortus*. *Parasitology*, **119**, 483–490.

50 Newlands, G.F., Skuce, P.J., Knox, D.P., and Smith, W.D. (2001) Cloning and expression of cystatin, a potent cysteine protease inhibitor from the gut of *Haemonchus contortus*. *Parasitology*, **122**, 371–378.

51 Skuce, P.J., Newlands, G.F., Stewart, E.M., Pettit, D., Smith, S.K., Smith, W.D., and Knox, D.P. (2001) Cloning and characterisation of thrombospondin, a novel multidomain glycoprotein found in association with a host protective gut extract from *Haemonchus contortus*. *Mol. Biochem. Parasitol.*, **117**, 241–244.

52 Smith, W.D., Skuce, P.J., Newlands, G.F., Smith, S.K., and Pettit, D. (2003) Aspartyl proteases from the intestinal brush border of *Haemonchus contortus* as protective antigens for sheep. *Parasite Immunol.*, **25**, 521–530.

53 Smith, W.D., Newlands, G.F., Smith, S.K., Pettit, D., and Skuce, P.J. (2003) Metalloendopeptidases from the intestinal brush border of *Haemonchus contortus* as protective antigens for sheep. *Parasite Immunol.*, **25**, 313–323.

54 Cachat, E., Newlands, G.F., Ekoja, S.E., McAllister, H., and Smith, W.D. (2010) Attempts to immunize sheep against *Haemonchus contortus* using a cocktail of recombinant proteases derived from the protective antigen. H-gal-GP. *Parasite Immunol.*, **32**, 414–419.

55 Smith, W.D., van Wyk, J.A., and van Strijp, M.F. (2001) Preliminary observations on the potential of gut membrane proteins of *Haemonchus contortus* as candidate vaccine antigens in sheep on naturally infected pasture. *Vet. Parasitol.*, **27**, 285–297.

56 LeJambre, L.F., Windon, R.G., and Smith, W.D. (2008) Vaccination against *Haemonchus contortus*: performance of native parasite gut membrane glycoproteins in Merino lambs grazing contaminated pasture. *Vet. Parasitol.*, **153**, 302–312.

57 Williamson, A.L., Lecchi, P., Turk, B.E., Choe, Y., Hotez, P.J., McKerrow, J.H., Cantley, L.C., Sajid, M., Craik, C.S., and Loukas, A. (2004) A multi-enzyme cascade of hemoglobin proteolysis in the intestine of blood-feeding hookworms. *J. Biol. Chem.*, **279**, 35950–35957.

58 Delcroix, M., Sajid, M., Caffrey, C.R., Lim, K.C., Dvorák, J., Hsieh, I., Bahgat, M., Dissous, C., and McKerrow, J.H. (2006) A multienzyme network functions in intestinal protein digestion by a platyhelminth parasite. *J. Biol. Chem.*, **281**, 39316–39329.

59 Liu, J., Istvan, E.S., Gluzman, I.Y., Gross, J., and Goldberg, D.E. (2006) *Plasmodium falciparum* ensures its amino acid supply with multiple acquisition pathways and redundant proteolytic enzyme systems. *Proc. Natl. Acad. Sci. USA*, **103**, 8840–8845.

60 Horn, M., Nussbaumerová, M., Sanda, M., Kovárová, Z., Srba, J., Franta, Z., Sojka, D., Bogyo, M., Caffrey, C.R., Kopácek, P., and Mares, M. (2009) Hemoglobin digestion in blood-feeding ticks: mapping a multipeptidase pathway by functional proteomics. *Chem. Biol.*, **16**, 1053–1063.

61 Jasmer, D.P., Mitreva, M.D., and McCarter, J.P. (2004) mRNA sequences for *Haemonchus contortus* intestinal cathepsin B-like cysteine proteases display an extreme in abundance and diversity compared with other adult mammalian parasitic nematodes. *Mol. Biochem. Parasitol.*, **137**, 297–305.

62 Boisvenue, R.J., Stiff, M.I., Tonkinson, L.V., Cox, G.N., and Hageman, R. (1992) Fibrinogen-degrading proteins from *Haemonchus contortus* used to vaccinate sheep. *Am. J. Vet. Res.*, **53**, 1263–1265.

63 Cox, G.N., Pratt, D., Hageman, R., and Boisvenue, R.J. (1990) Molecular cloning and primary sequence of a cysteine protease expressed by *Haemonchus contortus* adult worms. *Mol. Biochem. Parasitol.*, **41**, 25–34.

64 Pratt, D., Cox, G.N., Milhausen, M.J., and Boisvenue, R.J. (1990) A developmentally regulated cysteine protease gene family in *Haemonchus contortus. Mol. Biochem. Parasitol.*, **43**, 181–191.

65 Pratt, D., Armes, L.G., Hageman, R., Reynolds, V., Boisvenue, R.J., and Cox, G.N. (1992) Cloning and sequence comparisons of four distinct cysteine proteases expressed by *Haemonchus contortus* adult worms. *Mol. Biochem. Parasitol.*, **51**, 209–218.

66 Pratt, D., Boisvenue, R.J., and Cox, G.N. (1992) Isolation of putative cysteine protease genes of *Ostertagia ostertagi. Mol. Biochem. Parasitol.*, **56**, 39–48.

67 Knox, D.P., Smith, S.K., and Smith, W.D. (1999) Immunization with an affinity purified protein extract from the adult parasite protects lambs against infection with *Haemonchus contortus. Parasite Immunol.*, **21**, 201–210.

68 Ruiz, A., Molina, J.M., González, J.F., Conde, M.M., Martín, S., and Hernández, Y.I. (2004) Immunoprotection in goats against *Haemonchus contortus* after immunization with cysteine protease enriched protein fractions. *Vet. Res.*, **35**, 565–572.

69 Skuce, P.J., Redmond, D.L., Liddell, S., Stewart, E.M., Newlands, G.F., Smith, W.D., and Knox, D.P. (1999) Molecular cloning and characterization of gut-derived cysteine proteinases associated with a host protective extract from *Haemonchus contortus. Parasitology*, **119**, 405–412.

70 Redmond, D.L. and Knox, D.P. (2004) Protection studies in sheep using affinity-purified and recombinant cysteine proteinases of adult *Haemonchus contortus. Vaccine*, **22**, 4252–4261.

71 Redmond, D.L. and Knox, D.P. (2006) Further protection studies using recombinant forms of *Haemonchus contortus* cysteine proteinases. *Parasite Immunol.*, **28**, 213–219.

72 Schallig, H.D., van Leeuwen, M.A., and Cornelissen, A.W. (1997) Protective immunity induced by vaccination with two *Haemonchus contortus* excretory secretory proteins in sheep. *Parasite Immunol.*, **19**, 447–453.

73 Vervelde, L., Kooyman, F.N., Van Leeuwen, M.A., Schallig, H.D.,

MacKellar, A., Huntley, J.F., and Cornelissen, A.W. (2001) Age-related protective immunity after vaccination with *Haemonchus contortus* excretory/secretory proteins. *Parasite Immunol.*, **23**, 419–426.

74 Yatsuda, A., Bakker, N., Krijgsveld, J., Knox, D.P., Heck, A.J., and de Vries, E. (2006) Identification of secreted cysteine proteases from the parasitic nematode *Haemonchus contortus* detected by biotinylated inhibitors. *Infect. Immun.*, **74**, 1989–1993.

75 Bakker, N., Vervelde, L., Kanobana, K., Knox, D.P., Cornelissen, A.W., de Vries, E., and Yatsuda, A.P. (2004) Vaccination against the nematode *Haemonchus contortus* with a thiol-binding fraction from the excretory/secretory products (ES). *Vaccine*, **22**, 618–628.

76 De Vries, E., Bakker, N., Krijgsveld, J., Knox, D.P., Heck, A.J., and Yatsuda, A.P. (2009) An AC-5 cathepsin B-like protease purified from *Haemonchus contortus* excretory secretory products shows protective antigen potential for lambs. *Vet. Res.*, **40**, 41.

77 Geldhof, P., Claerebout, E., Knox, D., Vercauteren, I., Looszova, A., and Vercruysse, J. (2002) Vaccination of calves against *Ostertagia ostertagi* with cysteine proteinase enriched protein fractions. *Parasite Immunol.*, **24**, 263–270.

78 Geldhof, P., Vercauteren, I., Gevaert, K., Staes, A., Knox, D.P., Vandekerckhove, J., Vercruysse, J., and Claerebout, E. (2003) Activation-associated secreted proteins are the most abundant antigens in a host protective fraction from *Ostertagia ostertagi*. *Mol. Biochem. Parasitol.*, **128**, 111–114.

79 Meyvis, Y., Geldhof, P., Gevaert, K., Timmerman, E., Vercruysse, J., and Claerebout, E. (2007) Vaccination against *Ostertagia ostertagi* with subfractions of the protective ES-thiol fraction. *Vet. Parasitol.*, **149**, 239–245.

80 Dalton, J.P., Brindley, P.J., Knox, D.P., Brady, C.P., Hotez, P.J., Donnelly, S., O'Neill, S.M., Mulcahy, G., and Loukas, A. (2003) Helminth vaccines: from mining genomic information for vaccine targets to systems used for protein expression. *Int. J. Parasitol.*, **33**, 621–640.

81 Cai, G.B., Bae, Y.A., Kim, S.H., Na, B.K., Kim, T.S., Jiang, M.S., and Kong, Y. (2006) A membrane-associated metalloprotease of *Taenia solium* metacestode structurally related to the FACE-1/Ste24p protease family. *Int. J. Parasitol.*, **36**, 925–935.

82 Sajid, M., McKerrow, J.H., Hansell, E., Mathieu, M.A., Lucas, K.D., Hsieh, I., Greenbaum, D., Bogyo, M., Salter, J.P., Lim, K.C., Franklin, C., Kim, J.H., and Caffrey, C.R. (2003) Functional expression and characterization of *Schistosoma mansoni* cathepsin B and its trans-activation by an endogenous asparaginyl endopeptidase. *Mol. Biochem. Parasitol.*, **131**, 65–75.

83 Collins, P.R., Stack, C.M., O'Neill, S.M., Doyle, S., Ryan, T., Brennan, G.P., Mousley, A., Stewart, M., Maule, A.G., Dalton, J.P., and Donnelly, S. (2004) Cathepsin L1, the major protease involved in liver fluke (*Fasciola hepatica*) virulence: propetide cleavage sites and autoactivation of the zymogen secreted from gastrodermal cells. *J. Biol Chem.*, **279**, 17038–17046.

84 Ranjit, N., Zhan, B., Hamilton, B., Stenzel, D., Lowther, J., Pearson, M., Gorman, J., Hotez, P., and Loukas, A. (2009) Proteolytic degradation of hemoglobin in the intestine of the human hookworm *Necator americanus*. *J. Infect. Dis.*, **199**, 904–912.

85 Williamson, A.L., Brindley, P.J., Abbenante, G., Datu, B.J., Prociv, P., Berry, C., Girdwood, K., Pritchard, D.I., Fairlie, D.P., Hotez, P.J., Zhan, B., and Loukas, A. (2003) Hookworm aspartic protease, Na-APR-2, cleaves human hemoglobin and serum proteins in a host-specific fashion. *J. Infect. Dis.*, **187**, 484–494.

86 Hola-Jamriska, L., King, L.T., Dalton, J.P., Mann, V.H., Aaskov, J.G., and Brindley, P.J. (2000) Functional expression of dipeptidyl peptidase I (CathepsinC) of the oriental blood fluke *Schistosoma japonicum* in *Trichoplusia ni* insect cells. *Protein Expr. Purif.*, **19**, 384–392.

87 Brindley, P.J., Kalinna, B.H., Wong, J.Y., Bogitsh, B.J., King, L.T., Smyth, D.J., Verity, C.K., Abbenante, G., Brinkworth, R.I., Fairlie, D.P., Smythe, M.L., Milburn, P.J., Bielefeldt-Ohmann, H., Zheng, Y., and McManus, D.P. (2001) Proteolysis of human hemoglobin by schistosome cathepsin D. *Mol. Biochem. Parasitol.*, **112**, 103–112.

88 Williamson, A.L., Brindley, P.J., Abbenante, G., Prociv, P., Berry, C., Girdwood, K., Pritchard, D.I., Fairlie, D.P., Hotez, P.J., Dalton, J.P., and Loukas, A. (2002) Cleavage of hemoglobin by hookworm cathepsin D aspartic proteases and its potential contribution to host specificity. *FASEB J.*, **16**, 1458–1460.

89 De Maere, V., Vercauteren, I., Geldhof, P., Gevaert, K., Vercruysse, J., and Claerebout, E. (2005) Molecular analysis of astacin-like metalloproteases of *Ostertagia ostertagi*. *Parasitology*, **130**, 89–98.

90 Reszka, N., Rijsewijk., F.A., Zelnik., V., Moskwa., B., and Bieńkowska-Szewczyk, K. (2007) *Haemonchus contortus*: characterization of the baculovirus expressed form of aminopeptidase H11. *Exp. Parasitol.*, **117**, 208–213.

91 Loukas, A., Bethony, J.M., Williamson, A.L., Goud, G.N., Mendez, S., Zhan, B., Hawdon, J.M., Elena Bottazzi, M., Brindley, P.J., and Hotez, P.J. (2004) Vaccination of dogs with a recombinant cysteine protease from the intestine of canine hookworms diminishes the fecundity and growth of worms. *J. Infect. Dis.*, **189**, 1952–1961.

92 Loukas, A., Bethony, J.M., Mendez, S., Fujiwara, R.T., Goud, G.N., Ranjit, N., Zhan, B., Jones, K., Bottazzi, M.E., and Hotez, P.J. (2005) Vaccination with recombinant aspartic hemoglobinase reduces parasite load and blood loss after hookworm infection in dogs. *PLoS Med.*, **2**, e295.

93 Kwa, M.S., Veenstra, J.G., and Roos, M.H. (1994) Benzimidazole resistance in *Haemonchus contortus* is correlated with a conserved mutation at amino acid 200 in beta-tubulin isotype 1. *Mol. Biochem. Parasitol.*, **63**, 299–303.

94 Redmond, D.L., Clucas, C., Johnstone, I.L., and Knox, D.P. (2001) Expression of *Haemonchus contortus* pepsinogen in *Caenorhabditis elegans*. *Mol. Biochem. Parasitol.*, **112**, 125–131.

95 Britton, C. and Murray, L. (2002) A cathepsin L protease essential for *Caenorhabditis elegans* embryogenesis is functionally conserved in parasitic nematodes. *Mol. Biochem. Parasitol.*, **122**, 21–33.

96 Murray, L., Geldhof, P., Clark, D., Knox, D.P., and Britton, C. (2007) Expression and purification of an active cysteine protease of *Haemonchus contortus* using *Caenorhabditis elegans*. *Int. J. Parasitol.*, **37**, 1117–1125.

97 Kotze, A.C. and Bagnall, N.H. (2006) RNA interference in *Haemonchus contortus*: suppression of beta-tubulin gene expression in L3, L4 and adult worms *in vitro*. *Mol. Biochem. Parasitol.*, **145**, 101–110.

98 Knox, D.P., Geldhof, P., Visser, A., and Britton, C. (2007) RNA interference in parasitic nematodes of animals: a reality check? *Trends Parasitol.*, **23**, 105–107.

99 Geldhof, P., Murray, L., Couthier, A., Gilleard, J.S., McLauchlan, G., Knox, D.P., and Britton., C. (2006) Testing the efficacy of RNA interference in *Haemonchus contortus*. *Int. J. Parasitol.*, **36**, 801–810.

100 Visser, A., Geldhof, P., de Maere, V., Knox, D.P., Vercruysse, J., and Claerebout, E. (2006) Efficacy and specificity of RNA interference in larval life-stages of *Ostertagia ostertagi*. *Parasitology*, **133**, 777–783.

101 Samarasinghe, B., Knox, D.P., and Britton, C. (2011) Factors affecting susceptibility to RNA interference in *Haemonchus contortus* and *in vivo* silencing of an H11 aminopeptidase gene. *Int. J. Parasitol.*, **41**, 51–59.

102 Vervecken, W., Callewaert, N., Kaigorodov, V., Geysens, S., and

Contreras, R. (2007) Modification of the N-glycosylation pathway to produce homogeneous, human-like glycans using GlycoSwitch plasmids. *Methods Mol. Biol.*, **389**, 119–138.

103 Jacobs, P.P., Geysens, S., Vervecken, W., Contreras, R., and Callewaert, N. (2009) Engineering complex-type N-glycosylation in *Pichia pastoris* using GlycoSwitch technology. *Nat. Protoc.*, **4**, 58–70.

25
Schistosomiasis Vaccines – New Approaches to Antigen Discovery and Promising New Candidates

Alex Loukas[*], Soraya Gaze, Mark Pearson, Denise Doolan, Philip Felgner, David Diemert, Donald P. McManus, Patrick Driguez, and Jeffrey Bethony

Abstract

Vaccine development for schistosomiasis has had a chequered history. Many antigens that showed initial promise in murine models dropped by the wayside and only two vaccines are currently in clinical trials. In this chapter, we discuss antigen discovery in light of the "schistosomics" revolution, with a particular focus on immunomics, and undertake some crystal ball gazing on where all this information might lead us in the near future. We then discuss the transition of neglected tropical disease vaccines towards clinical trials via a public–private partnership model, using the discovery and preclinical development of the *Sm*-TSP-2 schistosomiasis vaccine as a case study.

Introduction

Schistosomes are some of the most important parasites of humans in terms of their global health impact on children, pregnant women, and people engaged in subsistence farming [1–3]. When the chronic morbidities due to schistosomiasis are fully considered, based on disability-adjusted life years (DALYs) lost, this disease ranks among the most important in developing countries, resulting in an annual loss of between 4.5 and 92 million DALYs [4, 5]. Schistosomiasis can be treated with anthelmintic drugs, but this approach does not protect against rapid and high-frequency reinfection with schistosome parasites [4]. The mainstay of control for schistosomiasis is the quinoline compound, praziquantel. There are concerns that mass administration of praziquantel is unsustainable because of lower-than-expected efficacies of single-dose praziquantel and high rates of post-treatment reinfection, pointing towards the potential emergence of drug resistance [6]. Indeed, praziquantel resistance has been generated in *Schistosoma mansoni* in the laboratory [7]. Mass drug administration (MDA) programs are, therefore, inadequate in isolation, and new tools and integrated approaches are needed to ensure long-term, sustainable control of schistosomiasis [8]. Among these, vaccines are an essential component. Herein,

[*] Corresponding Author

we describe the use of various "schistosomics" approaches to characterize the transcriptomes, genomes, and proteomes of schistosomes, as well as the postgenomic molecular applications of these datasets to identify the most suitable target antigens for vaccine development to combat the disease they cause.

Schistosomes

Schistosome flatworms (phylum Platyhelminthes), also known as trematodes or flukes, cause approximately 207 million cases of human schistosomiasis world-wide, mostly in sub-Saharan Africa [3]. However, some estimates indicate that as many as 400 million people may be affected [9]. In Africa, *Schistosoma haematobium* is the most prevalent human schistosome; it causes urinary tract schistosomiasis, which comprises approximately two-thirds of the world's cases of schistosomiasis. *Schistosoma mansoni* is the principal cause of intestinal schistosomiasis and is responsible for approximately one-third of all cases. *S. mansoni* also causes schistosomiasis in Latin America, with most of the cases occurring in Brazil, while *Schistosoma japonicum* and *Schistosoma mekongi* cause approximately 1 million cases of intestinal schistosomiasis in East Asia [3].

Schistosomes are transmitted through contact with freshwater containing the infective free-swimming microscopic cercariae, which actively penetrate the skin of their human host. Cercariae that have entered human skin shed their tails to become schistosomula, which enter the vasculature and lungs before relocating to the venous system where they become sexually mature adults, pair, then mate and egg production begins [10]. Adults of *S. haematobium* migrate to the venous plexus that drains the bladder and reproductive organs, whereas, for example, *S. mansoni* and *S. japonicum* migrate to the mesenteric veins draining the intestine [10]. Female schistosomes produce eggs, each equipped with a spine that helps penetration through blood vessels, and into the urinary tract and genitals (*S. haematobium*) or intestine and liver (*S. mansoni* and *S. japonicum*). Much of the pathological effects from schistosomiasis are a result of the immune response to parasite eggs trapped in host tissues during chronic infection. The resulting granulomata become fibrotic, which in turn results in severe circulatory impairment in affected organs [11].

Schistosome Genomics and Transcriptomics

Draft genome sequences were published for *S. mansoni* and *S. japonicum* [12, 13]. More recently the genome of S. haematobium was reported, a major milestone given that this species is widely considered as the most important of the schistosome species in terms of prevalence and pathogenicity [14]. For the purposes of this chapter, we will focus primarily on *S. mansoni*. The haploid *S. mansoni* genome is approximately 363 Mb in size and contains almost 12 000 genes, distributed across seven autosomal plus one sex chromosome pairs (ZW in the female and ZZ in the male) [12]. Prior to the sequencing of the genomes, comprehensive transcriptomic datasets [15] and genetic maps [16] were published, providing scaffolds with which to assemble the genome sequences. More recently, DNA microarrays have been generated by multiple groups, and utilized to explore transcriptional profiles of different developmental stages of the schistosome parasites [17–19] and the transcriptional effects of different treatments [20]. Fitzpatrick *et al.* [17] conducted a thorough characterization of schistosome development using statistical and network-based exploratory analyses, highlighted key transcriptional changes associated with life cycle progression, and identified numerous candidate molecules for drug and vaccine development, including membrane-spanning proteins, such as the G-protein-coupled receptors and tetraspanins.

Schistosomes are acoelomate organisms (i.e., they lack a defined body cavity), and have parenchymal tissues surrounding their organs, making the manual dissection of organs or organ systems difficult. Recent advances in laser microdissection microscopy (LMM), however, have allowed researchers to start to assemble a gene atlas for schistosomes, whereby the transcriptional profiles of defined schistosome tissues or organs have been delineated using a combination of LMM to isolate defined tissues for RNA extraction, followed by microarray analysis to specifically identify the most abundant transcripts in tissues of interest [21, 22]. This approach has proven particularly relevant for the selection of antigens for vaccine and drug development.

LMM has been used successfully to dissect the gut and other tissues of *S. mansoni* [21, 22], allowing for the identification of 393 contigs that were upregulated in the gastrointestinal tract of the adult female worm. Given that schistosomes reside in the vasculature and ingest blood as a source of nutrition, the gut of the parasite is considered to be a vulnerable tissue to target for vaccine development. Numerous proteolytic enzymes (proteases) were among the most highly expressed genes in gut tissues. Given their function in the proteolysis of hemoglobin and serum proteins [23–25], these enzymes are central to growth, reproduction, and survival, and are, thus, worthy of consideration as vaccine targets. Indeed, a number of these proteases have already been validated as drug targets [26] and/or by RNA interference (RNAi) shown to be important for worm development *in vitro* and *in vivo* [27, 28]. Recently, we used a microarray for *S. mansoni* to identify the most abundant transcripts in maturing schistosomula [20] – the developmental stage of the parasite that is considered to be particularly vulnerable to the immune response [29]. The most highly upregulated genes included a tetraspanin (*Sm-tsp-3* – one of the genes also highlighted by [17]) that is known to be expressed in the outer apical membrane of the parasite [30] and was 1600-fold upregulated during the first 5 days of schistosomulum development. Intestinal proteases were also highly upregulated, including orthologs of some *S. japonicum* proteases that were previously noted to be highly expressed in gut tissue [21].

Schistosome Proteomics

Various tissues and fluids from schistosomes have been characterized using a range of proteomic approaches. Of particular relevance to vaccine development is the elucidation of the tegument surface proteome of the adult blood fluke. The schistosome tegument is a syncytium, and acts as the direct interface between the host and the parasite, and as such, contains extracellular proteins; Skelly and Wilson [31] have provided a comprehensive review on the schistosome tegument. Many vaccine antigens that are located in the tegument have been tested in murine models of schistosomiasis [29], but only a few are likely to be available to antibodies on the surface of a live, intact parasite [30, 32]. DeMarco and Verjovski-Almeida [33] recently reviewed the use of proteomics to identify schistosome proteins for vaccine antigen and drug discovery. We have thus restricted our discussion to studies that focus on the outer membrane proteins of the schistosome tegument, primarily because we believe that exposed membrane proteins are likely to be the most efficacious as vaccine antigens [29, 34].

By labeling the surface of live adult *S. mansoni* with biotin, Braschi and Wilson showed that only primary amine groups that are exposed on the outer surface of the tegument incorporate the label, allowing for their purification via streptavidin affinity chromatography and characterization by liquid chromatography-tandem mass spectrometry [30]. Surprisingly, few proteins were detected on the surface of the live parasite using this approach, reflecting an epithelium that is relatively depauperate in surface-exposed proteins. This finding, however, limits the number of target vaccine antigens to a manageable number. Indeed, when tested, these outer membrane proteins have conferred good levels of protection in mice and are recognized preferentially by antibodies from resistant people in Brazil [35–37]. A similar study was conducted using biotinylated *S. japonicum*, but instead of excising bands from a one-dimensional gel for protein extraction, Mulvenna et al. used an off-gel electrophoresis technique to minimize protein loss during sample preparation and subsequently identified orthologs of the *S. mansoni*-labeled proteins as well as additional membrane-spanning proteins of interest [32].

After schistosome cercariae penetrate the skin and transform into schistosomula, they enter the vasculature and migrate (depending on species) to the portal or bladder vessels via the lungs. The first 3–5 days of this migratory process between the skin and the lungs is thought to represent the most susceptible stage to antibody-mediated killing [29, 38, 39]. Neither the tegument nor excreted/secreted proteins from *in vitro* cultured or *in vivo* obtained schistosomula have been characterized to date, primarily due to the difficulty in obtaining sufficient quantities of material for protein analysis, but such studies would be decidedly instructive for future selection of immunogens.

Schistosome Postgenomics

One of the most revolutionary advances in the postgenomic era for the study of parasitic helminths has been gene silencing by RNAi (see also Chapters 6 and 7). Parasitic helminths, by virtue of their often complex life cycles and large genomes, have generally rendered themselves refractory to many genetic manipulation tools that allow the exploration of gene function [40, 41]. However, RNAi is now widely used to assess gene function in schistosomes and appears to be particularly effective for genes expressed in tissues readily accessible to double-stranded RNA, such as the tegument and gastrodermis [42, 43]. RNAi has been used to confirm gene function for a number of potential schistosome vaccine antigens and drug targets, and helps explain how some vaccines, which are based on these proteins, might exert their efficacy. RNAi of a *S. mansoni* tetraspanin known as *Sm*-TSP-2 impacted on proper tegument development and decreased *S. mansoni* survival *in vivo* [44]. Also, RNAi of the genes encoding the gastrodermal proteases, cathepsins D [27], B, L, and an asparaginyl endopeptidase [25], has confirmed their respective contributions to substrate cleavage during the multienzyme process of hemoglobin digestion. The ability to silence schistosome genes and assess function *in vitro* and *in vivo* prompted us to suggest that lethality consequent on RNAi be taken as one of several critical criteria in ranking antigens for progress towards clinical trials as a vaccine for schistosomiasis [4].

Schistosome Immunomics

The availability of the three major human schistosome genomes, coupled with the proteomic characterization of the tegument and other tissues, has provided researchers with the tools required to apply postgenomic approaches to vaccine antigen discovery. High-throughput protein expression techniques, such as *in vitro* translation using prokaryotic or eukaryotic ribosomes, and sera from resistant humans and animals (e.g., hyperinfected rats or animals vaccinated with irradiated cercariae), means that schistosome researchers are now armed and ready to utilize immunomics approaches. Recently, we designed and manufactured the first *Schistosoma* immunomics protein microarray [45], and are currently using it as a vaccine discovery tool. The proteins selected for inclusion on the chip include those from previously published proteomic data and *in silico* screening of available sequences to identify potential immunogens based on protein location, with a particular emphasis on proteins expressed on/in the tegument. Following cloning, selected sequences were expressed in a cell-free expression system and contact-printed onto nitrocellulose-coated microscope slides to form microarrays. The arrays have been probed with IgG (different subclasses) and IgE from resistant and chronically infected humans and animals (Gaze *et al.*, unpublished). The approach will allow us to identify antigens that are the major target of protective IgG responses, while avoiding antigens that might induce potentially harmful IgE responses when administered as vaccines [4]. This innovative technology of reverse vaccinology has the potential to transform vaccine research for schistosomiasis and other parasitic diseases of humans and animals.

There are, of course, inherent problems with many high-throughput approaches and immunomics is no exception. One of the major challenges to developing vaccines against eukaryotic pathogens, such as helminths, is the faithful replication (e.g., domain structure, glycosylation, and post-translational processing) of vaccine antigens using recombinant technologies. Given that many helminth vaccine antigens are extracellular, they are processed through the secretory pathway, often undergo complex post-translational processing, and are extensively disulfide bonded.

We routinely express helminth secreted proteins in yeast or insect cells to obtain properly folded recombinant molecules. Cell-free protein expression systems, whether they be components of prokaryotic or eukaryotic cells, do not possess the cellular machinery to process secreted proteins and will not always faithfully reproduce the correct fold. Given the caveats, the high-throughput nature of this expression system, nonetheless, lends itself well to immunomic studies and has an excellent record of identifying antigens for a range of single-celled pathogens [46–48].

Case for a Schistosomiasis Vaccine

The justification for developing vaccines against schistosomiasis has been reviewed recently [4, 29, 49], and includes high disease burden [5, 50], high rates of post-treatment reinfection, the inability of chemotherapy-based morbidity control to interrupt transmission [51], and the exclusive reliance on praziquantel for control [29, 52]. An important additional stimulus to develop new preventive approaches to schistosomiasis control is the observation of so-called "rebound morbidity" (i.e., up to 80% of children living in high transmission areas can suffer recurrent aggressive inflammation following interrupted annual chemotherapy because of reinfection) [1].

The feasibility of developing vaccines for schistosomiasis has been reviewed extensively [4, 29, 53]. Humans living in endemic areas can become resistant or partially immune to reinfection over time [54]. Furthermore, irradiated larvae (cercariae) can elicit high levels of protective immunity in laboratory animals and several recombinant protein vaccines have been shown to elicit comparable levels of protective immunity in immunized animals that were subsequently challenged with cercariae [29].

Sm-TSP-2 Schistosomiasis Vaccine

The Sabin Vaccine Institute in partnership with the Fundação Oswaldo Cruz (FIOCRUZ) and Instituto Butantan is working to transition a *S. mansoni* vaccine into clinical testing in Brazil [4]. The primary targets of this vaccine development program are schistosome membrane proteins identified by combined genomic, postgenomic, and proteomic analyses of the adult *S. mansoni* outer surface, or tegument (Table 25.1). As indicated earlier, the tegument of adult schistosomes is a single syncytium covering the entire body and is a dynamic layer involved in several physiologic processes, including parasite nutrition, osmoregulation, and evasion of host immunity [34]. Hence, the schistosome tegument is a potentially vulnerable target for immunological attack by host antibodies. However, analysis of the schistosome proteome predicts that surprisingly few membrane-spanning proteins of the tegument are accessible to the host immune response [30]. They include a family of tetraspanin integral membrane proteins [37] and several outer membrane proteins of unknown function such as Sm29 [35, 55]. The tetraspanins are so-named

Table 25.1 Ranking table for prioritizing schistosomiasis vaccine antigens for progression towards clinical trials (adapted from [4]).

S. mansoni antigen	Target of IgE[a]	Reduced adult worm counts (mice)[b]	Reduced egg counts (mice)[c]	Preferential recognition by resistant humans[d]	Intramammalian stage targeted[e]	Ease of manufacture	Known structure /function	RNAi phenotype[f]	Final score
	NO = GO	1–5	1–5	1–3	1–3	0–3	0–2	0–2	maximum = 23
	Yes = STOP				Score				
Sm-TSP-2	no	4	4	3	3	3	1	2	20/23 (87%)
Sm29	ND	4	3	1	2	1	0	ND	11/21 (52%)
Sm-TSP-1	ND	3	3	0	2	3	1	2	14/23 (56%)

a) If individuals naturally infected with *S. mansoni* develop IgE to the protein, the antigen is immediately down-selected.
b) Reflects quintiles of reduced worm burdens in vaccinated mice challenged with infective larvae, compared to controls. Antigen formulated with an adjuvant approved (or under assessment) for human use.
c) Reflects reduced liver egg and/or fecal egg burdens in vaccinated mice challenged with infective larvae, compared to controls. Scoring as above for adult worm counts.
d) Reflects tertiles of the difference in mean IgG1 or IgG3 units between resistant and chronically infected groups.
e) Protein accessible to the immune system in intramammalian developmental stages: 1 = detected on the surface of fixed schistosomulum or adult; 2 = detected on the surface of live schistosomulum *or* live adult; 3 = detected on surface of live schistosomulum *and* live adult.
f) Reflects essential nature of the target protein for parasite survival based on RNAi experiments: 0 = RNAi results in no effect; 1 = RNAi results in deleterious *in vitro* phenotype; 2 = RNAi results in deleterious *in vitro* phenotype and affects survival *in vivo* (animal models) after transfer of double-stranded RNA-treated parasites into mice.

because they contain four transmembrane domains, with two extracellular loops that are predicted to interact with exogenous proteins or ligands [34]. The second extracellular domain fragment of a *S. mansoni* tetraspanin, *Sm*-TSP-2, has been selected for development as a human vaccine antigen (Figure 25.1a and b). When the extracellular domain was expressed in either *Pichia pastoris* or *Escherichia coli* and formulated with several different adjuvants, including Freund's complete adjuvant, aluminum hydroxide, or aluminum hydroxide together with CpGs, it provided 50–70% protection in mice vaccinated with the antigen followed by challenge with *S. mansoni* cercariae [37, 56]. In addition, evidence from human epidemiological studies indicates that putatively resistant individuals living in endemic areas of Brazil have elevated antibody responses to this protein compared with chronically infected individuals from the same endemic areas [37]. Recently, the ortholog of *Sm*-TSP-2 in *S. japonicum*, *Sj*-TSP-2, was described and resulted in protection in mice similar to that described of *Sm*-TSP-2, suggesting that this molecule may be effective against multiple human schistosome species [57].

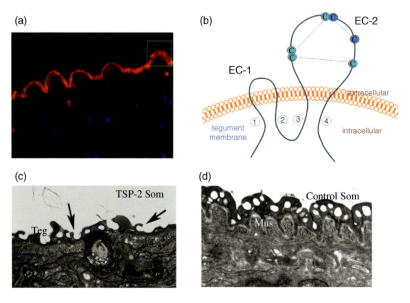

Figure 25.1 *S. mansoni* tegument. (a) Fluorescence micrograph of the tegument of an adult male *S. mansoni* probed with a mouse antibody raised to recombinant tetraspanin *Sm*-TSP-2 (red). Nuclei, stained with 4′,6-diamidino-2-phenylindole (DAPI), are blue. (b) Schematic representation of *Sm*-TSP-2 in the tegument plasma membrane. Extracellular loops (ECs) are indicated, cysteine residues are shown (the lines between them denote the disulfide bond pairing), and transmembrane domains are shown numbered from the N- to the C-terminus. (c) The tegument of a schistosomulum of *S. mansoni* that was incubated for 7 days with double-stranded RNA targeting either *Sm-tsp-2* or (d) luciferase (as a control). Digitate extensions (arrows) are more abundant on the surface of the tegument incubated with *tsp-2* double-stranded RNA. Mus, muscle; Som, schistosomulum; Teg, tegument. (Reproduced with permission from [4].)

The importance of tetraspanins in the proper development of the tegument and survival of worms has been highlighted by RNAi. Specifically, the ultrastructural morphology of adult worms and schistosomula treated *in vitro* with *Sm-tsp-2* double-stranded RNA displays a distinctly vacuolated and thinner tegument compared with controls, suggestive of impaired closure of tegumentary invaginations [44] (Figure 25.1c and d). Moreover, injection of mice with schistosomula that had been pretreated with *Sm-tsp-2* double-stranded RNA resulted in 83% fewer parasites recovered from the mesenteric veins 4 weeks later compared to mice that had been injected with schistosomula exposed to nonschistosome double-stranded RNA [44]. Other tegument tetraspanins are also attractive vaccine candidates; for example, *Sm-tsp-3* is the most highly upregulated mRNA in maturing schistosomula – a developmental stage widely accepted as susceptible to damage by the human immune system [17, 20]. In addition, *Sj23* is a tegument tetraspanin that is showing promise as a DNA vaccine aimed at water buffaloes, an important reservoir host for *S. japonicum* in China [58].

Conclusions

Administered in early childhood, a schistosomiasis vaccine could prevent the major pediatric sequelae of the disease, including anemia, malnutrition, slowed growth, and impaired cognitive development [4]. *Sm*-TSP-2 is being developed as a recombinant protein vaccine to prevent heavy infections with *S. mansoni* – the leading cause of intestinal schistosomiasis. Initially, a vaccine containing *Sm*-TSP-2 is being formulated with Alhydrogel® (aluminum hydroxide); however, it will also be evaluated with an additional immunostimulant such as a lipid A derivative. The vaccine will be given intramuscularly in one or two doses, depending on the number required to achieve a protective response. Extension of protection into adulthood would also prevent the severe anemia in pregnancy related to schistosome infection and reduce transmission. Such vaccines may also have an important impact on poverty reduction because of their anticipated effect on improving pediatric development and maternal health [59].

The *Sm*-TSP-2 vaccine candidate is being developed with the ultimate goal being that even the most impoverished populations will have access to it as soon as it is available. As such, a strategic roadmap is being followed to ensure that low-cost manufacturing processes are utilized and that vaccine manufacturers in middle-income, disease-endemic countries are involved from the start. In the Americas, Brazil is the furthest advanced with two major vaccine manufacturers (FIOCRUZ-Biomanguinhos and Instituto Butantan) actively engaged in development [60]. Accurate forecasting of the eventual demand for licensed vaccines is essential and is underway for an intestinal schistosomiasis vaccine.

Significant hurdles must be overcome during clinical development of the *Sm*-TSP-2 schistosomiasis vaccine, not least of which is securing adequate funding to conduct the clinical trials required for licensure. Additional obstacles include obtaining access to the novel adjuvants that may be required to induce an adequate immune response and the difficulty of conducting large-scale efficacy studies in endemic areas. As schistosomiasis is prevalent in predominantly resource-limited areas, phase III clinical trials will be logistically challenging. Furthermore, because the clinical effects of schistosomiasis are chronic, with sequelae such as iron-deficiency anemia often only appearing after months or years of infection [5], efficacy trials will, by necessity, be long in duration.

References

1 Hotez, P.J., Bethony, J.M., Oliveira, S.C., Brindley, P.J., and Loukas, A. (2008) Multivalent anthelminthic vaccine to prevent hookworm and schistosomiasis. *Expert Rev. Vaccines*, **7**, 745–752.

2 Hotez, P.J., Brindley, P.J., Bethony, J.M., King, C.H., Pearce, E.J., and Jacobson, J. (2008) Helminth infections: the great neglected tropical diseases. *J. Clin. Invest.*, **118**, 1311–1321.

3 Steinmann, P., Keiser, J., Bos, R., Tanner, M., and Utzinger, J. (2006) Schistosomiasis and water resources development: systematic review, meta-analysis, and estimates of people at risk. *Lancet Infect. Dis.*, **6**, 411–425.

4 Hotez, P.J., Bethony, J.M., Diemert, D.J., Pearson, M., and Loukas, A. (2010) Developing vaccines to combat hookworm infection and intestinal schistosomiasis. *Nat. Rev. Microbiol.*, **8**, 814–826.

5 King, C.H. and Dangerfield-Cha, M. (2008) The unacknowledged impact of chronic schistosomiasis. *Chronic. Illn.*, **4**, 65–79.

6 Clements, A.C., Bosque-Oliva, E., Sacko, M., Landoure, A., Dembele, R., Traore, M., Coulibaly, G., Gabrielli, A.F., Fenwick, A., and Brooker, S. (2009) A comparative study of the spatial distribution of schistosomiasis in Mali in 1984–1989 and 2004–2006. *PLoS Negl. Trop. Dis.*, **3**, e431.

7 Fallon, P. and Doenhoff, M. (1994) Drug-resistant schistosomiasis: resistance to praziquantel and oxamniquine induced in *Schistosoma mansoni* in mice is drug specific. *Am. J. Trop. Med. Hyg.*, **51**, 83–88.

8 Gray, D.J., McManus, D.P., Li, Y., Williams, G.M., Bergquist, R., and Ross, A.G. (2010) Schistosomiasis elimination: lessons from the past guide the future. *Lancet Infect. Dis.*, **10**, 733–736.

9 King, C.H. (2010) Parasites and poverty: the case of schistosomiasis. *Acta Trop.*, **113**, 95–104.

10 Gryseels, B., Polman, K., Clerinx, J., and Kestens, L. (2006) Human schistosomiasis. *Lancet*, **368**, 1106–1118.

11 Pearce, E.J. and MacDonald, A.S. (2002) The immunobiology of schistosomiasis. *Nat. Rev. Immunol.*, **2**, 499–511.

12 Berriman, M. *et al.* (2009) The genome of the blood fluke *Schistosoma mansoni*. *Nature*, **460**, 352–360.

13 The *Schistosoma japonicum* Genome Sequencing and Functional Analysis Consortium (2009) The *Schistosoma japonicum* genome reveals features of host–parasite interplay. *Nature*, **460**, 345–352.

14 Young, N.D., Jex, A.R., Li, B., Liu, S., Yang, L., Xiong, Z., Li, Y., Cantacessi, C., Hall, R.S., Xu, X., Chen, F., Wu, X., Zerlotini, A., Oliveira, G., Hofmann, A., Zhang, G., Fang, X., Kang, Y., Campbell, B.E., Loukas, A., Ranganathan, S., Rollinson, D., Rinaldi, G., Brindley, P.J., Yang, H., Wang, J., and Gasser, R.B. (2012) Whole-genome sequence of Schistosoma haematobium. *Nat. Genet.*, **44**(2), 221–225.

15 Verjovski-Almeida, S. *et al.* (2003) Transcriptome analysis of the acoelomate human parasite *Schistosoma mansoni*. *Nat. Genet.*, **35**, 148–157.

16 Criscione, C.D., Valentim, C.L., Hirai, H., LoVerde, P.T., and Anderson, T.J. (2009)

Genomic linkage map of the human blood fluke *Schistosoma mansoni*. *Genome Biol.*, **10**, R71.

17 Fitzpatrick, J.M., Peak, E., Perally, S., Chalmers, I.W., Barrett, J., Yoshino, T.P., Ivens, I.C., and Hoffmann, K.F. (2009) Anti-schistosomal intervention targets identified by lifecycle transcriptomic analyses. *PLoS Neglect. Trop. Dis.*, **3**, e543.

18 Gobert, G.N., Moertel, L., Brindley, P.J., and McManus, D.P. (2009) Developmental gene expression profiles of the human pathogen *Schistosoma japonicum*. *BMC Genomics*, **10**, 128.

19 Jolly, E.R., Chin, C.S., Miller, S., Bahgat, M.M., Lim, K.C., DeRisi, J., and McKerrow, J.H. (2007) Gene expression patterns during adaptation of a helminth parasite to different environmental niches. *Genome Biol.*, **8**, R65.

20 Gobert, G.N., Tran, M.H., Moertel, L., Mulvenna, J., Jones, M.K., McManus, D.P., and Loukas, A. (2010) Transcriptional changes in *Schistosoma mansoni* during early schistosomula development and in the presence of erythrocytes. *PLoS Neglect. Trop. Dis.*, **4**, e600.

21 Gobert, G.N., McManus, D.P., Nawaratna, S., Moertel, L., Mulvenna, J., and Jones, M.K. (2009) Tissue specific profiling of females of *Schistosoma japonicum* by integrated laser microdissection microscopy and microarray analysis. *PLoS Negl. Trop. Dis.*, **3**, e469.

22 Nawaratna, S.S., McManus, D.P., Moertel, L., Gobert, G.N., and Jones, M.K. (2011) Gene atlasing of digestive and reproductive tissues in *Schistosoma mansoni*. *PLoS Negl. Trop. Dis.*, **5**, e1043.

23 Brindley, P.J. et al. (2001) Proteolysis of human hemoglobin by schistosome cathepsin D. *Mol. Biochem. Parasitol.*, **112**, 103–112.

24 Caffrey, C.R., McKerrow, J.H., Salter, J.P., and Sajid, M. (2004) Blood 'n' guts: an update on schistosome digestive peptidases. *Trends Parasitol.*, **20**, 241–248.

25 Delcroix, M., Sajid, M., Caffrey, C.R., Lim, K.C., Dvorak, J., Hsieh, I., Bahgat, M., Dissous, C., and McKerrow, J.H. (2006) A multienzyme network functions in intestinal protein digestion by a platyhelminth parasite. *J. Biol. Chem.*, **281**, 39316–39329.

26 Abdulla, M.H., Lim, K.C., Sajid, M., McKerrow, J.H., and Caffrey, C.R. (2007) Schistosomiasis mansoni: novel chemotherapy using a cysteine protease inhibitor. *PLoS Med.*, **4**, e14.

27 Morales, M.E., Rinaldi, G., Gobert, G.N., Kines, K.J., Tort, J.F., and Brindley, P.J. (2008) RNA interference of *Schistosoma mansoni* cathepsin D, the apical enzyme of the hemoglobin proteolysis cascade. *Mol. Biochem. Parasitol.*, **157**, 160–168.

28 Correnti, J.M., Brindley, P.J., and Pearce, E.J. (2005) Long-term suppression of cathepsin B levels by RNA interference retards schistosome growth. *Mol. Biochem. Parasitol.*, **143**, 209–215.

29 McManus, D.P. and Loukas, A. (2008) Current status of vaccines for schistosomiasis. *Clin. Microbiol. Rev.*, **21**, 225–242.

30 Braschi, S. and Wilson, R.A. (2006) Proteins exposed at the adult schistosome surface revealed by biotinylation. *Mol. Cell Proteomics*, **5**, 347–356.

31 Skelly, P.J. and Wilson, R.A. (2006) Making sense of the schistosome surface. *Adv. Parasitol.*, **63**, 185–284.

32 Mulvenna, J., Moertel, L., Jones, M.K., Nawaratna, S., Lovas, E.M., Gobert, G.N., Colgrave, M., Jones, A., Loukas, A., and McManus, D.P. (2010) Exposed proteins of the *Schistosoma japonicum* tegument. *Int. J. Parasitol.*, **40**, 543–554.

33 DeMarco, R. and Verjovski-Almeida, S. (2009) Schistosomes – proteomics studies for potential novel vaccines and drug targets. *Drug Discov. Today*, **14**, 472–478.

34 Loukas, A., Tran, M., and Pearson, M.S. (2007) Schistosome membrane proteins as vaccines. *Int. J. Parasitol.*, **37**, 257–263.

35 Cardoso, F.C. et al. (2008) *Schistosoma mansoni* tegument protein Sm29 is able to induce a T_h1-type of immune response and protection against parasite infection. *PLoS Negl. Trop. Dis.*, **2**, e308.

36 Cardoso, F.C., Pacifico, R.N., Mortara, R.A., and Oliveira, S.C. (2006) Human antibody responses of patients living in endemic areas for

schistosomiasis to the tegumental protein Sm29 identified through genomic studies. *Clin. Exp. Immunol.*, **144**, 382–391.

37 Tran, M.H., Pearson, M.S., Bethony, J.M., Smyth, D.J., Jones, M.K., Duke, M., Don, T.A., McManus, D.P., Correa-Oliveira, R., and Loukas, A. (2006) Tetraspanins on the surface of *Schistosoma mansoni* are protective antigens against schistosomiasis. *Nat. Med.*, **12**, 835–840.

38 El Ridi, R. and Tallima, H. (2009) *Schistosoma mansoni ex vivo* lung-stage larvae excretory–secretory antigens as vaccine candidates against schistosomiasis. *Vaccine*, **27**, 666–673.

39 Mountford, A.P., Harrop, R., and Wilson, R.A. (1995) Antigens derived from lung-stage larvae of *Schistosoma mansoni* are efficient stimulators of proliferation and gamma interferon secretion by lymphocytes from mice vaccinated with attenuated larvae. *Infect. Immun.*, **63**, 1980–1986.

40 Mann, V.H., Morales, M.E., Kines, K.J., and Brindley, P.J. (2008) Transgenesis of schistosomes: approaches employing mobile genetic elements. *Parasitology*, **135**, 141–153.

41 Mann, V.H., Morales, M.E., Rinaldi, G., and Brindley, P.J. (2010) Culture for genetic manipulation of developmental stages of *Schistosoma mansoni*. *Parasitology*, **137**, 451–462.

42 Krautz-Peterson, G., Bhardwaj, R., Faghiri, Z., Tararam, C.A., and Skelly, P.J. (2010) RNA interference in schistosomes: machinery and methodology. *Parasitology*, **137**, 485–495.

43 Stefanic, S., Dvorak, J., Horn, M., Braschi, S., Sojka, D., Ruelas, D.S., Suzuki, B., Lim, K.C., Hopkins, S.D., McKerrow, J.H., and Caffrey, C.R. (2010) RNA interference in *Schistosoma mansoni* schistosomula: selectivity, sensitivity and operation for larger-scale screening. *PLoS Negl. Trop. Dis.*, **4**, e850.

44 Tran, M.H., Freitas, T.C., Cooper, L., Gaze, S., Gatton, M.L., Jones, M.K., Lovas, E., Pearce, E.J., and Loukas, A. (2010) Suppression of mRNAs encoding tegument tetraspanins from *Schistosoma mansoni* results in impaired tegument turnover. *PloS Pathol.*, **6**, e1000840.

45 Driguez, P., Doolan, D.L., Loukas, A., Felgner, P.L., and McManus, D.P. (2010) Schistosomiasis vaccine discovery using immunomics. *Parasites Vectors*, **3**, 4.

46 Crompton, P.D. et al. (2010) A prospective analysis of the Ab response to *Plasmodium falciparum* before and after a malaria season by protein microarray. *Proc. Natl. Acad. Sci. USA*, **107**, 6958–6963.

47 Davies, D.H., Wyatt, L.S., Newman, F.K., Earl, P.L., Chun, S., Hernandez, J.E., Molina, D.M., Hirst, S., Moss, B., Frey, S.E., and Felgner, P.L. (2008) Antibody profiling by proteome microarray reveals the immunogenicity of the attenuated smallpox vaccine modified vaccinia virus ankara is comparable to that of Dryvax. *J. Virol.*, **82**, 652–663.

48 Eyles, J.E. et al. (2007) Immunodominant *Francisella tularensis* antigens identified using proteome microarray. *Proteomics*, **7**, 2172–2183.

49 Bergquist, N.R., Leonardo, L.R., and Mitchell, G.F. (2005) Vaccine-linked chemotherapy: can schistosomiasis control benefit from an integrated approach? *Trends Parasitol.*, **21**, 112–117.

50 King, C.H., Dickman, K., and Tisch, D.J. (2005) Reassessment of the cost of chronic helmintic infection: a meta-analysis of disability-related outcomes in endemic schistosomiasis. *Lancet*, **365**, 1561–1569.

51 King, C.H., Sturrock, R.F., Kariuki, H.C., and Hamburger, J. (2006) Transmission control for schistosomiasis – why it matters now. *Trends Parasitol.*, **22**, 575–582.

52 Bergquist, R., Utzinger, J., and McManus, D.P. (2008) Trick or treat: the role of vaccines in integrated schistosomiasis control. *PLoS Negl. Trop. Dis.*, **2**, e244.

53 Oliveira, S.C., Fonseca, C.T., Cardoso, F.C., Farias, L.P., and Leite, L.C. (2008) Recent advances in vaccine research against schistosomiasis in Brazil. *Acta Trop.*, **108**, 256–262.

54 Correa-Oliveira, R., Caldas, I.R., and Gazzinelli, G. (2000) Natural versus drug-induced resistance in *Schistosoma*

mansoni infection. *Parasitol. Today*, **16**, 397–399.

55 Cardoso, F.C., Pinho, J.M., Azevedo, V., and Oliveira, S.C. (2006) Identification of a new *Schistosoma mansoni* membrane-bound protein through bioinformatic analysis. *Genet. Mol. Res.*, **5**, 609–618.

56 Pearson, M.S., Pickering, D.A., McSorley, H.J., Bethony, J.M., Tribolet, L., Dougall, A.M., Hotez, P., and Loukas, A. (2012) Enhanced Protective Efficacy of a Chimeric Form of the Schistosomiasis Vaccine Antigen *Sm*-TSP-2. *PLoS Negl. Trop. Dis.*, **6**(3), e1564.

57 Yuan, C., Fu, Y.J., Li, J., Yue, Y.F., Cai, L.L., Xiao, W.J., Chen, J.P., and Yang, L. (2010) *Schistosoma japonicum*: efficient and rapid purification of the tetraspanin extracellular loop 2, a potential protective antigen against schistosomiasis in mammalian. *Exp. Parasitol.*, **126**, 456–461.

58 Da'dara, A.A., Li, Y.S., Xiong, T., Zhou, J., Williams, G.M., McManus, D.P., Feng, Z., Yu, X.L., Gray, D.J., and Harn, D.A. (2008) DNA-based vaccines protect against zoonotic schistosomiasis in water buffalo. *Vaccine*, **26**, 3617–3625.

59 Hotez, P.J. and Ferris, M.T. (2006) The antipoverty vaccines. *Vaccine*, **24**, 5787–5799.

60 Morel, C.M. *et al.* (2005) Health innovation networks to help developing countries address neglected diseases. *Science*, **309**, 401–404.

26
Sm14 *Schistosoma mansoni* Fatty Acid-Binding Protein: Molecular Basis for an Antihelminth Vaccine

Miriam Tendler*, *Celso Raul Romero Ramos, and Andrew J.G. Simpson*

Abstract

Infections caused by soil-transmitted helminths and schistosomes afflict the largest number of humans world-wide. They are found throughout the developing world, particularly in sub-Saharan Africa, the Americas, China, and East Asia. Since the 1970s, these infections have been treated and controlled by chemotherapy. However, this strategy alone or in combination with health education and/or other associated measures has failed to control disease transmission despite continuous large-scale and massive treatment programs. In contrast, the most successful programs undertaken hitherto to control, and even eradicate, infectious diseases have employed vaccines. To date, however, vaccines are not available to control helminth infections. We discuss the accumulated data on the experimental vaccine incorporating the *Schistosoma mansoni* fatty acid-binding protein (Sm14) for human schistosomiasis and livestock fasciolosis. This vaccine is currently in clinical trials in humans and large animals in Brazil.

Schistosomiasis and Fascioliasis

Helminths are the most common parasites of humans and are disseminated throughout developing countries, particularly in Africa and South America. Helminth infections are arguably the most neglected of infectious (tropical) diseases. It is estimated that they afflict 3 billion people or half of the global human population. Fifty years after Stoll published his article "This wormy world" [1], the global prevalence of infections with intestinal nematodes remains virtually unchanged despite decades of continuous use of anthelmintic drugs in massive programs [2]. The time has come to change this scenario and focus on effective control measures employing vaccination.

Schistosomiasis is a chronic, debilitating disease affecting millions of people in poor countries targeted by the World Health Organization (WHO) for control efforts [3]. Morbidity is particularly pronounced in school-age children whose

---

* Corresponding Author

physical health and intellectual capacity are fundamental to national development in endemic countries. Due to the need for an intermediate snail host, the distribution of the infection is associated with lakes, rivers, and water development schemes, thus putting more than 600 million people at risk world-wide [3]. Despite control efforts, an estimated 200 million people are infected, of which 120 million are symptomatic and 20 million have severe disease symptoms. The majority of infected people (80–85%), including the most severely affected, are in Africa [4]. These figures may, in fact, turn out to be underestimates as a recent meta-analysis found the number of people at risk to be closer to 800 million [5]. Regardless of more than two decades of well-executed control activities based on large-scale chemotherapy, the disease is expanding in Brazil where, in recent years, new foci have been detected in areas previously free of infection [6, 7].

Chemotherapy is primarily directed against morbidity and does not influence transmission. This results in the continued presence of the disease. Moreover, an increased severity of morbidity can occur upon chemotherapy, as was first reported in 80% of children with schistosomiasis japonica subjected to drug treatment in high transmission areas in the Philippines [8, 9]. This undesired effect, termed "rebound morbidity," is thought to be due to an interruption of the natural downregulation of the specific immunological mechanisms typical of schistosomiasis. Such recurrent inflammation within 6 months of reinfection has also been reported following treatment of schistosomiasis mansoni in Sudan and West African countries [6]. This worrying aspect needs to be taken seriously as the aggravated gross symptoms cause long-term pathology that is difficult to remedy. In the 1990s, the WHO's Special Programme for Research and Training in Tropical Diseases (TDR) created a product development program and initiated collaborations with other major international donors to promote, among other tools, the rapid development of vaccines for the control of endemic diseases. This "push strategy" was chosen to achieve effective research projects fostering innovation in the context of rapid product development. In the field of vaccine development, the aim was to develop ways and means to immunize against the most important human parasite diseases. Although the malaria vaccine projects scored initial successes, further progress has been complicated. With regard to schistosomiasis, more than 10 important antigens with potential as vaccines candidates emerged from the several hundred scientific projects supported by international donor agencies and national research programs over the last few decades [10, 11]. Among those that are still being seriously pursued, the *Schistosoma mansoni* fatty acid-binding protein (FABP; Sm14) antigen stands out (i) due to the steady progress that has been achieved, including the field trials currently underway in Brazil, and (ii) because it is the only vaccine candidate to emerge from an endemic country for schistosomiasis. The very special feature of Sm14 is its strong immunological reactivity with an antigen shared by another helminth parasite, namely *Fasciola hepatica*, which gives this vaccine candidate the potential to be used against more than one infection. *F. hepatica* can cause disease in humans, but is primarily a problem for cattle and sheep, leading to annual losses over US$3 billion in the food industry world-wide [12]. The international patents for Sm14, granted to the Oswaldo Cruz Foundation

(FIOCRUZ), a Brazilian research institution associated with the Brazilian Ministry of Health, have been licensed to Alvos Biotecnologia SA that was recently acquired by OuroFino Animal Health Ltd, which is now leading the Sm14 vaccine project, both for veterinary and medical use.

Like other parasitic helminths, schistosomes are unable to synthesize long-chain fatty acids or sterols and hence are completely dependent on the host for these essential nutrients components [13]. FABPs are critical for the uptake of fatty acids from host blood, and are thus prime targets for both vaccine and drug development [14]. In parallel, market forces have emerged in North America and Europe where there is interest in developing safer methods, such as vaccines, for the control of veterinary diseases, which could gradually replace the use of antiparasitic drugs in livestock, and, thus, avoid chemical residues in milk, meat, and their derivatives. Indeed, immunoprophylaxis is regarded as the most promising avenue for effective control of parasitic infection in livestock world-wide as it safeguards food production and minimizes the use of drugs both at the environmental and individual levels (www.deliver-project.eu). The export value of European Union (EU) of ruminant livestock averages €2.3 (US$3) billion annually. This market depends on guarantees of quality and safety. Whether exports are in the form of meat or added-value meat and dairy products, the EU believes that they will only be accepted in markets if produced at a high standard ensuring freedom from zoonotic pathogens and from potentially harmful drug residues.

To date, the control of helminth infections in cattle has required chemical drugs considered to be unhealthy to animals, the environment, and consumers due to the risk associated with drug residues infiltrating milk and meat products. These concerns underlie the formal recommendation by the European Community (www.deliver-project.eu) for gradually reducing the use of chemical drugs in livestock and replacing them with vaccines. The drugs that are currently being discouraged for use in European cattle are essentially the same as those used to treat human helminth infections in endemic areas of developing countries.

Discovery of the Sm14 Vaccine Antigen

The search for a vaccine against schistosomiasis at FIOCRUZ started in the 1980s and originally focused on the development of an antischistosome vaccine in isolated products released into saline solution by adult *S. mansoni* worms [15, 16].

In the early 1990s, using molecular biological techniques, it became possible to identify and clone the genes of a number of antigenic components from the original mixture of released products and shown to protect mice against infection. Specifically, an expression cDNA library from mRNA of *S. mansoni* adult worms was constructed using the λgt11 phage vector and clones isolated using immune serum. This approach identified known antigens such as glutathione *S*-transferase (GST; Sm28) [17] and paramyosin [18]. However, other cDNA clones coding for antigens not yet studied were also identified. Using a strategy involving sera from individual experimental animals with high and low levels of protection, single-component vaccine candidates were identified. The DNA sequencing of one such clone encoded a protein with a theoretical molecular mass of 14 kDa (Sm14) [19]. The deduced amino acid sequence of Sm14 showed significant homology to the FABP family [20]. The Sm14 protein was produced in recombinant form (rSm14) and its lipid-binding properties demonstrated *in vitro* [19]. Thus, the first parasite FABP was isolated.

The recombinant antigen, rSm14, formed the basis of a long-term investigation that involved vaccination in out-bred animals, specifically, SW mice and NZ rabbits that have high and low susceptibility to cercarial infection, respectively. Vaccination parameters that influence protection were assessed to optimize the immunization route and scheme (number of doses, dosage of antigen protein, adjuvants). In addition, Sm14 peptide sequences associated with protection of mice against both fasciolosis and schistosomiasis were selected, and shall be assayed in the context of biological markers of vaccine-induced protection [21]. An innovative methodology, based on the population analysis of worm burden frequency distributions, was used to measure protection – an approach that we believe was critical for these experiments [22].

The FABPs of many helminth parasites of humans and animals have now been characterized, including those from *F. hepatica* [23], *Schistosoma japonicum* [24], *Fasciola gigantica* [25], and *Clonorchis sinensis* [26]. At FIOCRUZ, we considered rSm14 as a potential vaccine with wide antihelminth activity.

Function of Parasite FABPs

Numerous functions have been proposed for eukaryotic FABPs, including to (i) facilitate the uptake of fatty acids, their transport to intracellular organelles, or their delivery to specific metabolic pathways, (ii) protect cell membranes and enzymes from the effects of high concentrations of fatty acids and acyl-CoA derivatives, (iii) maintain a large deposit of intracellular fatty acids for rapid mobilization, and (iv) assist in differentiation [20, 27]. Also, FABPs contribute to host–parasite interactions [13].

In *S. mansoni*, the Sm14 protein was immunolocalized at the basal lamella of the tegument and gut epithelium [19, 28–30] (Figure 26.1). This supports the putative function of Sm14 in the transport of fatty acids from host cells. In *F. hepatica* and *F. gigantica*, FABPs are also located in the tegument and parenchymal cells [31], and, like Sm14 [32], are found in the excretory/secretory products [33]. As FABPs are intracellular proteins, the fact that these proteins are found in secreted material might be due to tegument exchange under stress conditions being employed as a strategy to protect the parasite from the immune system [34]. There is also the possibility of FABP secretion via nonclassical mechanisms (without the mediation of the endoplasmic reticulum and Golgi complex) as occurs with mammalian galectin-3 secretion [35].

Immunolocalization studies of antioxidant enzymes in *S. mansoni*, such as superoxide dismutase and glutathione peroxidase [36], showed that these enzymes have a similar localization as Sm14 in the tegument of schistosomes [28–30]. As immune attack is directed against the tegument with substances that generate free

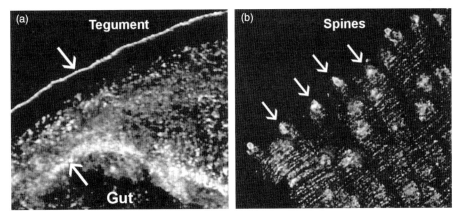

Figure 26.1 Immunolocalization of Sm14 protein in adult *S. mansoni*: (a) ×400, arrows indicate the Sm14 antibody depositions; (b) ×100, arrows indicate the spine structures at the parasite tegument. (Adapted from [30].)

radicals, enzymes and proteins with antioxidant function might be important for parasite survival within the host [36].

The Sm14 protein shows enhanced specificity for arachidonic acid [37]. The structure of Sm14 in complex with arachidonic acid was resolved at 2.4 Å resolution and showed that the aliphatic arachidonic acid chain adopts a stable hairpin-looped conformation in the protein cavity (Figure 26.2) [37]. Arachadonic acid is produced as part of the immune responses against helminths [38], and has been proposed as a safe and cost-effective antischistosomal agent [39]. El Ridi et al. [39] showed that the arachidonic acid activates the tegumental neutral sphingomyelinase. The activity of this enzyme results in the exposure of parasite surface membrane antigens to immune attack, and leads to the killing of *S. mansoni* and *S. haematobium* worms [39]. Microscopy revealed that arachidonic acid-mediated worm killing was associated with spine destruction, membrane blebbing, and disorganization of the apical membrane structure [39] – all sites where Sm14 is localized (Figure 26.1) [28–30]. In light of the functions proposed for arachidonic acid, Sm14 may help protect the parasite against the deleterious action of arachidonic acid as well as facilitate its metabolism [40].

The induction of *F. hepatica* FABP synthesis was characterized as a parasite antioxidant response [41]. This was established by a proteomic study of *F. hepatica* during its growth in the biliary ducts and is in keeping with the proposed antioxidant activity of Sm14, as stated above.

Proteomics has also been important in the study of action of anthelmintic drugs. In *F. hepatica*, this methodology was used to study the proteins that are induced by treatment with triclabendazole (TCBZ) in sensitive and resistant lineages [42]. FABPs, as well as GST, were identified as proteins specifically induced in the resistance to TCBZ lineage. Recombinant *F. hepatica* Fh15 (FABP) and GST proteins were able to bind the TCBZ, suggesting that these proteins participate in metabolism

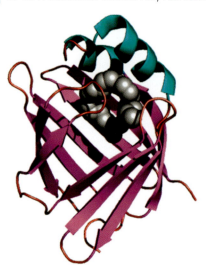

Figure 26.2 Ribbon representation of the crystal structure of Sm14 protein in complex with arachidonic acid shown in a space-fill representation (Protein Data Bank ID: 1VYG) Reprinted with permission from [37]© (2004) American Chemical Society. Figure prepared with PyMol software.

of TCBZ [42]. Timanova-Atanasova *et al.* [43] isolated a native protein from *F. hepatica*, called Fh13, with FABP activity that binds with high affinity to bithionol – a drug used against fascioliasis.

These results indicate that parasite FABPs are also associated with resistance to anthelmintics by sequestration and transport of drugs from the membrane to specific intracellular organelles [43]. The binding of drugs by FABPs may also buffer the intracellular levels of these chemicals since the proteins are found in abundance in the cytoplasm (the FABPs correspond to 2–5% of total intracellular protein) [20, 27].

As helminth FABPs are phylogenetically related yet distinct from those of other organisms, such as mammals [13], findings may be extrapolated from one parasite to another. The immunological cross-reactivity between Sm14 and FABPs of different species of flukes, roundworms, and tapeworms has been demonstrated [44], as well as cross-protective immunity against infection by F. hepatica in mice [45], sheep [46], and goats [47].

Development of Sm14: A FABP-Based Vaccine Against Helminths

The first immunization experiments with rSm14 protein were performed using a fusion protein construct with β-galactosidase formed in the λgt11 vector. Vaccinations of Swiss mice were performed with 10 µg of the semipurified recombinant antigens Sm14, and compared with GST and paramyosin that were also expressed as fusion proteins with β-galactosidase in the cDNA library.

Immunization with 300 μg of crude saline extract was used as control. The mice were challenged with cercariae 60 days after vaccination and worms perfused 45 days after challenge [48]. Sm14 induced levels of protection of approximately 60% in outbred mice. These results indicated that the Sm14 antigen had potential as a vaccine [48].

After this finding, several recombinant forms of the protein Sm14 were obtained. One of the first constructions was obtained using pGEMEX-Sm14 that expressed Sm14 fused with the major capsid protein of T7 phage with a molecular weight of approximately 45 kDa [45]. Also, pRSETA-Sm14 and pRSETA-6xHis-Sm14 constructs were obtained allowing purification of the antigen using immobilized metal-affinity chromatography [49]. Other groups expressed Sm14 in Escherichia coli as a fusion with maltose-binding protein [50] and tetanus toxin fragment C [51]. In *Mycobacterium bovis* BCG, Sm14 was expressed as a fusion with the *Mycobacterium fortuitum* β-lactamase protein [52]. Sm14 has also been expressed in a *Salmonella* vaccine strain [53]. In recent years we expressed and purified the Sm14 protein without any fusion in the *E. coli* and *Pichia pastoris* systems ([54, 55] and unpublished results). Regardless of the nature of the fusion protein or production platform used, or laboratory in which the protein was tested, Sm14 protein conferred protection (greater than 40% reductions in adult worm burdens) against *S. mansoni* infection. These data, collected over two decades of study, provide confidence in relation to the immunological properties of Sm14.

The FABP of others parasites including *S. japonicum* (*Sj*-FABP) [56], *F. hepatica* Fh-12 [57], *F. gigantica* (*Fg*-FABP) [58], *Echinococcus granulosus* (*Eg*-FABP) [59], and C. sinensis (*Cs*-FABP) [60] have also been used as vaccines with success. The cross-protection of Sm14 against infection by *F. hepatica* was demonstrated in mice [45] and sheep [46], as stated above. Likewise, immunization with *F. hepatica* Fh-12 induces protection against infection by schistosome species (87% reduction in adult worm burden [61, 62]). Peptides derived from Sm14 confer a greater than 40% of protection against fasciolosis in mice [21] and, to a lesser extent, in goats [63]. The parasite FABPs are highly conserved and this feature is important when choosing a drug or vaccine target.

Since the finding of Tendler *et al.* [45], Sm14 has been considered a bivalent vaccine against *S. mansoni* and *F. hepatica*. Fasciolosis results on average in losses of €2.5 (US$3.2) billion annually to the livestock and food industries worldwide (www.deliver-project.eu) [64, 65]. Human fascioliasis is also common in parts of South America, Africa, and Asia where over 17 million people are exposed to the disease [66].

Almeida *et al.* [46] formulated Sm14 with alum and Ribi adjuvants to immunize sheep. The Ribi adjuvant, which is no longer on the market, contains monophosphoril Lipid A (MPL), trehalose dimecolate, and *Mycobacterium* phlei cell wall skeleton. Immunization with this formulation resulted in high levels of protection against infection with *F. hepatica* in sheep [46]. Recently, goats that were immunized with Sm14 formulated with Quil A adjuvant recorded a significant reduction in gross hepatic lesions [47], but to a lesser extent (56% reduction in hepatic lesions) than that reported by Almeida *et al.* [46]. The importance of the adjuvant system was also established for immunization of sheep with *F. hepatica* FABP. Specifically, a protective immune response was only achieved by specific combinations of adjuvant and immunomodulators using a system called adjuvant adaptation [67].

The precise mechanism of anti-FABP immunity is still unknown. In people in endemic areas from Brazil and Egypt, a helper T cell T_h1 response associated with specific human IgG1 and IgG3 subclass antibodies correlates with resistance to infection [68–71].

The development of schistosomiasis vaccines received a boost in the 1990s, thanks to the creation of the WHO TDR that promoted vaccines for major human parasitic diseases, including malaria, leishmaniasis, and schistosomiasis. Based on published results from different protective antigens against schistosomes, TDR selected a total of six antigens and recommended their production under Good Manufacturing Practice (GMP) to facilitate clinical trials [72]. Sm14 is the only antigen of the six that is being developed in a country in which schistosomiasis is endemic.

Sm14 Protein Stability

To produce recombinant proteins under GMP conditions, it is first necessary to scale production from a bench to a pilot industrial scale. Such scaling is one of the most important and limiting stages in moving towards clinical trials and the eventual large-scale production of antigen. The production scale-up of Sm14 protein was initiated at the Molecular Biotechnology Laboratory of the Butantan Institute, Sao Paulo, Brazil. The work was subsequently moved to the Laboratory of Experimental Schistosomiasis at FIOCRUZ and finished at the GMP facility of the Ludwig Institute for Cancer Research (LICR), Cornell University, in the United States.

One of the problems faced in any scale-up process is the stability and solubility of the selected proteins. Initially, the Sm14 protein showed precipitation during storage at 4 °C and transport between laboratories. This problem was resolved in two stages. (i) The more stable variant with a M20T Sm14 polymorphism was selected [73]. (ii) A single amino acid substitution, C62V, was undertaken to obtain an even more stable product with enhanced thermal and chemical characteristics [74]. The Sm14-M20V62 protein was used to collect nuclear magnetic resonance (NMR) data [54] and solve the structure of Sm14 [74] (Figure 26.3).

There are no significant structural differences between the Sm14 crystal (Figure 26.2) [37] and NMR (Figure 26.3) [74] structures, and the Sm14-M20V62 variant presents the characteristic fold of the FABP protein family. It was, therefore, concluded that the epitopes in Sm14-M20V62 are exposed in the same way as on the wild-type Sm14-M20C62.

These structural data and the considerable information on immunoprotective activity, biochemical activity, immunolocalization, characterization of the polymorphism, gene sequence, transcriptome, and proteome render Sm14 one of the best-characterized *S. mansoni* proteins.

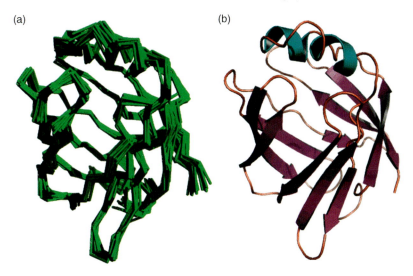

Figure 26.3 Solution structure of Sm14-M20V62 protein by NMR. (a) Overlap of the carbon skeletons of 20 structures deduced by NMR. (b) Ribbon diagram of the structure with lower free energy (Protein Data Bank ID: 2POA) [74] © (2009) Elsevier. Figure prepared with PyMol software.

Scaling-Up the Sm14 Production Process

The more stable, untagged Sm14-M20V62 protein, which does not precipitate during storage and transport, was chosen for GMP production. Over the last 5 years, high-level expression systems have been developed, both in E. coli, in which Sm14 is expressed as a soluble intracellular protein, and in P. pastoris, from which Sm14 can be either secreted or expressed intracellularly (unpublished data). In particular, methodologies have been tailored to facilitate high yield and purity at low cost bearing in mind the large populations that need to be served. The final process adopted is shown in Figure 26.4.

At each stage of the development process, quality control experiments are performed that include assessment of purity and identity by sodium dodecyl sulfate–polyacrylamide gel electrophoresis, Western blots, mass spectroscopy, protein sequencing, determination of the secondary structure by circular dichroism (because structure is important for the protective activity of Sm14), and immunization and challenge experiments in animals to verify the effectiveness of the product.

The production process of Sm14 has been successfully scaled-up to pilot-scale and pilot bulks have been obtained at the LICR-GMP facility of Cornell University (New York). The fill/finishing of bulk vialing was accomplished at Florida Biologix (Alachua, FL) – a contract manufacturing organization. An extensive grid of quality control tests and stability are underway at the contract research organization, PPD (Middleton, WI). All these steps take place in the United States [65].

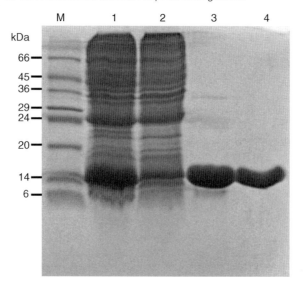

Figure 26.4 Process of purification of recombinant untagged Sm14-M20V62 protein from *E. coli* lysates. M, molecular weight standard; 1, clarified lysate of E. coli; 2, flow through; 3, elution from ion-exchange chromatograph; 4, protein after gel-filtration step.

The GMP production and fill/finish, as well as the quality controls, were achieved thanks to the support of FINEP (Financier of Studies and Projects of Brazilian Ministry of Science and Technology) for the public–private partnership between FIOCRUZ, Alvos Biotecnologia SA, and OuroFino Animal Health Ltd [65].

Clinical Trials

In parallel to the development and production of rSm14 protein, studies to find the appropriate adjuvant for vaccine formulation have been conducted. As stated above, the Ribi adjuvant, successfully used for a decade, is no longer on the market. Fortunately, a partnership was established between FIOCRUZ and the Infectious Disease Research Institute (IDRI) in Seattle, WA. IDRI is a nongovernment institution that supports the development of vaccines, diagnostics, and therapeutics for neglected diseases. This institution provided the synthetic lipid A adjuvant (called GLA), manufactured under GMP conditions, for the formulation of Sm14 for human vaccination. This adjuvant is currently being used in clinical trials for different vaccines. Both GLA and MPL, the critical component of the Ribi adjuvant, are agonists of Toll-like receptor 4 [75, 76]. Thus, it is expected that GLA will generate the same type of response that Ribi adjuvant.

Two adjuvant formulations have been tested in rabbits, mice, and cattle: GLA-AF (aqueous formulation) and GLA-SE (squalene oil-in-water emulsion). The protection against *S. mansoni* infection in mice was similar using both formulations to that achieved using Ribi. However, GLA-SE was selected for clinical trials as it produced the stronger immune response (data not shown). Toxicological studies of Sm14-GLA formulations did not show any hazards in tested animals. A dossier with the preclinical information was submitted in December 2009 to the Brazilian Sanitary Surveillance Agency (ANVISA) to request permission for phase I clinical safety trials. This permission was granted in December 2010 by ANVISA and a phase I clinical trial is presently ongoing, conducted by the Institute of Clinical Research Evandro Chagas (IPEC) on the FIOCRUZ campus in Rio de Janeiro, Brazil.

Conclusions

During the years of research with Sm14 as a vaccine candidate for schistosomiasis and fascioliasis, the Laboratory of Experimental Schistosomiasis at FIOCRUZ has been transformed, with the support of state and international funding sources, from a parasitological laboratory to a molecular biology and protein chemistry unit. An extensive scientific literature concerning the use of rSm14 protein as a vaccine, as well as the structure and function of Sm14, has been accumulated (56 PubMed hits using the search query "*Schistosoma* fatty acid binding protein"). In addition, partnerships between public and private entities have been established. At present, OuroFino Animal Health Ltd, which acquired Alvos Biotecnologia SA, holds the Sm14 patent licenses (www.ourofino.com). This project represents the first time that an antigen discovered by laboratory research undertaken in Brazil has been moved into clinical trials, and provides both experience for and a boost to the local biotechnology industry. We are optimistic that the project will continue to progress and eventually result in the production of a vaccine with real human benefits.

References

1. Stoll, N.R. (1947) This wormy world. *J. Parasitol.*, **33**, 1–18.
2. Chan, M.S. (1997) The global burden of intestinal nematode infections-fifty years on. *Parasitol. Today*, **13**, 438–443.
3. World Health Organization (2002) Expert Committee. Prevention and control of schistosomiasis and soil-transmitted helminthiasis. *WHO Tech. Rep. Ser.*, **912**, 1–57.
4. Chitsulo, L., Engels, D., Montresor, A., and Savioli, L. (2000) The global status of schistosomiasis and its control. *Acta Trop.*, **41**, 41–51.
5. King, C.H. (2010) Parasites and poverty: the case of schistosomiasis. *Acta Trop.*, **113**, 95–104.
6. World Health Organization (1996) *State of the World's Vaccines and Immunization*, WHO, Geneva.
7. World Health Organization (1998) *Report of the World Health Organization Informal Consultation on Schistosomiasis Control*, WHO, Geneva.
8. Olds, G.R., Olveda, R., Wu, G., Wiest, P., McGarvey, S., Aligui, G., Zhang, S. *et al.* (1996) Immunity and morbidity in schistosomiasis japonicum infection. *Am. J. Trop. Med. Hyg.*, **55**, 121–126.
9. Bergquist, N.R., Leonardo, L.R., and Mitchell, G.F. (2005) Vaccine-linked chemotherapy: can schistosomiasis control benefit from an integrated approach? *Trends Parasitol.*, **21**, 112–117.

10 Bergquist, N.R., Al Sherbiny, M., Barak, R., and Olds, R. (2002) Blueprint for schistosomiasis vaccine development. *Acta Trop.*, **82**, 183–192.

11 Bergquist, N.R. (2004) Prospects for schistosomiasis vaccine development. *TDR News*, 71.

12 Spithill, T.W., Smooker, P.M., and Copeman, D.B. (1999) Fasciola *gigantica*: epidemiology, control, immunology and molecular biology, in *Fasciolosis* (ed. J.P. Dalton), CABI, Wallingford, pp. 465–525.

13 Esteves, A., Joseph, L., Paulino, M., and Ehrlich, R. (1997) Remarks on the phylogeny and structure of fatty acid binding proteins from parasitic platyhelminths. *Int. J. Parasitol.*, **27**, 1013–1023.

14 McManus, D.P. and Loukas, A. (2008) Current status of vaccines for schistosomiasis. *Clin. Microbiol. Rev.*, **21**, 225–242.

15 Scapin, M. and Tendler, M. (1977) Immunoprecipitins in human schistosomiasis detected with adult worm antigens released by 3M KCl. *J. Helminthol.*, **51**, 71–72.

16 Tendler, M. and Scapin, M. (1981) *Schistosoma mansoni* antigenic extracts obtained by different extraction procedures. *Mem. Inst. Oswaldo. Cruz*, **76**, 103–109.

17 Balloul, J.M., Grzych, J.M., Pierce, R.J., and Capron, A. (1987) A purified 28,000 dalton protein from *Schistosoma mansoni* adult worms protects rats and mice against experimental schistosomiasis. *J. Immunol.*, **138**, 3448–3453.

18 Lanar, D.E., Pearce, E.J., James, S.L., and Sher, A. (1986) Identification of paramyosin as schistosome antigen recognized by intradermally vaccinated mice. *Science*, **234**, 593–596.

19 Moser, D., Tendler, M., Griffiths, G., and Klinkert, M.Q. (1991) A 14 kDa *Schistosoma mansoni* polypeptide is homologous to a gene family of fatty acid binding proteins. *J. Biol. Chem.*, **266**, 8447–8454.

20 Glatz, J.F.C. and Van der Vusse, G.J. (1990) Cellular fatty acid-binding proteins: current concepts and future directions. *Mol. Biochem. Parasitol.*, **98**, 237–251.

21 Vilar, M.M., Barrientos, F., Almeida, M., Thaumaturgo, N., Simpson, A., Garratt, R., and Tendler, M. (2003) An experimental bivalent peptide vaccine against schistosomiasis and fascioliasis. *Vaccine*, **22**, 137–144.

22 Tendler, M., Lima, A.O., Pinto, R.M., Cruz, M.Q., Brascher, H.M., and Katz, N. (1982) Immunogenic and protective activity of an extract of *Schistosoma mansoni*. *Mem. Inst. Oswaldo. Cruz*, **77**, 275–283.

23 Rodríguez-Pérez, J., Rodríguez-Medina, J.R., García-Blanco, M.A., and Hillyer, G.V. (1992) *Fasciola hepatica*: molecular cloning, nucleotide sequence, and expression of a gene encoding a polypeptide homologous to a *Schistosoma mansoni* fatty acid-binding protein. *Exp. Parasitol.*, **74**, 400–407.

24 Becker, M.M., Kalinna, B.H., Waine, G.J., and McManus, D.P. (1994) Gene cloning, overproduction and purification of a functionally active cytoplasmic fatty acid-binding protein (*Sj*-FABPC) from the human blood fluke *Schistosoma japonicum*. *Gene*, **148**, 321–325.

25 Smooker, P.M., Hickford, D.E., Vaiano, S.A., and Spithill, T.W. (1997) Isolation, cloning, and expression of fatty-acid binding proteins from *Fasciola gigantica*. *Exp. Parasitol.*, **85**, 86–91.

26 Lee, J.S. and Yong, T.S. (2004) Expression and cross-species reactivity of fatty acid-binding protein of *Clonorchis sinensis*. *Parasitol. Res.*, **93**, 339–343.

27 Storch, J. and Thumser, A.E. (2000) The fatty acid transport function of fatty acid-binding proteins. *Biochim. Biophys. Acta*, **1486**, 28–44.

28 Gobert, G.N. (1998) Immunolocalization of schistosome proteins. *Microsc. Res. Tech.*, **42**, 176–185.

29 Brito, C.F., Oliveira, G.C., Oliveira, S.C., Street, M., Riengrojpitak, S., Wilson, R.A., Simpson, A.J., and Correa-Oliveira, R. (2002) Sm14 gene expression in different stages of the *Schistosoma mansoni* life cycle and immunolocalization of the Sm14 protein within the adult worm. *Braz. J. Med. Biol. Res.*, **35**, 377–381.

30 Thaumaturgo, N. (2002) Immulocalization of Sm14 in adult worms of *Schistosoma mansoni* Sambon, 1907 (Digenea-Schistosomatidae), obtained in Swiss mice. Master's Thesis, FIOCRUZ, Rio de Janeiro.

31 Pankao, V., Sirisriro, A., Grams, R., Vichasri-Grams, S., Meepool, A., Kangwanrangsan, N., Wanichanon, C. et al. (2006) Classification of the parenchymal cells in *Fasciola gigantica* based on ultrastructure and their expression of fatty acid binding proteins (FABPs). *Vet. Parasitol.*, **142**, 281–292.

32 Thaumaturgo, N., Vilar, M.M., Diogo, C.M., Edelenyi, R., and Tendler, M. (2001) Preliminary analysis of Sm14 in distinct fractions of *Schistosoma mansoni* adult worm extract. *Mem. Inst. Oswaldo Cruz*, **96**, 79–83.

33 Jefferies, J.R., Campbell, A.M., van Rossum, A.J., Barrett, J., and Brophy, P.M. (2001) Proteomic analysis of *Fasciola hepatica* excretory–secretory products. *Proteomics*, **1**, 1128–1132.

34 Skelly, P.J. and Wilson, A.R. (2006) Making sense of the schistosome surface. *Adv. Parasitol.*, **63**, 185–284.

35 Hughes, R.C. (1999) Secretion of the galectin family of mammalian carbohydrate-binding proteins. *Biochim. Biophys. Acta*, **1473**, 172–185.

36 Mei, H. and LoVerde, P.T. (1997) *Schistosoma mansoni*: the developmental regulation and immunolocalization of antioxidant enzymes. *Exp. Parasitol.*, **86**, 69–78.

37 Angelucci, F., Johnson, K.A., Baiocco, P., Miele, A.E., Brunori, M., Valle, C., Vigorosi, F. et al. (2004) *Schistosoma mansoni* fatty acid binding protein: specificity and functional control as revealed by crystallographic structure. *Biochemistry*, **43**, 13000–13011.

38 Maizels, R.M. and Yazdanbakhsh, M. (2003) Immune regulation by helminth parasites: cellular and molecular mechanisms. *Nat. Rev. Immunol.*, **3**, 733–744.

39 El Ridi, R., Aboueldahab, M., Tallima, H., Salah, M., Mahana, N., Fawzi, S., Mohamed, S.H., and Fahmy, O.M. (2010) *In vitro* and *in vivo* activities of arachidonic acid against *Schistosoma mansoni* and *Schistosoma haematobium*. *Antimicrob. Agents Chemother.*, **54**, 3383–3389.

40 Abdel-Baset, H., O'Neill, G.P., and Ford-Hutchinson, A.W. (1995) Characterization of arachidonic-acid-metabolizing enzymes in adult *Schistosoma mansoni*. *Mol. Biochem. Parasitol.*, **73**, 31–41.

41 Morphew, R.M., Wright, H.A., LaCourse, E.J., Woods, D.J., and Brophy, P.M. (2007) Comparative proteomics of excretory–secretory proteins released by the liver fluke *Fasciola hepatica* in sheep host bile and during *in vitro* culture ex host. *Mol. Cell Proteomics*, **6**, 963–972.

42 Chemale, G., Perally, S., LaCourse, E.J., Prescott, M.C., Jones, L.M., Ward, D., Meaney, M. et al. (2010) Comparative proteomic analysis of triclabendazole response in the liver fluke *Fasciola hepatica*. *J. Proteome Res.*, **9**, 4940–4951.

43 Timanova-Atanasova, A., Jordanova, R., Radoslavov, G., Deevska, G., Bankov, I., and Barrett, J. (2004) A native 13-kDa fatty acid binding protein from the liver fluke *Fasciola hepatica*. *Biochim. Biophys. Acta*, **1674**, 200–204.

44 Thaumaturgo, N., Vilar, M.M., Edelenyi, R., and Tendler, M. (2002) Characterization of Sm14 related components in different helminths by sodium dodecyl sulphate–polyacrylamide gel electrophoresis and Western blotting analysis. *Mem. Inst. Oswaldo Cruz*, **1**, 115–116.

45 Tendler, M., Brito, C.A., Vilar, M.M., Serra-Freire, N., Diogo, C.M., Almeida, M.S., Delbem, A.C. et al. (1996) A *Schistosoma mansoni* fatty acid-binding protein, Sm14, is the potential basis of a dual-purpose anti-helminth vaccine. *Proc. Natl. Acad. Sci. USA*, **93**, 269–273.

46 Almeida, M.S., Torloni, H., Lee-Ho, P., Vilar, M.M., Thaumaturgo, N., Simpson, A.J., and Tendler, M. (2003) Vaccination against *Fasciola hepatica* infection using a *Schistosoma mansoni* defined recombinant antigen, Sm14. *Parasite Immunol.*, **25**, 135–137.

47 Mendes, R.E., Zafra, R., Pérez-Ecija, R.A., Buffoni, L., Martínez-Moreno, A.,

Tendler, M., and Pérez, J. (2010) Evaluation of local immune response to *Fasciola hepatica* experimental infection in the liver and hepatic lymph nodes of goats immunized with Sm14 vaccine antigen. *Mem. Inst. Oswaldo Cruz*, **105**, 698–705.

48 Tendler, M., Vilar, M.M., Brito, C.A., Freire, N.M., Katz, N., and Simpson, A. (1995) Vaccination against schistosomiasis and fascioliasis with the new recombinant antigen Sm14: potential basis of a multi-valent anti-helminth vaccine? *Mem. Inst. Oswaldo Cruz*, **90**, 255–256.

49 Ramos, C.R., Vilar, M.M., Nascimento, A.L., Ho, P.L., Thaumaturgo, N., Edelenyi, R., Almeida, M. et al. (2001) r-Sm14-pRSETA efficacy in experimental animals. *Mem. Inst. Oswaldo Cruz*, **96**, 131–135.

50 Brito, C.F., Fonseca, C.T., Goes, A.M., Azevedo, V., Simpson, A.J., and Oliveira, S.C. (2000) Human IgG1 and IgG3 recognition of *Schistosoma mansoni* 14 kDa fatty acid-binding recombinant protein. *Parasite Immunol.*, **22**, 41–48.

51 Abreu, P.A., Miyasato, P.A., Vilar, M.M., Dias, W.O., Ho, P.L., Tendler, M., and Nascimento, A.L. (2004) Sm14 of *Schistosoma mansoni* in fusion with tetanus toxin fragment C induces immunoprotection against tetanus and schistosomiasis in mice. *Infect. Immun.*, **72**, 5931–5937.

52 Varaldo, P.B., Leite, L.C., Dias, W.O., Miyaji, E.N., Torres, F.I., Gebara, V.C., Armôa, G. et al. (2004) Recombinant *Mycobacterium bovis* BCG expressing the Sm14 antigen of *Schistosoma mansoni* protects mice from cercarial challenge. *Infect. Immun.*, **72**, 3336–3343.

53 Pacheco, L.G., Zucconi, E., Mati, V.L., Garcia, R.M., Miyoshi, A., Oliveira, S.C., de Melo, A.L., and Azevedo, V. (2005) Oral administration of a live Aro attenuated *Salmonella* vaccine strain expressing 14-kDa *Schistosoma mansoni* fatty acid-binding protein induced partial protection against experimental schistosomiasis. *Acta Trop.*, **95**, 132–142.

54 Pertinhez, T.A., Sforça, M.L., Alves, A.C., Ramos, C.R., Ho, P.L., Tendler, M., Zanchin, N.I., and Spisni, A. (2004) ^{1}H, ^{15}N and ^{13}C resonance assignments of the apo Sm14-M20(C62V) protein, a mutant of *Schistosoma mansoni* Sm14. *J. Biomol. NMR*, **29**, 553–554.

55 Huang, C.J., Damasceno, L.M., Anderson, K.A., Zhang, S., Old, L.J., and Batt, C.A. (2011) A proteomic analysis of the *Pichia pastoris* secretome in methanol-induced cultures. *Appl. Microbiol. Biotechnol.*, **90**, 235–247.

56 Yuan, H., You-En, S., Long-Jiang, Y., Xiao-Hua, Z., Liu-Zhe, L., Cash, M., Lu, Z. et al. (2007) Studies on the protective immunity of *Schistosoma japonicum* bivalent DNA vaccine encoding Sj23 and Sj14. *Exp. Parasitol.*, **115**, 379–386.

57 Martínez-Fernández, A.R., Nogal-Ruiz, J.J., López-Abán, J., Ramajo, V., Oleaga, A., Manga-González, Y., Hillyer, G.V., and Muro, A. (2004) Vaccination of mice and sheep with Fh12 FABP from *Fasciola hepatica* using the new adjuvant/ immunomodulator system ADAD. *Vet. Parasitol.*, **126**, 287–298.

58 Nambi, P.A., Yadav, S.C., Raina, O.K., Sriveny, D., and Saini, M. (2005) Vaccination of buffaloes with *Fasciola gigantica* recombinant fatty acid binding protein. *Parasitol. Res.*, **97**, 129–135.

59 Chabalgoity, J.A., Harrison, J.A., Esteves, A., Demarco de Hormaeche, R., Ehrlich, R., Khan, C.M., and Hormaeche, C.E. (1997) Expression and immunogenicity of an *Echinococcus granulosus* fatty acid-binding protein in live attenuated *Salmonella* vaccine strains. *Infect. Immun.*, **65**, 2402–2412.

60 Lee, J.S., Kim, I.S., Sohn, W.M., Lee, J., and Yong, T.S. (2006) A DNA vaccine encoding a fatty acid-binding protein of *Clonorchis sinensis* induces protective immune response in Sprague-Dawley rats. *Scand. J. Immunol.*, **63**, 169–176.

61 Abán, J.L., Ramajo, V., Arellano, J.L., Oleaga, A., Hillyer, G.V., and Muro, A.A. (1999) fatty acid binding protein from *Fasciola hepatica* induced protection in C57/BL mice from challenge infection with *Schistosoma bovis*. *Vet. Parasitol.*, **83**, 107–121.

62 Hillyer, G.V. (2005) Fasciola antigens as vaccines against fascioliasis and

schistosomiasis. *J. Helminthol.*, **79**, 241–247.

63 Zafra, R., Buffoni, L., Pérez-Ecija, R.A., Mendes, R.E., Martínez-Moreno, A., Martínez-Moreno, F.J., and Pérez, J. (2009) Study of the local immune response to *Fasciola hepatica* in the liver and hepatic lymph nodes of goats immunised with a peptide of the Sm14 antigen. *Res. Vet. Sci.*, **87**, 226–232.

64 Piedrafita, D., Spithill, T.W., Smith, R.E., and Raadsma, H.W. (2010) Improving animal and human health through understanding liver fluke immunology. *Parasite Immunol.*, **32**, 572–581.

65 Tendler, M. and Simpson, A.J. (2008) The biotechnology-value chain: development of Sm14 as a schistosomiasis vaccine. *Acta Trop.*, **108**, 263–266.

66 Mas-Coma, M.S., Esteban, J.G., and Bargues, M.D. (1999) Epidemiology of human fascioliasis: a review and proposed new classification. *Bull. World Health Organ.*, **77**, 340–346.

67 López-Abán, J., Nogal-Ruiz, J.J., Vicente, B., Morrondo, P., Diez-Baños, P., Hillyer, G.V., Martínez-Fernández, A.R. *et al.* (2008) The addition of a new immunomodulator with the adjuvant adaptation ADAD system using fatty acid binding proteins increases the protection against *Fasciola hepatica*. *Vet. Parasitol.*, **153**, 176–181.

68 Brito, C.F., Fonseca, C.T., Goes, A.M., Azevedo, V., Simpson, A.J., and Oliveira, S.C. (2000) Human IgG1 and IgG3 recognition of *Schistosoma mansoni* 14 kDa fatty acid-binding recombinant protein. *Parasite Immunol.*, **22**, 41–48.

69 Brito, C.F., Caldas, I.R., Coura Filho, P., Correa-Oliveira, R., and Oliveira, S.C. (2000) CD4$^+$ T cells of schistosomiasis naturally resistant individuals living in an endemic area produce interferon-gamma and tumour necrosis factor-alpha in response to the recombinant 14 kDa *Schistosoma mansoni* fatty acid-binding protein. *Scand. J. Immunol.*, **51**, 595–601.

70 Al-Sherbiny, M., Osman, A., Barakat, R., El Morshedy, H., Bergquist, R., and Olds, R. (2003) *In vitro* cellular and humoral responses to *Schistosoma mansoni* vaccine candidate antigens. *Acta Trop.*, **88**, 117–130.

71 Fonseca, C.T., Cunha-Neto, E., Kalil, J., Jesus, A.R., Correa-Oliveira, R., Carvalho, E.M., and Oliveira, S.C. (2004) Identification of immunodominant epitopes of *Schistosoma mansoni* vaccine candidate antigens using human T cells. *Mem. Inst. Oswaldo Cruz*, **99**, 63–66.

72 Bergquist, N.R. (1998) Schistosomiasis vaccine development: progress and prospects. *Mem. Inst. Oswaldo Cruz*, **93**, 95–101.

73 Ramos, C.R., Figueredo, R.C., Pertinhez, T.A., Vilar, M.M., do Nascimento, A.L., Tendler, M., Raw, I. *et al.* (2003) Gene structure and M20T polymorphism of the *Schistosoma mansoni* Sm14 fatty acid-binding protein. Molecular, functional, and immunoprotection analysis. *J. Biol. Chem.*, **278**, 12745–12751.

74 Ramos, C.R., Spisni, A., Oyama, S. Jr, Sforça, M.L., Ramos, H.R., Vilar, M.M., Alves, A.C. *et al.* (2009) Stability improvement of the fatty acid binding protein Sm14 from *S. mansoni* by Cys replacement: structural and functional characterization of a vaccine candidate. *Biochim. Biophys. Acta*, **1794**, 655–662.

75 Coler, R.N., Baldwin, S.L., Shaverdian, N., Bertholet, S., Reed, S.J., Raman, V.S., Lu, X. *et al.* (2010) A synthetic adjuvant to enhance and expand immune responses to influenza vaccines. *PLoS One*, **5**, e13677.

76 Coler, R.N., Bertholet, S., Moutaftsi, M., Guderian, J.A., Windish, H.P., Baldwin, S.L., Laughlin, E.M. *et al.* (2011) Development and characterization of synthetic glucopyranosyl lipid adjuvant system as a vaccine adjuvant. *PLoS One*, **6**, e16333.

27
Mechanisms of Immune Modulation by *Fasciola hepatica*: Importance for Vaccine Development and for Novel Immunotherapeutics

Mark W. Robinson[*], *John P. Dalton, Sandra M. O'Neill, and Sheila M. Donnelly*

Abstract

The liver fluke *Fasciola hepatica* can live for long periods in its definitive mammalian host. This longevity is related to the parasite's ability to modulate host immune responses to benefit its survival (i.e., suppression of T_h1/T_h17 responses and the promotion of strong T_h2/T_{reg}-mediated responses). Various reports indicate that this immune regulation may reduce the capacity of animals to resist other bystander infections (e.g., *F. hepatica*-infected mice exhibit reduced protective immune responses to the respiratory bacterium, *Bordetella pertussis*). Experiments in cattle infected with *F. hepatica* revealed reductions in interferon-γ responses to coinfections with *Mycobacterium bovis*. Molecules secreted by the parasite such as cathepsin L cysteine peptidases, the antioxidant peroxiredoxin, and a cathelicidin-like defense molecule play central roles in manipulating the function of host innate immune cells, and thus the development of protective adaptive immune responses. While these molecules influence innate immune cells in distinct ways, they likely function in concert to establish the potent T_h2/T_{reg}-mediated immune environment in the host. Vaccines that prevent the action of these immunomodulatory molecules may not only protect animals against liver fluke disease, but reduce their susceptibility to coincident parasitic or microbial infections. Taking a broader view, understanding how the liver fluke influences host immunity via specific cell surface receptors and intracellular signaling pathways could reveal strategies to selectively suppress certain inflammatory processes, and eventually lead to immunotherapeutic treatments for conditions such as arthritis, inflammatory bowel disease, and diabetes.

Introduction

Fasciola hepatica is the causative agent of liver fluke disease (fasciolosis) in domestic animals, predominantly sheep and cattle, in regions with temperate climates. The global economic loss due to this parasite is difficult to estimate, but, along with the related tropical parasite, *F. gigantica*, could be over US$3 billion each year [1]. Human fasciolosis is now a major food-borne zoonosis in many countries including Iran,

[*] Corresponding Author

Parasitic Helminths: Targets, Screens, Drugs and Vaccines, First Edition. Edited by Conor R. Caffrey
© 2012 Wiley-VCH Verlag GmbH & Co. KGaA. Published 2012 by Wiley-VCH Verlag GmbH & Co. KGaA.

Peru, Cuba, Bolivia and Egypt. Each year an estimated 2.4 million people are infected world-wide and 180 million people are at risk of infection [1].

Fluke eggs, released by adult parasites residing in the bile ducts of the mammalian host, are carried into the intestine and are passed with the feces. The eggs hatch and release free-swimming miracidia that find and penetrate the tissues of their molluscan intermediate hosts: *F. hepatica* typically infects the freshwater snail *Galba truncatula* (formerly known as *Lymnaea truncatula*). Within the digestive gland of the infected snail, the parasite undergoes a series of developmental changes and multiplications that ends in the release of thousands of free-swimming cercariae. These adhere to, and encyst as metacercariae, on vegetation and are infective to the definitive mammalian host. Following ingestion of the vegetation contaminated with metacercaria, the parasites excyst in the small intestine. The newly excysted juvenile (NEJ) flukes penetrate through the gut wall and enter the peritoneal cavity, where flukes spend a period of time wandering over the viscera before locating and penetrating the liver parenchyma. After about 10–12 weeks, they enter the bile ducts where they become obligate blood feeders, complete their development, and produce eggs [1, 2]. Current treatments rely on anthelmintics, such as triclabendazole, but parasites resistant to these have emerged in Europe and Australia making the development of a vaccine more urgent [3].

F. hepatica can live for long periods in its host – typically 1–2 years in cattle, but up to 20 years in sheep [2]. This longevity is related to the parasite's ability to modulate host immune responses to benefit its survival (i.e., suppression of helper T cell T_h1/T_h17 responses and the promotion of strong T_h2/regulatory T cell (T_{reg})-mediated responses). Experiments in mice have shown that infection with *F. hepatica* induces potent T_h2/Treg responses, characterized by the production of interleukin (IL)-4, -5, and -10, and transforming growth factor (TGF)-β [4–6]. At the same time, the parasite suppresses the generation of the T_h1-associated cytokines, interferon (IFN)-γ and IL-2 [4, 5]. As a consequence of the reduced T_h1 immune responses, mice coinfected with *F. hepatica* and *Bordetella pertussis* (causative agent of whooping cough) exhibit a significant delay in clearing the bacterial infection from the lungs [7, 8]. In addition, mice immunized with the whooping cough vaccine exhibited a similar reduction in T_h1 responses when infected with *F. hepatica*, thereby impacting vaccine efficacy [7, 8]. Studies by Mulcahy, Dalton and colleagues using cattle and sheep also found that *F. hepatica* induced potent T_h2-driven immune responses [9, 10], and that vaccine efficacy was dependent on the promotion of strong T_h1 responses [9–11]. The T_h2 responses induced by the parasite in cattle are sufficiently potent to suppress delayed-type hypersensitivity reactions and IFN-γ production to coinfecting *Mycobacterium bovis* [12].

Those molecules that most likely influence the immune system of the host are secreted or shed by the parasite into the tissues and circulation, and are considered prime candidates for vaccine development [1]. The major molecules so far isolated from medium in which *F. hepatica* is cultured (commonly referred to as excretory/secretory (ES) products) and their demonstrated immunomodulatory properties are summarized in Table 27.1. Here, we focus on three of these molecules (i.e., cathepsin L, peroxiredoxin, and a cathelicidin-like defense molecule), and show how each of

Introduction

Table 27.1 Major secreted molecules from F. hepatica, immunomodulatory effects, and efficacy as anti-Fasciola vaccines.

Fasciola molecule	Effect on immune system	Protection in vaccine trial (%)[a]
Cathepsin L1 and cathepsin L2	degrades endosomal TLR3 cleaves hinge region of IgG inhibits the differentiation of T_h17 cells by dendritic cells	68.5 (native CL1/CL2 combination)
Peroxiredoxin	induces M2 macrophages	52.0 (recombinant)
Helminth defense molecule	modulates LPS-mediated response in macrophages	not tested
Leucine aminopeptidase	unknown	89.6 (native) 81.0 (recombinant)
Glutathione S-transferase	inhibits proliferation of spleen cells and production of nitric oxide by macrophages inhibits differentiation of T_h17 cells by dendritic cells	69.0 (native)
Fatty acid-binding protein	unknown	76.0 (recombinant)

[a] Only the highest level of protection obtained in the various trials for each antigen is shown (summarized from [1] and Dalton, unpublished data).

these alters innate immune cell function and influences host immune responses to the parasite.

Cathepsin L Cysteine Peptidases

Cathepsin L cysteine peptidases (Clan CA, family C1 [13]) are major components of the ES products of all stages of F. hepatica that develop in the mammalian host [14]. These enzymes are stored as inactive zymogens or proenzymes in secretory vesicles of the gastrodermal epithelial cells before secretion in large quantities into the lumen of the parasite gut and then externally into the host tissues [15, 16]. The secreted cysteine peptidases degrade host interstitial matrix proteins, such as collagen, laminin, and fibronectin, and are central to the acquisition of nutrients by digesting host proteins to peptides [17, 18]. The peptidases also have a range of systemic effects on the host immune response that help prevent immune-mediated elimination of the parasite [19].

Mammalian hosts infected with F. hepatica develop specific antibodies [20] and yet no evidence exists of antibody-mediated eosinophil damage to NEJs in nonpermissive bovine hosts [21]. Although effector cells readily adhered to NEJs in the presence of immune sera, they failed to do so if the parasite's ES products were added, which indicated that the contents of ES products can prevent interaction between immune serum antibodies and eosinophils. In the presence of leupeptin, the effector cells remained attached to the NEJs, thus identifying the active component within ES products as a cysteine peptidase [22]. Subsequently, in vitro studies confirmed that papain-like cathepsin L peptidases secreted by F. hepatica cleaved all IgG subclasses at the same peptide bond located within the hinge region [23], thus preventing the interaction of IgG with immune effector cells and the development of antibody-dependent cellular cytotoxicity (ADCC). This restricted proteolytic activity suggests a conserved mechanism used by the parasite to evade the host immune response.

Analyses of the subclasses of cathepsin L-specific antibodies produced during human fasciolosis reveal the predominance of an IgG4 isotype [24]. In addition, studies examining the immune responses of cattle that were either experimentally or naturally infected with F. hepatica metacercariae showed that animals generated IgG1 antibodies (equivalent to human IgG4) specific for cathepsin L and little or no IgG2 antibodies [25, 26]. Production of these isotypes correlates with the absence of T_h1-type responses and the induction of potent T_h2-type immune response by the parasite.

It has been previously suggested that the strong polarized T_h2 environment promoted by helminth parasites prevents the development of T_h1/T_h17 immune responses [27]. However, our data indicate that secreted F. hepatica cysteine peptidases directly suppress the differentiation of T_h1 and T_h17 cells, independently of T_h2-type cytokines, by altering the function of innate immune cells critical in the priming of naïve T cells [4, 5]. In response to invading pathogens, dendritic cells express surface molecules and produce cytokines that modulate the effector functions of responding T cells. For example, the secretion of IL-12 and IL-23 from dendritic cells is necessary to promote the differentiation of T_h1 and T_h17 cells, respectively. Stimulation of murine bone marrow-derived dendritic cells with cathepsin L induced elevated levels of surface-expressed CD40, but not CD80, CD86, or major histocompatibility complex class II. This partial activation of dendritic cells was dependent on Toll-like receptor (TLR) 4 and the phosphorylation of the intracellular mitogen-activated protein kinase, p38. Exposure of dendritic cells to cathepsin L resulted in the secretion of IL-6 and IL-12p40, but neither IL-12p70 or IL-23 were produced, and these cytokines were also suppressed by cathepsin L when dendritic cells were stimulated with lipopolysaccharide (LPS). The absence of these cytokines explains why cathepsin L-stimulated dendritic cells do not promote T_h17 responses from naive $CD4^+$ T cells following antigenic stimulation [28].

Like dendritic cells, secretion of cytokines by macrophages in response to pathogen recognition influences the phenotype of developing T-cells. Similar to the effect on dendritic cells, cathepsin L prevented the secretion of the T_h1-associated inflammatory cytokine IL-12 [29] and the T_h17-associated cytokine IL-23 (Donnelly, unpublished data) as well as IL-6, tumor necrosis factor (TNF)-α, and nitric oxide from macrophages in response to TLR ligands [29]. Inactivation of macrophages is a result of the specific inhibition of MyD88-independent TRIF-dependent signaling pathways of TLR4 and TLR3 [29]. As a consequence of this, activation of both T_h1 and T_h17 responses to antigenic stimulation is inhibited in mice given *F. hepatica* cathepsin L ([20] and Donnelly, unpublished data).

These data detail the mechanisms by which parasite secreted cysteine peptidases alter immune cell function and prevent the establishment of potent T_h1-driven inflammatory responses that would lead to parasite elimination. The critical function of cysteine peptidases in immunomodulation, tissue penetration, and prevention of ADCC suggests that the *F. hepatica* cathepsin L peptidases could be exploited as potential vaccines [19]. Supporting this proposition, *in vitro* analyses demonstrated that neutralization of cathepsin L by specific antibodies allowed eosinophil attachment to the parasite and thus the initiation of ADCC [30]. In addition, silencing cathepsin L gene expression in *F. hepatica* NEJs by RNA interference significantly reduced penetration of the rat intestinal wall [31]. Furthermore, the ability of *Fasciola* ES products to inhibit development of T_h1 immune responses was abrogated by specific cysteine peptidase inhibitors [8].

Vaccine trials using *F. hepatica* cathepsin L have shown reductions in fluke burdens in the range of 55–72% compared to unvaccinated controls, and a marked reduction in parasite fecundity and/or egg viability [11, 32]. As expected, given that cathepsin L suppresses T_h1 immune responses, vaccine-induced protection was associated with a high parasite-specific IgG2 titer and avidity [9], and the induction of a T_h1 response or a mixed T_h1/T_h2 response [9–11]. Correlating with this switch in adaptive immune responses, macrophages isolated from vaccinated animals showed an increase in the ratio of nitric oxide to arginase production, reflecting the induction of a T_h1-associated phenotype [11]. Thus, the cathepsin L-blocking antibodies elicited by the vaccine prevent the parasite from suppressing the T_h1 response of the host and establishing a T_h2-mediated milieu that is typical of natural infections.

A correlation exists between T_h1/T_h17 immune responses and the development of severe inflammation-mediated pathology in helminth-infected mice [33, 34]. Regulation of both is critical to the control of inflammatory pathology associated with helminth infection. The development of autoimmune diseases also involves both T_h17 and T_h1 immune responses [35, 36]. Current strategies in the development of immune therapies for these diseases are aimed at using molecules that prevent innate immune cell activation of adaptive T cell responses. Thus, the study of how helminth-derived cysteine peptidases alter innate immune responses may aid the development of novel therapeutic approaches for the treatment of T_h1/T_h17-mediated inflammatory disorders.

Peroxiredoxin

Helminth parasites undergo rapid growth phases, produce numerous offspring, and, hence, their tissues and cells exist in an environment of high oxidative stress. Within their vertebrate hosts, the parasites are also exposed to reactive oxygen species (ROS) released from immune effector cells such as eosinophils, macrophages, and neutrophils. Despite such potent oxidative assaults, helminths possess the necessary armory to defend against ROS and survive in their hosts for many years. *F. hepatica* expresses abundant levels of superoxide dismutase to reduce superoxide to H_2O_2, and peroxiredoxin to eliminate toxic levels of H_2O_2 [37–41].

Although peroxiredoxin is constitutively expressed throughout the life cycle of *F. hepatica*, a differential level of expression is observed during distinct stages of parasite development. The highest level of peroxiredoxin protein expression is found in the infective stage of the parasite that traverses the host intestine. Expression of peroxiredoxin protein is upregulated by almost 50% in this stage compared with both the immature stage flukes that migrate through the liver tissues and the adult parasites that reside within the bile ducts [42]. Tissue invasion and penetration is a vulnerable time in the parasite life cycle, and undoubtedly attracts considerable attention from the cellular arm of the host immune system. During this time the parasite likely requires increased protection against ROS, which is reflected by the increase in peroxiredoxin expression. Proteomics and molecular studies show that peroxiredoxin is secreted by adult *F. hepatica* and immunocytochemical studies have revealed that peroxiredoxin is located in the gut epithelium of adult worms (Dalton, unpublished data). Strikingly, peroxiredoxin lacks a predicted N-terminal signal peptides required for classical endoplasmic reticulum/Golgi secretion implying that peroxiredoxin molecules can be exported via noncanonical secretory pathways in helminths [42].

Given their extracorporeal secretion by helminth parasites, we first proposed that the primary function of peroxiredoxin molecules was in the inactivation of ROS released by the host's immune effector cells [40, 41]. However, as we have recently demonstrated that helminth peroxiredoxin can influence the immune responses of the host by altering the function of macrophage cells, we now believe that they also contribute to immune modulation. Macrophages respond with remarkable plasticity to different stimuli by altering their phenotype. These "activated" macrophages have been generally classified as M1 (classically activated) and M2 (alternatively activated) populations [43]. The alternatively activated macrophages are found in all T_h2 cytokine environments regardless of whether activation is induced by parasitic, asthmatic, or tumor-associated inflammation [44], and have therefore been classified as a phenotype of macrophage induced by IL-4 and/or IL-13. Several markers have been identified as characteristic of this IL-4/IL-13 activated phenotype, such as Arg-1, mannose receptor, Fizz1, and Ym1 [44]. During helminth infections, M2 macrophages not only help enhance T_h2 cell differentiation [45], but also suppress T_h1 inflammatory responses [46]. Therefore, one strategy by which parasitic worms regulate the immune response is by modifying macrophage function.

F. hepatica induces the activation of M2 macrophages within 24 h and a strongly biased T_h2 immune response within 7 days [4, 5, 47]. Coinciding with this rapid immune modulation is the abundant secretion of peroxiredoxin from the juvenile parasite worms [42]. Administration of *F. hepatica* ES products can induce alternative activation of macrophages and T_h2 responses in mice that are as potent as infection with parasites [4, 5]. The active T_h2-inducing protein fraction of ES contains peroxiredoxin and functionally active recombinant *F. hepatica* peroxiredoxin also induces the activation of M2 macrophages, as indicated by the expression of Ym1 and Arg1, when administered intraperitoneally into immune competent BALB/c mice and IL-4- or IL-13-deficient mice [5]. In the absence of exogenous cytokine stimulation, recombinant peroxiredoxin induced the expression of Ym1 in peritoneal macrophages *in vitro*, suggesting that parasite peroxiredoxin directly alters the characteristics of macrophage populations independently of IL-4 and IL-13. The modulating capacity of peroxiredoxin was independent of its antioxidant activity as an inactive recombinant variant of *F. hepatica* peroxiredoxin also induced the expression of Ym1 and Arg1 in macrophages both *in vivo* and *in vitro* [5]. We have proposed that peroxiredoxin-mediated activation of macrophages probably involves direct interaction of a conserved peroxiredoxin structural motif with an, as yet unknown, receptor.

As expected for an M2 macrophage, peroxiredoxin-activated macrophages promote the differentiation of T_h2 cells and suppress the development of T_h1 cells from naive $CD4^+$ T cells in a coculture [5]. In addition, the adoptive transfer of peroxiredoxin-activated macrophages to naive murine recipients results in the polarization of T-cells towards a T_h2 phenotype in response to stimulation with anti-CD3 (Donnelly, unpublished data). Our data showing that administration of peroxiredoxin-specific antibodies during infection of *F. hepatica* blocked the expression of Ym1 in peritoneal macrophages and significantly reduced the development of T_h2 responses support the potential of exploiting a peroxiredoxin-based vaccine strategy to prevent the parasite establishing a favorable immune environment.

The neutralization of parasite-secreted peroxiredoxin and, therefore, prevention of the development of T_h2 immune responses may well have been the mechanism by which vaccination with a high molecular mass fraction of *Fasciola* ES products (which we now know contains peroxiredoxin) protected 42% of cattle against a challenge infection [32]. Supporting these initial observations, we have subsequently found that delivery of recombinant peroxiredoxin to sheep provided high levels of protection (52%) against a heterologous challenge with *F. hepatica* parasites (Dalton, unpublished data). In addition, protection of goats following immunization with recombinant peroxiredoxin was associated with a reduction in the levels of IL-4 secreted by cells of the hepatic draining lymph node [48].

Our discovery of peroxiredoxin as a molecule that instructs T_h2 responses via Ym1-expressing macrophages provides a model that can be used to dissect the mechanisms behind T_h2-driven immune responses. Characterization of the structural motif (s) on peroxiredoxin that binds to and activates macrophages and the elucidation of the cognate receptor has implications not only for the development of antihelminth treatments, but also as prospective immuno- or chemotherapeutics for human inflammatory disorders.

Cathelicidin-Like Helminth Defense Molecule

It has been demonstrated experimentally that intestinal injury and systemic endotoxemia are two factors leading to morbidity during helminth infection of mice [46, 49]. Indeed, translocation of intestinal bacteria and their toxins into circulation is common during many helminth infections due to disruption of the barrier function of the intestinal epithelium. Even nonenteric helminths, such as

F. hepatica that reside in the bile ducts, cause biliary obstruction, which increases intraductal pressure leading to the disruption of hepatocellular tight junctions and subsequent translocation of *Escherichia coli* and enterococcus [50, 51]. Despite such bacterial colonization, potent host responses such as septicemia are not common events during helminth infections [52]. While the mechanism of resistance to septicemia during helminth infection is poorly understood, it is known that innate immune cells rather than those of the adaptive immune system play an essential protective role. For example, mice deficient in the IL-4α receptor specifically on macrophages and neutrophils, but not T-cells, experienced high mortality (100%) associated with increased sepsis following infection with *Schistosoma mansoni* [46, 49]. We have shown that protection against harmful inflammatory responses is due, in part, to the inhibition of proinflammatory cytokine release (including IL-12) from macrophages by secreted helminth cathepsin peptidases [29]. However, our recent discoveries suggest that *F. hepatica* liberates specific defense molecules/peptides that are also central players in this process.

Host defense (also termed antimicrobial) peptides represent an evolutionarily conserved component of innate immunity [53]. They are potent signaling molecules released by cells of the innate immune system in response to cellular stimulation by microbes and proinflammatory mediators [54]. Multiple peptides are simultaneously secreted at the site of inflammation and work cooperatively to protect against the detrimental effects of an excessive innate inflammatory response. Thus, defense peptides have been shown to suppress LPS-mediated responses [55, 56], promote phagocytosis while inhibiting oxidant responses of neutrophils or monocytes [57, 58], and inhibit proinflammatory cytokine secretion by macrophages in the presence of bacteria or other nonspecific inflammatory stimuli [58, 59].

Using an integrated transcriptomics and proteomics platform we have recently identified a novel 8-kDa *F. hepatica* secretory protein (termed *F. hepatica* helminth defense molecule (HDM)-1) that exhibits similar structural characteristics to the human cathelicidin-derived host defense peptide, LL-37 [42, 60]. Circular dichroism spectroscopy analysis has shown that both native and recombinant HDM-1 have predominantly α-helical secondary structure. Additionally, secondary structure predictions and helical wheel analysis have shown that, like LL-37, the C-terminal of HDM-1 forms a distinct amphipathic α-helix [60].

Human LL-37 dampens initial innate immune responses to prevent excessive inflammation and also strongly impacts on the adaptive immune response in a manner independent of conditioning dendritic cells [61]. Specifically, LL-37 modulates the activity of IFN-γ on a variety of cell types, including monocytes, macrophages, and B-lymphocytes. LL-37 also strongly inhibits the IFN-γ priming of LPS responses and the synergistic responses to a combined treatment with IFN-γ and LPS. Given the central function of IFN-γ in innate and adaptive immunity, this modulation of IFN-γ responses has important implications for both types of immune responses.

F. hepatica HDM-1 and a peptide corresponding to the C-terminus of the protein protect mice against LPS-induced inflammation by significantly reducing the release of inflammatory mediators (TNF and IL-1β) from macrophages [60]. The C-terminal peptide is specifically released from the parent HDM-1 by cleavage with a cathepsin L protease. Thus, the secretion of HDM-1 and the cathepsin L-mediated processing of this molecule by *F. hepatica* may ensure that potentially lethal LPS, either from intestinal flora or from microbial coinfections, is neutralized and that activation of macrophages by LPS is controlled. Consequently, excessive inflammatory responses are avoided and the survival of the host, and therefore the parasite, are prolonged. In addition, the secretion of HDM-1/C-terminal peptide would help explain the potent suppression of immune responses directed against bacterial or viral infections that can occur during *F. hepatica* infection.

Conclusions

The liver fluke *F. hepatica* secretes various molecules that function to create an immunological environment in the host that allows its successful migration through host tissues and establishment in the bile ducts. The manipulation of the host immune response begins within hours of the parasite penetrating the intestinal wall through the interaction of parasite antigens with innate immune cells, dendritic cells, and macrophages, so that within days a robust but nonprotective T_h2 response has been established and protective T_h1 responses have been suppressed. As infection progresses towards chronicity, T_h2 regulatory cytokines (IL-4 and IL-10) persist, thereby maintaining the T_h2 phenotype. However, *F. hepatica* also modulates the function of dendritic cells to induce parasite-specific T_{reg}s, which secrete IL-10 and TGF-β, and express CTLA-4 [6]. These regulatory cells help suppress T_h1/T_h17 cell development and limit the magnitude of T_h2 responses, thus preventing fibrosis, which damages the host. Vaccination studies have shown that overcoming the parasite requires the induction of antibodies that neutralize the parasites ability to activate and maintain long-term suppression of host immune responses [9–11]. We have, therefore, focused our attention on identifying those molecules that modulate the host immune response for potential inclusion in vaccine formulations (i.e., adjuvant–antigen mixes) that block their function.

Over the last century there have been marked improvements in social and economic conditions in the developed world [62]. This has led to reduced exposure to a range of infectious agents, including helminth parasites, which has dramatically altered the balance of our immune systems. It has been proposed that reduced exposure to certain helminths might be responsible for the increased incidence of autoimmune conditions such as type 1 diabetes, arthritis, multiple sclerosis, and inflammatory bowel disease (IBD) [62–65]. Indeed, the incidence of several autoimmune diseases is inversely correlated with the occurrence of endemic helminth infections [62, 63]. These observations have led to the idea of "worm therapy," or the proposal that the anti-inflammatory T_h2/T_{reg} responses induced by helminth parasites would control the excessive T_h1/T_h17 immune responses in human inflammatory diseases. Infections with live worms have been carried out in the treatment of IBD and have produced improvement in the clinical condition [63–65]. The use of live parasites as therapeutic agents is problematic due to uncontrolled tissue damage and pathology. A more desirable option would be to mimic the beneficial effects of helminth infection by using the molecules the parasite employs to modulate host responses. Treatment with helminth molecules, or their synthetic analogs, would not only be safer, but would allow for a finer level of treatment and control, and a better understanding of their immunomodulatory mechanisms.

In this chapter we have described the mechanisms with which various *F. hepatica* secretory molecules exert their distinct effects on innate immune cells. Cathepsin L is taken into the endosomes of macrophages where it cleaves TLR3 and suppresses the intracellular signals required for the production of T_h1-inducing cytokines [29]; peroxiredoxin induces the alternative activation of macrophages that facilitate T_h2-mediated responses [4, 5] and HDM-1 prevents the stimulation of innate cells by bacterial pathogen-associated molecular pattern molecules, such as LPS, that may enter the circulatory system due to damage to the intestine or bile ducts caused by the parasite [60]. These mechanisms not only teach us fundamental lessons about how helminth parasites can intervene in host inflammatory processes, but also offer an improved understanding of inflammatory diseases in general and, possibly, new treatments for these common autoimmune conditions.

References

1 McManus, D.P. and Dalton, J.P. (2006) Vaccines against the zoonotic trematodes *Schistosoma japonicum, Fasciola hepatica* and *Fasciola gigantica. Parasitology*, **133**, S43–S51.

2 Andrews, S.J. (1999) The life cycle of *Fasciola hepatica*, in *Fasciolosis* (ed. J.P. Dalton), CABI, Wallingford, pp. 1–30.

3 Brennan, G.P., Fairweather, I., Trudgett, A., Hoey, E., Mccoy, M., Mcconville, M., Meaney, M. *et al.* (2007) Understanding triclabendazole resistance. *Exp. Mol. Pathol.*, **82**, 104–109.

4 Donnelly, S., O'Neill, S.M., Sekiya, M., Mulcahy, G., and Dalton, J.P. (2005) Thioredoxin peroxidase secreted by *Fasciola hepatica* induces the alternative activation of macrophages. *Infect. Immun.*, **73**, 166–173.

5 Donnelly, S., Stack, C.M., O'Neill, S.M., Sayed, A.A., Williams, D.L., and Dalton, J.P. (2008) Helminth 2-Cys peroxiredoxin drives T_h2 responses through a mechanism involving alternatively activated macrophages. *FASEB J.*, **22**, 4022–4032.

6 Walsh, K.P., Brady, M.T., Finlay, C.M., Boon, L., and Mills, K.H.G. (2009) Infection with a helminth parasite attenuates autoimmunity through TGF-β-mediated suppression of T_h17 and T_h1 responses. *J. Immunol.*, **183**, 1577–1586.

7 Brady, M.T., O'Neill, S.M., Dalton, J.P., and Mills, K.H. (1999) *Fasciola hepatica* suppresses a protective T_h1 response against *Bordetella pertussis*. *Infect. Immun.*, **67**, 5372–5378.

8 O'Neill, S.M., Mills, K.H., and Dalton, J.P. (2001) *Fasciola hepatica* cathepsin L cysteine proteinase suppresses *Bordetella pertussis*-specific interferon-gamma production *in vivo*. *Parasite Immunol.*, **23**, 541–547.

9 Mulcahy, G., O'Connor, F., McGonigle, S., Dowd, A., Clery, D.G., Andrews, S.J., and Dalton, J.P. (1998) Correlation of specific antibody titre and avidity with protection in cattle immunized against *Fasciola hepatica*. *Vaccine*, **16**, 932–939.

10 Mulcahy, G., O'Connor, F., Clery, D., Hogan, S.F., Dowd, A.J., Andrews, S.J., and Dalton, J.P. (1999) Immune responses of cattle to experimental anti-*Fasciola hepatica* vaccines. *Res. Vet. Sci.*, **67**, 27–33.

11 Golden, O., Flynn, R.J., Read, C., Sekiya, M., Donnelly, S.M., Stack, C., Dalton, J.P., and Mulcahy, G. (2010) Protection of cattle against a natural infection of *Fasciola hepatica* by vaccination with recombinant cathepsin L1 (rFhCL1). *Vaccine*, **28**, 5551–5557.

12 Flynn, R.J., Mannion, C., Golden, O., Hacariz, O., and Mulcahy, G. (2007) Experimental *Fasciola hepatica* infection alters responses to tests used for diagnosis of bovine tuberculosis. *Infect. Immun.*, **75**, 1373–1381.

13 Rawlings, N.D., Barrett, A.J., and Bateman, A. (2010) MEROPS: the peptidase database. *Nucleic Acids Res.*, **38**, D227–D233.

14 Tort, J., Brindley, P.J., Knox, D., Wolfe, K.H., and Dalton, J.P. (1999) Proteinases and associated genes of parasitic helminths. *Adv. Parasitol.*, **43**, 161–266.

15 Dalton, J.P. and Heffernan, M. (1989) Thiol proteases released *in vitro* by *Fasciola hepatica*. *Mol. Biol. Parasitol.*, **35**, 161–166.

16 Collins, P.R., Stack, C.M., O'Neill, S.M., Doyle, S., Ryan, T., Brennan, G.P., Mousley, A. *et al.* (2004) Cathepsin L1, the major protease involved in liver fluke (*Fasciola hepatica*) virulence: propetide cleavage sites and autoactivation of the zymogen secreted from gastrodermal cells. *J. Biol. Chem.*, **279**, 17038–17046.

17 Berasaín, P., Goñi, F., McGonigle, S., Dowd, A., Dalton, J.P., Frangione, B., and Carmona, C. (1997) Proteinases secreted by *Fasciola hepatica* degrade extracellular matrix and basement membrane components. *J. Parasitol.*, **83**, 1–5.

18 Robinson, M.W., Dalton, J.P., and Donnelly, S. (2008) Helminth pathogen cathepsin proteases: it's a family affair. *Trends Biochem. Sci.*, **33**, 601–608.

19 Donnelly, S., Dalton, J.P., and Robinson, M.W. (2011) How pathogen-derived cysteine proteases modulate host immune responses. *Adv. Exp. Med. Biol.*, **712**, 192–207.

20 O'Neill, S.M., Parkinson, M., Strauss, W., Angles, R., and Dalton, J.P. (1998) Immunodiagnosis of *Fasciola hepatica* infection (fascioliasis) in a human population in the Bolivian Altiplano using purified cathepsin L cysteine proteinase. *Am. J. Trop. Med. Hyg.*, **58**, 417–423.

21 Duffus, W.P. and Franks, D. (1980) *In vitro* effect of immune serum and bovine granulocytes on juvenile *Fasciola hepatica*. *Clin. Exp. Immunol.*, **41**, 430–440.

22 Carmona, C., Dowd, A.J., Smith, A.M., and Dalton, J.P. (1993) Cathepsin L proteinase secreted by *Fasciola hepatica in vitro* prevents antibody-mediated eosinophil attachment to newly excysted juveniles. *Mol. Biochem. Parasitol.*, **62**, 9–17.

23 Berasain, P., Carmona, C., Frangione, B., Dalton, J.P., and Goñi, F. (2000) *Fasciola hepatica*: parasite-secreted proteinases degrade all human IgG subclasses: determination of the specific cleavage sites and identification of the immunoglobulin fragments produced. *Exp. Parasitol.*, **94**, 99–110.

24 Hassan, M.M., Abbaza, B.E., El-Karamany, I., Dyab, A.K., El Sharkawy, E.M., Ismail, F., and Asal, K.H. (2004) Detection of anti-*Fasciola* isotypes among patients with fascioliasis before and after treatment with Mirazid. *J. Egypt. Soc. Parasitol.*, **34**, 857–864.

25 Mulcahy, G., Joyce, P., and Dalton, J.P. (1999) Immunology of *Fasciola hepatica* infection, in *Fasciolosis* (ed. J.P. Dalton), CABI, Wallingford, pp. 341–376.

26 Hoyle, D.V., Dalton, J.P., Chase-Topping, M., and Taylor, D.W. (2002) Pre-exposure of cattle to drug-abbreviated *Fasciola hepatica* infections: the effect upon subsequent challenge infection and early immune response. *Vet. Parasitol.*, **111**, 65–82.

27 Maizels, R.M., Balic, A., Gomez-Escobar, N., Nair, M., Taylor, M.D., and Allen., J.E. (2004) Helminth parasites – masters of regulation. *Immunol. Rev.*, **201**, 89–116.

28 Dowling, D.J., Hamilton, C.M., Donnelly, S., La Course, J., Brophy, P.M., Dalton, J., and O'Neill, S.M. (2010) Major secretory antigens of the helminth *Fasciola hepatica* activate a suppressive dendritic cell phenotype that attenuates T_h17 cells but fails to activate T_h2 immune responses. *Infect. Immun.*, **78**, 793–801.

29 Donnelly, S., O'Neill, S.M., Stack, C.M., Robinson, M.W., Turnbull, L., Whitchurch, C., and Dalton, J.P. (2010) Helminth cysteine proteases inhibit TRIF-dependent activation of macrophages via degradation of TLR3. *J. Biol. Chem.*, **285**, 3383–3392.

30 Smith, A.M., Carmona, C., Dowd, A.J., McGonigle, S., Acosta, D., and Dalton, J.P. (1994) Neutralization of the activity of a *Fasciola hepatica* cathepsin L proteinase by anti-cathepsin L antibodies. *Parasite Immunol.*, **16**, 325–328.

31 McGonigle, L., Mousley, A., Marks, N.J., Brennan, G.P., Dalton, J.P., Spithill, T.W., Day, T.A., and Maule, A. (2008) The silencing of cysteine proteases in *Fasciola hepatica* newly excysted juveniles using RNA interference reduces gut penetration. *Int. J. Parasitol.*, **38**, 149–155.

32 Dalton, J.P., McGonigle, S., Rolph, T.P., and Andrews, SJ. (1996) Induction of protective immunity in cattle against infection with *Fasciola hepatica* by vaccination with cathepsin L proteinases and with hemoglobin. *Infect. Immun.*, **64**, 5066–5074.

33 Babu, S., Bhat, S.Q., Pavan Kumar, N., Lipira, A.B., Kumar, S., Karthik, C., Kumaraswami, V., and Nutman, T.B. (2009) Filarial lymphedema is characterized by antigen-specific T_h1 and T_h17 proinflammatory responses and a lack of regulatory T cells. *PLoS Negl. Trop. Dis.*, **3**, e420.

34 Rutitzky, L.I., Smith, P.M., and Stadecker, M.J. (2009) T-bet protects against exacerbation of schistosome egg-induced immunopathology by regulating T_h17-mediated inflammation. *Eur. J. Immunol.*, **39**, 2470–2481.

35 Langrish, C.L., Chen, Y., Blumenschein, W.M., Mattson, J., Basham, B., Sedgwick, J.D., McClanahan, T. *et al.* (2005) IL-23 drives a pathogenic T cell population that induces autoimmune inflammation. *J. Exp. Med.*, **201**, 233–240.

36 Luger, D., Silver, P.B., Tang, J., Cua, D., Chen, Z., Iwakura, Y., Bowman, E.P. *et al.* (2008) Either a T_h17 or a T_h1 effector response can drive autoimmunity: conditions of disease induction affect dominant effector category. *J. Exp. Med.*, **205**, 799–810.

37 Barrett, J. (1980) Peroxide metabolism in the liver fluke. *J. Parasitol.*, **66**, 697.

38 Callahan, H.L., Crouch, R.K., and James, E.R. (1988) Helminth anti-oxidant enzymes – a protective mechanism against host oxidants. *Parasitol. Today*, **4**, 218–225.

39 McGonigle, S. and Dalton, J.P. (1995) Isolation of *Fasciola hepatica* haemoglobin. *Parasitology*, **111**, 209–215.

40 McGonigle, S., Curley, G.P., and Dalton, J.P. (1997) Cloning of peroxiredoxin, a novel antioxidant enzyme, from the helminth parasite *Fasciola hepatica*. *Parasitology*, **115**, 101–104.

41 McGonigle, S., Dalton, J.P., and James, ER. (1998) Peroxidoxins: a new antioxidant family. *Parasitol. Today*, **14**, 139–145.

42 Robinson, M.W., Menon, R., Donnelly, S.M., Dalton, J.P., and Ranganathan, S. (2009) An integrated transcriptomics and proteomics analysis of the secretome of the helminth pathogen *Fasciola hepatica*: proteins associated with invasion and infection of the mammalian host. *Mol. Cell. Proteomics*, **8**, 1891–1907.

43 Gordon, S. (2003) Alternative activation of macrophages. *Nat. Rev. Immunol.*, **3**, 23–35.

44 Edwards, J.P., Zhang, X., Frauwirth, K.A., and Mosser, D.M. (2006) Biochemical and functional characterization of three activated macrophage populations. *J. Leukoc. Biol.*, **80**, 1298–1307.

45 Loke, P., MacDonald, A.S., and Allen, J.E. (2000) Antigen-presenting cells recruited by *Brugia malayi* induce T_h2 differentiation of naïve $CD4^+$ T cells. *Eur. J. Immunol.*, **30**, 1127–1135.

46 Herbert, D.R., Holscher, C., Mohrs, M., Arendse, B., Schwegmann, A., Radwanska, M., Leeto, M. *et al.* (2004) Alternative macrophage activation is essential for survival during schistosomiasis and downmodulates T helper 1 responses and immunopathology. *Immunity*, **20**, 623–635.

47 O'Neill, S.M., Brady, M.T., Callahan, J.J., Mulcahy, G., Joyce, P., Mills, K.H., and Dalton, JP. (2000) Fasciola hepatica infection downregulates T_h1 responses in mice. Parasite Immunol., 22, 147–155.

48 Mendes, R.E., Pérez-Ecija, R.A., Zafra, R., Buffoni, L., Martínez-Moreno, A., Dalton, J.P., Mulcahy, G., and Pérez, J. (2010) Evaluation of hepatic changes and local and systemic immune responses in goats immunized with recombinant peroxiredoxin (Prx) and challenged with Fasciola hepatica. Vaccine, 28, 2832–2840.

49 Leeto, M., Herbert, D.R., Marillier, R., Schwegmann, A., Fick, L., and Brombacher, F. (2006) T_H1-dominant granulomatous pathology does not inhibit fibrosis or cause lethality during murine schistosomiasis. Am. J. Pathol., 169, 1701–1712.

50 Ogunrinade, A. and Adegoke, G.O. (1982) Bovine fascioliasis in Nigeria – intercurrent parasitic and bacterial infections. Trop. Anim. Health Prod., 14, 121–125.

51 Valero, M.A., Navarro, M., Garcia-Bodelon, M.A., Marcilla, A., Morales, M., Hernandez, J.L., Mengual, P., and Mas-Coma, S. (2006) High risk of bacterobilia in advanced experimental chronic fasciolosis. Acta Trop., 100, 17–23.

52 Onguru, D., Liang, Y., Griffith, Q., Nikolajczyk, B., Mwinzi, P., and Ganley-Leal, L. (2011) Human schistosomiasis is associated with endotoxemia and Toll-like receptor 2- and 4-bearing B cells. Am. J. Trop. Med. Hyg., 84, 321–324.

53 Boman, H.G. (1995) Peptide antibiotics and their role in innate immunity. Annu. Rev. Immunol., 13, 61–92.

54 Hirsch, T., Metzig, M., Niederbichler, A., Steinau, H.U., and Eriksson, E. (2008) Role of host defense peptides of the innate immune response in sepsis. Shock, 30, 117–126.

55 Giuliani, A., Pirri, G., and Rinaldi, A.C. (2010) Antimicrobial peptides: the LPS connection. Methods Mol. Biol., 618, 137–154.

56 Murakami, T., Obata, T., Kuwahara-Arai, K., Tamura, H., and Hiramatsu, K. (2009) Antimicrobial cathelicidin polypeptide CAP11 suppresses the production and release of septic mediators in D-galactosamine-sensitized endotoxin shock mice. Int. Immunol., 21, 905–912.

57 Tecle, T., White, M.R., Gantz, D., Crouch, E.C., and Hartshorn, K.L. (2007) Human neutrophil defensins increase neutrophil uptake of influenza A virus and bacteria and modify virus-induced respiratory burst responses. J. Immunol., 178, 8046–8052.

58 Miles, K., Clarke, D.J., Lu, W., Sibinska, Z., and Beaumont, P.E. (2009) Dying and necrotic neutrophils are anti-inflammatory secondary to the release of alpha-defensins. J. Immunol., 183, 2122–2132.

59 Tecle, T., Tripathi, S., and Hartshorn, K.L. (2010) Review: defensins and cathelicidins in lung immunity. Innate Immun., 16, 151–159.

60 Robinson, M.W., Donnelly, S., Hutchinson, A.T., To, J., Taylor, N.L., Norton, R.S., Perugini, M.A., and Dalton, J.P. (2011) A family of helminth molecules that modulate innate cell responses via molecular mimicry of host antimicrobial peptides. PLoS Pathog., 7, e1002042.

61 Nijnik, A., Pistolic, J., Wyatt, A., Tam, S., and Hancock, R.E. (2009) Human cathelicidin peptide LL-37 modulates the effects of IFN-gamma on APCs. J. Immunol., 183, 5788–5798.

62 Dunne, D.W. and Cooke, A. (2005) A worm's eye view of the immune system: consequences for evolution of human autoimmune disease. Nat. Rev. Immunol., 5, 420–426.

63 Elliott, D.E. and Weinstock, J.V. (2009) Helminthic therapy: using worms to treat immune-mediated disease. Adv. Exp. Med. Biol., 666, 157–166.

64 McKay, D.M. (2009) The therapeutic helminth? Trends Parasitol., 25, 109–114.

65 Broadhurst, M.J., Leung, J.M., Kashyap, V., McCune, J.M., Mahadevan, U., McKerrow, J.H., and Loke, P. (2010) IL-22$^+$ CD4$^+$ T cells are associated with therapeutic Trichuris trichiura infection in an ulcerative colitis patient. Sci. Transl. Med., 2, 60ra88.

28
Prospects for Immunoprophylaxis Against *Fasciola hepatica* (Liver Fluke)

Terry W. Spithill*, *Carlos Carmona, David Piedrafita, and Peter M. Smooker*

Abstract

Despite considerable research focused on the development of vaccines for *Fasciola* (liver fluke) infections in ruminants, there is still no commercial vaccine. Development of vaccines has been hindered both by our lack of insight into natural acquired immune mechanisms expressed by ruminants against fluke infection as well as a lack of immune correlates on hosts that are protected by experimental vaccines. In this chapter, we review the prospects and challenges we face regarding the development of experimental fluke vaccines, the nature of immune responses associated with host resistance, the potential for combination vaccines, and the criteria for commercial interest in a vaccine, including the minimal efficacy necessary to produce economic benefits in ruminants. Due to the widespread resistance of *Fasciola* to triclabendazole, we also discuss the potential demand for a human vaccine.

Introduction

Liver fluke infection (fasciolosis) is a major parasitic disease caused by *Fasciola hepatica* and *Fasciola gigantica* – flatworm parasites transmitted following ingestion of herbage carrying infective cysts. Liver flukes cause serious economic losses to Australian (A$60–90 million/year) and global (more than US$3 billion/year) livestock production [1–3]. Fasciolosis is a significant constraint on ruminant productivity in Southeast Asia, Asia, Africa, and the Middle East, with prevalences of 80–100% and more than 600 million animals at risk of infection [1, 2]. Infected animals suffer a 15–20% reduced weight gain, anemia, decreased fertility, milk production, and feed conversion efficiency, and a diminished work capacity that impacts crop production in Southeast Asia and Africa [2]. Moreover, the World Health Organization (WHO) recognizes *Fasciola* as a significant food-borne zoonosis, with high infection rates observed in Bolivia (more than 1 million cases; prevalences of 72–100%), Peru, Africa, and the Middle East, with up to 830 000 people infected in Egypt alone and 180 million at risk of disease world-wide [3].

* Corresponding Author

Triclabendazole (TCBZ) is the drug of choice for treatment of fasciolosis, but resistance to this drug is now widespread in Europe [4]. This highlights the urgent need for research into alternative control methods, including production of an effective vaccine as an attractive and sustainable control strategy. However, current experimental vaccines have three problems: (i) none have been chosen on the basis that they are known targets of acquired immunity, rather they were selected either as cross-reacting with antisera raised against *Schistosoma* antigens (e.g., fatty acid-binding protein) or rationally as molecules considered to be important in fluke biology (e.g., glutathione S-transferase (GST) and secreted cathepsin proteases) [5, 6]; (ii) vaccine efficacy is variable between animals (e.g., [7]); and (iii) with the exception of the leucine amino peptidase (LAP) vaccine (see below), the general level of efficacy achieved to date (38–72%) falls short of the greater than 80% level of protection required for a commercially viable product in cattle [5, 6]. We believe that a better understanding of the targets of acquired immunity in cattle is required if we are to devise a commercial livestock vaccine.

There is good evidence that cattle can acquire moderate to high levels of resistance to *F. hepatica* or *F. gigantica* following experimental vaccination with irradiated metacercariae (48–89% reductions in fluke burdens) [8] or single antigens [5, 6], suggesting that a commercial vaccine is achievable – the key step now is to identify the antigens targeted by acquired immunity. In terms of mechanisms of acquired immunity, we showed that juvenile *F. hepatica* are susceptible to antibody-dependent cell cytotoxicity (ADCC) *in vitro* that was mediated by nitric oxide released by *rat* peritoneal macrophages bound to the parasite surface [1, 9]. We extended our studies to the resistant Indonesian thin tail (ITT) breed of sheep and identified an ADCC immune mechanism in *sheep* effective against juvenile *F. gigantica in vitro*; notably, killing was mediated by superoxide radicals (not nitric oxide) produced by macrophages [1, 2, 10]. This is consistent with observations that sheep lung and peritoneal lavage macrophages do not produce nitric oxide [1, 9], and only low levels of nitrite are detected in culture supernatants of alveolar macrophages from sheep or peripheral blood mononuclear cells from sheep, goat, and cattle (reviewed in [9]).

The *F. gigantica*–sheep system that we have defined extensively since 1997 [1, 2, 10, 11] has led to fundamental new insights into how the ruminant immune system responds to *Fasciola* infection (reviewed in [1, 2]) and is an excellent model for understanding *F. hepatica*–host interactions. Although the immune mechanisms that kill *Fasciola* in cattle have not yet been resolved, we hypothesize that they may involve an ADCC mechanism similar to that observed against *F. gigantica* in sheep. Our results suggest the important conclusion that antigens on the surface tegument of juvenile/immature flukes are recognized by immune sera and are likely targets of ADCC. We need to identify and characterize these surface antigens as they represent novel vaccine candidates.

In addition to various chapters in this volume, recent reviews have summarized the progress with several *Fasciola* vaccine candidates [5, 6]. Here, we focus on the prospects and challenges we face to develop lead experimental vaccines for ruminants, and to understand the nature of immune responses associated with host resistance and the potential for combination vaccines. We also discuss the criteria required for commercial interest in a vaccine, including the threshold level of efficacy necessary to produce economic benefits in ruminants. Due to the widespread emergence of TCBZ resistance in *Fasciola* and the extent of human infection, we also discuss the potential demand for a human vaccine.

Secreted Cysteine Proteases as Vaccines

Liver flukes secrete a variety of proteases over their life cycle in the definitive host. These include several cathepsin B and cathepsin L proteases of which the liver fluke genome encodes at least 10 copies of each [12]. Expression of these proteases can be temporally regulated with different secreted cathepsins B and L being expressed in newly excysted juveniles (NEJs), immature, and adult flukes or expressed somatically throughout the life cycle (Figure 28.1) [12–14]. These proteases are considered to be virulence factors, and digest a wide range of host substrates that presumably facilitate feeding, immune evasion, and migration [12–17]. As found for *Schistosoma mansoni* [18], small-molecule inhibitors of *F. hepatica* cathepsins B are cidal and highlight the central function of these proteases in fluke biology [19]. Furthermore, RNA

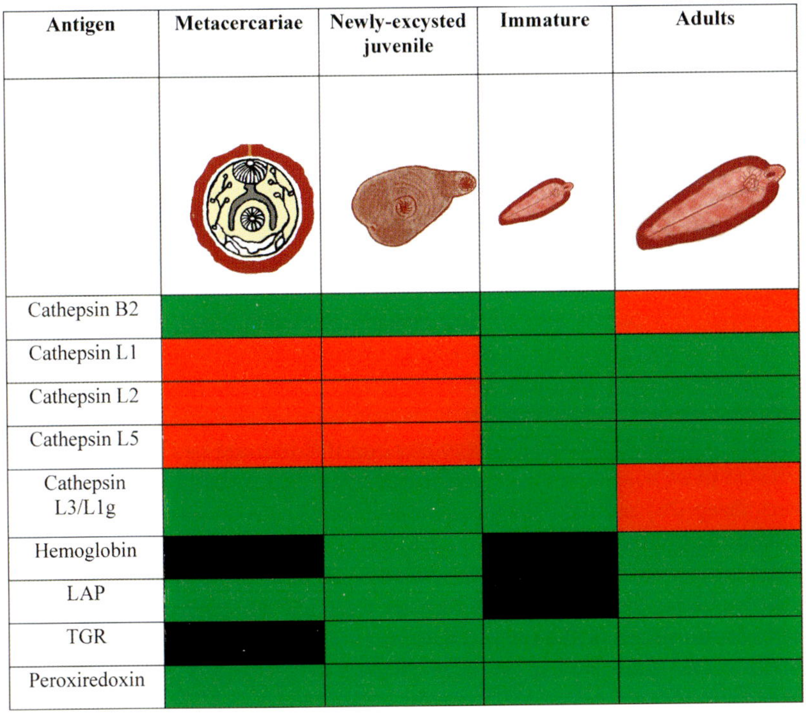

Antigen	Metacercariae	Newly-excysted juvenile	Immature	Adults
Cathepsin B2	green	green	green	red
Cathepsin L1	red	red	green	green
Cathepsin L2	red	red	green	green
Cathepsin L5	red	red	green	green
Cathepsin L3/L1g	green	green	green	red
Hemoglobin	black	green	black	green
LAP	green	green	black	green
TGR	black	green	green	green
Peroxiredoxin	green	green	green	green

Figure 28.1 Expression profile for vaccine candidates against *F. hepatica*. Green, present; red, absent; black, not known.

interference of either cathepsin L1 or cathepsin B2 diminishes the ability of NEJs to penetrate rat intestine *in vitro* [20].

Cathepsins L (FhcatL) secreted by adult flukes were the first cysteine proteases to be tested as a liver fluke vaccine and over the years there have been many examples of this molecule being evaluated in a variety of animals [5, 6, 21–27]. Theoretically, FhcatL has potential advantages as a vaccine target. They are secreted in relatively large amounts, are highly immunogenic, contribute to the digestion of host substrates, and various forms are expressed at all stages of the life cycle in the definitive host (Figure 28.1) [12–14]. However, despite 15 years of vigorous research, there is as yet no cathepsin L vaccine available for *Fasciola*. Certainly, efficacy has been observed. In an early study in cattle, vaccination with FhcatL1 resulted in a 38–69% reduction in fluke burdens [21], whereas in sheep, FhcatL1 and FhcatL2 elicited 33–34% protection [22]. Trials have also been carried out in rats using baculovirus-expressed cathepsin L that resulted in a 52% reduction in fluke burden after challenge [23]. In an unusual experiment also performed in rats, immunization using bacterial inclusion bodies that contained FhcatL1 produced a 70–80% protection [24].

The Freund's adjuvant used in cattle trials [21] is not suitable for routine use in the veterinary sector. This was a stumbling block for some time, but a recent publication has shown a potential way forward. Recombinant FhcatL1 was used to vaccinate cattle in oil-based adjuvants that are suitable for veterinary use [25]. Cattle were vaccinated twice and then allowed to graze for 13 weeks on pasture known to contain metacercariae. This study therefore replicates the natural form of infection, compared with an experimental challenge trial where a fixed dose of metacercariae is delivered. Animals that had been vaccinated with recombinant FhcatL1 were significantly protected, with a 48.2% mean reduction in fluke burden [25]. This is a very promising result as it demonstrates that some protection against natural challenge can be induced in cattle using acceptable adjuvants and a recombinant protease.

Yet, the level of protection achieved with FhcatL1 is not sufficient for a commercial vaccine. In three cattle trials with native or recombinant FhcatL1 involving eight experimental groups, the level of efficacy achieved ranged between 38 and 69.5% (mean 50.6%) [21, 25], which is clearly less than the greater than 80% generally considered necessary for commercial development (see below). The challenge is now to identify adjuvant/antigen combinations that improve protection or other molecules that increase the protective responses over that induced by FhcatL1 alone. In contrast to these positive results, a mixture of native *F. hepatica* cathepsin L did not protect sheep [26] and native *F. gigantica* cathepsin L did not protect cattle using acceptable adjuvants [27].

Overall, these results suggest that *F. hepatica* cathepsin L alone may not provide sufficient efficacy for a commercial vaccine. It should be noted that FhcatL1 and FhcatL2 are only expressed by adult parasites, so that the question remains whether juvenile-specific cathepsins L, such as FhcatL3 or FhcatL4 [13], offer superior protection.

Cathepsin B2 (termed FhCB2 and originally reported as FhcatB1) [28, 29] has recently been evaluated for efficacy as a vaccine against liver fluke. Again, we can

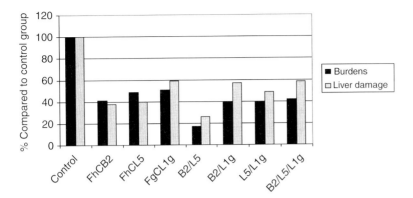

Figure 28.2 Multivalent cathepsin vaccine elicits better protection than single-component vaccines. Rats were vaccinated with the proteases indicated, alone and in combination. Adult fluke burdens and liver damage were assessed and compared to nonvaccinated controls (as a percentage with control value set at 100%). All fluke burden reductions were significant ($P<0.05$). Fh, *F. hepatica*; Fg, *F. gigantica*; CB, cathepsin B; CL cathepsin L. (Data from [30].)

speculate as to the advantages of FhCB2 as a target. (i) It is predominately expressed in the early stages of the parasite life cycle in the host and may therefore attract immune responses to flukes before they become established. (ii) This protease may be involved in excystment and tissue invasion, and therefore vaccine-induced responses may target the fluke as it emerges in the host gut and enters the peritoneum. (iii) It has been demonstrated that FhCB2 is immunogenic in a natural infection [29]. Subsequently, FhCB2 was tested in a vaccine trial in rats in which three cathepsins were evaluated: two cathepsins L (FhcatL5 and FgcatL1g) and one cathepsin B (FhCB2) [30]. FhCB2 induced a high level of protective immunity, as measured by both liver damage scores and fluke burdens after challenge (Figure 28.2). The adjuvant used was Quil A, which is acceptable for veterinary use. Interestingly, however, FhCB2 offered better protection (60%) than the two variants of cathepsin L (FhcatL1g, 43%; FhcatL5, 51%). Indeed, a combination of the FhCB2 and FhcatL5 gave the highest levels of protection (83%) [30], and, thus, passes the benchmark protection level required for commercial acceptance. The evaluation of combination vaccines in cattle and/or sheep is now warranted.

LAP Vaccine

FhLAP (EC 3.4.11.1) was isolated and purified from a detergent soluble extract of adult worms [31]. By specific histochemistry and immunoelectron microscopy it was preferentially localized inside the epithelial cells that line the alimentary tract of the adult worm; hence, a participation in the last stages of host protein digestion was proposed. FhLAP showed broad activity against fluorogenic substrates at pH 8.0, and its activity was enhanced by the divalent metal cations Zn^{2+}, Mn^{2+}, and Mg^{2+}. Native FhLAP was used as a vaccine in Corriedale sheep with Freund's adjuvant and induced high levels of protection, alone or in combination with FhCatL1 and FhCatL2 [22]. Vaccinated animals in the FhLAP group had an 89% decrease in worm burden compared to the control group. Those sheep that received a trivalent mixture of FhLAP, FhCatL1, and FhCatL2 also showed a significant protection level (79%) which was higher than the *nonsignificant* protection observed with the divalent FhcatL1/FhcatL2 mixture (60%) [22]. In both the LAP vaccine groups, four out of six sheep harbored no flukes in their livers, which is unusual for liver fluke vaccine trials and highlights the striking efficacy of LAP. Moreover, analysis of serum aspartate aminotransferase (AST) and γ-glutamyl transferase (GGT) levels revealed that AST levels were elevated in the LAP group (i.e., evidence of damage to liver cells), but GGT levels were normal (i.e., no evidence to suggest damage to the bile ducts in this group). These data strongly suggest that immune killing of migrating flukes occurred in the parenchyma before the immature flukes reached the bile ducts. Thus, a LAP vaccine appears to have efficacy against early immature flukes.

More recently, a fully functional recombinant FhLAP (rFhLAP) expressed in *Escherichia coli* as a thioredoxin fusion protein was molecularly characterized and the enzyme activity found to be identical to the previously isolated native immunogen [32]. FhLAP is a homohexameric enzyme and binds two cations – characteristics of the M17 family in the MEROPS peptidase database (merops.sanger.ac.uk). A phylogenetic comparison with homologous enzymes from diverse species demonstrates that all metazoan LAPs constitute a well-defined group that diverges from similar enzymes from bacteria, plants, and unicellular eukaryotes. In addition, FhLAP and its orthologs in flatworms constitute a well-defined cluster within vertebrate enzymes. When subcutaneously inoculated with Freund's adjuvant, rFhLAP induced a strong (78%) protective immune response in rabbits orally challenged with *F. hepatica* metacercariae [32].

Although the anti-FhLAP IgG antibodies elicited in sheep inhibited enzymatic activity, there was no statistically significant correlation between antibody titers against LAP and worm burdens in any of the groups [22]. The protective mechanism induced by the LAP vaccine is difficult to explain due to the intracellular localization of the enzyme. In agreement with the "hidden antigen" status, very low anti-FhLAP titers were detected in naturally infected animals and only traces of LAP activity are found in excretory/secretory (ES) products of adult *F. hepatica*. In contrast, FhLAP was strongly recognized by a group of sera from confirmed human patients in a two-dimensional electrophoresis analysis of ES products [33]. An explanation for this apparent paradox could be that, during fluke development in humans, the parasite is more stressed and a portion of the aminopeptidase leaks from gastrodermal cells into the fluke's lumen, and from there into the human host to elicit a greater immune response.

In a recent large vaccination trial in Corriedale sheep [34], rFhLAP was formulated with five different adjuvants. Immunization with rFhLAP induced a significant 49–87% reduction of fluke burdens in all vaccinated groups compared to adjuvant control groups. Interestingly, all vaccine preparations elicited specific mixed IgG1/IgG2 responses independently of the adjuvant used. Morphometric analysis of recovered liver flukes showed no significant size modifications in the different vaccinated groups, suggesting that the flukes that survived the protective immune response developed at a normal rate in the host [34]. It will be of interest to determine why a small proportion of flukes (10–20%) can escape the highly protective immune response induced by the LAP vaccine – it is possible that divergence in the LAP sequence may occur within the challenge fluke population and that the surviving flukes may express a variant LAP enzyme that is unaffected by the induced anti-LAP IgG response.

In contrast to the promising data with *F. hepatica* LAP in sheep, a recent trial in buffalo evaluating a homologous LAP sequence from *F. gigantica* failed to elicit protection [35]. The basis for the different results is not clear. The *F. gigantica* sequence differs in seven positions from the *F. hepatica* sequence, but it is not known whether these particular positions are critical for vaccine efficacy. It is also possible that induction of effector responses (or the response mechanisms themselves) differs between sheep and buffalo such that a LAP vaccine may induce a less-effective response in buffaloes.

Antioxidant Vaccines

Thioredoxin Glutathione Reductase

In platyhelminths, thioredoxin glutathione reductase (TGR) appears to be the only enzyme responsible for recycling both thioredoxin and GSH as these parasites lack glutathione reductase and thioredoxin reductase. The crucial function of TGR in parasite redox homeostasis was confirmed when potent TGR inhibitors induced the in vitro killing of *S. mansoni* schistosomula and *Echinococcus granulosus* protoscoleces [36, 37]. Indeed, TGR is now a lead target for development of novel antischistosomal drugs [38]. A thioredoxin reductase activity from a *F. hepatica* detergent-soluble extract was initially isolated and characterized [39]. Due to its glutaredoxin activity it was suggested that the purified protein could in fact be a TGR showing glutathione and thioredoxin specificities. More recently, a *F. hepatica* TGR was cloned and functionally expressed in *E. coli*, and found to be identical to the enzyme originally labeled as thioredoxin reductase [40]. In a preliminary trial rFhTGR inoculated with Freund's adjuvant in rabbits induced nearly 100% protection (96.7%) compared to the adjuvant control group [40]. However, two consecutive trials conducted in Hereford calves subcutaneously inoculated with 500 µg rFhTGR in one- and two-booster schedules failed to demonstrate a significant protection against metacercarial challenge (Maggioli *et al.*, unpublished data).

Peroxiredoxin

Peroxiredoxin – a hydrogen peroxide scavenger secreted by NEJ and adult flukes that also induces alternative activation of macrophages in the murine model [41] – was tested as a vaccine in goats (see Chapter 27 for more information on immunomodulatory effector mechanisms in *Fasciola*). The recombinant peroxiredoxin mixed with Quil A as adjuvant showed 34% (not significant) protection in goats compared to the adjuvant control, although pathological analysis of the livers found reduced gross and microscopic damage and decreased infiltration by competent immune cells in the peroxiredoxin group [42]. Furthermore, a recent trial in buffaloes that tested recombinant peroxiredoxin from *F. gigantica* also failed to induce protection alone or combined with FgLAP delivered in Montanide M70 [35]. The vaccine potential of peroxiredoxin therefore remains open.

Way Forward: Combination Vaccines

The most successful vaccines are multivalent. For example, attenuated viral and bacterial vaccines are generally more potent than individual subunit vaccines derived from the pathogens, and the same is true for attenuated malaria vaccines [43]. However, for helminths, generating large quantities of attenuated parasites is not practical, as the parasites cannot be easily cultured or attenuated in a cost-effective manner. Furthermore, an experiment conducted in sheep in which an irradiated *F. hepatica* metacercariae vaccine did not induce protective responses suggests that an attenuated vaccine is not appropriate in all cases (reviewed in [44, 45]). Therefore, it may be that a judicious selection of two or more *F. hepatica* antigens for a combination vaccine will be more effective.

The question then becomes which antigens to choose for a multivalent vaccine? Clearly, combining those antigens that alone have some efficacy would be a starting point. In fact, this was undertaken in the first demonstration of FhcatL1 as an immunogen [21]. In this report, FhcatL1 or FhcatL2 was combined with fluke hemoglobin (FhHb), with the highest protection (72%) elicited by FhcatL2 plus FhHb. Unfortunately, FhcatL2 was not tested alone so it cannot be certain that the protection was due to a synergistic effect; however, the observation that immunization with FhHb alone led to lower protection (44%) suggests that the higher level of protection observed after vaccination with the dual-component vaccine results from the combination inducing an additive or synergistic immunity. FhcatL1 and FhcatL2 have been tested alone, as a bivalent combination, and as a trivalent vaccine with FhLAP in sheep [22]. The bivalent FhCatL1 and FhCatL2 combination showed a nonsignificant efficacy of 60% compared to 34 and 33% for the separate enzymes, respectively; however, significant protection was *only* observed with FhcatL1 alone (34%) and the trivalent vaccine (79%), but the trivalent vaccine was less efficacious than FhLAP alone (89%). Therefore, these data do not support a synergistic effect of FhcatL1 and FhcatL2 in combination with FhLAP.

As stated above, we have tested two cathepsin Ls and FhCB2 in a vaccine trial to determine the relative effectiveness of the combination versus single-component vaccine [30]. The results obtained indicated that a combination of two components in the vaccine was optimal (Figure 28.2). Interestingly, the dual-component vaccine induced greater protection than a vaccine comprising all three components, indicating that "more may sometimes be less" and lead to antagonistic effects. One possible explanation for this is that relative antigen dosage of each individual protective antigen was lowered in the triple combination (the total amount of protein delivered was fixed at 20 μg/dose). Alternatively, antigenic competition may have reduced the induction of appropriate effector responses in the trivalent vaccine. We speculate that an ideal vaccine for testing should comprise a cathepsin B such as FhCB2 and the highly efficacious FhLAP, as discussed above.

It is important to consider how these multivalent vaccines are constructed and delivered. Screening of combination vaccines could be done in model systems, such as the rat infection model. This was the reasoning behind the recent FhCB2 and FhcatL5 or FgcatL1g combination trials in rats [30]. In these experiments, the absolute levels of protection are not the real aim – it is the relative performance of the different combinations that is of interest. In most experiments to date individual recombinant proteins have been expressed and then mixed. Theoretically, it should be possible to simplify this process by creating fusion proteins, perhaps with a flexible linker joining them to ensure independent folding of each antigen. Hybrid vaccines for cestodes have recently been produced [46]. Once such experiments are performed, the best combination or fusion vaccines will need to be tested in target species.

It is prudent to undertake the testing of adjuvants that are acceptable to the industry. There is a wealth of data demonstrating the efficacy of individual liver fluke vaccines delivered in Freund's adjuvant and now the relative performance of these antigens needs to be tested in acceptable adjuvants. Morrison *et al.* [7] performed such an extensive analysis of 10 adjuvants with the native GST vaccine of *F. hepatica* and showed that Quil A in Squalene Montanide 80 was the most efficacious with that antigen, inducing a mean 43% reduction in fluke burdens. Further evaluation of adjuvants for use in livestock is clearly warranted.

Recent Advances in Understanding Immunity to Liver Fluke Infection

The genetic heterogeneity of *Fasciola* spp., their large proteome, broad range of antigens, different life cycle stages, and our limited understanding of immunological responses in natural ruminant hosts challenge the development of reproducible and efficacious vaccines. Recent concerted efforts studying protective immune responses in ruminants have led to greater insights of the importance of the rejection processes in the definitive host–parasite system, some of which are highlighted below.

Requirements for the induction of specific phenotypes, such as helper T cell T_h1/T_h2-type responses, are considered key in the development of protective immunity by the host. The typical allergic- or T_h2-type immune responses that are induced by helminth infections have been well characterized and extensively studied in murine model systems [47]. Most helminth parasite infections induce a strong type 2 immune response, with early production of interleukin (IL)-4 over interferon (IFN)-γ that is considered important in the protective immunity of the host, and is associated with a reduction in both worm burdens and disease severity [48, 49]. Whereas this paradigm seems to hold for most nematode infections, it is less clear for trematode infections such as the commonly studied *Schistosoma* parasites, where both type 1 and 2 responses have been associated with protection [50, 51].

Immune responses to *Fasciola* spp. have almost exclusively been studied in goats, sheep, and cattle in which a strong but nonprotective immune response to liver fluke infection occurs that is highly biased towards a type 2 response [1]. Until recently it was considered that sheep were unable to develop a natural immunity to *Fasciola* [1, 52]; however, several studies have suggested that some sheep breeds do resist a natural *F. gigantica* infection [53–56]. ITT sheep have an innate and adaptive protective response to *F. gigantica* infection, but are nonetheless susceptible to *F. hepatica* [1, 2, 11, 53]. This has allowed studies focusing on the inherent differences between the tropical and temperate parasites, and their ability to modulate the immune response that contributes to either host-protective immune responses (*F. gigantica*) or immune evasion (*F. hepatica*). These studies revealed a significant difference in the cytokine and antibody profiles of ITT sheep infected with *F. gigantica* compared to *F. hepatica*, with a higher ratio of IL-4/IFN-γ mRNA expression and specific IgG1/IgG2 antibodies strongly correlating with pathology [57]. Interestingly, the significant type 1 cytokine profile occurred in the lymph node closest to the site of infection at the time (3 weeks postinfection) when the effective immune response against *F. gigantica* liver flukes occurs. When the same *F. gigantica* infection in the resistant ITT sheep was compared with the susceptible Merino breed, the resistant type 1 phenotype against liver fluke infection was only observed in the ITT sheep [57]. These studies provide the first evidence to suggest that the induction of an early type 1 immune response in this natural sheep host may be responsible for the ability to resist liver fluke infection.

These studies are intriguing since the requirement for a type 1 immune response to resist *F. hepatica* infections has been alluded to in sheep and cattle as IgG2 antibody levels were associated with lower liver fluke recoveries [58, 59]. Similarly, experimental vaccination studies have shown an association between parasite-specific IgG2 antibody titers and vaccine-induced protection against *F. hepatica* infection in cattle [25, 60]. These results suggest that protective responses against liver fluke infection are associated with type 1 immune responses, but it is likely these responses are also required to be induced in a site-specific and in a time-dependent manner. Thus, although early expression of IFN-γ has been detected in sheep and cattle infected with *F. hepatica*, suggesting a T_h1/T_h0 phenotype, this has only been observed transiently and not generally correlated in the local draining lymph nodes with parasite migration [61]. This is also reflected in liver fluke-resistant ITT sheep, where only local draining lymph nodes showed such a type 1 immune response and, furthermore, surviving parasites induce type 2 responses later in the infection [57]. This suggests that type 2 responses are necessary to maintain parasite survival.

How does the parasite induce dominant type 2 immune responses to survive? A large number of potential *F. hepatica* proteins may be involved in inducing type 2 immune responses [62–64], and a small number of tegumental and ES molecules have been investigated [2, 65, 66] (see also Chapter 27). These include various *Fasciola* proteases, GSTs, and peroxidases, which have been hypothesized to interact with immune cells to drive type 2 responses. Classically activated macrophages are usually associated with type 1 responses and thereby combat bacterial infections, via free radical production. Alternatively activated macrophages (AAMFs) are linked to T_h2 responses. The functions of these cells are not completely understood, but they may prime T_h2 cell differentiation or suppression of type 1 responses through IL-10 expression. AAMFs are induced by several *Fasciola* proteins [61, 66, 67]. A strong correlation can be made between the presence of these suppressor cells and susceptibility during secondary infection [68]. All of these findings are based on animals susceptible to *Fasciola* infection. The corollary finding that AAMFs do not operate in resistant animals, such as ITT sheep with natural immunity to *F. gigantica*, or an immunologically resistant model, such as rats, would need to be demonstrated in order to confirm a contribution by AAMFs to susceptibility to liver fluke infection.

It is curious that the parasite defense proteins purported to drive type 2 responses are also induced in response to cytotoxic molecules, including free radicals generated by the host to kill helminth parasites. These parasite defense molecules against free radicals may contribute to the differential resistance observed in ITT sheep against *F. gigantica* and *F. hepatica*. Cells from infected *F. gigantica* sheep were able to mediate ADCC against newly excysted juvenile *F. gigantica in vitro* [10] and this was dependent on the production of superoxide free radicals. In contrast, these cytotoxic mechanisms were ineffective against juvenile *F. hepatica* parasites, suggesting that this species expresses some form of defense against killing by superoxide. This hypothesis is supported by the observation that inhibition of several *F. hepatica* defense enzymes rendered *F. hepatica* susceptible to free radical killing *in vitro* [69].

The preceding sections highlight the integrated immune response in natural hosts during the development of immunity to liver fluke infection. These studies suggest differential resistance to *Fasciola* infection is determined in part by biochemical differences between species of *Fasciola*, possibly via controlling susceptibility to ADCC killing. The results imply that molecules that help regulate and accentuate T_h2 responses, such as ES defense proteins and tegumental antigens, may also be good vaccine targets.

Surface Tegument Proteins as Proposed New Candidate Vaccines

The tegument is a syncytial layer of cytoplasm covering the fluke that is rich in secretory inclusions and bounded externally by a plasma membrane bearing a dense glycocalyx. Important tegumental functions include renewal of the surface plasma membrane and uptake of nutrients [70]. The combined plasma membrane and its glycocalyx interacts directly with the immune system, and proteins and glycan epitopes exposed on the tegument surface represent likely targets of ADCC that we reported with sheep and rats [9, 10]. However, few studies have analyzed fluke tegument proteins. Early studies using radiolabeling identified up to 14 surface labeled proteins of size from 10 to more than 200 kDa in juvenile *F. hepatica*, and showed that the surface profile varied between juvenile, immature, and adult flukes [71, 72]. None of these tegument proteins has been further characterized. One study identified a fluke protein showing a repetitive sequence [73].

It is likely that surface glycan epitopes are immunoreactive in fasciolosis, but are they immunoprotective? In schistosomiasis, glycans are hyper-reactive, but not protective [74, 75]. The IgG responses to schistosome secretions are overwhelmingly directed to glycans as shown by loss of reactivity upon periodate treatment of antigens. Though there is one report of vaccination with keyhole limpet hemacyanin eliciting 50–70% protection in the laboratory rat, anti-keyhole limpet hemacyanin serum from a rabbit failed to passively protect mice (cited in [75]). These observations challenge the concept that antiglycan responses are protective while suggesting that glycan epitopes are a parasite-protective "smoke-screen" [74, 75]. Several studies suggest that glycans from parasitic helminths are involved in host immune evasion and modulation [76]. This suggests that the focus for vaccine developers should be the identification of surface protein antigens.

The total tegument proteome of the flatworm *S. mansoni* has been defined [77, 78]. Subsequently, Braschi and Wilson [79] applied surface biotinylation of live worms (using impermeant reagents) to identify 24 schistosome surface-exposed proteins. Similar analysis of the surface proteome of *Schistosoma japonicum* [80] and *Opisthorchis viverrini* [81] identified 54 and 25 proteins, respectively. Wilson et al. [82] have now developed enzymatic shaving methods to selectively release surface components that are accessible to proteases (e.g., trypsin) and phospholipases (e.g., phosphatidylinositol-specific phospholipase C) to create a comprehensive picture of the schistosome surface.

Recently, we have begun an exploration of the tegument proteome of adult flukes applying techniques developed by Wilson et al. [83]. The method for isolation of the tegument surface membranes of adult *F. hepatica* was derived from the freeze/thaw/vortex method used for the blood fluke *S. mansoni* [78]. The proteins were reduced, alkylated, trypsinized overnight, and the resulting peptides purified and analyzed [79]. A total of 229 proteins were identified from the fluke tegument. We functionally annotated 24 proteins predicted to be membrane-associated, based either on the known biochemistry of *Schistosoma* orthologs or the presence of signal sequences and transmembrane domains. Three appear to be distinct annexins, one (FhAnx-1) a major constituent as judged by its exponentially modified protein abundance index score. A single tetraspanin (FhTSP-1) was also identified. Three transport proteins – two of them anion-selective channels and the third a glucose transporter – were detected plus three membrane enzymes, a carbonic anhydrase, and two calpain proteases. A CD59 ortholog (FhCD59-1) was identified, which in humans is an inhibitor of complement fixation. Four *F. hepatica*-specific proteins (FhMP1–4) were predicted to encode one to three membrane-spanning regions and so were assigned to the membrane category. Nine of the membrane-associated proteins are known to be surface exposed in *S. mansoni* [79], *S. japonicum* [80], and *O. viverrini* [81]. These data provide new insights into the *F. hepatica* tegument proteome, and reveal a group of candidate proteins that may represent targets for ADCC that is active in rats and sheep against *Fasciola* juvenile flukes *in vitro*. A comparative analysis of proteins on the surface tegument of juvenile and immature flukes is clearly warranted, and may identify potential new vaccine candidates for downstream analysis.

Criteria Needed for Development of a Commercial Liver Fluke Vaccine

The key question confronting commercial fluke vaccine producers is the level of efficacy required to elicit production benefits in sheep and cattle. Several studies have shown that production losses in cattle are observed once fluke burdens exceed 30–40 parasites [84, 85]. If we take 30 flukes as being the threshold for economic loss in cattle we then ask what is the known intensity of fluke infections in cattle as this will determine the level of efficacy required for economic benefit. Thus, vaccines such as FhGST or FhcatL1, inducing a mean protective effect as low as 43% [7] and 52% [21], respectively, will reverse economic loss only in herds exposed to burdens of around 52–62 flukes, whereas a FhLAP vaccine (efficacy 89%) will reduce losses in animals with burdens of 272 flukes. Although intensity of infection will vary between regions, fluke burdens of 40–140 have been reported in cattle in United States [86], and in the United Kingdom, only 3% of cattle livers had more than 50 flukes [87]. In Iran and Nigeria, mean fluke burdens of 68–99 were reported in cattle (reviewed in [88]). These data suggest that experimental vaccines with efficacy of about 50% are commercially viable in the United Kingdom, whereas FhLAP would appear to be the best vaccine in most regions.

Prospects for a Human Vaccine

Human fasciolosis caused by *F. hepatica* is an important food-borne zoonosis emerging in many countries, particularly in Peru, Bolivia, Egypt, and Iran [3]. The highest recorded prevalence corresponds to rural communities in the Bolivian and Peruvian Altiplano, close to Lake Titicaca, where up to 60% of the population in some areas is infected [89]. As with other food-borne trematodiasis, liver fluke disease caused by *F. hepatica* is focally distributed, and related to physiographic, socioeconomic, and behavioral factors. In this sense, the highest prevalence (up to 75%) observed in school-age children in Andean communities [90] is strongly associated with livestock minding, eating of aquatic plants, and contaminated water drinking.

Although bithionol is still used in some countries (e.g., the United States), the only drug currently recommended for the treatment of human fasciolosis is TCBZ; however, it has been registered for this use in only four countries [91]. This drug is effective and usually well tolerated, causing only minor adverse effects. Moreover, there are no reports of *F. hepatica* resistant to TCBZ in human infections. In addition, a program based on mass screening and selective chemotherapy in school-age children from highly infected populations of the Nile Delta in Egypt was effective in reducing prevalence from 5.6% in 1998 to 1% in 2003 [92]. However, the introduction of this control strategy raises the possibility of resistance to TCBZ emerging in these human populations, as has occurred in production animals [4], which emphasizes the need to discover and develop novel flukicides. With the exceptions of the peroxidic compounds artemisinins and trioxolanes, these efforts have been sparse in the last few decades [91].

Among other control measures such as health education programs and improved farming practices, an effective and commercially available vaccine for fasciolosis aimed at domestic ruminants would provide the opportunity for a human vaccine, particularly in highly endemic situations. The WHO has estimated that 180 million people are at risk of fluke infection [3]. Given the recent widespread emergence of TCBZ-resistant fluke populations in the United Kingdom, Europe, and Australia, there is an increasing risk of transmission of drug-resistant fluke infections to humans. Given the dearth of research into new flukicides, it would be prudent to consider a vaccine-based strategy for control of human infections once an efficacious veterinary vaccine is commercially available.

Conclusions

We are optimistic that a commercial vaccine to control liver fluke infection in ruminants is feasible. If the high efficacy achieved in sheep with rFhLAP is confirmed in cattle, this molecule may represent a "stand-alone" vaccine that would reduce fluke burdens below the threshold level required for economic benefit in most regions of the world. We also suggest that it is worthwhile investigating the commercial development of combination vaccines using molecules with distinct functions and expressed at different times during fluke development, such as a juvenile cathepsin B (e.g., FhCB1, FhCB2, or FhCB3) combined with FhLAP or a cathepsin B combined with an immature/adult stage cathepsin L (e.g., FhcatL1, FhcatL2, or FhcatL5). Such FhLAP-based combination vaccines could potentially be produced as hybrid fusion proteins to simplify commercial production and delivery. Recent insights into the mechanisms of immunity in sheep to *F. gigantica* have revealed that T_h1-type immune responses and ADCC contribute to protection against juvenile/immature liver flukes in ruminants. Accordingly, these observations suggest that adjuvants such as Quil A that can induce type 1 responses would enhance fluke vaccine efficacy [93]. Moreover, if ADCC directed at the surface of juvenile/immature flukes is a key effector mechanism operating *in vivo*, we hypothesize that the characterization of surface exposed tegument proteins on juvenile/immature flukes should be a priority in order to harness ADCC and enhance efficacy. If a commercial vaccine with an efficacy greater than 80% in livestock is established, applying such a vaccine for human prophylaxis in highly endemic regions would avoid the significant risk of human infections with TCBZ-resistant flukes.

References

1 Piedrafita, D., Raadsma, H.W., Prowse, R., and Spithill, T.W. (2004) Immunology of the host–parasite relationship in fasciolosis (*Fasciola hepatica* and *Fasciola gigantica*). *Can. J. Zool.*, **82**, 233–250.

2 Piedrafita, D., Spithill, T.W., Smith, R.E., and Raadsma, H.W. (2010) Improving animal and human health through understanding liver fluke immunology. *Parasite Immunol.*, **32**, 572–581.

3 Mas-Coma, S., Bargues, M.D., and Valero, M.A. (2005) Fascioliasis and other plant-borne trematode zoonoses. *Int. J. Parasitol.*, **35**, 1255–1278.

4 Fairweather, I. (2005) Triclabendazole: new skills to unravel an old(ish) enigma. *J. Helminthol.*, **79**, 227–234.

5 Hillyer, G.V. (2005) Fasciola antigens as vaccines against fascioliasis and schistosomiasis. *J. Helminthol.*, **79**, 241–247.

6 McManus, D.P. and Dalton, J.P. (2006) Vaccines against the zoonotic trematodes *Schistosoma japonicum*, *Fasciola hepatica* and *Fasciola gigantica*. *Parasitology*, **133** (Suppl.), S43–S61.

7 Morrison, C.A., Colin, T., Sexton, J.L., Bowen, F., Wicker, J., Friedel, T., and Spithill, T.W. (1996) Protection of cattle against *Fasciola hepatica* infection by vaccination with glutathione S-transferase. *Vaccine*, **14**, 1603–1612.

8 Haroun, E.M. and Hillyer, G.V. (1986) Resistance to fascioliasis – a review. *Vet. Parasitol.*, **20**, 63–93.

9 Piedrafita, D., Parsons, J.C., Sandeman, R.M., Wood, P.R., Estuningsih, S.E., Partoutomo, S., and Spithill, T.W. (2001) Antibody-dependent cell-mediated cytotoxicity to newly excysted juvenile *Fasciola hepatica in vitro* is mediated by reactive nitrogen intermediates. *Parasite Immunol.*, **23**, 473–482.

10 Piedrafita, D., Estuningsih, E., Pleasance, J., Prowse, R.K., Raadsma, H.W., Meeusen, E.N.T., and Spithill, T.W. (2007) Peritoneal lavage cells of Indonesian thin-tail sheep mediate antibody-dependent superoxide radical cytotoxicity *in vitro* against newly excysted juvenile *Fasciola gigantica* but not juvenile *Fasciola hepatica*. *Infect. Immun.*, **75**, 1954–1963.

11 Pleasance, J., Raadsma, H.W., Estuningsih, S.E., Widjajanti, S., Meeusen, E., and Piedrafita, D. (2011) Innate and adaptive resistance of Indonesian Thin Tail sheep to liver fluke: a comparative analysis of *Fasciola gigantica* and *Fasciola hepatica* infection. *Vet. Parasitol.*, **178**, 264–272.

12 Smooker, P.M., Jayaraj, R., Pike, R.N., and Spithill, T.W. (2010) Cathepsin B proteases of flukes – the key to facilitating parasite control? *Trends Parasitol.*, **26**, 506–514.

13 Cancela, M., Acosta, D., Rinaldi, G., Silva, E., Durán, R., Roche, L., Zaha, A. *et al.* (2006) A distinctive repertoire of cathepsins is expressed by juvenile invasive *Fasciola hepatica*. *Biochimie*, **90**, 1461–1475.

14 Robinson, M.W., Dalton, J.P., and Donnelly, S. (2008) Helminth pathogen cathepsin proteases: it's a family affair. *Trends Biochem. Sci.*, **33**, 601–608.

15 Tort, J., Brindley, P.J., Knox, D., Wolfe, K.H., and Dalton, J.P. (1999) Proteinases and associated genes of parasitic helminths. *Adv. Parasitol.*, **43**, 161–266.

16 Norbury, L.J., Beckham, S., Pike, R.N., Grams, R., Spithill, T.W., Fecondo, J.V., and Smooker, P.M. (2011) Adult and juvenile Fasciola cathepsin L proteases: different enzymes for different roles. *Biochimie*, **93**, 604–611.

17 Berasaín, P., Goñi, F., McGonigle, S., Dowd, A., Dalton, J.P., Frangione, B., and Carmona, C. (1997) Proteinases secreted by *Fasciola hepatica* degrade extracellular matrix and basement membrane components. *J. Parasitol.*, **83**, 1–5.

18 Abdulla, M.H., Lim, K.C., Sajid, M., McKerrow, J.H., and Caffrey, C.R. (2007) Schistosomiasis mansoni: novel chemotherapy using a cysteine protease inhibitor. *PLoS Med.*, **4**, e14.

19 Beckham, S.A., Piedrafita, D., Phillips, C.I., Samarawickrema, N., Law, R.H.P., Smooker, P.M., Quinsey, N.S. *et al.* (2009) A major

cathepsin B protease from the liver fluke *Fasciola hepatica* has atypical active site features and a potential role in the digestive tract of newly excysted juvenile parasites. *Int. J. Biochem. Cell Biol.*, **41**, 1601–1612.

20 McGonigle, L., Mousley, A., Marks, N.J., Brennan, G.P., Dalton, J.P., Spithill, T.W., and Maule, A.G. (2008) The silencing of cysteine proteases in *Fasciola hepatica* newly excysted juveniles using RNA interference reduces gut penetration. *Int. J. Parasitol.*, **38**, 149–155.

21 Dalton, J.P., McGonigle, S., Rolph, T.P., and Andrews, S.J. (1996) Induction of protective immunity in cattle against infection with *Fasciola hepatica* by vaccination with cathepsin L proteinases and with hemoglobin. *Infect. Immun.*, **64**, 5066–5074.

22 Piacenza, L., Acosta, D., Basmadjian, I., Dalton, J.P., and Carmona, C. (1999) Vaccination with cathepsin L proteinases and with leucine aminopeptidase induces high levels of protection against fascioliasis in sheep. *Infect. Immun.*, **67**, 1954–1961.

23 Reszka, N., Cornelissen, J.B., Harmsen, M.M., Bieńkowska-Szewczyk, K., de Bree, J., Boersma, W.J., and Rijsewijk, F.A. (2005) *Fasciola hepatica* procathepsin L3 protein expressed by a baculovirus recombinant can partly protect rats against fasciolosis. *Vaccine*, **23**, 2987–2993.

24 Kesik, M., Jedlina-Panasiuk, L., Kozak-Cieszczyk, M., Płuciennczak, A., and Wedrychowicz, H. (2007) Enteral vaccination of rats against *Fasciola hepatica* using recombinant cysteine proteinase (cathepsin L1). *Vaccine*, **25**, 3619–3628.

25 Golden, O., Flynn, R.J., Read, C., Sekiya, M., Donnelly, S.M., Stack, C., Dalton, J.P., and Mulcahy, G. (2010) Protection of cattle against a natural infection of *Fasciola hepatica* by vaccination with recombinant cathepsin L1 (rFhCL1). *Vaccine*, **28**, 5551–5557.

26 Wijffels, G.L., Salvatore, L., Dosen, M., Waddington, J., Wilson, L., Thompson, C., Campbell, N. *et al.* (1994) Vaccination of sheep with purified cysteine proteinases of *Fasciola hepatica* decreases worm fecundity. *Exp. Parasitol.*, **78**, 132–148.

27 Estuningsih, S.E., Smooker, P.M., Wiedosari, E., Widjajanti, S., Vaiano, S., Partoutomo, S., and Spithill, T.W. (1997) Evaluation of antigens of *Fasciola gigantica* as vaccines against tropical fasciolosis in cattle. *Int. J. Parasitol.*, **27**, 1419–1428.

28 Wilson, L.R., Good, R.T., Panaccio, M., Wijffels, G.L., Bozas, S.E., Sandeman, R.M., and Spithill, T.W. (1998) *Fasciola hepatica*: characterization and cloning of the major cathepsin B protease secreted by newly excysted juvenile liver fluke. *Exp. Parasitol.*, **88**, 85–94.

29 Law, R.H., Smooker, P.M., Irving, J.A., Piedrafita, D., Ponting, R., Kennedy, N.J., Whisstock, J.C. *et al.* (2003) Cloning and expression of the major secreted cathepsin B-like protein from juvenile *Fasciola hepatica* and analysis of immunogenicity following liver fluke infection. *Infect. Immun.*, **71**, 6921–6932.

30 Jayaraj, R., Piedrafita, D., Dynon, K., Grams, R., Spithill, T.W., and Smooker, P.M. (2009) Vaccination against fasciolosis by a multivalent vaccine of stage-specific antigens. *Vet. Parasitol.*, **160**, 230–236.

31 Acosta, D., Goñi, F., and Carmona, C. (1998) Characterization and partial purification of a leucine aminopeptidase from *Fasciola hepatica*. *J. Parasitol.*, **84**, 1–7.

32 Acosta, D., Cancela, M., Piacenza, L., Roche, L., Carmona, C., and Tort, J.F. (2008) *Fasciola hepatica* leucine aminopeptidase, a promising candidate for vaccination against ruminant fasciolosis. *Mol. Biochem. Parasitol.*, **158**, 52–64.

33 Marcilla, A., De la Rubia, J.E., Sotillo, J., Bernal, D., Carmona, C., Villavicencio, Z., Acosta, D. *et al.* (2008) Leucine aminopeptidase is an immunodominant antigen of *Fasciola hepatica* excretory and secretory products in human infections. *Clin. Vaccine Immunol.*, **15**, 95–100.

34 Maggioli, G., Acosta, D., Silveira, F., Rossi, S., Giacaman, S., Basika, T., Gayo, V., Rosadilla, D., Roche, L., Tort, J., and Carmona, C. (2011) The recombinant

35 Raina, O.K., Nagar, G., Varghese, A., Prajitha, G., Alex, A., Maharana, B.R., and Joshi, P. (2011) Lack of protective efficacy in buffaloes vaccinated with *Fasciola gigantica* leucine aminopeptidase and peroxiredoxin recombinant proteins. *Acta. Trop.*, **118**, 217–222.

34 gut-associated M17 leucine aminopeptidase in combination with different adjuvants confers a high level of protection against *Fasciola hepatica* infection in sheep. *Vaccine*, **29**, 9057–9063.

36 Simeonov, A., Jadhav, A., Sayed, A.A., Wang, Y., Nelson, M.E., Thomas, C.J., Inglese, J. *et al.* (2008) Quantitative high-throughput screen identifies inhibitors of the *Schistosoma mansoni* redox cascade. *PloS Negl. Trop. Dis.*, **2**, e127.

37 Bonilla, M., Denicola, A., Novoselov, S.V., Turanov, A.A., Protasio, A., Izmendi, D., Gladyshev, V.N., and Salinas, G. (2008) Platyhelminth mitochondrial and cytosolic redox homeostasis is controlled by a single thioredoxin glutathione reductase and dependent on selenium and glutathione. *J. Biol. Chem.*, **283**, 17898–17907.

38 Rai, G., Sayed, A.A., Lea, W.A., Luecke, H.F., Chakrapani, H., Prast-Nielsen, S., Jadhav, A. *et al.* (2009) Structure mechanism insights and the role of nitric oxide donation guide the development of oxadiazole-2-oxides as therapeutic agents against schistosomiasis. *J. Med. Chem.*, **52**, 6474–6483.

39 Maggioli, G., Piacenza, L., Carambula, B., and Carmona, C. (2004) Purification, characterization, and immunolocalization of a thioredoxin reductase from adult *Fasciola hepatica*. *J. Parasitol.*, **90**, 205–211.

40 Maggioli G., Silveira, F., Martín-Alonso, J.M., Salinas, G., Carmona, C., and Parra, F. (2011) A recombinant thioredoxin-glutathione reductase from *Fasciola hepatica* induces a protective response in rabbits. *Exp. Parasitol.*, **129**, 323–330.

41 Donnelly, S., O'Neill, S.M., Sekiya, M., Mulcahy, G., and Dalton, J.P. (2005) Thioredoxin peroxidase secreted by *Fasciola hepatica* induces the alternative activation of macrophages. *Infect. Immun.*, **73**, 166–173.

42 Mendes, R.E., Pérez-Ecija, R.A., Zafra, R., Buffoni, L., Martínez-Moreno, A., Dalton, J.P., Mulcahy, G., and Pérez, J. (2010) Evaluation of hepatic changes and local and systemic immune responses in goats immunized with recombinant peroxiredoxin (Prx) and challenged with *Fasciola hepatica*. *Vaccine*, **28**, 2832–2840.

43 Good, M.F. (2011) A whole parasite vaccine to control the blood stages of Plasmodium – the case for lateral thinking. *Trends Parasitol.*, **27**, 335–340.

44 Spithill, T.W., Smooker, P.M., Sexton, J.L., Bozas, E., Morrison, C.A., and Parsons, J.C. (1999) The development of vaccines against fasciolosis, in *Fasciolosis* (ed. J.P. Dalton), CABI, Wallingford, pp. 377–410.

45 Creaney, J., Spithill, T.W., Thompson, C.M., Wilson, L.R., Sandeman, R.M., and Parsons, J.C. (1995) Attempted immunisation of sheep against *Fasciola hepatica* using γ-irradiated metacercariae. *Int. J. Parasitol.*, **25**, 853–856.

46 Gauci, C., Jenkins, D., and Lightowlers, M.W. (2011) Strategies for optimal expression of vaccine antigens from taeniid cestode parasites in *Escherichia coli*. *Mol. Biotechnol.*, **48**, 277–289.

47 Anthony, R.M., Rutitzky, L.I., Urban, J.F. Jr, Stadecker, M.J., and Gause, W.C. (2007) Protective immune mechanisms in helminth infection. *Nat. Rev. Immunol.*, **7**, 975–987.

48 Hewitson, J.P., Grainger, J.R., and Maizels, R.M. (2009) Helminth immunoregulation: the role of parasite secreted proteins in modulating host immunity. *Mol. Biochem. Parasitol.*, **167**, 1–11.

49 Moreau, E. and Chauvin, A. (2010) Immunity against helminths: interactions with the host and the intercurrent infections. *J. Biomed. Biotech.*, **2010**, 428593.

50 Dessein, A., Kouriba, B., Eboumbou, C., Dessein, H., Argiro, L., Marquet, S., Elwali, N.E. *et al.* (2004) Interleukin-13 in

the skin and interferon-gamma in the liver are key players in immune protection in human schistosomiasis. *Immunol. Rev.*, **201**, 180–190.

51 McManus, D.P. and Loukas, A. (2008) Current status of vaccines for schistosomiasis. *Clin. Microbiol. Rev.*, **21**, 225–242.

52 Mulcahy, G., Joyce, P., and Dalton, J.P. (1999) Immunology of *Fasciola hepatica* infection, in *Fasciolosis* (ed. J.P. Dalton), CABI, Wallingford, pp. 341–376.

53 Roberts, J.A., Estuningsih, S.E., Wiedosari, E., and Spithill, T.W. (1997) Acquisition of resistance against *Fasciola gigantica* by Indonesian thin tail sheep. *Vet. Parasitol.*, **73**, 215–224.

54 Hansen, D.S., Clery, D.G., Estuningsih, S.E., Widjajanti, S., Partoutomo, S., and Spithill, T.W. (1999) Immune responses in Indonesian thin tail and Merino sheep during a primary infection with *Fasciola gigantica*: lack of a specific IgG2 antibody response is associated with increased resistance to infection in Indonesian sheep. *Int. J. Parasitol.*, **29**, 1027–1035.

55 Waweru, J.G., Kanyari, P.W., Mwangi, D.M., Ngatia, T.A., and Nansen, P. (1999) Comparative parasitological and haematological changes in two breeds of sheep infected with *Fasciola gigantica*. *Trop. Anim. Health Prod.*, **31**, 363–372.

56 Zhang, W., Moreau, E., Huang, W., and Chauvin, A. (2004) Comparison of humoral response in sheep to *Fasciola hepatica* and *Fasciola gigantica* experimental infection. *Parasite*, **11**, 153–159.

57 Pleasance, J., Wiedosari, E., Raadsma, H.W., Meeusen, E., and Piedrafita, D. (2011) Resistance to liver fluke infection in the natural sheep host is correlated with a type-1 cytokine response. *Parasite Immunol.*, **33**, 495–505.

58 Wiedosari, E., Hayakawa, H., and Copeman, B. (2006) Host differences in response to trickle infection with *Fasciola gigantica* in buffalo, Ongole and Bali calves. *Trop. Anim. Health Prod.*, **38**, 43–53.

59 Raadsma, H.W., Kingsford, N.M. Suharyanta, Spithill, T.W., and Piedrafita., D. (2007) Host responses during experimental infection with *Fasciola gigantica* or *Fasciola hepatica* in Merino sheep I. Comparative immunological and plasma biochemical changes during early infection. *Vet. Parasitol*, **143**, 275–286.

60 Mulcahy, G., O'Connor, F., McGonigle, S., Dowd, A., Clery, D.G., Andrews, S.J., and Dalton, J.P. (1998) Correlation of specific antibody titre and avidity with protection in cattle immunized against *Fasciola hepatica*. *Vaccine*, **16**, 932–939.

61 Flynn, R.J. and Mulcahy, G. (2008) The roles of IL-10 and TGF-beta in controlling IL-4 and IFN-gamma production during experimental *Fasciola hepatica* infection. *Int. J. Parasitol.*, **38**, 1673–1680.

62 Morphew, R.M., Wright, H.A., LaCourse, E.J., Woods, D.J., and Brophy, P.M. (2007) Comparative proteomics of excretory–secretory proteins released by the liver fluke *Fasciola hepatica* in sheep host bile and during *in vitro* culture ex host. *Mol. Cell. Proteomics*, **6**, 963–972.

63 Young, N.D., Hall, R.S., Jex, A.R., Cantacessi, C., and Gasser, R.B. (2010) Elucidating the transcriptome of *Fasciola hepatica* – a key to fundamental and biotechnological discoveries for a neglected parasite. *Biotechnol. Adv.*, **28**, 222–231.

64 Young, N.D., Jex, A.R., Cantacessi, C., Hall, R.S., Campbell, B.E., Spithill, T.W., Tangkawattana, S. *et al.* (2011) A portrait of the transcriptome of the neglected trematode, *Fasciola gigantica* – biological and biotechnological implications. *PloS Negl. Trop. Dis.*, **5**, e1004.

65 Flynn, R.J., Mulcahy, G., and Elsheikha, H.M. (2010) Coordinating innate and adaptive immunity in *Fasciola hepatica* infection: implications for control. *Vet. Parasitol.*, **169**, 235–240.

66 Hacariz, O., Sayers, G., and Mulcahy, G. (2011) A preliminary study to understand the effect of *Fasciola hepatica* tegument on naive macrophages and humoral responses in an ovine model. *Vet. Immunol. Immunopathol.*, **139**, 245–249.

67 Flynn, R.J., Irwin, J.A., Olivier, M., Sekiya, M., Dalton, J.P., and Mulcahy, G.

(2007) Alternative activation of ruminant macrophages by *Fasciola hepatica*. *Vet. Immunol. Immunopathol.*, **120**, 31–40.

68 Flynn, R.J., Mannion, C., Golden, O., Hacariz, O., and Mulcahy, G. (2007) Experimental *Fasciola hepatica* infection alters responses to tests used for diagnosis of bovine tuberculosis. *Infect. Immun.*, **75**, 1373–1381.

69 Piedrafita, D., Spithill, T.W., Dalton, J.P., Brindley, P.J., Sandeman, M.R., Wood, P.R., and Parsons, J.C. (2000) Juvenile *Fasciola hepatica* are resistant to killing *in vitro* by free radicals compared with larvae of *Schistosoma mansoni*. *Parasite Immunol.*, **22**, 287–295.

70 Dalton, J.P., Skelly, P., and Halton, D.W. (2004) Role of the tegument and gut in nutrient uptake by parasitic platyhelminths. *Can. J. Zool.*, **82**, 211–232.

71 Lammas, D.A., Duffus, W.P., and Taylor, D.W. (1985) Identification of surface proteins of juvenile stages of *Fasciola hepatica*. *Res. Vet. Sci.*, **38**, 248–249.

72 Dalton, J.P. and Joyce, P. (1987) Characterization of surface glycoproteins and proteins of different developmental stages of *Fasciola hepatica* by surface radiolabeling. *J. Parasitol.*, **73**, 1281–1284.

73 Trudgett, A., McNair, A.T., Hoey, E.M., Keegan, P.S., Dalton, J.P., Rima, B.K., Miller, A., and Ramasamy, P. (2000) The major tegumental antigen of *Fasciola hepatica* contains repeated elements. *Parasitology*, **121**, 185–191.

74 Eberl, M., Langermans, J.A., Vervenne, R.A., Nyame, A.K., Cummings, R.D., Thomas, A.W., Coulson, P.S., and Wilson, R.A. (2001) Antibodies to glycans dominate the host response to schistosome larvae and eggs: is their role protective or subversive? *J. Infect. Dis.*, **183**, 1238–1247.

75 Kariuki, T.M., Farah, I.O., Wilson, RA., and Coulson, P.S. (2008) Antibodies elicited by the secretions from schistosome cercariae and eggs are predominantly against glycan epitopes. *Parasite Immunol.*, **30**, 554–562.

76 Thomas, P.G. and Harn, D.A. Jr (2004) Immune biasing by helminth glycans. *Cell Microbiol.*, **6**, 13–22.

77 van Balkom, B.W., van Gestel, R.A., Brouwers, J.F., Krijgsveld, J., Tielens, A.G., Heck, A.J., and van Hellemond, J.J. (2005) Mass spectrometric analysis of the *Schistosoma mansoni* tegumental sub-proteome. *J. Proteome Res.*, **4**, 958–966.

78 Braschi, S., Curwen, R.S., Ashton, P.D., Verjovski-Almeida, S., and Wilson, A. (2006) The tegument surface membranes of the human blood parasite *Schistosoma mansoni*: a proteomic analysis after differential extraction. *Proteomics*, **6**, 1471–1482.

79 Braschi, S. and Wilson, R.A. (2006) Proteins exposed at the adult schistosome surface revealed by biotinylation. *Mol. Cell. Proteomics*, **5**, 347–356.

80 Mulvenna, J., Moertel, L., Jones, M.K., Nawaratna, S., Lovas, E.M., Gobert, G.N., Colgrave, M. *et al.* (2010) Exposed proteins of the *Schistosoma japonicum* tegument. *Int. J. Parasitol.*, **40**, 543–554.

81 Mulvenna, J., Sripa, B., Brindley, P.J., Gorman, J., Jones, M.K., Colgrave, M.L., Jones, A. *et al.* (2010) The secreted and surface proteomes of the adult stage of the carcinogenic human liver fluke *Opisthorchis viverrini*. *Proteomics*, **10**, 1063–1078.

82 Castro-Borges, W., Dowle, A., Curwen, R., Thomas-Oates, J., and Wilson, R.A. (2011) Mass spectrometric identification of exposed proteins on the surface of the *Schistosome* tegument released by enzymatic shaving: a rational approach for selection of vaccine candidates. *PLoS Negl. Trop. Dis.*, **5**, e993.

83 Wilson, R.A., Wright, J.M., de Castro-Borges, W., Parker-Manuel, S.J., Dowle, A.A., Ashton, P.D., Young, N.D., Gasser, R.B., and Spithill, T.W. (2011) Exploring the *Fasciola hepatica* tegument proteome. *Int. J. Parasitol.*, **41**, 1347–1359.

84 Hope Cawdery, M.J., Strickland, K.L., Conway, A., and Crowe, P.J. (1977) Production effects of liver fluke in cattle. 1. The effects of infection on liveweight gain, feed intake and food conversion efficiency in beef cattle. *Br. Vet. J.*, **133**, 145–159.

85 Vercruysse, J. and Claerebout, E. (2001) Treatment vs non-treatment of helminth

infections in cattle: defining the threshold. *Vet. Parasitol.*, **98**, 195–214.

86 Malone, J.B., Loyacano, A., Armstrong, D.A., and Archibald, L.F. (1982) Bovine fascioliasis: economic impact and control in Gulf Coast cattle based on seasonal transmission. *Bovine Pract.*, **17**, 126–133.

87 Dargie, J.D. (1986) The impact on production and mechanisms of pathogenesis of trematode infections in cattle and sheep, in *Parasitology – Quo Vadit? Proceedings of the 6th International Congress of Parasitology* (ed. M.J. Howell), Australian Academy of Science, Canberra, pp. 453–463.

88 Spithill, T.W. and Dalton, J.P. (1998) Progress in development of liver fluke vaccines. *Parasitol. Today*, **14**, 224–228.

89 Parkinson, M., O'Neill, S.M., and Dalton, J.P. (2007) Endemic human fasciolosis in the Bolivian Altiplano. *Epidemiol. Infect.*, **135**, 669–674.

90 Mas Coma, S., Anglés, R., Esteban, J.G., Bargues, M.D., Buchon, P., Franken, M., and Strauss, W. (1999) The Northern Bolivian Altiplano: a region highly endemic for human fascioliasis. *Trop. Med. Int. Health*, **4**, 454–467.

91 Keiser, J. and Utzinger, J. (2007) Food-borne trematodiasis: current chemotherapy and advances with artemisinins and synthetic trioxolanes. *Trends Parasitol.*, **23**, 555–562.

92 Curtale, F., Hassanein, Y.A., and Savioli, L. (2005) Control of human fascioliasis by selective chemotherapy: design, cost and effect of the first public health, school-based intervention implemented in endemic areas of the Nile Delta. *Egypt. Trans. R. Soc. Trop. Med. Hyg.*, **99**, 599–609.

93 Haçariz, O., Sayers, G., McCullough, M., Garrett, M., O'Donovan, J., and Mulcahy, G. (2009) The effect of Quil A adjuvant on the course of experimental *Fasciola hepatica* infection in sheep. *Vaccine*, **27**, 45–50.

29
Vaccines Against Cestode Parasites

Marshall W. Lightowlers[*], *Charles G. Gauci, Abdul Jabbar, and Cristian Alvarez*

Abstract

Extraordinary success has been achieved in the development of vaccines for the prevention of infection with cestode parasites in their intermediate hosts. The key to this success was the identification of a brief period in the parasites' development during which they are susceptible to immune attack. In common with other eukaryotic parasites, cestode parasites are relatively insusceptible to the hosts' immune response; however, for a period of a few days or, at most, weeks, the early developing metacestode is susceptible to antibody and complement-mediated attack. Evidence of this susceptibility is clear from the occurrence of concomitant immunity to most, if not all, species of taeniid cestode parasite in their intermediate hosts. Antigens associated with antioncosphere immunity were identified, cloned, and have been used as effective vaccines against experimentally administered challenge infections. Vaccines against *Echinococcus granulosus* and *Taenia solium* are currently undergoing field trials, and have great potential for reducing transmission of these important zoonotic parasites, thereby reducing the incidence of hydatid disease and neurocysticercosis in humans. Here, the development of these vaccines is reviewed and consideration given to the challenges that lie ahead as these vaccines begin to be used in disease control programs.

Introduction

Cestodes are a group of obligate flatworm parasites. Their life cycles typically involve two hosts – definitive and intermediate hosts. A single family of cestodes, the Taeniidae, has been the subject of investigations into vaccine development. Several taeniid species are common or obligate hosts for humans and domestic livestock species, causing morbidity, mortality, and economic loss. Other species are natural parasites of rodents and lagomorphs, and these have been used extensively as models in immunological investigations and studies on the development of vaccines (Table 29.1).

Unlike the vast majority of eukaryotic parasites of medical and veterinary significance, the taeniid cestode parasites provide striking examples where host immune

[*] Corresponding Author

Parasitic Helminths: Targets, Screens, Drugs and Vaccines, First Edition. Edited by Conor R. Caffrey
© 2012 Wiley-VCH Verlag GmbH & Co. KGaA. Published 2012 by Wiley-VCH Verlag GmbH & Co. KGaA.

Table 29.1 Principal medically and economically important taeniid species and those used extensively in laboratory studies.

Species	Obsolete synonyms	Principal intermediate hosts	Metacestode type	Principal definitive host
Taenia solium	Cysticercus cellulosae	pig (man)	cysticercus	man
Taenia saginata	Cysticercus bovis	cattle	cysticercus	man
Taenia hydatigena	Cysticercus tenuicollis	sheep	cysticercus	dog
Taenia ovis	Cysticercus ovis	sheep	cysticercus	dog
Taenia multiceps	Multiceps multiceps	sheep, goats, cattle (man)	coenurus	dog
Taenia pisiformis	Cysticercus pisiformis	rabbit	cysticercus	dog
Taenia taeniaeformis	Cysticercus fasciolaris	rodents	strobilocercus	cat
Taenia crassiceps		rodents	cysticercus (proliferative)	dog
Echinococcus granulosus		sheep, goats, cattle, pigs, and other herbivores (man)	unilocular hydatid cyst	dog
Echinococcus multilocularis		microtine rodents (man)	multilocular hydatid cyst	fox (dog)

responses can be completely effective in preventing a challenge infection. This phenomenon applies particularly to infections in the intermediate hosts, but not the definitive hosts. By capitalizing on the nature of the naturally occurring effective immune responses, several defined antigen vaccines have been developed for this group of pathogens that have no parallel in any other eukaryotic parasite [1].

Vaccine Development in Definitive Hosts

In seeking to control the transmission of medically and economically important taeniid cestodes, vaccines for use in the definitive hosts would be valuable because typically there are fewer definitive hosts involved in the parasites' transmission than intermediate hosts; also, the definitive hosts are often more easily accessed. In the case of *Echinococcus granulosus*, which causes cystic hydatid disease in humans and domestic livestock species world-wide, the parasite is commonly transmitted by sheep and goats, with domestic dogs playing a dominant role in disease transmission. Farmers generally have fewer dogs than sheep and also the dogs congregate around dwellings, making them readily available for interventions such as vaccination.

Two publications describe effective vaccines against *E. granulosus* infection in dogs [2, 3]. Neither has been validated independently nor has there been any published extension of the available data from the research groups involved. Concerns have been raised about the quality of the evidence to support the claimed vaccine effects [4]. There have also been descriptions of some level of vaccine-induced protection against infection with adults of the tapeworm *Taenia solium* in laboratory animal model models [5, 6]. However, the prospects for successful vaccine development in the definitive hosts of taeniid cestode parasites are not promising. There is no clear evidence to support the existence of effective immunological responses against taeniid cestodes in their definitive hosts. The host does certainly produce specific immunological responses to the adult worm parasites [7]; however, these are either entirely ineffective or at least poorly effective in expelling the parasites or in preventing the establishment of new infections. Gemmell *et al.* [8] undertook heroic studies on the influence of infections with *E. granulosus* on susceptibility to subsequent rounds of challenge infection. Although they observed a gradual decline in the number of worms establishing, as well as a decrease in the size and fecundity of worms in challenge infections, dogs that had experienced multiple rounds of infection and anthelmintic treatment remained susceptible to the establishment of fertile parasites from challenge infections. Any effective vaccine for dogs would need to induce a more substantial degree of immunity than that which occurs naturally against the parasite.

Vaccines Against Cestode Infections in Intermediate Hosts

Whereas little progress has been made in studies of immunity and vaccine development in definitive hosts, better advances have been made in vaccine development against taeniid cestode infections in their intermediate hosts. These developments were based on a sound understanding of the immune mechanisms operating against the early developing metacestode.

Clear Evidence for Protective Immune Responses

In contrast to the situation in definitive hosts, clear evidence of immunologically based protective immune responses against taeniid cestode parasites became evident soon after the first experimental investigations were undertaken. A strong suggestion of the development of immunity following an initial exposure to a taeniid metacestode was provided by Miller [9] while investigating infections with the parasite *Taenia taeniaeformis* in rats. He found that occasionally some animals that he had obtained from his supplier were completely refractory to an experimental infection. These animals invariably had one or a small number of mature, pre-existing strobilocerci in their livers as a result of exposure to the parasite prior to the animals being provided to him by his supplier. Two points became immediately apparent. The previous exposure to infection had rendered the host immune to a challenge infection; however, the immune responses that were capable of preventing a secondary infection were incapable of eliminating parasites that had established as metacestodes from the initial exposure. The term concomitant immunity was appropriated from the field of cancer immunology [10] in the 1960s to describe this type of immunity, first for the schistosomes, for which the phenomenon exists, but is only partially effective, then to the taeniid cestodes, but with up to 100% efficacy [11].

The weight of evidence supports the hypothesis that concomitant immunity to taeniid cestodes relates to immune responses induced against the oncosphere and the very early developing metacestode [12]. Although metacestodes continue to raise specific immune responses in infected hosts, these are neither effective against the metacestode itself nor do they maintain protection against a challenge infection as antioncosphere-specific responses wane.

Vaccine Development – Overall Strategy

Early research using *T. taeniaeformis* in rats and *Taenia pisiformis* in rabbits established the clear potential for development of vaccines against parasites belonging to the cestode family, Taeniidae. Subsequently, immunological investigations by Michael Gemmell, David Heath, Michael Rickard, and Graham Mitchell established the basis upon which subsequent practical vaccine developments were based [11]. Over the past 30 years, the principal targets of vaccine-related research were the parasites causing cystic hydatidosis and neurocysticercosis in humans, *E. granulosus* and *T. solium*, respectively. A number of research groups have undertaken vaccine-related research on these parasites with the most effective and independently validated approach being through the characterization of antigens from the oncosphere life cycle stage. Both *E. granulosus* and *T. solium* are, however, relatively difficult to manipulate in a research environment because of difficulties in obtaining and handling infective eggs. The strategy which was adopted towards the development of oncosphere antigen based vaccines was, in sequential order:

- Establish the basic parameters surrounding vaccine-induced immunity using parasite species that are readily manipulated in the laboratory, particularly *T. taeniaeformis, T. pisiformis,* and *Taenia ovis.*
- Develop a practical vaccine against a commercially significant parasite, but one relatively easily manipulated in the laboratory (*T. ovis*).
- Use the knowledge gained in developing a *T. ovis* vaccine to demonstrate that the tools and knowledge could be applied in the development of an effective vaccine against a related species (*Taenia saginata*).
- Adopt these successful strategies, with confidence, in the development of vaccines against *E. granulosus* and *T. solium*.

Existing, Effective, Recombinant Vaccines

The strategy adopted towards the development of practical vaccines against taeniid cestode parasites has been extraordinarily successful. The *Escherichia coli*-expressed 45W vaccine against *T. ovis* infection in sheep was the first effective, defined antigen vaccine against any parasitic organism and has been recognized as a milestone in the history of parasitology [13]. This discovery has formed the basis for the subsequent development of effective vaccines against *T. saginata* in cattle, *T. solium* in pigs, and *E. granulosus* in sheep and other hosts (Table 29.2). Using the same foundations, progress has also been made in vaccination against *Echinococcus multilocularis* in rodents and against *Taenia multiceps* in sheep. The vaccines utilize recombinant proteins that are expressed uniquely in the oncosphere and early developing parasite [14]. Either 50 (*T. ovis, E. granulosus*) or 200 µg (*T. saginata, T. solium*) recombinant protein together with the adjuvant Quil A is injected subcutaneously or intramuscularly on two occasions 1 month apart. Protective immunity is associated with the development of complement-fixing circulating antibodies capable of killing oncospheres in a challenge infection. Immunity is apparent following the second immunization, and appears to remain relatively effective for at least 6 months in the case of *T. ovis* [15] and at least 1 year in the case of *E. granulosus* [16]. The level of protection afforded by the vaccines exceeds 90% and commonly is of the order of 99–100% (Table 29.2).

Characteristics of Host-Protective Antigens

The taeniid cestode vaccines are the most effective defined antigen vaccines against parasitic infections. Studies into the immune mechanisms that render these parasites susceptible to host immune responses and the characteristics of the target antigens may provide insights that could be valuable in the development of other antiparasite vaccines, particularly vaccines against other helminths.

Table 29.2 Recombinant oncosphere antigens of taeniid cestodes that induce host-protective immune responses.

Species	Antigen	Protein ID	GenBank accession	Homology group[a]	Protection (%)[b]	Reference
Taenia ovis	To45W	CAA33300	X15228	45W	94	[34]
	To45S	AAC46952	U20640	45W	87	[46]
	To16K	AAB49687	U89944	16K	92	[47]
	To18K	AAB49686	U89943	18K	99	[47]
Taenia multiceps	Tm16	ABV25964	EF672036	16K	74	[48]
Taenia saginata	TSA-9[c]	CAA67185	X98576	45W	99	[49]
	TSA-18[c]	CAA67186	X98577	18K	99	[49]
Taenia solium	TSOL18	AAD09326	AF017788	18K	100	[50]
	TSOL45	AAK31940	AF267115	45W	97	[50]
Echinococcus granulosus	EG95	CAA62433	X90928	EG95	100	[51]
Echinococcus multilocularis	EM95	AAL51153	AY062921	EG95	83	[52]

a) Assignment to a particular homology group, designated by the abbreviation used for the first antigen of the group to be characterized, indicates a high level of amino acid homology between antigens.
b) Indicates the optimum level of protection achieved in vaccination and challenge trials in the parasite's natural intermediate host species compared to challenge controls.
c) TSA-9 and TSA-18 were found to act synergistically; results represent those of vaccination trials using the two antigens together.

Protective Antigens are Secreted
Early research on the characterization of protective antigens of taeniid cestode parasites sparked controversy about whether the host was required to be exposed directly to the living parasite in order to develop immunity to a subsequent challenge infection. Rickard and Bell [17] provided the first demonstration that direct contact between the parasite and host was not required for the induction of protective immune responses; protective antigens were capable of diffusing through a membrane-bound chamber (0.22 μm pore size) implanted intraperitoneally in which living parasites were enclosed. Subsequently, Rickard's research group showed that host-protective antigens could be collected from the parasites maintained in *in vitro* culture [12]. The situation as to the precise origin of the host-protective antigens was somewhat complicated by the discovery that the nonactivated oncosphere contains protective antigens [12]. Both the parasite cultures that had been used to collect excreted/secreted antigens and the parasite diffusion chambers used by Rickard and Bell [17] could not exclude the possibility of their being contaminated with somatic antigens arising from the death and disintegration of parasites. Definitive proof that the parasites do indeed secrete host-protective antigens, at least in *in vitro* culture, was provided recently by Jabbar *et al.*, who demonstrated the presence of specific protective antigens within secretory blebs extruded from cultured parasites [18]. In keeping with the secreted nature of the antigens is the presence of a predicted secretory signal sequence at the N-terminal of the full-length protein sequences. [14].

Stage-Specific Expression
All of the protective oncosphere antigens that have been investigated are expressed uniquely in the oncosphere and early developing parasite [14]. No evidence has been found that the proteins are present or expressed in mature metacestodes, or in those parts of the adult tapeworm that do not contain developing or mature oncospheres. The precise timing of the initiation of expression of the proteins in the ontogeny of the oncosphere is not known nor is the timing of the cessation of expression during the development of the metacestode. Studies undertaken on the ultrastructure of the developing metacestode of *T. taeniaeformis* describe a dramatic transformation of the parasite tegument at around 7 days development from one covered in microvilli to one covered in microtriches typical of the mature metacestode [19, 20]. It is tempting to associate this change in the parasite's tegument structure with the marked change that occurs in the early parasite's susceptibility to antibody and complement-mediated attack early in the development of the metacestode [21]; however, there is no direct evidence to support this hypothesis. It appears that other, and perhaps all, taeniid species may follow a similar pattern whereby the developing parasite changes from being susceptible to immune attack to being relatively or completely insusceptible. The precise timing of these events does apparently differ between the species because, in the case of *T. pisiformis* in rabbits, the parasite appears to remain susceptible to immune attack for a longer period [22] than does *T. taeniaeformis* [21].

Presence of One or Two Fibronectin Type III Domains
Bioinformatic analyses of the amino acid sequences of all of the host-protective oncosphere antigens have identified conserved features within the proteins. A fibronectin type III (FnIII) domain is one feature that was first identified in the To45W vaccine antigen from *T. ovis* and in the oncA antigen from *T. taeniaeformis* [23]. The domain is also present in receptor protein tyrosine phosphatases of lymphocytes [23]. All of the host-protective oncosphere antigens contain one or two FnIII domains (Figure 29.1).

The FnIII domain consists of approximately 90 amino acids and occurs in proteins involved in specific molecular recognition, such as in cell surface hormone and cytokine receptors, cell adhesion molecules, extracellular matrix proteins, chaperonins, and carbohydrate-binding proteins [24]. Proteins containing multiple tandem repeats of the FnIII domain include tenascins and fibronectins [25], which are proteins involved in cell proliferation, adhesion, and migration, and are associated with embryonic development, wound healing, and tumorigenesis [26]. The three-dimensional structure of the 10th FnIII module of fibronectin has been determined [27]. It consists of seven β-strands forming a sandwich of two antiparallel β-sheets of three and four strands. Although the amino acid sequence homology between FnIII domains from different proteins is low, the tertiary structures are similar [28].

Many FnIII domain-containing proteins are often large proteins consisting of multiple FnIII repeats and other protein domain types [25]. In comparison, the taeniid oncosphere proteins are much smaller and quite simple, containing only one

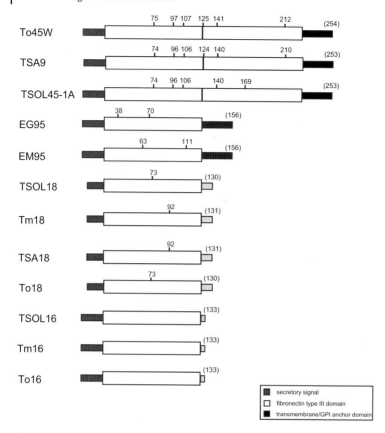

Figure 29.1 Schematic illustration showing the locations of secretory signals, FnIII domains, and transmembrane/GPI anchor domains of taeniid vaccine antigens. Numbers indicate amino acid position of predicted N-linked glycosylation sites and numbers in brackets represent the length of the predicted full-length protein from the initiator methionine. (Reproduced with permission and modifications from Lightowlers et al. [14].)

or two FnIII domains. The short isoforms of prolactin receptors are among the few nontaeniid proteins that are also composed essentially of only one or two extracellular FnIII domains (as well as a secretory signal, single transmembrane domain and a short intracellular domain) [29]. Prolactin receptors, belonging to the class 1 cytokine receptor superfamily, are involved in signal transduction mechanisms, and have been associated with cell proliferation, differentiation, and development, as well as tumor growth [29].

In addition to the FnIII domain, all of the taeniid antigens contain a predicted secretory signal at the N-terminus (Figure 29.1). The EG95 and 45W antigen groups also contain a predicted transmembrane domain or potential glycosylphosphatidylinositol (GPI) anchor at the C-terminus. These features provide further evidence to indicate that the oncosphere antigens are possibly secreted or membrane-associated.

Oncosphere Structure and Localization of the Protective Antigens

Recently, Jabbar et al. published a series of papers describing the localization of various host-protective antigens of a number of taeniid cestodes [18, 30–32]. The work was preceded by the researchers undertaking a description of the basic ultrastructure of the organism itself since this information was not available [33].

From a structural point of view, oncospheres are bilaterally symmetrical, spherical, or oval-shaped embryos armed with three pairs of hooks, containing pair(s) of glands and surrounded by embryonic envelopes. Prior to hatching and activation, the oncosphere is surrounded by a keratinous shell composed of tapering hexagonal blocks as well as a thin protective amorphous layer composed of two closely apposed double-unit membranes and referred to as the oncospheral membrane. Both the shell and the oncospheral membrane are discarded during the hatching and activation of the parasite under the influence of bile salts. The cellular features of the parasite are three pairs of hooks interconnected by a complex hook muscle system that is responsible for coordination of their synchronized movements, a unique hook region membrane that covers the somatophoric (anterior) pole of the oncosphere, a tegument having filamentous processes/microvilli of various lengths, and various somatic cell types (Figure 29.2). The cell types comprising the oncosphere in *T. ovis* are: (i) a penetration gland type 1 (PG1) containing two to four cell bodies interconnected by narrow cytoplasmic bridges, (ii) a syncytium structure referred to as a PG type 2 (PG2) containing four nuclei, (iii) a uninucleated median mesophoric gland cell, (iv) somatic cells representing myocytons, (v) germinative cells, (vi) a pair of nerve cells, and (vii) a pair of median somatophoric cells. The cell types and their number vary slightly among the different species; in the case of *T. ovis*, the oncosphere is composed of a total of 19 cells.

Jabbar et al. [18, 30–32] investigated the localization of host-protective antigens using both light microscopy and immunogold methods in transmission electron microscopy (TEM). The investigations involving TEM included careful quantification of labeling density for all oncospheral cell types and major structures with the data analyzed statistically. Using light microscopy techniques, the antigens of *T. ovis* (To16, To18, and To45W) were seen in the cytoplasm of two to four distinct cells [32]. Confocal immunofluorescence microscopy reveals that each of the antigens colocalizes within the same cells in the oncosphere (Figure 29.3, first two rows). Like *T. ovis*, the EG95 protein in *E. granulosus* is present predominantly in the cytoplasm of two to four distinct cells. The location of the host-protective antigens seems to vary slightly in *T. saginata* and *T. solium*, in which different antigens have a tendency to predominate in different cell types [31]. In contrast, for *T. ovis*, the various antigens colocalize in the same cell types. Specific staining for TSA9 in *T. saginata* and for TSOL45 in *T. solium* shows a similar pattern to that seen in *T. ovis* and *E. granulosus*. Positive staining for TSA18 in *T. saginata* oncospheres and for TSOL16 and TSOL18 in *T. solium* is evident in a different cell type (Figure 29.3, third row: note that TSOL16 and TSOL45 antigens are present in two different cell types, which is different to their homologs in *T. ovis* (first two rows)). The staining seen in particular cell types in nonactivated oncospheres is also present in activated oncospheres, together with a

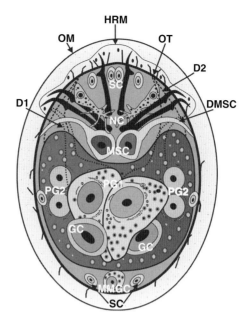

Figure 29.2 Schematic diagram of the *T. ovis* oncosphere illustrating the symmetry and cellular organization. D1, duct-like structures of penetration gland type 1; D2, duct-like structures of penetration gland type 2; DMSC, duct of median somatophoric cell; GC, germinative cell; HRM, hook region membrane; MMGC, median mesophoric gland cell; MSC, median somatophoric cell; Mv, microvilli; NC, nerve cell; OM, oncospheral membrane; OT, oncospheral tegument; PG1, penetration gland type 1; PG2, penetration gland type 2; SC, somatic cell. (Reproduced from Jabbar et al. [33] with permission.)

more generalized staining of the oncospheral parenchyma in activated oncospheres. This is the situation for all species and antigens examined, except for TSA9 in *T. saginata* in which staining is restricted to particular cells even in activated oncospheres [30, 31]. Although there is generalized antigen-specific staining seen throughout the parenchyma of activated oncospheres (Figure 29.3, fourth row), no positive staining is observed on the surface of nonactivated or recently activated oncospheres in all of the species investigated.

The staining pattern for host-protective antigens seen in the parasites changes as the parasites began to develop in culture (Figure 29.3, last two rows). During the first few days of culture, a generalized staining pattern is found throughout the parasite parenchyma, but without obvious staining of the oncospheral surface (To16 and To45W). After 7–9 days of development, the metacestodes become enlarged, and antigen-specific staining is evident both on the surface and in the cells within the developing metacestode (Figure 29.3, bottom row). In *T. ovis*, all three host-protective antigens are absent in parasites by 15 days of culture [30]. In subsequent studies using TEM, all three antigens of *T. ovis* and EG95 in *E. granulosus* were present predominantly in the secretory granules and cytoplasm of the PG1 and PG2

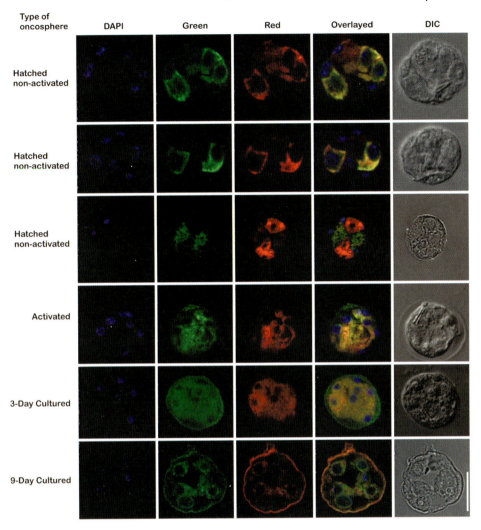

Figure 29.3 Confocal immunofluorescence images of sectioned *T. ovis* and *T. solium* oncospheres showing the localization of various host-protective antigens in different combinations. The first and second rows show hatched nonactivated *T. ovis* oncospheres that were reacted with antisera to To18 and To45W and to To16 and To18, respectively. The third row shows a nonactivated *T. solium* oncosphere that was reacted with TSOL16 and TSOL45 antisera. The fourth row shows an activated oncosphere of *T. ovis* that was reacted with To18 and To45W antisera. The last two rows show colocalization in *T. ovis* metacestodes that were cultured *in vitro* for 3 (fifth row) and 7–9 days (bottom row); the former was treated with To18 and To45W antisera, and the latter with To16 and To45W antisera. Each row of images shows the same oncosphere imaged so as to reveal 4′,6-diamidino-2-phenylindole-stained nuclei, green and/or red fluorescence, and a visible light image obtained via a differential interference contrast filter. The yellow/orange color in the overlaid image represents combined localization of the green (To18, To16, or TSOL16) and red (To18 (just second row), To45W, or TSOL45) fluorescence associated with the localization of individual antigens. Scale bar, 10 μm. (Reproduced from Jabbar *et al.* [30, 31] with permission.)

cells [18, 32]. Examination of *T. ovis* oncospheres that had been activated *in vitro* revealed that each of the three host-protective antigens was found in the penetration gland secretion "blebs" following the activation of the oncospheres [18].

One interesting outcome of these studies is the realization that invading oncospheres appear not to be susceptible to vaccine-induced antibody and complement-mediated attack because there is no evidence to indicate that any of the protective antigens is present on the parasite surface. Nevertheless, the antigens are being secreted by the freshly activated oncosphere within membrane-enclosed cytoplasmic blebs. As the parasite develops further, the antigens become associated with the tegument, presumably rendering them susceptible to immune attack. It would be interesting to discover precisely when the host-protective antigens become associated with the oncospheral surface and to determine the origin of the tegument-associated proteins (i.e., whether they are derived somatically or, somehow, come to coat the tegument). It would also be important to show that the developmental characteristics seen *in vitro* are similar in parasites developing *in vivo*.

Prospects for Practical Application of Anticestode Vaccines

It is now more than 20 years since the description of the 45W vaccine for *T. ovis* [34]. There were two complementary incentives for those involved in development of the *T. ovis* vaccine: a commercial incentive on the part of the company funding the work, and the potential for *T. ovis* to act as a model for the development of vaccines against the parasite species causing neurocysticercosis and hydatid disease in humans. The *T. ovis* vaccine development program was an extraordinary success; all safety, efficacy, and commercial production work was completed, and the vaccine received registration for use as a commercial product. Nevertheless, the product has not been marketed. Much the same also holds true for the other vaccines against *T. saginata*, *T. multiceps*, *T. solium*, and *E. granulosus*. The basic difficulty with achieving commercialization has been a lack of sufficient commercial incentive for these products to be manufactured, distributed, and used. With the exception of *T. multiceps*, infections in the animal hosts of these parasites do not cause dramatic production loss or death. Problems with *T. ovis*, *T. saginata*, and *T. solium* infections typically only occur when the animals are slaughtered and the infected meat is downgraded in value or designated as unfit for consumption. By the time the animal is found to be infected at the abattoir, it may have changed owners and the individual who suffers the financial loss due to parasite infection of the carcass may not be the person who owned the animal at the time it was infected. Commonly, farmers are oblivious to their animals being infected with cestode parasites. Hence, there is little direct economic incentive for livestock owners to spend time or money to prevent taeniid cestode infections. Schemes could be imagined whereby a premium was paid for animals that were certified as being vaccinated; however, the practicalities of implementing such schemes have inhibited commercial livestock vaccine manufacturers from marketing these products. Potential exists for these vaccines to be incorporated together with other, existing commercial vaccines (e.g., the clostridial vaccines commonly used in livestock). However, the significant cost involved in registering a new combination vaccine product and the unclear economic benefit for vaccine manufacturers have meant that this option has not been adopted to date. In the case of *E. granulosus*, no economic losses can be ascribed clearly and directly to infection in livestock, and hence there is little or no economic incentive for farmers to control the disease.

The potential value of the vaccines against *T. solium* and *E. granulosus* is in their ability to reduce the transmission of the parasites, and the resultant incidence of neurocysticercosis and hydatid disease in humans. Had these parasites caused substantial economic losses directly in the livestock animals involved, it is likely that the TSOL18 and EG95 vaccines would have been adopted enthusiastically by livestock owners. However, the lack of economic incentives for the livestock owners to do anything about transmission of the associated parasites will require other approaches to be used if the vaccines are to be adopted as aids to the prevention of neurocysticercosis and hydatid disease. Substantial effort and funding has been invested over the past 50 years towards control of hydatid disease [35, 36], and in many situations the efforts have been relatively unsuccessful because of the limitations in the use or effectiveness of the methods that were available. The EG95 vaccine now offers a powerful new tool to assist with future hydatid disease control campaigns. Hydatid disease control programs have been, and will be, implemented by governments with the support of agencies such as the World Health Organization, the Food and Agriculture Organization, and the Panamerican Health Organization. Modeling of the likely value of the hydatid vaccine to control disease transmission suggests that it would improve the effectiveness of control programs and reduce the duration required for a control program to achieve a substantial reduction in disease transmission [37, 38]. Currently, relatively small-scale vaccine programs are underway in the Chubut and Rio Negro provinces in Argentina, in China, and in Sardinia; however, these are unlikely to provide clear evidence concerning the practicality and effectiveness of vaccination for control of *E. granulosus* transmission. It would be valuable to implement a medium-scale hydatid control program incorporating livestock in a region where information could be first obtained on the baseline disease prevalence and then adequately monitor disease status during the program to provide definitive data on its cost-effectiveness.

Many of the factors that limit the adoption of disease control measures for *T. solium* are the same as those for *E. granulosus*. Most importantly, there is a lack of economic incentive for pig owners to prevent the disease in their animals. There is, however, another major factor that imposes a greater limitation on the prospects for *T. solium* control. That is, the full life cycle of the parasite's transmission is restricted almost entirely to some of the poorest, least educated, and often remote people in the world. The reason for this is apparent from the mode of transmission of *T. solium*. The parasite is normally transmitted when pigs have access to human feces. The only significant variation to this pattern may be the involvement of dogs as intermediate hosts in certain parts of the world [39], although even in these places, pigs are likely to be the dominant species involved as intermediate hosts. For these reasons, the places where transmission of *T. solium* is of most importance are also those where disease control activities are limited by poor public education and community infrastructure, and weak local and national government. In addition, people in these regions typically have health problems that include malnutrition, diarrheal diseases, malaria, tuberculosis, HIV, and so on. In such situations, neurocysticercosis due to *T. solium* pales into insignificance on a population basis, even if it does not for those individuals affected. A critical factor affecting the perceived relative importance of *T. solium* is the paucity of data about the prevalence and impact of the disease. Even today, there is little quantitative information available (e.g., disability life-adjusted years), regarding the impact of neurocysticercosis that can inform governmental and nongovernmental agencies [40].

One factor that encourages control measures for *T. solium*, and hence the prospects for implementation of the TSOL18 vaccine, is the potential for the disease to be eradicated [41, 42]. The parasite's life cycle is restricted almost entirely to domestic pigs and humans. There are effective anthelmintics to remove the adult tapeworm from infected humans and now the TSOL18 vaccine provides an efficient measure for limiting or preventing transmission by pigs. Logically, implementation of control measures in both humans and pigs would eliminate the parasite [42]. Another factor that favors implementation of *T. solium* control is that the intermediate hosts do not live for long periods. Except for breeder animals, most pigs are consumed within approximately the first year of life; hence, for most animals it is not necessary to provide booster vaccinations to maintain life-long immunity. These attributes of *T. solium* suggest that investment in control measures would be likely to decrease disease transmission and, consequently, the incidence of human neurocysticercosis.

Unique Combination of Vaccination and Chemotherapy

The taeniid cestode vaccines act against the early developing metacestode; they do not affect established metacestodes. This potentially limits the value of the vaccines in areas where the parasites are hyperendemic because of the possibility that neonate animals are infected before they can be vaccinated. Theoretically, it could be possible to protect neonates via specific antibody in colostrum from vaccinated dams; however, high levels of maternally derived specific antibodies in neonates could be expected to inhibit active immunization of the young animals, as is the case with other animal and human vaccines.

In the case of *T. solium*, Gonzalez et al. discovered that a single oral treatment of pigs with 30 mg/kg of oxfendazole kills all cysticerci in the muscles of an infected pig [43]. This offers an opportunity to overcome the problem of neonatal infection with *T. solium* in pigs raised in areas where parasite transmission is hyperendemic. Pigs can be treated with oxfendazole at the time they are vaccinated, thereby removing viable, mature muscle parasites that may be pre-existing at the time of vaccination. This hypothesis was tested in a recent field trial of the TSOL18 vaccine that was carried out in Cameroon [44]. At the time when the young pigs received their second vaccination, after which they would be immune to *T. solium* infection, they were given an oral dose of 30 mg/kg oxfendazole. When the animals were assessed for *T. solium* infection at approximately 12 months of age, there was a high level of viable infection in the muscles of control pigs; however, the animals that had received both TSOL18 vaccination and oxfendazole treatment had no viable parasites in their muscles [44]. The control animals in this field trial also received oxfendazole treatment as neonates, so the difference between the treatment groups was due entirely to TSOL18 vaccination. The complete absence of any viable parasites in the vaccination-plus-oxfendazole treatment group indicated that, had any of the animals been infected prior to vaccination, the treatment combination had been effective in eliminating them.

Benzimidazole drugs are used for the treatment of hydatidosis in humans; however, they are used over long periods and are often ineffective [45]. A number of studies on the effects of various anthelmintics on hydatid disease in animals have failed to identify an effective single-dose treatment. Hence, there is no option available for an anthelmintic combination with the EG95 vaccine for young livestock animals that could eliminate established hydatid cysts existing at the time the animals were first vaccinated. Most investigations of the effects of anthelmintics on hydatid cysts in animals have used naturally infected animals that have had mature hydatid cysts. If a strategy were to be used involving vaccination plus chemotherapy against *E. granulosus* in young animals, any cysts existing at the time of vaccination could only be quite immature. The potential for single-dose treatment of immature hydatid cysts in sheep is currently under investigation using oxfendazole, albendazole, and/or praziquantel in animals having 2- to 3-month-old experimentally induced infections with *E. granulosus* (Lightowlers and Gauci, unpublished). Initially two anthelmintic treatments are being given 1 month apart at the highest nontoxic dose known for these chemicals. Two treatments are being used because if the treatment were to be incorporated as part of a vaccination program, animals are required to receive two immunizations, hence there are two opportunities to give anthelmintic without requiring any corralling or handling of the animals beyond what would already be taking place as part of the vaccination program. The results of this initial experiment will be known at the end of 2012.

Conclusions

Experience with the development of anticestode vaccines offers a number of lessons, both practical and salutary, for those interested in vaccination against other parasitic diseases. Most importantly, the effectiveness of the anticestode vaccines indicates unequivocally that it is possible to achieve a high level of protection against a complex eukaryotic parasite using a simple, defined antigen vaccine. Somewhat surprisingly, however, the principal hurdles on the path to implementing a vaccine control strategy for cysticercosis and hydatid disease are commercial, political, and practical, rather than issues associated with developing effective vaccines *per se*. As outlined in this volume, many research programs are underway for vaccines for other parasitic diseases, for which the major hurdle is achieving a reliable and significant level or protection. More attention may be warranted by researchers and funding agencies about the attributes of a vaccine that would be required for it to be a practical success against the various parasitic diseases being investigated. In cases where these attributes are unattainable or extremely unlikely to be attained, it may be useful to reassess research priorities and question whether vaccine-related research is a worthwhile investment.

The TSOL18 vaccine against *T. solium* and the EG95 vaccine against *E. granulosus* are almost 100% effective, provide an effective duration of protection, and can be manufactured inexpensively. Whether these attributes will ever overcome the lack of a strong economic incentive for livestock owners to use the vaccines remains to be seen. Certainly, the vaccines have the potential to contribute to disease control programs leading to a substantial reduction in human morbidity and mortality due to neurocysticercosis and cystic hydatid disease. It is to be hoped that this potential is realized through the investment by philanthropic and development agencies, and by the governments of those countries for which these diseases are major public health problems.

Acknowledgments

The authors wish to acknowledge research support from the National Health and Medical Research Council of Australia and the Wellcome Trust.

References

1 Lightowlers, M.W. (2006) Cestode vaccines: origins, current status and future prospects. *Parasitology*, **133**, S27–S42.

2 Petavy, A.F., Hormaeche, C., Lahmar, S., Ouhelli, H., Chabalgoity, A., Marchal, T., Azzouz, S., Schreiber, F. *et al.* (2008) An oral recombinant vaccine in dogs against *Echinococcus granulosus*, the causative agent of human hydatid disease: a pilot study. *PLoS Negl. Trop. Dis.*, **2**, e125.

3 Zhang, W., Zhang, Z., Shi, B., Li, J., You, H., Tulson, G., Dang, X., Song, Y. *et al.* (2006) Vaccination of dogs against *Echinococcus granulosus*, the cause of cystic hydatid disease in humans. *J. Infect. Dis.*, **194**, 966–974.

4 Torgerson, P.R. (2008) Dogs, vaccines and *Echinococcus*. *Trends Parasitol.*, **25**, 57–58.

5 Sciutto, E., Rosas, G., Cruz-Revilla, C., Toledo, A., Cervantes, J., Hernandez, M., Hernandez, B., Goldbaum, F.A. *et al.* (2007) Renewed hope for a vaccine against the intestinal adult *Taenia solium*. *J. Parasitol.*, **93**, 824–831.

6 León-Cabrera, S., Cruz-Rivera, M., Mendlovic, F., Ávila-Ramírez, G., and Flisser, A. (2009) Standardization of an experimental model of human taeniosis for oral vaccination. *Methods*, **49**, 346–350.

7 Jenkins, D.J. and Rickard, M.D. (1985) Specific antibody responses to *Taenia hydatigena*, *Taenia pisiformis* and *Echinococcus granulosus* infection in dogs. *Aust. Vet. J.*, **62**, 72–78.

8 Gemmell, M.A., Lawson, J.R., and Roberts, M.G. (1986) Population dynamics in echinococcosis and cysticercosis: biological parameters of *Echinococcus granulosus* in dogs and sheep. *Parasitology*, **92**, 599–620.

9 Miller, H.M. Jr (1931) Immunity of the albino rat to superinfestation with

Cysticercus fasciolaris. J. Prev. Med., **5**, 453–464.

10 Mitchell, G.F. (1990) A note on concomitant immunity in host–parasite relationships: a successfully transplanted concept from tumor immunology. *Adv. Cancer Res.*, **54**, 319–332.

11 Rickard, M.D. and Williams, J.F. (1982) Hydatidosis/cysticercosis: immune mechanisms and immunization against infection. *Adv. Parasitol.*, **21**, 229–296.

12 Lightowlers, M.W. (2010) Fact or hypothesis: concomitant immunity in taeniid cestode infections. *Parasite Immunol.*, **32**, 582–589.

13 Cox, F.E.G. (1993) Milestones in parasitology. *Parasitol. Today*, **9**, 347–348.

14 Lightowlers, M.W., Gauci, C.G., Chow, C., Drew, D.R., Gauci, S.M., Heath, D.D., Jackson, D.C., Dadley-Moore, D.L. *et al.* (2003) Molecular and genetic characterisation of the host-protective oncosphere antigens of taeniid cestode parasites. *Int. J. Parasitol.*, **33**, 1207–1217.

15 Harrison, G.B., Shakes, T.R., Robinson, C.M., Lawrence, S.B., Heath, D.D., Dempster, R.P., Lightowlers, M.W., and Rickard, M.D. (1999) Duration of immunity, efficacy and safety in sheep of a recombinant *Taenia ovis* vaccine formulated with saponin or selected adjuvants. *Vet. Immunol. Immunopathol.*, **70**, 161–172.

16 Heath, D.D., Jensen, O., and Lightowlers, M.W. (2003) Progress in control of hydatidosis using vaccination – a review of formulation and delivery of the vaccine and recommendations for practical use in control programmes. *Acta Trop.*, **85**, 133–143.

17 Rickard, M.D. and Bell, K.J. (1971) Immunity produced against *Taenia ovis* and *T. taeniaeformis* infection in lambs and rats following *in vivo* growth of their larvae in filtration membrane diffusion chambers. *J. Parasitol.*, **57**, 571–575.

18 Jabbar, A., Crawford, S., Gauci, C.G., Walduck, A.K., Anderson, G.A., and Lightowlers, M.W. (2010) Oncospheral penetration glands and secretory blebs are the source of *Taenia ovis v*accine antigens. *Infect. Immun.*, **78**, 4363–4373.

19 Engelkirk, P.G. and Williams, J.F. (1982) *Taenia taeniaeformis* (Cestoda) in the rat: ultrastructure of the host–parasite interface on days 1 to 7 postinfection. *J. Parasitol.*, **68**, 620–633.

20 Engelkirk, P.G. and Williams, J.F. (1983) *Taenia taeniaeformis* (Cestoda) in the rat: ultrastructure of the host–parasite interface on days 8 to 22 postinfection. *J. Parasitol.*, **69**, 828–837.

21 Mitchell, G.F., Goding, J.W., and Rickard, M.D. (1977) Studies on immune responses to larval cestodes in mice. Increased susceptibility of certain mouse strains and hypothymic mice to *Taenia taeniaeformis* and analysis of passive transfer of resistance with serum. *Aust. J. Exp. Biol. Med. Sci.*, **55**, 165–186.

22 Heath, D.D. (1973) Resistance to *Taenia pisiformis* larvae in rabbits. II. Temporal relationships and the development phase affected. *Int. J. Parasitol.*, **3**, 491–498.

23 Bork, P. and Doolittle, R.F. (1993) Fibronectin type III modules in the receptor phosphatase CD45 and tapeworm antigens. *Protein Sci.*, **2**, 1185–1187.

24 Koide, A., Bailey, C.W., Huang, X., and Koide, S. (1998) The fibronectin type III domain as a scaffold for novel binding proteins. *J. Mol. Biol.*, **284**, 1141–1151.

25 Tucker, R.P. and Chiquet-Ehrismann, R. (2009) Evidence for the evolution of tenascin and fibronectin early in the chordate lineage. *Int. J. Biochem. Cell. Biol.*, **41**, 424–434.

26 Bencharit, S., Cui, C.B., Siddiqui, A., Howard-Williams, E.L., Sondek, J., Zuobi-Hasona, K., and Aukhil, I. (2007) Structural insights into fibronectin type III domain-mediated signaling. *J. Mol. Biol.*, **367**, 303–309.

27 Main, A.L., Harvey, T.S., Baron, M., Boyd, J., and Campbell, I.D. (1992) The three-dimensional structure of the tenth type III module of fibronectin: an insight into RGD-mediated interactions. *Cell*, **71**, 671–678.

28 Potts, J.R. and Campbell, I.D. (1996) Structure and function of fibronectin modules. *Matrix Biol.*, **15**, 313–320.

29 Bole-Feysot, C., Goffin, V., Edery, M., Binart, N., and Kelly, P.A. (1998) Prolactin (PRL) and its receptor: actions, signal transduction pathways and phenotypes observed in PRL receptor knockout mice. *Endocrinol. Rev.*, **19**, 225–268.

30 Jabbar, A., Kyngdon, C.T., Gauci, C.G., Walduck, A.K., McCowan, C., Jones, M.K., Beveridge, I., and Lightowlers, M.W. (2010) Localisation of three host-protective oncospheral antigens of *Taenia ovis*. *Int. J. Parasitol.*, **40**, 579–589.

31 Jabbar, A., Verastegui, M., Lackenby, J.A., Walduck, A.K., Gauci, C.G., Gilman, R.H., and Lightowlers, M.W. (2010) Variation in the cellular localization of host-protective oncospheral antigens in *Taenia saginata* and *Taenia solium*. *Parasite Immunol.*, **32**, 684–695.

32 Jabbar, A., Jenkins, D.J., Crawford, S., Walduck, A.K., Gauci, C.G., and Lightowlers, M.W. (2011) Oncospheral penetration glands are the source of the EG95 vaccine antigen against cystic hydatid disease. *Parasitology*, **138**, 89–99.

33 Jabbar, A., Crawford, S., Mlocicki, D., Swiderski, Z.P., Conn, D.B., Jones, M.K., Beveridge, I., and Lightowlers, M.W. (2010) Ultrastructural reconstruction of *Taenia ovis* oncospheres from serial sections. *Int. J. Parasitol.*, **40**, 1419–1431.

34 Johnson, K.S., Harrison, G.B., Lightowlers, M.W., O'Hoy, K.L., Cougle, W.G., Dempster, R.P., Lawrence, S.B., Vinton, J.G. *et al.* (1989) Vaccination against ovine cysticercosis using a defined recombinant antigen. *Nature*, **338**, 585–587.

35 Murrell, K.D.E. (2005) *WHO/FAO/OIE Guidelines for the Surveillance, Prevention and Control of Taeniasis/Cysticercosis*, WHO/FAO/OIE, Paris.

36 Craig, P.S., McManus, D.P., Lightowlers, M.W., Chabalgoity, J.A., Garcia, H.H., Gavidia, C.M., Gilman, R.H., Gonzalez, A.E. *et al.* (2007) Prevention and control of cystic echinococcosis. *Lancet Infect. Dis.*, **7**, 385–394.

37 Torgerson, P.R. (2003) The use of mathematical models to simulate control options for echinococcosis. *Acta Trop.*, **85**, 211–221.

38 Torgerson, P.R. (2006) Mathematical models for the control of cystic echinococcosis. *Parasitol. Int.*, **55**, S253–S258.

39 Ito, A., Putra, M.I., Subahar, R., Sato, M.O., Okamoto, M., Sako, Y., Nakao, M., Yamasaki, H. *et al.* (2002) Dogs as alternative intermediate hosts of *Taenia solium* in Papua (Irian Jaya), Indonesia confirmed by highly specific ELISA and immunoblot using native and recombinant antigens and mitochondrial DNA analysis. *J. Helminthol.*, **76**, 311–314.

40 Bern, C., Garcia, H.H., Evans, C., Gonzalez, A.E., Verastegui, M., Tsang, V.C., and Gilman, R.H. (1999) Magnitude of the disease burden from neurocysticercosis in a developing country. *Clin. Infect. Dis.*, **29**, 1203–1209.

41 Lightowlers, M.W. (1999) Eradication of *Taenia solium* cysticercosis: a role for vaccination of pigs. *Int. J. Parasitol.*, **29**, 811–817.

42 Lightowlers, M.W. (2010) Eradication of *Taenia solium* cysticercosis: a role for vaccination of pigs. *Int. J. Parasitol.*, **40**, 1183–1192.

43 Gonzales, A.E., Garcia, H.H., Gilman, R.H., Gavidia, C.M., Tsang, V.C., Bernal, T., Falcon, N., Romero, M. *et al.* (1996) Effective, single-dose treatment or porcine cysticercosis with oxfendazole. *Am. J. Trop. Med. Hyg.*, **54**, 391–394.

44 Assana, E., Kyngdon, C.T., Gauci, C.G., Geerts, S., Dorny, P., De Deken, R., Anderson, G.A., Zoli, A.P. *et al.* (2010) Elimination of *Taenia solium* transmission to pigs in a field trial of the TSOL18 vaccine in Cameroon. *Int. J. Parasitol.*, **40**, 515–519.

45 Brunetti, E. and Junghanss, T. (2009) Update on cystic hydatid disease. *Curr. Opin. Infect. Dis.*, **22**, 497–502.

46 Lightowlers, M.W., Waterkeyn, J.G., Rothel, J.S., Gauci, C.G., and Harrison, G.B. (1996) Host-protective fragments and antibody binding epitopes

of the *Taenia ovis* 45W recombinant antigen. *Parasite Immunol.*, **18**, 507–513.

47 Harrison, G.B., Heath, D.D., Dempster, R.P., Gauci, C., Newton, S.E., Cameron, W.G., Robinson, C.M., Lawrence, S.B. *et al.* (1996) Identification and cDNA cloning of two novel low molecular weight host-protective antigens from *Taenia ovis* oncospheres. *Int. J. Parasitol.*, **26**, 195–204.

48 Gauci, C., Vural, G., Oncel, T., Varcasia, A., Damian, V., Kyngdon, C.T., Craig, P.S., Anderson, G.A. *et al.* (2008) Vaccination with recombinant oncosphere antigens reduces the susceptibility of sheep to infection with *Taenia multiceps*. *Int. J. Parasitol.*, **38**, 1041–1050.

49 Lightowlers, M.W., Rolfe, R., and Gauci, C.G. (1996) *Taenia saginata*: vaccination against cysticercosis in cattle with recombinant oncosphere antigens. *Exp. Parasitol.*, **84**, 330–338.

50 Flisser, A., Gauci, C.G., Zoli, A., Martinez-Ocana, J., Garza-Rodriguez, A., Dominguez-Alpizar, J.L., Maravilla, P., Rodriguez-Canul, R. *et al.* (2004) Induction of protection against porcine cysticercosis by vaccination with recombinant oncosphere antigens. *Infect. Immun.*, **72**, 5292–5297.

51 Lightowlers, M.W., Lawrence, S.B., Gauci, C.G., Young, J., Ralston, M.J., Maas, D., and Health, D.D. (1996) Vaccination against hydatidosis using a defined recombinant antigen. *Parasite Immunol.*, **18**, 457–462.

52 Gauci, C., Merli, M., Muller, V., Chow, C., Yagi, K., Mackenstedt, U., and Lightowlers, M.W. (2002) Molecular cloning of a vaccine antigen against infection with the larval stage of *Echinococcus multilocularis*. *Infect. Immun.*, **70**, 3969–3972.

Index

a

AAD-1566. *See* monepantel
AAD sensitivity   289, 294
abamectin   238, 239, 285, 302, 305
ABCG2 transporter   245
ABC transport proteins   33
abomasum   294, 303, 409
Acanthocheilonema viteae jird model   378
ACC-1. *See* acetylcholine-gated chloride channel
acetylcholine (ACh)   4, 234, 237, 293
acetylcholine-gated chloride channel   8, 11, 12
AC2 gene   28
acoelomate   106, 423
Acrobeles   26
activation-associated secreted protein (ASP)   409
adjuvants block copolymer (BC)   387
adult worm motility (AWM) assays   141
albendazole   185, 192, 220, 222, 241, 255, 268, 273, 276, 358, 364, 380, 499
Alhydrogel®   429
alternatively activated macrophages (AAMFs)   475
aluminum hydroxide   428
amidantel   206
amino-acetonitrile derivatives (AADs)   4, 32, 137, 234, 283
– biological target of   286
– chemical structure of   284
– mis-splicing mutations   292
γ-aminobutyric acid (GABA)   4
aminolevulinic acid dehydratase (ALAD)   260
aminopeptidase   412
4-aminopiperidine   149
aminotransferase (AST)   470
amoscanate   243
Ancylostoma caninum   34, 46, 243, 365, 401
Ancylostoma ceylanicum   271, 349

Ancylostoma duodenale   25, 46, 61, 184, 271, 347, 364
anthelmintics   3, 234, 421
– adoption of mechanism-based screens   125
– agents   24
– approval, by WHO   268
– benzimidazole   222
– chitinase inhibitor/ionophore   241, 242
– cholinergic agonists   243–245
– cholinergic antagonists   238
– compound screening   144
– Cry protein   269
– drug discovery (*See also* drug development process)
– GABA agonist   240
– gene carrying resistance   244
– glutamate-gated chloride ion channels (GluCls)   239, 240
– on hydatid disease in animals   499
– innate immune response inhibitor   242
– isothiocyanate-ATP inhibition   243
– mechanism-based screens for   126
– modes of action   234, 235
– – AADs (monepantel)   237, 238
– – cholinergic agonists   234–237
– optimization   148–152
– pharmacokinetics   211
– postinfection and efficacy   192
– potency of Cry5B   273
– resistance to   5, 244
– SH ligand   242
– SLO-1 potassium channel activator   240
– target sites   5, 6
– trematocidal drugs, development   326
– triclabendazole   452
– types of   233, 234
– veterinary   220, 223, 229
antibody-dependent cellular cytotoxicity (ADCC)   379, 384, 454, 455, 466, 475, 477

anticancer drugs 125
antifilarial therapy
– anti-*Wolbachia* treatment 252–254
– doxycycline, indications 254, 255
antifilarial vaccine development 377–391
– animal models 383, 384
– – for lymphatic filariae vaccine studies 384–387
– – for *Onchocerca volvulus* vaccine studies 387, 388
– – using nonhuman parasites in rodents 388
– antipathology vaccine 382, 383
– antitransmission vaccine 383
– bovine onchocerciasis 380, 381
– comparative vaccine studies 388, 389
– current status 383
– feline filariasis 381
– immunity 378, 379
– multivalent vaccines 389
– new vaccine candidates, discovery 389–391
– panhelmintic vaccine 383
– prophylactic vaccines 382
anti-fluke vaccines 74
antigen
– complex 404
– production and delivery approaches 409
antihelminth vaccines, candidates development 367
anti-HIV therapy 275
anti-L3 vaccine 381
antioxidant enzymes, immunolocalization studies 438
antioxidants 80
– vaccines 471
antipathology vaccine 382, 383
antiprotozoals 327
antitransmission vaccine 383
anti-*Wolbachia* consortium (A·WOL) 251, 252
– assay development/screening strategy 256, 257
– drug regimen refinement 256
– effective antifilarial therapy 252–254
– library screening
– – anti-infective 259
– – diversity-based 259
– – registered drug 257, 258
– – target discovery 259–262
– lipid II biosynthesis 261
– new chemical entities (NCEs) 259
– screening strategy 257
– second-generation 256
– treatment
– – cost- and time-effective strategy 257
– – stunted *L. sigmodontis* larvae 258

aquaporin (Ce-AQP-2) 96
Artemisia cina 233
artemisinin 77
Ascaridia galli 25, 33, 141–143
Ascaridida 67
Ascaris lumbricoides 233
Ascaris suum 13, 26, 61, 128, 234
aspartic protease (APR) 365, 401, 405
Aspergillus niger 128
Asu-unc-8 237
Asu-unc-63 237
autoimmune diseases 455
automated phenotype analysis 166–168
– for drug screening against 168
avermectins 32, 239, 240
avr-15 gene 32
avr-14 mutant 33
axon terminal 287
Aztecs 234

b
Babesia bovis 107
Bacillus thuringiensis crystal (Cry) proteins 267–276
– antiroundworm activity 274
– for *C. elegans* to resist 275, 276
– Cry21A protein in mice 273, 274
– free-livingroundworms, intoxicate 270
– hookworm parasite, *in vitro* and *in vivo* 271–273
– hypersusceptibility studies 274, 275
– intoxicate animal-parasitic roundworms *ex vivo* 270, 271
– intoxicate plant-parasitic roundworms 270
– mechanism of action 269, 270
– and nAChR agonists, synergy 275
– plant-parasitic nematodes feed 270
– safety of 268, 269
– single-dose therapy of *H. bakeri* 273
– therapeutic activity 271
1,3-benzenedioic acid 149
benzimadazoles 92
benzimidazole-bound αβ-heterodimers 241
benzimidazoles 24, 29, 136, 139, 150, 241, 245, 284, 285, 346, 499
bioinformatics, recent developments in 14, 53, 62
biological image analysis 162
– algorithmic approach 173
– CART algorithm 175
– image capture 163
– image segmentation 163–166
– – algorithms for schistosome 168–172
– – for filarial parasites for HTS 172, 173

- parasite tracking   164
- quantitative phenotyping   164, 165, 173–175
- resources   162
- results from classifier using data from videos   175
- tracking algorithm   173–175
- workflow for drug screening   162, 163
BLAST   47, 63, 288
bovine abomasum   409
bovine onchocerciasis   380, 381
Brugia malayi   5, 45, 92, 128, 136, 252
- heat-shock protein   128, 129
- image segmentation of   172
- recombinant myosin   384
- target prioritization, using TDR targets database   54
Brugia pahangi   381
β-tubulin ligands   92, 245
- benzimidazole resistance   245

c

Caenorhabditis briggsae   13, 27, 63
Caenorhabditis elegans   4, 24, 63, 161, 234, 269, 285, 298, 329, 399
- acr-23, discovery of   294
- *ben-1* mutant   29
- chloride currents in   32
- cholinergic receptor of   236
- comparative pharmacology of   30
- functional genomics using   90, 91
- genetic screening   289
- genome encodes   241
- GluCl genes   240
- glutamate-gated chloride channels   92
- gut and secretory system   401
- high-throughput chemical screening and   203
- lat-1/lat-2 genes   33
- levamisole receptor channels   31
- macrocyclic lactone sensitivity   245
- mutagenesis screen   240
- mutants resistant   276
- orthology-based RNAi phenotype data mapping   50–52
-- OrthoMCL database   50
-- TDR Targets database   51
-- WormBase database   51
- parasitic nematode genes, expressed in   28
- PF1022A and emodepside inhibited locomotion of   33
- as platform
-- for anthelmintic characterization   202, 203
-- for anthelmintic drug discovery   203–205
-- for target discovery   34, 35
- to resist   275, 276
- sensitive to thiabendazole   29
- as tool to understand mode of   31–34
- vaccine antigens expression   410–412
- wild-type   275
- xenobiotics   205–207, 212, 213
calcium antagonists   313
calcium blockers   314
calcium channel hypothesis   313
calcium signaling cascade   236, 243
calpain   111
carcinogens   74
cathelicidin-like helminth defense molecule   452, 457–459
cathepsin B   478
- like cysteine protease genes   402
- vaccine   406
cathepsin B2   468
- advantages   469
cathepsins L   468, 469
- cysteine peptidases   453–455
cDNA library   66, 389, 437
Cel-ACR-23 receptor   290, 291
cell-free protein expression systems   425, 426
Cephalobidae   26
Ce-PHI-10   96
cestode infection
- in humans and livestock   191
- hybrid vaccines for   473, 485, 487, 488
- infection models   189
- RNAi   113, 332
- selected compounds in rodent models   192
- taeniid cestode vaccines   498
cestode parasites vaccines   485–500
- against cestode infections in intermediate hosts   487, 488
- development, strategy   488, 489
- existing, effective, recombinant vaccines   489
- fibronectin type III domains   491, 492
- host-protective antigens characteristics   489, 490
- practical application prospects   496–498
- protective antigens   490
-- oncosphere structure and localization   493–496
- protective immune responses, evidence for   488
- stage-specific expression   491
- vaccination and chemotherapy, combination   498, 499
- vaccine development in definitive hosts   487
chemistry-to-gene screens   14, 15

chemotherapy 357–369, 436
– based morbidity control 426
Chenopodium ambrosioides 233, 234
chitinase 128
cholangiocarcinoma (CCA) 74
choline concentration–response curve 290
cholinergic agonists 235
cloning vaccine candidates 390
clonorchiasis 324
Clonorchis sinensis 74, 79, 80, 189, 324
closantel 241, 242
cofactor-dependent phosphoglycerate mutase (dPGM) 261
cofactor-independent PGM (iPGM) 261
combination vaccines 472, 473
combinatorial chemistry 125
commercial vaccine, development 477
comparative genome analyses 25, 44, 67
complement-fixing circulating antibodies 489
complex eukaryotic expression vectors 366
concomitant immunity 485
Cooperia oncophora 34, 46, 140
CoPs 348, 349, 354
– reproducibility 354
crop protection 24
Cry21A protein 273
Cry6A proteins 270
Cry5B proteins 270, 272, 273
Cry5B–TBD 275
Cry proteins 268–271, 274, 275
Cryptosporidium 242
Cry6 subfamily protein (Cry6A) 270
current Good Manufacturing Practice (cGMP) 343, 344, 350
cyclo-octadepsipeptide 33
cyclooxygenase pathway 242
Cys-Loop LGIC Complex 4, 5, 15
– *Drosophila melanogaster* 12
– eukaryotic 15
– first crystal structure of 15
– LGC-44, represent ancestral 12
– superfamilies of other nematodes 13, 14
Cys-loop LGIC gene superfamily 13
Cys-loop superfamily 287
cysteine peptidase inhibitors 455
cysteine proteases 330, 365, 406–408, 409
cysticercosis 106
cystic hydatidosis 488
cyst nematodes 35
cytochalasin D (CyD) 314
cytochrome P450 (CYP) 329
cytotoxic drugs 125
cytotoxicity 152

d
daf-16 gene 30
Danio rerio 161
Database of Essential Genes (DEG) 259
DEG-3/DES-2 oligomer 293
2-deoxy-paraherquamide 297, 299
– animal safety studies, pivotal target 303–305
– commercialization 305
– – derquantel scale-up 305
– – registration/launch 305
– mode of action 301, 302
– PNU-141962, characterization 298–301
– *in vivo* (Jird)/*in vitro* effects against 300
depsipeptides 137
derquantel 206, 238
– toxicity of 300
dicarboxylic acid 149
Dicrocoeliidae 74
diethylcarbamazine 123, 125, 242
– contraindications 380
Digenea 73
Diphyllobothrium latum 315
Diplogasterida 25
Dirofilaria immitis 14, 254, 377
disrupted phenotype 148
dithiothreitol (DTT) 408
DNA
– damage 74
– immunization 387
– microarrays 423
– sequencing 438
– vaccination 409
– vaccines 409, 410, 429
DNA-directed RNA polymerase 260
dog heart worm 254
dominant type 2 immune responses 474
dopamine 4
dose-reduction index (DRI) values 275
dose–response curves 350
double-stranded RNAi 14
doxycycline 255, 256
draft genome sequences 422
Drosophila melanogaster 7, 63, 161
– Cys-loop LGICs 12
DrugBank database 260
drug development process 125, 220
– chemistry, manufacturing, and controls (CMC) aspect 225, 226
– clinical trials 226, 227
– CROs, role of 228
– discovery of hit molecule against 223, 224
– drug development program and amendments 229

– funding   228
– nonprofit organizations, role in (*See* product development partnerships (PDPs))
– NTD drug development   228
– preclinical studies   224, 225
– regulatory considerations   227, 228
– stages   223, 224
drug–pathogen interactions   160
drug resistance   298, 316
dual-component vaccine   472
Dugesia japonica   313
dyf genes   239

e

Echinococcus granulosus   46, 191, 441, 471, 485, 486, 487, 490
Echinococcus multilocularis   46, 113, 191, 326, 486, 489, 490
Echinostoma caproni   189, 191, 192, 327
egg hatch test (EHT)   138, 139
egg reduction rates (ERRs)   328
EG95 vaccine   497, 499, 500
electroporation   97, 111
ELT-2 polypeptide   29
emodepside   33, 137, 240
endoplasmic reticulum   237, 244
– degeneration of   241
– receptor protein   244
enzyme-linked immunosorbent assay analyses   406
epitopes   383
– prediction algorithms   390
Escherichia coli   91, 126, 140, 261, 270, 344, 405, 428, 441, 458, 470, 489
EST and genome sequence data   403
ethyl methane sulfonate   8
eukaryotic parasites   485
EuPathDB   44
excretory/secretory (ES) products   390, 452, 470
exogenous proteins   428
expressed sequence tag (EST) sequences   26, 44, 62
expression system   410, 411

f

Fasciola gigantica   74, 75, 191, 438, 466
Fasciola hepatica   74, 189, 191, 241, 327, 436
Fascioliasis   191, 435–437
Fasciolidae   74
fasciolid liver flukes, life cycles   76
fasciolosis   465
fatty acid-binding protein (FABP)   436, 437
– binding of drugs   440

fecal egg count reduction test   303, 304
feline filariasis   381
fenbendazole   24, 136
fibronectin type III (FnIII) domain   491
filamentous processes   493
filarial-infected vectors   378
filarial nematodes   92, 251–262
– disease-causing species   252
– first-stage larvae of   254
– macrofilaricidal drug for   252
filariasis
– automated phenotype analysis for drug   168
– causing organisms (*See Wuchereria bancrofti*)
– chemotherapy of   128
– lymphatic   187, 188, 254–256, 262, 360–362, 378–389
Filarioidea   160
fktf-1 gene   29
flatworms. *See Clonorchis sinensis; Onchocerca volvulus*
flubendazole   157, 233, 241
FMRFamide   129
food-borne zoonosis   477
Freund's Complete adjuvant (FCA)   384, 468, 473
fusion proteins   440, 441

g

GABA-gated chloride channels   9, 32
GABA receptor cation channels   11
Galba truncatula   452
gastrointestinal nematode parasites of humans   184
– disease and impact   184, 186
– hookworm infection
– – Rockefeller Sanitary Commission for eradication   220
– – and rodent models   186, 187
gastrointestinal parasites of livestock   61
GeneDB   44
gene silencing   14
– by RNAi   412
genetic heterogeneity   473
genetic manipulation tools   424
gene-to-gene variability   111
genome-sequencing projects   13
genomics   14
genotoxicity   152
Global Access Strategy   362, 367
Global Network for Neglected Tropical Disease Control   367
Globodera rostochiensis   29
GluCl genes   8, 240, 245
GluCl modulators   244, 245

glutamate-gated chloride channels
  (GluCls)   4, 32, 92
γ-glutamyl transferase (GGT)   470
glutathione S-transferase (GST)   361, 384,
  408, 437, 439, 466
glyceraldehyde-3-phosphate dehydrogenase
  (GAPDH) gene   29
Glycine max   35
glycosylphosphatidylinositol (GPI)   492
gpd gene   29
gpd-3 gene   29
G-protein-coupled receptors (GPCRs)   127,
  330, 331
granulin   79
green fluorescent protein (GFP)   29, 289
growth factor receptor-binding protein 2
  (GRB2)   79

h

Haemonchus contortus   25, 26, 61, 90,
  124, 136, 143, 237, 271, 283, 291, 399,
  403, 404, 411
– cysteine proteases   406–408
– microsomal aminopeptidase from
  403, 404
hamster model   271, 349
H. bakeri   272–274
Hco-acr-8   237
Hco-AVR-14   14
Hco-deg-2   237
Hco-deg-3   237
Hco-deg-3H   244
Hco-des-2H   244
Hco-GGR-3 (dopamine)   14
Hco-lgc-38   26
Hco-LGC-55 (tyramine)   14
Hco-mptl-1   237, 244, 292
H. contortus   13, 14, 28, 29, 33, 34, 64, 91, 96,
  97, 126, 140, 144, 184, 237, 243, 244, 284,
  291, 294, 402, 403, 406, 411, 412
– *acr-23*   237
Hco-unc-29.1   237
Hco-unc-38   237
Hco-unc-63a   237
Hco-unc-63b   243
healthcare delivery systems   369
heat-shock protein   128
– neuromuscular targets in   129, 130
helical wheel analysis   458
helminth defense molecule (HDM)-1   458
Hereford calves   471
Heterodera glycines   35
H-gal-GP   404, 405
high-throughput screening (HTS)   160

hookworm vaccine
– bioassay for potency   349
– human immune response   347–349
– infection, natural history   347
– NTD vaccines   346, 347, 349–354
– potency assay   344–346
– preclinical development   343–354
– preclinical testing   349
– valley of darkness   350, 351
host immune effector molecules   390
host immune responses   426, 459
host immune system   402
host–parasite systems   388
host-protective antigens   490, 494
host's immune effector cells   456
H. polygyrus   273
H11 protein   97
5-HT channels   11
human drug pharmacopeia screen   258
human ether-a-go-go related gene
  (hERG)   329
human hookworm vaccine   369
– PDP strategy   368
human papilloma virus (HPV) vaccines   368
hydatid disease   497, 499
hyperpolarization   240
hypersusceptibility   275

i

IgE-mediated disorders   349
IgG antibody   348, 365, 470
– cleavage   402
IgG4 isotype   454
Illumina technology   66, 78
image analysis workflow, for drug
  screening   162. *See also* biological image
  analysis
imidazolides   298
imidazothiazoles   24, 136, 234
immobilized metal-affinity
  chromatography   441
immune modulation mechanisms   451–460
immune regulatory networks   379
immune responses   488
– kinetics   380
– level and type   382
immunity   378, 379, 473–475
immunization challenge model   345
– requirements   345
immunization experiments   440
immunization protocols   388, 389
immunoelectron microscopy   469
immunogold methods   493
immunolocalization, of Sm14 protein   439

immunoprophylaxis   437, 465–478
individual drug administration (IDA)   255
– current recommended treatment strategies for   253
Indonesian thin tail (ITT)   466
inflammatory bowel disease (IBD)   459
innovative developing countries (IDCs)   367
interferon (IFN)-γ   473
intestinal fluke infections   324
intestinal schistosomiasis   422
intracellular protein   438
investigational new drug (IND)   327
in vivo biological assays   351
in vivo RNAi, development   410
iron deficiency anemia (IDA)   347
ivermectin   7, 15, 24, 137, 297
– *Hcavr-14* (*HcGluCla3*), involved in   33
– to nematode Cys-loop LGICs   15
– resistance   360
– sensitivity in *C. elegans*   7
– triple mutant, avr-14/avr-15/glc-1, resistant to   32
– use in onchocerciasis   359

k

Kato–Katz diagnostic technique   310
KCNMA1 gene   34

l

LAP vaccine   469–471
larval development assay (LDA)   283
larval migration inhibition test (LMIT)   139
larval paralysis test (LPT)   140
laser microdissection microscopy (LMM)   423
latrophilin receptor *(lat-2)*   33, 240
Leishmania major   107
leucine amino peptidase (LAP) vaccine   401, 466, 469–471
lev-1   236
lev-8   236
lev-9   237
lev-10   237
LEV-11   15, 236, 243
levamisole   8, 24, 31, 136, 236, 237, 285
– resistance   236, 243, 244
– targets   288
levamisole receptors   31, 236, 243
– UNC-22   15, 236
– *unc-29*   236, 243
– *unc-38*   236, 243
– *unc-50*   237
– *unc-63*   236, 243
– UNC-68   15, 236, 243
– *unc-74*   237

levant wormseed   233
L-glutamate   7
ligand-gated anion channels   7, 26
– LGC-32   12
– LGC-33   12
– LGC-34   12, 14
– LGC-35   11
– LGC-40   12
– LGC-42   12
– LGC-45   12
– LGC-50   11
– LGC-53   12
lipooxygenase   242
lipophilicity   151
lipopolysaccharide (LPS)   454
lipoproteins   261
liquid chromatography-tandem mass spectrometry   424
Litomosoides carinii   188
Litomosoides sigmodontis   255, 383
liver flukes   73, 74, 324, 451. *See also Fasciola hepatica*; fasciolosis
– life cycles   76
– omics research of   79–81
– signs and pathological changes associated with   75
– socioeconomic importance   75
– transcriptomic studies   77–79
– – resources   79
L3 surface-specific antibodies   379
lung fluke. *See Paragonimus westermani*
Lymnaea stagnalis   12
Lymnaea truncatula   452
lymphatic filariasis   187, 188, 256, 360–362, 378, 382
– natural host–parasite systems   380
– vaccine   361, 385, 386

m

macrocyclic lactones   24, 136, 137, 239, 244
macrofilaricidal activity   254
macrophages   456, 459
– endosomes   460
– populations characteristics   457
Malachite Green   128
Manduca sexta   161
Mansonella perstans   254
marcfortine A   298, 299
marcfortine G ring   298
mass drug administration (MDA)   186, 221, 251, 357, 358, 361, 369, 377, 380, 382, 391, 421
– strategies for   253
mebendazole   241

median effective dose (ED$_{50}$) method 351
mefloquine 328, 329
meiosis 285
melarsamine 242
Meloidogyne arenaria 25, 26
Meriones unguiculatus 283
MEROPS peptidase database 470
metacercariae vaccine 472
metacestodes 494
micro agar larval development test (MALDT) 140
microarray analysis 44
microfilariae 378
microfilaricidal drugs 254
microtubules 92, 241
miracidium 107
MOD-1 (modulation of locomotion defective) 11
modified T$_h$2 response 347, 348
monepantel 137, 283–294
– acetylcholine receptors 294
– ACR-23 channel modulator 291
– amino-acetonitrile derivatives, discovery of 283, 284
– commercial formulation 284
– efficacy of 284, 285
– hypothetical interaction 294
– interference, hypothetical model of 293
– mode of action 285–288
– – *Cel*-ACR-23 receptor, functional characterization 290, 291
– – *C. elegans*, use of 289
– – *H. contortus* monepantel-1 gene, discovery 291–293
– – model for 294
– molecular mechanism 291
– optical *R*-enantiomer 291
– resistance 244
– selection of 284, 285
– tolerability of 285
monophosphoril lipid A (MPL) 441
motility tests 141
moxidectin 245
mptl-1 gene 244
multivalent cathepsin vaccine 469
multivalent vaccines 389, 391, 473
– approach 389
– cathepsin vaccine 389
murine model systems 473
Mus musculus 63, 161
mutation 91, 92
– in the β-tubulin isotype I 245
– of genes required for *C. elegans* cuticle integrity 212
– of GluCla1–3 8
– *tub-1* gene 29
Mycobacterium fortuitum 441

n

nAChR agonists 274
– antiroundworm activity 274
– Cry Proteins, synergy 275
– hypersusceptibility studies 274, 275
nAChR gene families 8, 9
N-acyl amino-acetonitriles 283
national immunization programs 368
native proteins
– protective effects 413
– vaccine, impact 407
Necator americanus 13, 25, 46, 61, 62, 346, 364
neglected tropical disease (NTD) vaccines 159, 219, 220, 343, 350, 351, 354
– adverse consequences 366
– candidate antigens, discovery 343
– cautionary tale for 346, 347
– challenge for 344
– potency assays 350, 351–354
– potency testing for 349, 350
Nematoda 127
nematode-induced immune regulatory system 379
nematode infection models 182
– *Haemonchus* rodent models 183, 184
– nematode infections in livestock 182, 183
– other nematode species for 184
– – efficacious doses of selected compounds against 185, 186
– *Trichostrongylus* rodent models 183
nematode infections in livestock 182, 183
nematode screening, *in vitro* 256
nematode-specific nAChRs 11
Nematospiroides dubius 273
neurocysticercosis 497, 500
neuron-specific antibodies 289
neurotransmitter-gated ion channels 286
neurotransmitters 12
newly excysted juveniles (NEJs) 467
new vaccine candidates, discovery 389–391
NGS datasets 63
nicardipine 313, 314
nickel chelation chromatography 411
nicotinic acetylcholine receptors (nAChRs) 26, 286, 301
– agonists 268
– DEG-3 subfamily 288
– homopentameric 235
– N-, L-, and B-subtypes of 301
– types of 301

nifedipine 313
Nippostrongylus brasiliensis 25, 92, 271
nitazoxanide 242, 243, 268
4-nitrophenylpiperidine 149
nitroscanate 243
nonhomologous isofunctional enzymes (NISEs) 261
nonhuman test systems 343
nontaeniid proteins 492
N-type nAChRs 11

o

Oesophagostomum dentatum 13, 144, 243
– anthelmintic bioassays 146
off-gel electrophoresis technique 424
oig-4 237
Onchocerca gutturosa 257, 259
Onchocerca volvulus 28, 45, 91, 92, 128, 136, 188, 189, 241, 252, 254, 359, 360, 361, 379, 381, 383, 387, 388, 389, 390
– cellular immune response to 379
– vaccine candidates 385, 386
– – Ov-CPI-2 (Ov7) 381
onchocerciasis 188, 255, 256
– control programs 359
– ivermectin use 359
– natural host–parasite systems 380
oogenesis 254
open reading frames (ORFs) 63
opisthorchiasis 324
Opisthorchiidae 74
opisthorchiid flukes. *See Opisthorchis viverrini*
Opisthorchis viverrini 74, 324, 327
ornithine decarboxylase (ODC) 126
Ostertagia circumcincta 28, 271
Ostertagia ostertagi 25, 61, 96, 300, 399, 407
– cysteine proteases 409
Ov-GST-3 gene 29
oxibendazole 241

p

p-amino-phenethyl-*m*-trifluoromethylphenyl piperazine (PAPP) 129
Panagrellus redivivus 270
panhelminthic vaccines 383
paragonimiasis 324
Paragonimus westermani 189, 315
paraherquamide 92, 298, 299
parasite antigens 459
parasite defense proteins 475
parasite tracking 174

parasitic helminths
– genome sequence information 45, 46
– orthology-based RNAi phenotype data mapping 50–52
– unavailable genomic datasets 55, 56
– – targeted gene disruptions 55
parasitic nematode neurotransmitter receptors 30
parasitic nematodes 25, 61, 240
parasitic worms 233
penetration gland
– type 1 (PG1) 493
– type 2 (PG2) 493
Penicillium simplicissimum 297
pep-1 gene 28
peptides, annotation of 66
– public databases 66
peroxidic compounds 478
peroxiredoxin 112, 455–457, 471, 472
– activated macrophages 457
– protein expression 456
– specific antibodies
– – administration 457
PF1022A 33
P-glycoproteins 33, 239
phenothiazine 238
phenylacetylglycine (PAG) 333
phosphoenolpyruvate carboxykinase (PEPCK) 126
phosphofructokinase (PFK) 126
phylogenomics 14
physiology-based assays 138, 139
– on L3 and adult helminths 140, 141
– on nematode
– – egg hatch test (EHT) 139
– – larval development test (LDT) 140
– screening, using parasitic nematode stages 141–144
picrotoxin 5
piperazine 235, 240
– targets for 9–11
Plasmodium falciparum 107
Platyhelminthes 106
PNU-141962. *See* 2-deoxy-paraherquamide
PNU-105775, synthesis 298
polar surface area (PSA) 149
polymerase chain reaction (PCR) 289, 387
porcine vaccine 366
pore-forming toxins (PFTs) 270
potency assays 344–346
potency testing program 344, 352, 353
praziquantel (PZQ) 74, 309–316, 362
– chemotherapy 310
– cure rates (CRs) 324

– inositol phosphates 315
– juvenile worms 311
– limitations 310
– mass distribution 311
– mechanism of action 312–315
– paragonimiasis therapy 324
– performance improvement 315, 316
– resistance 311, 312
– schistosomiasis 315
– therapeutic success 325
– upstream 313
Pristionchus pacificus 26, 32, 270
product development partnerships (PDP) 219, 220, 228, 363
proinflammatory cytokines 380
prolactin receptors 492
prophylactic vaccines 382
protective adaptive immune responses
– development 451
protective immune response 350
protective oncosphere antigens 491
protein abundance index score 476
protein arrays 390
protein-coding expressed sequence tags (ESTs) 402
Protein Data Bank 55, 56
protein kinase C (PKC) signaling pathways 240
proteolytic enzymes 423
proteomics 44
proton ionophore effect 242
putative ligand-gated ion channel genes
– phylogenetic tree 288
pyrantel 24, 237
– resistance 243, 244
pyrazino isoquinoline ring system 310
pyruvate phosphate dikinase (PPDK) 261

q

quantitative polymerase chain reaction (qPCR) 256

r

rapid nutrient turnover 401
Ras-related C3 botulinum toxin substrate 1 (RAC1) 79
rational drug design (RDD) 326
reactive oxygen species (ROS) 80, 455
rebound morbidity 362
recombinant nematode proteases production 410
recombinant proteins 381, 473, 489
revitalizing concept 357

Rhabditida 25
ric-3 237
rifampicin 255, 256
RNA interference (RNAi) 35, 44, 67, 91, 326, 363, 412, 413, 423, 425, 429
– calcium channel β-subunit 314
– as discovery tool 110–112
– drugs, based on 113
– gene silencing 412
– induced phenotypes and identifying essential genes 112
– lead to, suppression of genes 110
– in other parasitic platyhelminths 113, 114
– in parasitic nematodes 92–96
– – improving 97, 98
– in platyhelminths 106
– in Schistosomes 108, 109
– – pathway 109, 110
– *in vivo* 96, 97
Rockefeller Sanitary Commission 220
rodent models
– for developments of anthelmintics 181
– *Haemonchus* rodent models 183, 184
– important translation step 182
– of lymphatic filarial infection 188
– of Onchocerciasis 189
– of other STH infections 187
– for schistosome infection 189, 191
– for *Strongyloides stercoralis* 187
– *Trichostrongylus* rodent models 183
roundworms. *See* Ascaris

s

Sabin Vaccine Institute 426
Saccharomyces cerevisiae 63, 107, 126
Sanger sequencing 63
Schistosoma 106
Schistosoma haematobium 11, 189, 312, 327, 362, 363
Schistosoma japonicum 77
– vaccine, advantage 364
Schistosoma mansoni 45, 77, 92, 107, 161, 189, 311
– activity of selected compounds 192
– fatty acid-binding protein 435, 436
– genome information 331
– increased sepsis following infection 458
– infection 333
– inhibitors of thioredoxin glutathione reductase in 92
– mouse model 329, 333
– purine nucleoside phosphorylase in 126
– *Sm28-GST* and *Sh28-GST* 362
– suppression of genes in 110

– target prioritization, using TDR Targets Database 54, 55
– tegumental surface tetraspanin (Sm-TSP-2) 363
– tegument, fluorescence micrograph 428
schistosomes 55, 330
– drug sensitivity 312
– gene suppression in 109
– genome sequences 330
– genomics, and transcriptomics 422, 423
– helper T cell T_h2 responses 348
– immunomics 425, 426
– postgenomics 424, 425
– proteomics 423, 424
– protocol for RNAi in 332
– quantitative whole-organism screens for 161
– RNAi in 108, 109
– – pathway 109, 110
– *Sm-tsp-2* transcript fail to generate 363
– TGR and peroxiredoxin for 112
– transient RNAi and its application in 111, 112
– transmitted through 423
schistosomiasis vaccines 106, 362–364, 421–430, 435–437, 445
– antigens ranking table for 427
– automated phenotype analysis for drug screening 168
– cases for 426
– schistosomes 422
– – genomics and transcriptomics 422, 423
– – immunomics 425, 426
– – postgenomics 424, 425
– – proteomics 423, 424
– Sm-TSP-2 vaccine 426–429
Schmidtea mediterranea 107
secreted cysteine proteases
– as vaccines 467–469
secretory blebs 490
secretory signals 492
Sequence Read Archive (SRA) 63
serotonin receptor, screen for ligands 129
sex chromosome 422
Sigmodon hispidus 188
signal-to-noise ratio 165
silence schistosome genes 425
slo-1 mutants 34
small interfering RNA (siRNA) 97
small-scale vaccine programs 497
SmAP gene 111
Sm14-M20V62 protein 443
– process of purification 444
– solution structure, by NMR 443

smoke-screen 476
Sm14 protein stability 442, 443
Sm-TSP-2 vaccine 429
Sm14 vaccine antigen, discovery 437, 438
soil transmitted helminthiases (STHs) 61, 220, 267, 357, 364, 435
spiroindole (2-desoxyparaherquamide) 238
Spirurida 67
sporocyst 107
SPRM1hc gene 111
Startect 302, 303–305
Stilbamidine 127
Strongylida 25, 67
Strongyloides ratti 32
Strongyloides stercoralis 25, 29, 187, 205
– rodent models 187
structure–activity relationship (SAR) models 161
superoxide radicals 466
surface teguent proteins, as candidate vaccines 475–477
S581Y 245

t
Taenia ovis 486, 489, 490
– confocal immunofluorescence images 495
– oncosphere schematic diagram 494
– vaccine development program 496
Taenia solium 313, 485, 486
– confocal immunofluorescence images 495
– control measures 498
– metacestode 410
Taenia taeniaeformis 486, 488
taeniid cestode
– definitive hosts 487
– protective antigens 490
– recombinant oncosphere antigens 490
– vaccines 489
tapeworms. *See* cestodes
target product profile (TPP) 221–223
target protein 413
tct-1 gene 30
TDR Targets Database 52–54
– strategies employed to prioritize targets using 53
tegument-associated proteins 476, 496
Teladordagia circumcincta 13, 237, 301
– impact 400
– scanning electron micrograph 400
Teladorsagia trifurcata 303
tetrahydropyrimidines 24
T_h1-associated phenotype 455
T_h2-driven immune responses 387, 452

Therapeutics for Rare and Neglected Diseases (TRND) program 328
thiabendazole 241
thiol-Sepharose-binding proteins (TSBPs) 407
– protein components 408
thioredoxin glutathione reductase 92, 112, 127, 329, 471
thioredoxin reductase 471
thiourea 243
T_h2/T_{reg}-mediated immune environment 451
T_h1-type immune responses 478
toll-like receptor (TLR) 4 454
Torpedo marmorata 7
toxin neutralization 344
transcriptomes 62
– of parasitic nematodes 67
– of strongylid nematodes 63–65
transcriptome sequencing projects 413
transferrin 98
transforming growth factor (TGF)-β 452
transient RNAi 332
translational science 182
transmission-blocking veterinary product 364
T regulatory cells 379
trematocidal drugs 326
Trematoda 73
trematodes 55
– infections in humans and livestock 189
– parasites 4
trematodiases 323
– challenges confronting drug discovery for 325, 326
– current therapy 324, 325
– disability-adjusted life years (DALYs) 324
– food-borne 324
– genomics tools 330–332
– metabolic profiling 332, 333
– phenotypic screening 329, 330
– reinvigorate trematode drug discovery 326–328
– repurposing drugs 328, 329
– schistosomiasis 323
– target validation through reverse genetics 332
tribendimidine (TBD) 77, 268
Trichostrongylus colubriformis 92, 271, 283
Trichuris trichiura 61, 268
triclabendazole (TCBZ) 74, 324, 325, 439, 466, 477
– resistance 467

Trypanosoma cruzi 107
TSOL18 vaccine 498, 499, 500
tub-1(iSE) gene 29
tubulin-binding genes 245
tumor-associated inflammation 456
tumor necrosis factor (TNF)-α 454
Tylenchida 26
tyramine 4

u

UniGene 63
US Code of Federal Regulations (CFRs), for potency testing 345
US Food and Drug Administration (FDA) 223, 260, 327, 350

v

vaccination-plus-oxfendazole treatment 499
vaccines
– antigens 424
– product development strategies 366–368, 377
vaccinology 381, 382
vermifuges 234
verticipyrone 128
Voronoi tessellation 166

w

Western blot analysis 409
whole organism in culture strategy 124
Wolbachia bacterial endosymbionts 251–262
Wolbachia depletion 254
World Health Assembly resolution 368
World Health Organization (WHO) 44, 358, 367, 378, 435, 465, 478
– Training in Tropical Diseases (TDR) 436, 442
WormBase 14
worm therapy 459
Wuchereria bancrofti 45, 50, 136, 252, 361, 377

x

xenobiotic resistance, circumventing 207
– modifying chemistry 208–212
– modifying screening paradigm 207, 208
xenobiotics 205–207, 212, 213
Xenopus laevis 32
Xenopus oocytes 236, 237, 243, 290, 313
– expression 237
xL3-vaccine model 387

z

Zeldia 26
Zolvix 90